The Journal of Infectious Diseases

Published by the John McCormick Institute for Infectious Diseases

EDITED BY

LUDVIG HEKTOEN AND EDWIN O. JORDAN

IN CONJUNCTION WITH

FRANK BILLINGS F. G. NOVY
W. T. SEDGWICK H. GIDEON WELLS

Volume 26

1920

Chicago, 1920

Composed and Printed by
American Medical Association Press
Chicago, Illinois, U. S. A.

ULTRASPECTROSCOPIC STUDIES ON BLOOD SERUM

I. THE ANTAGONISTIC ACTION OF SALT IN BLOOD SERUM

T. TADOKORO

From the Kent Chemical Laboratory, University of Chicago

Spectroscopic studies of colloidal solutions have been made by several investigators in the last ten years, but the experimental data have not been sufficient to show the real value of the application of the spectroscope in this field.

Zsigmondy and Ostwald[1] explained that the absorption band of any colloidal solution moves to the shorter wave length with increasing dispersion. The optical character of the colloidal solution depends not only on the material and degree of dispersion, but also on the form and surface of the particles.

Svedberg[2] who studied the relation of colloidal and molecular solution in gold, selenium, indigo, anilin blue, indophenol and azobenzol states that if the absorption of light of a very disperse colloidal solution is quite similar to that of the molecular solution of the same substance, it is conceivable that the discrete particles of the colloidal solution are molecules.

K. Voit[3] studied the color and degree of dispersion of colloidal suspensions and emulsions and found that the color depends on the degree of disperson in colloidal solution of suspensoid character and is independent of the degree of dispersion in emulsoid solution.

J. Lifschitz[4] states that the light absorption of colloidal solution depends on five factors: 1. The chemical nature of the dispersion phase; 2. its concentration; 3. the degree of dispersion; 4. the form of the particles; 5. the inner structure and the character of the surface of particles. As the light absorption of colloidal solutions is governed by many physicochemical factors, it is almost impossible to determine the effect of single physicochemical factors on light absorption. But

Received for publication Aug. 15, 1919.

[1] Zur Erkenntniss der Kolloide, 1905, p. 112; Koll. chem., Beitr. 3, 1910, 2, p. 409; Grundriss der Kolloidchemie, 1909, p. 222.
[2] Die Existenz der Moleküle, 1912.
[3] Koll. Ztschr., 1914, 15, p. 84.
[4] Koll. Ztschr., 1918, 22, p. 53.

in the comparative study of two colloidal solutions of the same nature and the same concentration, it is not difficult to determine changes in the degree of dispersion and in the inner and outer structure of the particles. Changes in the colloidal state, which are governed by many physicochemical factors, may occur in many different ways, because the colloidal state may be changed in all cases by qualitative and quantitative combinations of these factors.

On account of the great differences between all organic colloidal solutions of different origin, it is possible to identify the natural organic colloidal solutions of the same origin.

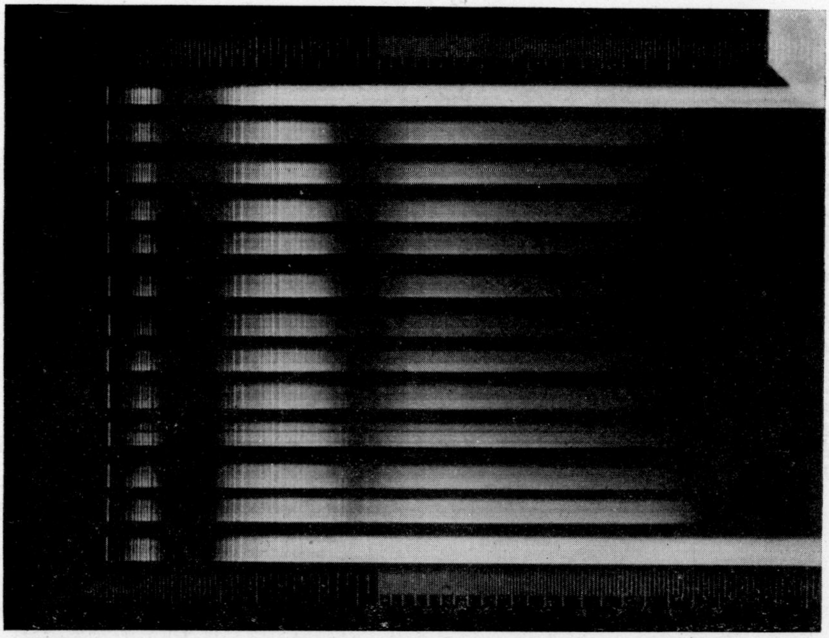

Fig. 1.—$CaCl_2$ and NaCl solutions.

If we compare the results of ultraspectroscopic investigations of colloidal solutions with the results using the ultramicroscope which investigates only the qualitative characteristics of the particles of the colloidal solution, we shall see that the former investigations have greater significance than the latter.

Last year I[5] studied the antagonistic action of salt in organic colloidal solutions, i.e., eggwhite, milk, plant juice and blood serum,

[5] Tokyo Chem. Jour., 1918.

and observed that the diffusion of an ion of one salt through the colloidal solution was antagonized by the presence of another salt of different ion. Now I intend to show the change in the colloidal state of serum by using an ultraspectroscope (1.D.15. London) during the antagonistic action of salt. In these experiments I used a hydrogen tube with a capillary 5 cm. long which was filled with hydrogen at 8 mm. pressure. For the illumination of the hydrogen lamp an alter-

TABLE 1

THE ANTAGONISTIC ACTION BETWEEN $CaCl_2$ AND NaCl SOLUTION (FIG. 1)

	Quantity and Concentration of Goat Serum and Salt Solution	Wave Length of Boundary Line of Absorption Band in Millimikrons
1	Hydrogen lamp control + H_2O only	2,150
2	8.0 c c 1:5 dilution of original serum + 2 c c H_2O	3,072
3	8.0 c c 1:5 dilution + 0.1 c c ½ normal $CaCl_2$ + 1.9 c c H_2O	3,072
4	8.0 c c 1:5 dilution + 0.2 c c ½ normal $CaCl_2$ + 1.8 c c H_2O	3,085
5	8.0 c c 1:5 dilution + 0.3 c c ½ normal $CaCl_2$ + 1.7 c c H_2O	3,090
6	8.0 c c 1:5 dilution + 0.4 c c ½ normal $CaCl_2$ + 1.6 c c H_2O	3,125
7	8.0 c c 1:5 dilution + 0.5 c c ½ normal $CaCl_2$ + 1.5 c c H_2O	3,140
8	8.0 c c 1:5 dilution 0.5 c c ½ normal $CaCl_2$ + 0.25 c c normal NaCl + 1.25 c c H_2O	3,085
9	8.0 c c 1:5 dilution 0.5 c c ½ normal $CaCl_2$ + 0.5 c c normal NaCl + 1.0 c c H_2O	3,065
10	8.0 c c 1:5 dilution 0.5 c c ½ normal $CaCl_2$ + 0.75 c c normal NaCl + 0.75 c c H_2O	3,065
11	8.0 c c 1:5 dilution 0.5 c c ½ normal $CaCl_2$ + 1.0 c c normal NaCl + 0.5 c c H_2O	3,050
12	8.0 c c 1:5 dilution 0.5 c c ½ normal $CaCl_2$ + 1.5 c c normal NaCl + 0.5 c c H_2O	3,035
13	8.0 c c H_2O + 0.5 c c ½ normal $CaCl_2$ + 1.5 c c normal NaCl	2,165

TABLE 2

THE ANTAGONISTIC ACTION BETWEEN $ZnSO_4$ AND $CaCl_2$ SOLUTION

	Quantity and Concentration of Rabbit Serum and Salt Solution (Fig. 2)	Wave Length of Boundary Line of Absorption Band in Millimikrons
1	Hydrogen lamp control + H_2O only	2,100
2	8.0 c c 1:8 dilution of original serum + 2.0 c c H_2O	2,950
3	8.0 c c 1:8 dilution + 0.1 c c 1/50 normal $ZnSO_4$ + 1.9 c c H_2O	2,995
4	8.0 c c 1:8 dilution + 0.2 c c 1/50 normal $ZnSO_4$ + 1.8 c c H_2O	3,050
5	8.0 c c 1:8 dilution + 0.25 c c 1/50 normal $ZnSO_4$ + 1.75 c c H_2O	3,310
6	8.0 c c 1:8 dilution + 0.5 c c 1/50 normal $ZnSO_4$ + 1.5 c c H_2O	2,985
7	8.0 c c 1:8 dilution + 0.5 c c 1/50 normal $ZnSO_4$ + 0.5 c c ½ normal $CaCl_2$ + 1.0 c c H_2O	2,960
8	8.0 c c 1:8 dilution + 0.5 c c 1/50 normal $ZnSO_4$ + 1.0 c c ½ normal $CaCl_2$ + 0.5 c c H_2O	2,960
9	8.0 c c 1:8 dilution + 0.5 c c 1/50 normal $ZnSO_4$ + 2.5 c c ½ normal $CaCl_2$	2,951
10	8.0 c c 1:8 dilution + 0.5 c c 1/50 normal $ZnSO_4$ + 2.5 c c ½ normal $CaCl_2$	2,950
11	8.0 c c 1:8 dilution + 0.5 c c 1/50 normal $ZnSO_4$ + 3.0 c c ½ normal $CaCl_2$	2,945
12	8.0 c c H_2O + 0.5 c c 1/50 normal $ZnSO_4$ + 3.0 c c ½ normal $CaCl_2$	2,135

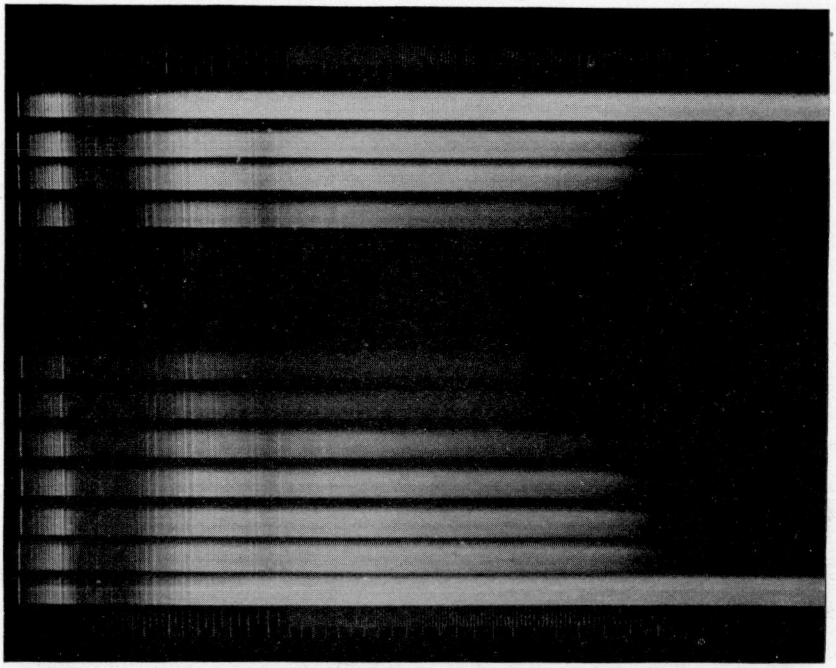

Fig. 2.—$ZnSo_4$ and $CaCl_2$ solutions.

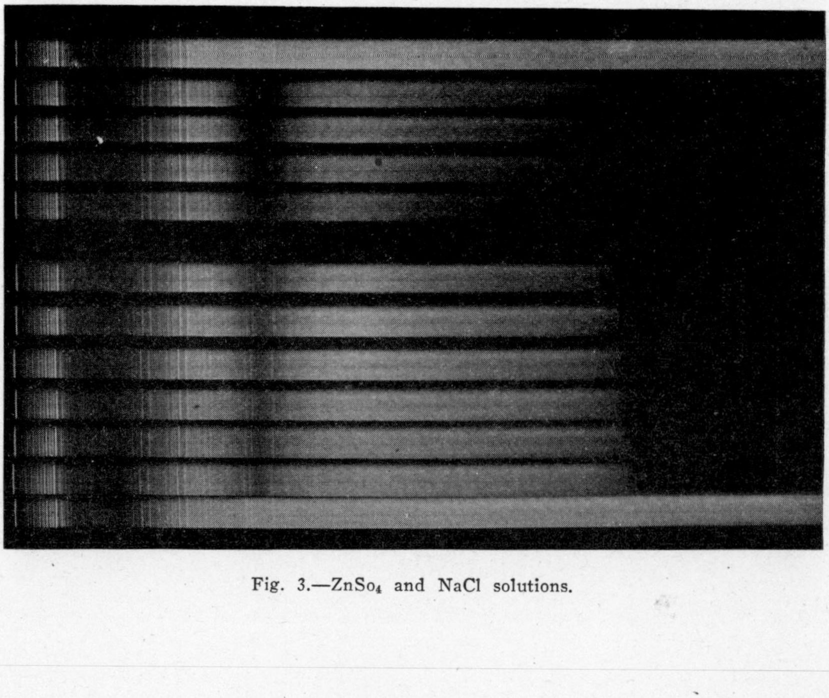

Fig. 3.—$ZnSo_4$ and NaCl solutions.

nating current of 220 volts was used and in the circuits was placed an induction coil and a resistance box to get 1,100 volts in the secondary circuit with a current of 4 amperes in the primary. A quartz cell 12 mm. thick was filled with a mixture of serum and salt solutions. All photographs were taken with 7 minute exposures using an Eastman panchromatic dry plate. The results are given in the tables and photographs.

TABLE 3

THE ANTAGONISTIC ACTION BETWEEN $ZnSO_4$ AND $NaCl_2$ SOLUTION (FIG. 3)

	Quantity and Concentration of Rabbit Serum and Salt Solution	Wave Length of Boundary Line of Absorption Band in Millimikrons
1	Hydrogen lamp control + H_2O only	2,100
2	8.0 c c 1:8 dilution of original serum + 2.0 c c H_2O	2,941
3	8.0 c c 1:8 dilution + 0.5 c c 1/50 normal $ZnSO_4$ + 1.5 c c H_2O	2,950
4	8.0 c c 1:8 dilution + 0.75 c c 1/50 normal $ZnSO_4$ + 1.25 c c H_2O	2,975
5	8.0 c c 1:8 dilution + 1.0 c c 1/50 normal $ZnSO_4$ + 1.0 c c H_2O	3,350
6	8.0 c c 1:8 dilution + 1.0 c c 1/50 normal $ZnSO_4$ + 0.5 c c normal NaCl + 0.5 c c H_2O	3,605
7	8.0 c c 1:8 dilution + 1.0 c c 1/50 normal $ZnSO_4$ + 0.5 c c normal NaCl + 0.25 c c H_2O	3,125
8	8.0 c c 1:8 dilution + 1.0 c c 1/50 normal $ZnSO_4$ + 1.0 c c normal NaCl	3,045
9	8.0 c c 1:8 dilution + 1.0 c c 1/50 normal $ZnSO_4$ + 1.0 c c normal NaCl	2,985
10	8.0 c c 1:8 dilution + 1.0 c c 1/50 normal $ZnSO_4$ + 1.5 c c normal NaCl	2,945
11	8.0 c c 1:8 dilution + 1.0 c c 1/50 normal $ZnSO_4$ + 2.0 c c normal NaCl	2,940
12	8.0 c c H_2O + 1.0 c c 1/50 normal $ZnSO_4$ + 2.0 c c normal NaCl	2,135

From these experiments we see that the following salts act antagonistically toward each other: $CaCl_2$ and NaCl, $ZnSO_4$ and $CaCl_1$ or $ZnSO_4$ and NaCl; that is the change in state of a colloidal serum produced by one salt was reversed by the other salt. This change must depend on the dispersion, the form or the structure of the particles, because in our experiments we used the same serum of the same concentration.

In order to explain this phenomenon the changes were observed under an ultramicroscope and the following results were obtained (Figs. 4 and 5):

1. The dilute serum showed mikrons which had Brownian movement.

2. If the serum was mixed with $ZnSO_4$ or $CaCl_2$, its particles formed aggregates and became heterogeneous and their movements stopped.

Fig. 4.—Serum plus $ZnSo_4$

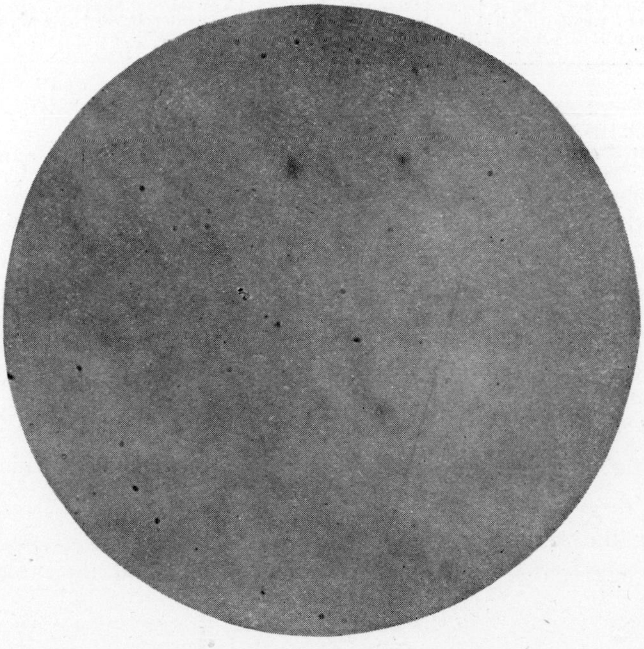

Fig. 5.—Serum plus $ZnSo_4$ with addition of NaCl solution.

3. If a serum containing $ZnSO_4$ or $CaCl_2$ was treated with $CaCl_2$ or NaCl, the aggregated particles became free and homogeneous as in the original serum.

SUMMARY

From the results I conclude that the antagonistic action of two salts on blood serum is caused by a reversal of the dispersion of the serum and of the change of the form and structure of particles.

ULTRASPECTROSCOPIC STUDIES ON BLOOD SERUM

II. THE DIFFERENCE IN THE COLLOIDAL STATE OF NORMAL AND IMMUNE SERUM

T. Tadokoro and Y. Nakayama

From the Kent Chemical Laboratory, University of Chicago, and the John McCormick Institute for Infectious Diseases, Chicago

As reported in the previous paper, the antagonistic action of different salts causes a change in the colloidal state of blood serum. The ultraspectroscopic investigation of the serum showed clearly the changes of the degree of dispersion and of the structures of the particles.

In the literature on immunization many reports are found which state that the actions of immune serum are intimately related to the colloidal state of the serum. For example, in the agglutination of blood corpuscles of a number of animals by ricin and other toxins there is a change in the colloidal state of the serum. A curious occurrence which seems to show the toxin-antitoxin reaction to be closely related to colloidal reactions in general is seen in the so-called Danysz[1] phenomenon. Bordet,[2] Joos,[3] have interpreted in different ways the fact that the presence of salt is necessary for agglutination by a serum. The colloidal explanation of the precipitin reaction is most reasonable. Bruck has shown that in the Wassermann reaction a precipitation takes place which is visible under the ultramicroscope. Weichhard's epiphanin reaction, i. e., the diffusion of methylene blue across the tube in which antigen and antibody are present and not in the control, seems to be a method for the determination of the degree of dispersion of blood serum. These interesting observations have prompted a study of the change in the colloidal state of blood serum with an ultraspectroscope. We omit the description of the ultraspecroscope illuminated by a hydrogen lamp and the explanation of the apparatus, because already explained in the previous paper. In this work we took photographs in the same way.

Received for publication Aug. 15, 1919.

[1] Ann. de l'Inst. Pasteur, 1902, 16, p. 331.
[2] Ann. de l'Inst. Pasteur, 1899, 13, p. 225.
[3] Centralbl. f. Bacteriol., I, O., 1903, 33, p. 762.

THE DIFFERENCE BETWEEN THE SERUMS OF DIFFERENT ANIMALS

To examine the difference in the serums of different animals, we used 7 samples of normal serum from different animals: 2 samples from rabbits, 2 from dogs, 2 from guinea-pigs and 1 from a horse; these samples were diluted with distilled water in different concentrations as shown. The photographs were taken and the position of the boundary lines of the absorption bands were measured on the plate. The results are given in table 1.

From these results it can be observed that in the original serum and the 1:2 or 1:4 dilution it was difficult to distinguish between the

TABLE 1

WAVE LENGTH IN MILLIMIKRONS OF BOUNDARY LINE OF ABSORPTION BAND OF NORMAL SERUMS

Concentration of Serum	Wave Length of Boundary Line of Absorption Band						
	Dog Serum		Guinea-Pig Serum		Rabbit Serum		Horse Serum
	A	B	A	B	A	B	
Original	4,275-3,880-3,625-3,360	5,600	5,750	5,750	4,350	5,800	4,250-3,880-3,135
2	4,150-4,050-3,065	5,350-4,950-4,200	5,625-5,125-4,375	5,700-5,050-4,500	4,250-3,950-3,060	5,650-5,450-5,200-5,150-4,350	3,070
4	3,040	4,050-3,965-3,280-3,145-3,085	4,225-3,880-3,450-3,125	5,650-5,350-4,350-3,890-3,500-3,115	4,180-4,052-3,025	4,300-3,900-3,310	3,040
6	.....	.....	.....	.....	4,080-2,985	4,180-4,040-3,020	
8	2,960	3,055	2,985	4,250-3,880-3,065	2,935	2,955	3,020
10	.....	.....	.....	.....	2,915	2,925	
12	.....	.....	2,915	4,180-3,980-2,970			
16	2,930	2,930	2,880	4,180-3,980-2,935	2,860-2,625-2,455	.....	3,990
24	.....	.....	.....	.....	.....	2,890-2,545-2,470	
32	2,810-2,575-2,480	2,850-2,585-2,465	2,425	2,825-2,790-2,425	2,780-2,410	2,840-2,655-2,430	2,955
64	2,425	2,420	2,375	2,410	2,383	2,395	2,925-2,560-2,470
128	2,385	2,365	2,345	2,380	2,359	2,365	2,895-2,615-2,450
256	2,345	2,330	2,315	2,335	2,330	2,325	2,410
512	2,325	2,305	2,280	2,305	2,282	2,295	
1,024	2,280	2,275	2,235	2,255	2,255		

A = straight line; B = dotted line.

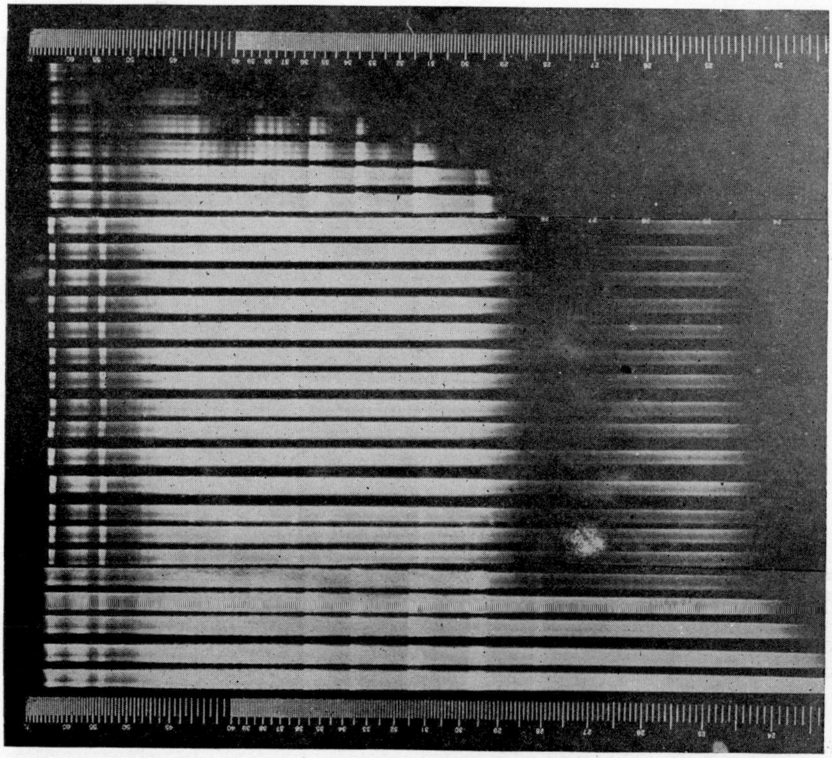

Fig. 1.—The special absorption band between 2,950-2,400 mikrons of normal rabbit serum.

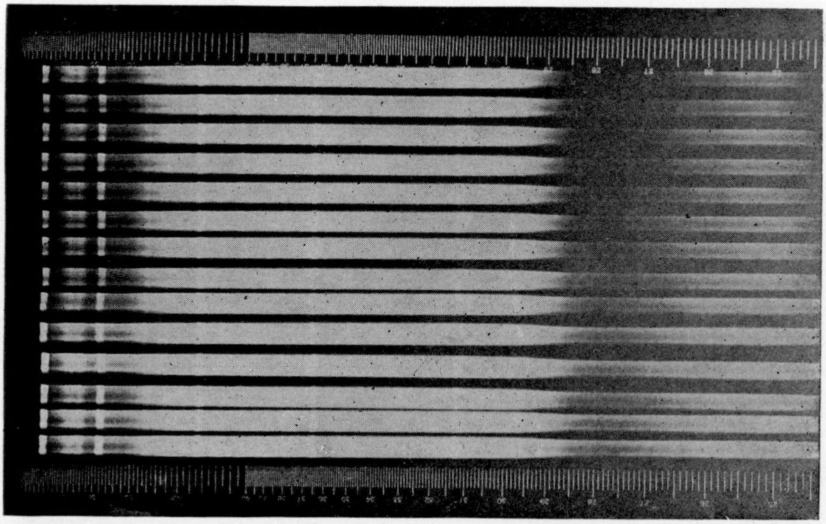

Fig. 2.—Serum of a normal rabbit.

kinds of animals because the absorption band of the serum was influenced by contamination with coloring matter from the blood corpuscles. Therefore we compared the samples between the wave lengths of 2,950 and 2,400 mikrons where every kind of blood serum shows a special absorption band (figure 1).

From the comparison of this part of the spectrum of different samples we observe a clear difference in the position of these absorption bands:

1. Dog serum has a large absorption band in a dilution of 1:32 and the illuminated part of the short wave length is small. Therefore this absorption band appears in a little higher dilution than 1:32 but disappears in a dilution of 1:64.

2. Guinea-pig serum shows this absorption band in solutions between 1:16 and 1:32 dilution, because in the 1:16 dilution, no absorption band is observed and in 1:32 dilution the band almost disappears.

3. Rabbit serum shows this absorption band in 1:16 dilution and it still appears in 1:32 dilution, but it is not continued in still higher dilutions as in the case of the dog, because the absorption band in 1:32 dilution is smaller than the illuminated part.

4. Horse serum shows this absorption band in dilutions of from 1:64 to 1:128 and still higher because the band in the 1:128 dilution is larger than the illuminated part.

THE DIFFERENCE BETWEEN NORMAL AND IMMUNE SERUM

In the next experiment we used immune serums of different animals.

1. Horse, 2 samples of normal and 2 samples of immune antistreptococcus serum.

2. Rabbit, 6 normal and 7 immune serums:

a. Antistreptococcus serum

b. Antistreptococcus serum; agglutinin titer, 1,280

c. Antistreptococcus serum; agglutinin titer, 1,600

d. Anti-egg serum, precipitin titer, 24,000

e. Anti-egg serum, precipitin titer, 24,000

f. Antimilk serum, precipitin titer, 200

g. Antiplatelet (dog) serum, precipitated in milk dilution, 1:200

3. Dog, one normal and two immune serums:

a. Antirat serum, agglutinin titer, 1:1,536

b. Antirat serum, agglutinin titer, 1:3,072

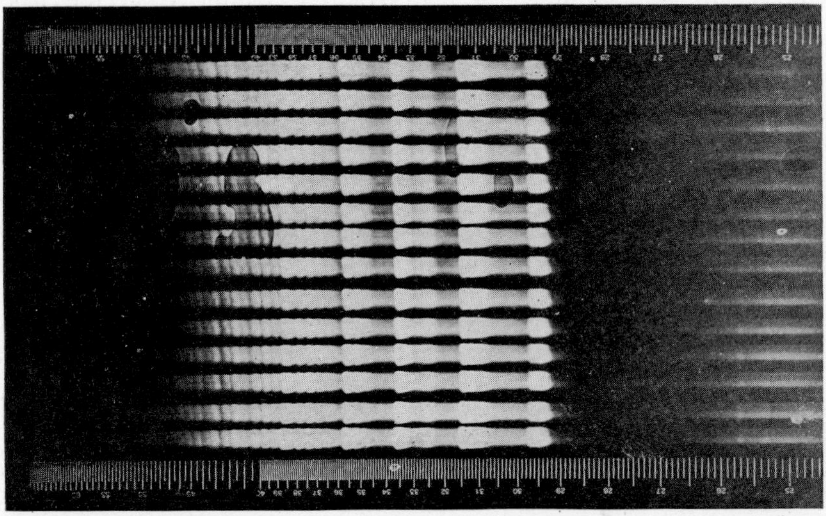

Fig 3.—Serum of rabbit injected with cow's milk.

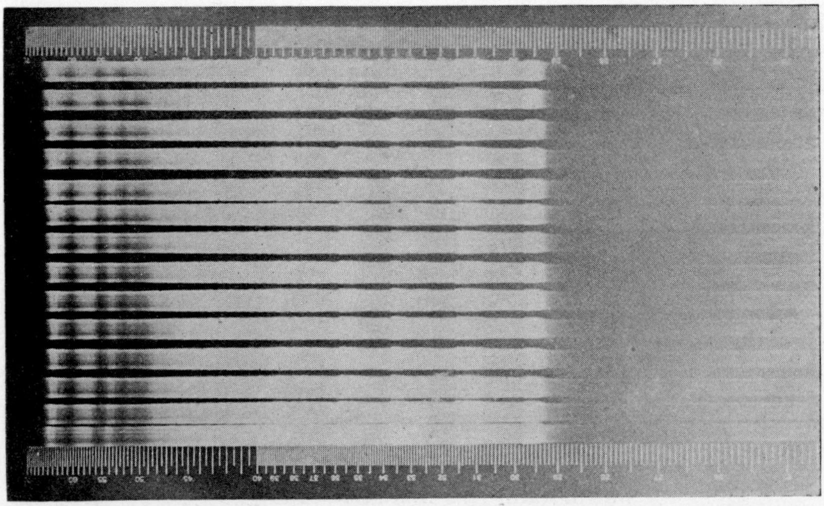

Fig. 4.—Serum of rabbit injected with dog platelets.

To dilute the serum we used always 0.9% sodium chlorid solution and as a preliminary experiment we examined 4 normal and immune serums in different dilutions with results as shown in tables 2, 3, 4, and 5.

TABLE 2

HORSE SERUM

Concentration of Serum	Wave Length in Millimikrons of Boundary Line of Absorption Band	
	Normal Serum	Immune Serum (Antistreptococcus)
Original	4,500-4,330-3,900-2,620-3,570-3,340	4,625-4,300-3,930-3,610-3,570-3,510-3,350
2	3,105	3,100
4	3,050	3,060
8	3,030	3,030
16	3,005	2,990
32	2,930	2,940
64	2,910-2,510-2,480	2,925-2,510-2,553
128	2,860-2,710-2,480	2,850-2,620-2,425
256	2.400	2,380

TABLE 3

HORSE SERUM

Concentration of Serum	Wave Length in Millimikrons of Boundary Line of Absorption Band	
	Normal Serum	Immune Serum (Antistreptococcus)
32	2,935	2,955
47	2,930	2,920
70	2,885-2,605-2,455	2,895-2,585-2,470
105	2,810-2,670-2,435	2,875-2,645-2,465
150	2,405	2,850-2,670-2,425
225	.....	2,400

TABLE 4

RARRIT SERUM

Concentration of Serum	Wave Length in Millimikrons of Boundary Line of Absorption Band	
	Normal Serum	Immune Serum (Antistreptococcus a)
32	2,925-2,565-2,500	2,980-2,540-2,510
46	2,800-2,600-2,490	2,880-2,585-2,470
69	2,425	2,810-2,710-2,425

TABLE 5

RARRIT SERUM

Concentration of Serum	Wave Length in Millimikrons of Boundary Line of Absorption Band	
	Normal Serum	Immune Serum (Antistreptococcus b)
30	2,910-2,501-2,495	2,910-2,610-2,470
36	2,865-2,660-2,455	2,875-2,655-2,455
43	2,795-2,665-2,450	2,810-2,660-2,445
51	2,425	2,765-2,710-2,435
61	2,410	2,410
47	2,395	2,390
89	2,375	2,380

TABLE 6

NORMAL RABBIT SERUM

Wave Length in Millimikrons of Boundary Line of Absorption Band			
Rabbit 1	Rabbit 2	Rabbit 3	Rabbit 4
2,920-2,610-2,480	2,920-2,610-2,460	2,840-2,750-2,460	2,850-2,740-2,445
2,815-2,660-2,480	2,890-2,650-2,450	2,820-2,735-2,465	2,840-2,750-2,445
2,810-2,665-2,460	2,810-2,655-2,450	2,800-2,730-2,465	2,815-2,760-2,435
2,805-2,665-2,460	2,800-2,650-2,450	2,460	2,435
2,805-2,675-2,450	2,800-2,695-2,445	2,455	2,435
2,800-2,675-2,450	2,765-2,715-2,445	2,445	2,435
2,445	2,440	2,445	2,430
2,445	2,440	2,440	2,430
2,440	2,440	2,440	2,420
2,430	2,430	2,430	2,415
2,435	2,427	2,425	2,415
2,430	2,427	2,425	2,410
2,424	2,424	2,425	2,400
2,415	2,408	2,415	2,400

TABLE 7

IMMUNE RABBIT SERUM

Wave Length in Millimikrons of Boundary Line of Absorption Band				
Anti-egg Serum	Antimilk Serum	Anti-egg Serum	Antiplatelet Serum	Antistreptococcus Serum
2,875-2,630-2,430	2,885-2,605-2,445	2,880-2,630-2,455	2,900-2,605-2,459	2,890-2,535-2,465
2,860-2,660-2,430	2,875-2,675-2,440	2,860-2,640-2,445	2,875-2,605-2,455	2,885-2,540-2,460
2,860-2,665-2,430	2,855-2,660-2,430	2,860-2,645-2,445	2,855-2,615-2,455	2,880-2,545-2,455
2,850-2,668-2,425	2,855-2,660-2,430	2,845-2,670-2,445	2,850-2,630-2,450	2,875-2,550-2,455
2,835-2,710-2,422	2,855-2,655-2,425	2,825-2,715-2,440	2,850-2,630-2,450	2,865-2,560-2,455
2,790-2,720-2,420	2,855-2,655-2,425	2,810-2,730-2,440	2,850-2,635-2,440	2,865-2,580-2,455
2,790-2,725-2,420	2,845-2,660-2,420	2,800-2,730-2,440	2,840-2,650-2,435	2,860-2,595-2,455
2,780-2,745-2,420	2,830-2,660-2,420	2,785-2,730-2,440	2,840-2,655-2,430	2,860-2,605-2,455
2,415	2,815-2,665-2,420	2,785-2,740-2,435	2,835-2,670-2,430	2,855-2,605-2,450
2,415	2,815-2,675-2,420	2,430	2,820-2,680-2,430	2,855-2,615-2,450
2,415	2,815-2,685-2,420	2,430	2,805-2,690-2,430	2,850-2,640-2,450
2,415	2,810-2,700-2,415	2,425	2,790-2,600-2,420	2,845-2,650-2,450
2,410	2,805-2,700-2,410	2,420	2,780-2,725-2,420	2,840-2,680-2,440
2,405	2,805-2,700-2,405	2,415	2,415	2,835-2,695-2,440
	2,805-2,705-2,405			
	2,805-2,630-2,405			
	2,805- -2,405			

TABLE 8

DOG, NORMAL AND IMMUNE SERUM

Wave Length in Millimikrons of Boundary Line of Absorption Band		
Normal Serum	Immune (Antirat) Serum	Immune (Antirat) Serum
2,890-2,535-2,465	2,870-2,680-2,460	2,900-2,610-,2480
2,885-2,540-2,460	2,850-2,690-2,450	2,900-2,620-2,460
2,880-2,545-2,455	2,845-2,700-2,445	2,880-2,625-2,460
2,875-2,550-2,455	2,845-2,715-2,440	2,880-2,625-2,460
2,865-2,560-2,455	2,845-2,720-2,435	2,875-2,630-2,455
2,865-2,580-2,455	2,835-2,720-2,430	2,870-2,640-2,450
2,860-2,595-2,455	2,830-2,720-2,425	2,865-2,650-2,445
2,860-2,605-2,455	2,820-2,720-2,425	2,860-2,660-2,440
2,855-2,605-2,450	2,800-2,725-2,425	2,855-2,670-2,440
2,855-2,615-2,450	2,800-2,740-2,425	2,855-2,680-2,435
2,850-2,460-2,450	2,800-2,750-2,420	2,850-2,685-2,428
2,845-2,650-2,450	2,790-2,765-2,420	2,840-2,690-2,425
2,840-2,680-2,440	2,415	2,835-2,690-2,425
2,835-2,695-2,440	2,415	2,830-2,720-2,420

From these results it is seen that the absorption band of immune serum is always larger and longer than that of normal serum. Therefore it is necessary to compare the position of the absorption band of normal and immune serum more exactly and accurately. The two kinds of serum were diluted as follows: one c c of serum diluted to 30.0 c c with 0.9% salt solution and 6.0 c c of this dilution was taken and diluted progressively with 0.25 c c of 0.9% sodium chlorid each time:

(1) 6.0 c c of diluted serum 1.0 c c serum with 29.0 c c NaCl-sol.
(2) 6.0 c c of diluted serum + 0.25 c c NaCl sol.
(3) 6.0 c c of diluted serum + 0.50 c c NaCl sol.
(4) 6.0 c c of diluted serum + 0.75 c c NaCl sol.
(5) 6.0 c c of diluted serum + 1.0 c c NaCl sol.
(6) 6.0 c c of diluted serum + 1.25 c c NaCl sol.
(7) 6.0 c c of diluted serum + 1.50 c c NaCl sol.
(8) 6.0 c c of diluted serum + 1.75 c c NaCl sol.
(9) 6.0 c c of diluted serum + 2.00 c c NaCl sol.
(10) 6.0 c c of diluted serum + 2.25 c c NaCl sol.
(11) 6.0 c c of diluted serum + 2.50 c c NaCl sol.
(12) 6.0 c c of diluted serum + 2.75 c c NaCl sol.
(13) 6.0 c c of diluted serum + 3.00 c c NaCl sol.
(14) 6.0 c c of diluted serum + 3.25 c c NaCl sol.

On the examination of diluted serum by the ultraspectroscope we obtained the results given in tables 6, 7, and 8.

From these results we secure a clear idea of the difference between normal and immune serum. The absorption band of immune serum between the wave length 2,950-2,400 mikrons is much larger and longer than that of normal serum. If we compare both kinds of serums with respect to the area occupied by the absorption band, the area of the absorption band of the immune serum is from two to ten times greater than that of normal serum.

SUMMARY

The difference between the serums of different animals, i. e., dog, guinea-pig, rabbit and horse, was observed in the position and the extent of the absorption band between the wave lengths 2,950-2,400 mikrons.

The absorption band of immune serum between the wave lengths 2,350-2,400 mikrons is much larger and longer than that of normal serum.

NONLACTOSE FERMENTING ORGANISMS FROM THE FECES OF INFLUENZA PATIENTS

N. P. Sherwood, C. M. Downs, and J. B. McNaught

From the Department of Bacteriology, University of Kansas, Lawrence

Leichtenstern[1] mentions that during the pandemic of 1889-1890, at least one fourth of the cases showed no respiratory complications and were frequently confused with typhoid. Differentiation was made, however, clinically on the basis of the short incubation period, sudden onset, and comparatively short duration of the disease. Such was the condition of affairs in many parts of the United States during the pandemic of 1918. Since there seemed to be no published data showing that careful laboratory methods had been used to differentiate mild typhoid and paratyphoid—enteritidis infections from influenza, it seemed worth while to make bacteriologic examinations of feces in recurring epidemics. This seemed more warranted after looking over the reports of the Kansas state epidemiologist, which showed a marked drop over previous years in reported cases of typhoid and paratyphoid fever.

The first cases studied were a few of typical influenzal pneumonia at Lawrence, Kan., during Dec., 1918. Relatively large recurring epidemics occurred at Wichita, in February and at Topeka, McPherson and other points in Kansas during March and April. Fecal examinations and in many instances blood cultures, blood counts and agglutination tests were made on typical cases in the isolation hospitals of these places. A series of control cases was studied at Topeka and also at Lawrence.

The technic of the fecal examination was: Samples were obtained as early as possible in the disease and wherever possible repeated examinations were made. In cases of constipation, the first fecal masses were discarded, and the more fluid portion containing some mucus was used for plating. Eosin-methylene blue agar plates, as suggested by Holt-Harris and Teague[2] were used. Four plates for undiluted feces and four plates for broth dilution were streaked. After 24 hours' incubation, colonies were fished and were customarily restreaked on eosin-blue plates and from these cultures were obtained for study. At first, several colonies of each type were picked but our experience at Lawrence and Wichita caused us to pick, if possible, a minimum of 15 colonies from any resembling typhoid or paratyphoid types and 2 or 3 of each of the other kinds. Suspicious colonies of the former types were, after replating, inoculated in new Russell's medium, morphology studied and

Received for publication Aug. 28, 1919.

[1] Nothnagels Encylopedia, Practical Medicine, 1905, p. 591.

[2] Jour. Infect. Dis., 1916, 18, p. 596.

Gram's stains made, and then tested out if necessary in litmus milk, gelatin and the following sugars and alcohols: dextrose, mannite, lactose, saccharose, arabinose, dulcite, xylose, rhamnose and salacin. New York Board of Health and American Museum strains of paratyphoid A, paratyphoid B, enteritidis and typhoid were used as control organisms. In addition, blood from a number of convalescent patients was obtained for agglutination tests. None of these patients had been vaccinated against any of these groups.

A summary of the results is shown in table 1.

TABLE 1

SUMMARY OF RESULTS

Source	Number of Samples from Typical Cases	Number of Samples from Control Cases	Kind of Organisms Found in Feces and Number of Samples Showing Same				
			Morgan's Bacillus	Enteritidis-like Organisms	B. typhosus	Percentages of Cases Showing: Typhoid or Enteritidis-like Organisms	Percentages of Cases Showing: Enteritidis-like Organisms
Isolation Hospital, Wichita	9	..	1	3	1	44%	33%
Isolation Hospital, Topeka	15	..	2	10	1	73%	66%
Noninfluenza cases, Topeka	..	12	None	None	None	None	None
Private cases, McPherson...	2	..	None	1	None	50%	50%
Private cases, Lawrence.....	6	..	None	3	1	66%	50%
Noninfluenzal private cases, Lawrence.................	..	10	None	None	1	10%	None

From table 1 it will be observed that at Wichita the feces from 9 cases were examined and enteritidis-like organisms found in 3, and B. typhosus in a fourth case. Morgan's bacillus was also found in one case associated with enteritidis-like organisms.

In the Topeka epidemic the feces from 15 cases were examined with the result that 10 were positive for enteritidis-like organisms and 1 for B. typhosus. Morgan's bacillus was found associated with other enteritidis-like organisms in 2 of the 10 positive cases. The 12 noninfluenza control cases were negative.

At Lawrence, enteritidis-like organisms were obtained from 3 of 6, and B. typhosus from a fourth case of influenza. None were obtained from 10 control cases, such as mumps, abscesses, 1 of typical typhoid fever, 2 cases of measles, 3 cases of tonsillitis and several cases of lobar pneumonia. Neither Morgan' bacillus nor paracolon bacilli were found.

The 2 cases at McPherson were mild ones. Enteritidis-like organisms were obtained from 1 of the 2 cases in children under 12 years of age. At McPherson a large epidemic was just ending when the work was done.

In view of the fact that enteritidis-like organisms were isolated in 33-1/3% of the cases at Wichita, 66% of those at Topeka, 50% of those at Lawrence, and 50% of those at McPherson, Kansas, most of them widely separated points, it seems worth while to state the cultural characteristics of these strains (table 2).

According to Jordan's[3] studies on this group, the organisms we have described would be classified as B. paratyphosus B, or B. enteritidis, showing some variation in dulcite. Strain 12 is atypical in xylose, while strain 3 gave no acid or gas in rhamnose. In regard to strain 10 which ferments salicin, it is of interest that a second sample of feces from this case gave us a number of salicin negative strains. Strain 11 showed some gas after 36 hours.

Krumwiede, Kohn and Valentine[4] observed variation in dulcite fermentation in their studies on the paratyphoid enteritidis group and summarize their findings as follows: "Evidently no one characteristic has served to differentiate between all strains of the B. suis and B. paratyphosus 'B' strains. Dulcite fermentation, as with most other members of the group, varies according to sub-group avidity, and has differential value only in so far as a low avidity indicates that a strain does not belong to the 'B' group."

It will be noted further from table 2 that all of our strains blackened lead acetate agar. According to Jordan,[5] B. suipestifer and B. paratyphosus A, consistently fail to do this, while B. paratyphosus B, and B. enteritidis uniformly blacken this medium. Since table 2 does not show the length of time the litmus milk cultures were kept under observation, it may be of interest to note that this was for a period of 3 weeks. Alkalinity persisted and no saponification occurred.

After we had obtained a number of strains at Topeka, it was decided to make agglutination tests using blood from convalescent patients and several strains from both Wichita and Topeka. The results were not at all consistent. Some tests were entirely negative with all strains, some negative with their own strains and positive with others, while some were positive with their own strains as well as a few of the others. A 1:60 dilution of serum was used. It was decided to check up the relationship by agglutination and absorption tests.

[3] Jour. Infect. Dis., 1917, 20, p. 457.
[4] Jour. Med. Research, 1918, 38, p. 89.
[5] Jour. Infect. Dis., 1917, 21, p. 554.

TABLE 2

Gram-Negative, Nonlactose Fermenting Bacilli Isolated from Supposedly True Influenza Cases

City	Organism Number	Gelatin Liquefaction	Motility	Litmus Milk 24 Hours	Litmus Milk 48 Hours	Litmus Milk 72 Hours	Litmus Milk 5 Days	Fermenting Acid and Gas, 24 Hours: Dextrose	Mannite	Saccharose	Arabinose	Dulcite 30 Hours	Xylose	Rhamnose	Salicin	Indol	Blackening of Lead Acetate Agar
Wichita................	1	—	+	A	al	al	al	⊕	⊕	—	⊕	—	⊕	⊕	—	—	+
	2	—	+	A	al	al	al	⊕	⊕	—	⊕	⊕	⊕	⊕			
	3	—	+	A	al	al	al	⊕	⊕	—	⊕	—	⊕	—	—	—	+
Topeka.................	4	—	+	A	al	al	al	⊕	⊕	—	⊕	—	⊕	⊕	—	—	+
	5	—	+	A	al	al	al	⊕	⊕	—	⊕	—	⊕	⊕	—	—	+
	6	—	+	A	al	al	al	⊕	⊕	—	⊕	—	⊕	⊕	—	—	+
	7	—	+	A	al	al	al	⊕	⊕	—	⊕	—	⊕	⊕	—	—	+
	8	—	+	A	al	al	al	⊕	⊕	—	⊕	⊕	⊕	⊕	—	—	+
	9	—	+	A	al	al	al	⊕	⊕	—	⊕	—	⊕	⊕	—	—	+
	10	—	+	A	al	al	al	⊕	⊕	—	⊕	⊕	⊕	⊕	⊕	—	+
	11	—	+	A	al	al	al	⊕	⊕	—	⊕	⊕	⊕	⊕	—	—	+
	12	—	+	A	al	al	al	⊕	⊕	—	⊕	—	—	—	—	—	+
	13	—	+	A	al	al	al	⊕	⊕	—	⊕	⊕	⊕	⊕	—	—	+
Lawrence...............	14	—	+	A	al	al	al	⊕	⊕	—	⊕	⊕	⊕	⊕	—	—	+
	15	—	+	A	al	al	al	⊕	⊕	—	⊕	⊕	⊕	⊕	—	—	+
	16	—	+	A	al	al	al	⊕	⊕	—	⊕	⊕	⊕	⊕	—	—	+
McPherson.............	17	..	+	A	al	al	al	⊕	⊕	—	⊕	⊕	⊕	⊕	—	—	+
Chicago University......	B. suipestifer	—	+	A	A	A	al	⊕	⊕	—	—	—	⊕	⊕	..	..	—
New York Health Laboratory Strains of....	Paratyphoid A	—	+	A	A	A	A	⊕	⊕	—	⊕	—	—	⊕	—	—	—
	Paratyphoid B	—	+	A	A	al	al	⊕	⊕	—	⊕	⊕	⊕	⊕	—	—	+
	B. Enteritidis	—	+	A	A	al	al	⊕	⊕	—	⊕	⊕	⊕	⊕	—	—	+

Acid and gas indicated by ⊕.

The results of cross agglutination and absorption tests may be summarized as follows:

Rabbits were tested for normal agglutinins and then immunized and specific immune serum for each of the strains isolated was obtained. In addition, immune serum was produced for our laboratory strains of B. enteritidis, B. paratyphosus A and B, and for two strains of B. suipestifer. Cultures of B. typhimurium and B. cavipesticus were obtained from the New York City Health Laboratory. Other strains of members of this group were supplied by the University of Chicago and by the Iowa State Agricultural College. In addition, immune serums for paratyphoid A and B were obtained from one of the commercial supply houses.

The strains of enteritidis-like organisms isolated from influenza cases showed practically the same slight amount of cross agglutination with paratyphoid B immune serum as the known strains of B. enteritidis we used. None showed any relationship to paratyphoid B by absorption tests. None showed any relationship by absorption tests to B. suipestifer, typhimurium, cavipesticus or paratyphoid A.

Many of them showed decided cross-agglutination with each other and with B. enteritidis. The absorption tests apparently divided them into the groups shown in table 3.

TABLE 3

SHOWING POSSIBLE TYPING OF ENTERITIDIS GROUP BY AGGLUTINATION AND ABSORPTION TESTS

	Classification of Strains According to Type				
	1 B. enteritidis	2	3	3 Atypical	4 Heterogeneous Group
	13	7 9	5 6 10 12 16 17	3 14	1 2 4 8 11
Total in each type*..	1	2	6	2	5

* Strain Number 15 was lost before typing was done.

It will be observed from table 3 that 1 strain was found to be identical with our laboratory strain of B. enteritidis, 2 strains fell into type 2, and 6 strains into type 3, and 2 into atypical type 3. By absorption the atypical type 3 strains reduced the titre of type 3 immune serum from 1-8000 to 1-160. These 3 types are well marked and specific groups; type 4 is a heterogeneous group the members of which show very little if any relationship with each other by absorption tests, and each member is agglutinated strongly by its serum only. This is analogous to the type of pneumococci. It may well be that with a larger series of organisms, the division might be extended to include one or more additional specific types.

There was no apparent correlation between the presence of these organisms and the type of stools, e. g., strain 13 in type 1 was apparently a case of influenzal pneumonia of the constipated type.

The 2 cases in type 2 were mild uncomplicated cases of influenza with constipation.

The 8 strains falling in type 3 were associated with cases as follows: Strains 5, 6, 10 and 12 were from mild, constipated cases of influenza, while strain 16 was from a severe case associated with diarrhea without pneumonia and strains 17 and 3 from influenzal-pneumonias of the diarrheal type. Strain 14 was from a case of constipated influenzal-pneumonia.

In the heterogeneous group, or type 4, strains 1 and 8 were associated with influenzal pneumonia, one case being of the diarrheal type and the other of the constipated; strain 2 came from an uncomplicated influenza with diarrhea, while 4 and 11 came from uncomplicated influenza, with constipation.

SUMMARY AND CONCLUSIONS

Bacteriologic examinations of the feces of 32 patients with influenza showed the presence of B. typhosus in 3 and of enteritidis-like organisms in 17 others. Examination in control cases (1 case of typhoid and 1 of mumps, 2 of measles, 3 of tonsillitis, several of lobar pneumonia and several surgical cases) yielded B. typhosus in the case of typhoid, but no enteritidis-like organisms in any of the other cases.

The presence of B. typhosus in three of the cases of influenza may be interpreted as influenza cases among typhoid carriers or mild cases of typhoid resembling influenza.

The significance of the enteritidis-like organisms is unknown.

The 17 strains of enteritidis-like organisms would be classified according to Jordan as either B. paratyphosus B, or B. enteritidis, with several of the strains atypical in dulcite. The relationship established by absorption tests shows that dulcite fermentation is variable in apparently identical strains.

By agglutination and absorption tests, these strains seem to show no relationship to B. paratyphosus A or B, B. suipestifer, B. typhimurium and B. cavipesticus. Many of them show relationship to our laboratory strain of B. enteritidis and one strain was found to be identical with it. This suggests that B. enteritidis may be typed similarly to the pneumococci. Our strains seemed to fall into 4 types, 3 specific and 1 heterogeneous group. We feel that this is more rational than calling them new organisms.

There seemed to be no correlation between the nature of stools and the presence of these organisms. They were found in both diarrheal and constipated stools, in mild and severe cases of influenza.

If these organisms have no clinical significance in these cases, it would seem to raise the question as to the value of much of the published work on epidemics of food poisoning, supposedly due to enteritidis-like organisms where the mere presence in feces coupled with more or less vague clinical pictures quite similar to many cases of influenza have been assumed to prove the enteritidis-like organisms as the causative factor.

Our results would seem to warrant more work being done on the gastro-intestinal tract in influenza.

HEMOLYTIC STREPTOCOCCI IN THE THROAT IN CERTAIN ACUTE INFECTIOUS DISEASES

Andrew Otteraaen

From the John McCormick Institute for Infectious Diseases, Chicago

To determine the prevalence of hemolytic streptococci in the throat of patients with acute infectious diseases some 300 patients have been examined.

Swabs were taken from the mouth and nose, as well as from the throat, of each patient. In swabbing the throat the tonsils and pharynx were always touched. The mouth included the cheeks, gums and the floor, also of course bringing along more or less saliva. In the nose attempts were made to reach the nasopharynx, but these were not always successful, many of the patients being very young children. After the swabs were taken, the methods adopted by the Medical Department of the United States Army for the isolation and identification of hemolytic streptococci[1] were followed with the exception that goat's blood was used for blood agar instead of horse, rabbit or human blood. The surface inoculation of blood agar plates was used and the organisms that answered to the current descriptions of hemolytic streptococci on blood agar plates, formed chains in broth, did not dissolve in bile and laked a 5% suspension of rabbit corpuscles in 2 hours, were considered as such.

The organisms in question, as usually described, formed small, grayish, shiny, moist, elevated, round colonies, surrounded by a clear zone of hemolysis about 2-4 mm. in diameter. Most of the strains of streptococci obtained in my work answered to this description, but all the strains were not exactly alike on blood agar plates. In general, strains obtained from healthy persons seemed like those obtained from patients, and no difference was noticed in strains from different sources in the same individual. On surface plates the colonies of some strains were very small in size, dense, opaque and of a grayish white color, surrounded by a comparatively large, completely cleared zone. The colonies of other strains were as large as 8 mm. in diameter, flat, slightly elevated, of a light grayish color, dull and finely granular. Other strains showed a rather small hemolytic zone compared to the size of the colony. All strains produced complete hemolysis, yet there was a difference in the clearness of the laked area, although the microscope revealed that all cells within the hemolytic zone had been laked. The colonies of most strains were round and convexly elevated, but some were lobulated or irregularly outlined; others were larger in size, flat, elevated; while still others showed a rounded raised edge with a slight central flattened depression. Most of the deep colonies were biconvex, but lobulated or irregularly outlined and triangular colonies were also seen. The color of the colonies varied from brownish to whitish.

Received for publication Aug. 11, 1919.

[1] Recommendations of the Committee on a Standard Routine Method for the Isolation and Identification of Hemolytic Streptococci from Throats, Sputa, and Pathologic Exudates, Jour. Lab. and Clin. Med., 1918, 3, p. 618; Jour. Med. Research, 1915, 31, p. 455.

The differences noted in the appearance of the colonies of different strains could not well be due to the blood agar as this was always fresh and plates of uniform thickness were used.

In the corpuscle suspension a few strains caused complete hemolysis in one hour. There was a tendency in certain strains of the stock culture to lose some of the hemolytic properties, this being more marked in the 5% suspension of rabbit corpuscles than on blood-agar plates. In most strains no difference was noticed. Fermentation tests of 50 strains gave results (table 1) showing that, according to Holman's classification,[2] the strains fall into the pyogenes and anginosus groups.

TABLE 1

SUGAR REACTION OF FIFTY STRAINS

Sugar	Lactose		Saccharose		Raffinose		Mannite		Inulin		Salicin	
	+	—	+	—	+	—	+	—	+	—	+	—
Number of strains....	50	0	50	0	0	50	4	46	0	50	2	48

In 140 of the 300 patients, or 46.6%, examined by the methods outlined, hemolytic streptococci were present at the time of entrance into the hospital; 40 more became positive during their stay in the hospital, making a total of 180 or 60% giving positive cultures. Of the 180 positive cases, 96 or 53.3% became negative while in the hospital, 84 or 46.6% remained positive. In 160 patients, or 53.3%, the cultures gave a negative result and 120, or 75%, of these remained negative while 40, or 25%, became positive while in the hospital. Of the 300 patients, 130 had diphtheria, of whom 58 or 46.6% gave positive cultures, and 125 had scarlet fever, of whom 98 or 78.4% gave hemolytic streptococci. The remaining 45 had miscellaneous diseases with 20 or 44.4% positive cultures. From a very small number of the patients would be obtained a positive culture from all three sources—mouth, throat and nose. Positive cultures were obtained from the mouth and throat of a larger number of patients, and from the throat and nose of a still larger number, while positive cultures were taken from the throat of all patients with positive cultures. Patients from the nose of whom positive cultures were obtained did not as a rule have streptococci in the mouth, and vice versa. In all, 50 positive cultures, or 16.3%, were obtained from the nose, and 33 positive cultures, or 11%, from the mouth. In the scarlet fever patients 20.8% positive cultures were obtained from the nose, and 12.8% from the mouth. Of the diphtheria patients 10% positive cultures were obtained from the nose and 4.6% from the mouth. The percentage of positive cultures in the miscellaneous diseases was alike for mouth and nose, being 11% from both sources. Apparently, the throat is the area of predilection while the nose, and especially the mouth, do not seem to harbor the organisms frequently. When hemolytic streptococci were present in the nose, they were very often the predominating organisms there; this was not true in the mouth where, as a rule, they were found in small numbers. The nasal secretions apparently furnish a good medium for the development of the streptococcus. In the throat the plates would give from a few colonies to an almost pure growth, but the streptococcus was never found in pure culture in any of the three sources. The great majority of these patients were children, most of whom had more or

[2] Jour. Med. Research, 1916, 34, p. 377.

less enlarged tonsils. Swabs were also taken, in the manner described, from 33 nurses on duty and 7 of these, or 21.2%, proved to be carriers of hemolytic streptococci—a rather low percentage, due perhaps to the protection afforded by the wearing of masks. Of a class of average healthy medical students, 57% gave positive cultures of streptococci.

It was noticed that a large number of the negative cases which later became positive did so after being placed with a carrier or carriers of the organism in question. This was not always true as some patients persisted in giving negative cultures although they were in a room with carriers. When several members of one family are ill, it is the rule to place these patients together as much as circumstances permit, and in my experience all became carriers of hemolytic streptococci. In only a few instances was this not true. The best example is that of a family of six in a ward: One patient gave a positive culture from the beginning, while in the remaining five the organisms could not be demonstrated at any time during the illness. Patients giving a positive culture at the time of their entrance into the hospital and later becoming negative would usually become so gradually, although the decrease in the number of streptococci was not parallel with the recovery of the patient. Nor did the number of organisms in patients that did not become negative always seem to be influenced by recovery. Many patients showed as large a number of organisms in their throats when well and ready to be discharged as they did at any time during their sickness.

The virulence for animals of the organisms I studied was low: 1 c c of a fresh broth culture did not seem to affect rabbits and 0.5 c c did not always kill a mouse. If phagocytability can be used as a guide to virulence, the hemolytic streptococci in question were not very virulent. Nearly all the strains tested were taken up by the human leukocytes in the presence of normal human serum in large numbers. In order to test the organisms as soon as possible after their removal from the body, swabs were inoculated into broth, incubated for from 4-6 hours, then phagocytosis experiments made. No chains of cocci were seen within the leukocytes. Diplococci and masses of individual cocci were seen, but it was not possible to say whether these cocci were hemolytic streptococci or pneumococci and staphylococci. As soon as pure cultures of hemolytic streptococci could be secured marked phagocytosis resulted. Strains obtained from other sources were not so uniform in this respect. Two strains from suppurating glands of the neck in scarlet fever patients did not give any phagocytosis at the end of 4 hours' cultivation in broth, but they did after the first subtransfer. Another strain which had been passed through mice was not taken up by leukocytes after being transferred directly from the mouse to serum broth, but it was taken up on the first subtransfer from the serum broth to a blood-agar slant. Several strains from cases of erysipelas were phagocytable as was one strain from a severe case of streptococcic septicemia. Several strains from pleural exudates from influenzae-pneumonia patients, one strain from a peritonsillar abscess, and one from the suppurating ear of a scarlet fever patient gave no phagocytosis when tested in the manner indicated, but they all soon became phagocytable on artificial growth. One strain from the spinal fluid of a case of streptococcic meningitis was nonphagocytable. This strain was not tested after growth on artificial medium. One strain obtained from the blood of a scarlet fever patient shortly before death of the patient was nonphagocytable after the eleventh subtransfer. Whether or not phagocytosis took place, there seemed to be no destruction or change of the leukocytes that came in contact with the streptococci. In pus and other exudates examined phagocytosis (by the patient's pus cells) was noted in many instances, so also in the leukocytes of mice that had been killed by the streptococcus. In the exudates there was also a destruction of leukocytes, but whether or not this was caused by the organisms present, could not be said. Pus cells are always more or less degenerated even in the absence of organisms. The report of the empyema commission of the U. S. Army states that in smears of fluid obtained by aspiration of the pleural cavity the majority of leukocytes present had undergone degeneration; also that in many cases there was no evidence of phagocytosis. In other, but fewer cases, phagocytosis was very marked. It seems that the resistance of hemolytic streptococci to opsonins may be lost rapidly on artificial cultivation; also that in some individuals opsonins are either absent or not present in a large enough amount to produce phagocytosis.

Comparison of Results Obtained by Different Methods

According to the committee on standard methods,[1] if streptococci are being sought for in material in which they may be quite rare, a preliminary growth in serum broth, glucose blood broth or cooked meat medium will serve to encourage this more than that of other organisms. If, on the other hand, it is desired to know the relative numbers of streptococci and other organisms present in the original material, it should be plated directly without preliminary enrichment. The recommendations also state that for routine examination of swabs in large numbers surface inoculation only of blood agar plates is sufficient. As stated, the latter method was followed in my work, and many of the recent investigators have also followed this method. As will be seen from tables 2 and 3, the percentage of streptococci obtained from various sources by different investigators, varies considerably. Some observers have found hemolytic streptococci in a much lower percentage from the same source. One reason for this is that different observers used different methods. Some followed the enrichment method, others washed the swab in a tube of melted blood agar and poured this on plates, while still others used the surface inoculation method.

After most of my observations had been made, the work was repeated on a small number of cases, using both the surface inoculation method and the enrichment method, in order to determine which method gave the highest number of positive cultures. Of 20 cases of scarlet fever, 19 or 95% gave positive cultures by the enrichment method, while 16 or 80% did so when the surface plate method was followed. Of 9 healthy individuals, one showed hemolytic streptococci by the latter method and 3 by the enrichment method. The class of medical students mentioned gave 46% by the surface plate method. According to these results, surface inoculation only of blood-agar plates as recommended is not sufficient for accurate work. A very small number of streptococci may have been picked up by the swab and in the process of inoculation of the plate the area of the swab containing the streptococci may not touch the blood agar at all, or the colonies may be so few in number that a hemolytic zone of a hemolytic staphylococcus, diphtheria bacillus or some other hemolytic organism may enclose and therefore obscure the small streptococcus colony that might be present. Also, the better growing organisms may entirely outgrow and cover the streptococci making it impossible to determine

[8] The Empyema Commission: Cases of Empyema at Camp Lee, Va., Jour. Am. Med. Assn., 1918, 71, p. 443.

their presence. We do not, as a rule, know whether the streptococci sought for are rare or numerous in the material to be examined, and the preliminary enrichment method certainly seems to yield more accurate results than the surface inoculation. The swab should be incubated in a liquid medium for a few hours, then inoculated into a tube of melted blood agar and poured in a plate. In this way the streptococci present will have become more numerous, and as the other organisms present do not grow as rapidly as on a surface plate, they will not interfere with the growth of hemolytic streptococci to such an extent that the latter are crowded over.

TABLE 2

INCIDENCE OF HEMOLYTIC STREPTOCOCCI FROM VARIOUS SOURCES IN VARIOUS DISEASES

Disease	Mouth		Throat		Nose		Sputum		Investigators
	No. of Cases	% Positive	No. of Cases	% Positive	No. of Cases	% Positive	No. of Cases	% Positive	
Influenza and pneumonia	....	....	....	....	....	4	....	20	Nuzum and others[4]
Measles	....	....	388	77.1	....	....	....	....	Levy and Alexander[5]
Influenzal bronchopneumonia	....	....	....	4	....	....	....	....	Keegan[6]
Influenza	....	....	....	4	....	....	....	....	Friedlander and others[7]
Bronchopneumonia	....	....	159	12.2	....	....	....	....	Hirsch and McKinney[8]
Tonsillitis	9	33.3	9	88.2	9	66.6	....	....	Nichols and Bryan[9]
Influenzal pneumonia	....	....	79	5	....	....	302	0	Hall, Stone and Simpson[10]
Influenzal pneumonia	....	....	366	34	....	....	740	17	Blanton and Irons[11]
Influenza	....	....	....	....	....	....	20	65	Davis[12]
Influenza	....	....	....	....	....	....	42	31	Davis[12]
Arthritis, nephritis, myocarditis	....	....	48	94	....	....	....	....	Davis[12]
Influenzal pneumonia	....	....	....	....	....	....	69	4.3	Opie, Freeman et al.[13]
Bronchopneumonia	....	....	....	....	....	....	43	14	Opie, Freeman et al.[13]
Measles	....	....	857	35	....	....	....	....	Cumming and others[14]
Lobar pneumonia	....	....	165	69	....	....	92	41	Cumming and others
Scarlet fever	....	....	192	87	....	....	....	....	Cumming and others
Otitis media	....	....	204	74	....	....	....	....	Cumming and others
Mumps	....	....	147	37	....	....	....	....	Cumming and others
Tonsillitis	....	....	79	54	....	....	....	....	Cumming and others
Pneumonia	....	....	....	....	....	....	156	30	Lamb[15]
Pneumonia and measles	....	....	....	5.7 to 20	....	....	....	....	Beals and others[16]
Pneumonia empyema	....	....	....	33 to 40	....	....	....	....	Beals and others
Acute infectious disease	300	11	300	60	300	16.3	....	....	Otteraaen
Diphtheria	130	4.6	130	46.6	130	10	....	....	Included in 300 cases of acute infectious diseases
Scarlet fever	125	12.8	145	82	125	20.8	....	....	

[4] Ibid., p. 1562.
[5] Ibid., 1918 70, p. 1827.
[6] Ibid., 1918, 71, p. 1051.
[7] Ibid., p. 1652.
[8] Ibid., p. 1735.
[9] Ibid., 1918, 71, p. 1813.
[10] Ibid., p. 1986.
[11] Ibid., p. 1988.
[12] Ibid., 1919, 72, p. 819.
[13] Ibid., 1919, 72, p. 108 and p. 556.
[14] Ibid., p. 704.
[15] Ibid., p. 1133.
[16] Jour. Infect. Dis., 1918, 23, p. 475.

TABLE 3

INCIDENCE OF HEMOLYTIC STREPTOCOCCI FROM VARIOUS SOURCES IN HEALTHY PERSONS AND FROM EXCISED TONSILS

Throat		Nose		Excised Tonsils		
Number of Cases	Percentage Positive	Number of Cases	Percentage Positive	Number of Cases	Percentage Positive	Investigators
489	14.8	....	....	....	....	Levy and Alexander[5]
95	83.2	....	....	....	....	Levy and Alexander
50	28	....	....	100 pairs	75	Nichols and Bryan[9]
		357	75	....	....	Blanton and Irons[11]
284	26	....	....	....	....	Opie, Freeman and others[13]
4,743	1	....	....	....	....	Hamilton and Havens[17]
42	60	....	....	61 pairs	97	Davis[12]
168	6	69	55	142	82	Cumming, Spruit and Aten[14]
308	1.6	....	....	....	....	Bunce, Berlin and Lawrence[18]
35	57	....	....	....	....	Otteraaen
33	21.2	....	....	....	....	Otteraaen

CONCLUSIONS

Hemolytic streptococci are frequent inhabitants of the throats of normal individuals and of persons suffering from acute infectious diseases. These streptococci are not virulent so far as indicated by the results of animal inoculations and phagocytoses experiments. The enrichment method should be used in preference to the surface plate method in examinations for streptococci.

[17] Jour. Am. Med. Assn., 1972, p. 272.
[18] Ibid., p. 782.

THE BACTERIOLOGY OF CHRONIC EMPYEMA

J. E. Gordon

From the Laboratory of the Base Hospital, Camp Gordon, Ga.

The development in the treatment of empyema from a purely surgical procedure to one involving the postoperative use of antiseptic solutions, has caused an increased interest in the bacteriology of that condition. Accurate bacteriologic information is recognized as of importance both from the standpoint of etiology and prognosis, and in the subsequent control of treatment.

The bacteriology of initial empyema, in civil practice, indicates that the pneumococcus is the organism most commonly involved as the causative agent, with the ordinary pus organisms next in importance, and finally the tubercle bacillus.[1] In the reports of various series of cases from army camps, however, a number of instances are recorded in which no case of pneumococcal origin has been observed. In general, the average incidence of pneumococcus empyema throughout the service will probably not be more than 20% of reported cases.

The unusual occurrence of streptococcus pneumonia during the past two winters, especially that of 1917-1918, has undoubtedly accounted for the fact that the predominating organism in empyema, as occurring in military practice, has been the streptococcus. In the majority of cases, the streptococcus has been of the hemolytic variety.[2]

In addition to the two main bacteriologic types of the infection, pneumococcus and streptococcus empyema, scattering reports are found in the literature in which the etiology is ascribed to a variety of organisms; to B. paratyphosus A,[3] B. paratyphosus B,[4] the meningococcus,[5] the gonococcus,[6] the staphylococcus,[7] and to actinomyces.[8] In addition, empyema due to B. influenzae of Pfeiffer, and to psorosperms are on record. Thus it must be recog-

Received for publication Aug. 11, 1919.

1 Osler: The Principles and Practice of Medicine, 1918.

2 Dunham and others: Jour. Am. Med. Assn., 1918, 71, p. 366; Hamburger and Mayers: ibid., 70, p. 915; Miller and Lusk: ibid., p. 702; Beals, Zimmerman and Marlow: J. Infect. Dis., 1918, 23, p. 475.

3 Weeks, C. C.: Lancet, 1916, 2, p. 433.

4 Roussel, Miramond de la Roquette and Fourcade: Bull. med. de l'Algérie, 1914, 25, p. 349.

5 Rubenstone, A. I.: New York Med. Jour., 1914, 100, p. 975.

6 Woodbury: Surg., Gynec. and Obst.: 1918, 27, p. 601.

7 Harrigan, A. H.: Med. Rec., 1915, 88, p. 629.

8 Shurly, B. R.: Tr. Climat. and Clin. Assn., 1914, 30, p. 196.

nized that while the common infecting agent in civil empyemas seems to be the pneumococcus, and the hemolytic streptococcus in the empyemas following the interstitial bronchopneumonia of the past two years, still empyema may on occasion be due to a wide variety of organisms.

BACTERIOLOGY OF CHRONIC EMPYEMA

Empyema must be recognized as a condition which may readily develop into the chronic state. Not only is the primary infection difficult to overcome, but secondary bacterial invasion is prone to ensue. With the opening of the chest cavity, the probability of secondary infection becomes almost assured. There is probably more gross infection in those cases of open pneumothorax which follow rib resection, than where thoracotomy with insertion of a relatively small tube is followed. But in either instance, it is evident that organisms may readily be aspirated into the pleural cavity. It is likewise evident that the flora thus introduced is likely to be diverse, and often representative of the saprophytic bacteria.

The presence of these secondary invaders has been recorded in the literature of empyema in several instances, without any direct reference to their nature except as "putrefactive bacteria."[9] Cole and MacCallum,[10] quote a particular case which at necropsy showed hemolytic streptococci in all cultures, as well as a gram-negative bacillus producing a putrefactive odor. They denote this putrefactive organism as being undoubtedly a terminal invader.

It seems clear that primary empyemic infection is in general due to one of two infecting micrococci, the pneumococcus and the streptococcus. And further, that following operation the bacterial flora is liable to undergo alteration, the pleura, already infected, being subjected to secondary invasion by organisms which confer on the discharge the fetid and putrescent odor so frequently observed in old empyema cases. A determination of the progressive bacterial picture or flora of these cases, as they develop chronicity, has formed the basis of this study.

CHRONIC EMPYEMA AT CAMP GORDON

The opportunity was afforded at this hospital of studying some 25 cases of empyema which had run a clinical course of from 2 months to as long as 17 months. Table 1 summarizes the histories

[9] Graham and Bell: Am. Jour. Med. Sc., 1918, 156, p, 839; Bel, G. S.: New Orleans Med. & Surg. Jour., 1917, 70, p. 33. Goltman, M.: Memphis Med. Month., 1916, 37, p. 127.

[10] Jour. Am. Med. Assn., 1918, 70, p. 1146.

of these cases. The date of admission, with the initial diagnosis, is given chronologically. A history of pneumonia, either primary or following measles or influenza (nasopharyngitis) is found to have preceded all cases with one exception. This case gave no history of an intercurrent pneumonia. The patient was admitted with measles, later developed a purulent otitis media, which was followed shortly

TABLE 1
PROGRESS RECORDS OF EMPYEMA CASES

Case No.	Date Admitted	Diagnosis on Admission	Pneumonia	Empyema	Status 4/1/19
1	12/23/17	Lobar pneumonia	12/23/17 Lobar, pneumo. 1	1/ 3/18 Hemolytic strep.	Free drainage
2	1/13/18	Measles, purulent otitis media 1/22/18	No history	1/23/18 Hemolytic strep.	Free drainage
3	4/ 5/18	Lobar pneumonia	4/ 5/18 Lobar, no culture	4/28/18 Hemolytic strep.	Discharged 2/24/19
4	7/16/18	Lobar pneumonia	7/16/18 Lobar, pneumo. I	7/27/18 Hemolytic strep.	Discharged 3/31/19
5	9/ 1/18	Measles	9/16/18 Lobar, streptoc.	9/24/18 Streptococcus	Closure 3/18/19
6	9/ 9/18	Measles	10/12/18 Lobar, hemolytic strep.	10/20/18 Hemolytic strep.	Free drainage
7	9/10/18	Measles	10/ 6/18 Lobar, hemolytic strep., pnc. IV	10/ 7/18 Hemolytic strep.	Discharged 3/15/19
8	9/18/18	Nasopharyngitis, acute	10/ 4/18 Lobar, hemolytic strep., pnc. IV	1/ 8/19 Hemolytic strep.	Discharged 3/23/19
9	9/23/18	Nasopharyngitis, acute bilateral	10/ 3/18 Bronchopneumonia, no culture	10/23/18 Hemolytic strep.	Free drainage
10	9/26/18	Nasopharyngitis	10/ 3/18 Lobar, hemolytic strep.	10/10/18 Hemolytic strep.	Free drainage
11	9/26/18	Nasopharyngitis, acute	10/ 9/18 Lobar, pneumo. II	10/27/18 Pneumococcus II	Free drainage
12	9/30/18	Lobar pneumonia	9/30/18 Lobar, no culture	10/29/18 Hemolytic strep.	Closure 3/24/19
13	10/ 2/18	Nasopharyngitis, acute	10/ 4/18 Lobar, hemolytic strep.	10/11/18 Hemolytic strep.	Closure 3/28/19
14	10/ 6/18	Nasopharyngitis, acute	10/ 7/18 Lobar, no culture	10/25/18 Hemolytic strep.	Closure 3/18/19
15	10/16/18	Lobar pneumonia	10/16/18 Lobar, pneumo. IV	10/24/18 Hemolytic strep.	Free drainage
16	10/18/18	Measles	10/29/18 Broncho., hemolytic strep.	11/ 5/18 Hemolytic strep.	Free drainage
17	10/23/18	Measles	11/ 1/18 Broncho., hemolytic strep.	11/ 4/18 Hemolytic strep.	Discharged 3/14/19
18	12/ 6/18	Tonsillitis	Jan. 1918 at Camp Meade, empyema 3/18/18	12/10/18 Recurrent emp., hem. strep.	Discharged 3/3/19
19	1/ 3/19	Bronchopneumonia	1/ 3/19 Broncho., streptococcus	1/15/19 Hemolytic strep.	Free drainage
20	1/14/19	Nasopharyngitis, tonsillitis	1/22/19 Broncho, pneumo. IV	2/ 6/19 Hemolytic strep.	Free drainage
21	1/15/19	Lobar pneumonia	1/15/19 Lobar, B. influenzae	1/23/19 Hemolytic strep.	Free drainage
22	1/18/19	Convalescent sup. pleurisy	Overseas history of influenzal pneumonia	10/28/18 Thoracotomy, Brest, France	Closure 3/25/19
23	1/27/19	Nasopharyngitis	1/28/19 Lobar, hemolytic strep.	2/ 2/19 Hemolytic strep.	Free drainage
24	1/28/19	Convalescent sup. pleuritis	Mumps, influenza, pneumonia, empyema October, 1918	11/11/18 Thoracotomy, Camp Merritt	Free drainage
25	2/ 6/19	Convalescent sup. pleuritis	10/18/18 Lobar (overseas)	11/19/18 Thoracotomy, Liverpool, Eng.	Free drainage

by a suppurative pleuritis. In all cases giving a history of pneumonia, the date on which the condition developed is accompanied by a statement of the diagnosed clinical type, together with the laboratory findings. The date of onset of the empyema, with the infecting organism, is followed by a statement of the status of the case, three months after the start of the investigation.

BLOOD PICTURE IN CHRONIC EMPYEMA

Before undertaking the bacteriologic study of these cases, it was deemed advisable to ascertain if this continued chronic condition had caused noticeable changes in the blood picture.

The blood in acute cases, which have been studied, shows invariably a leukocytosis varying from 15,000 to as high as 35,000 cells per c.mm. The average is about 20,000. In the acute condition, the differential count shows a neutrophilia of from 75% to 85%, small mononuclears representing 5% to 10% of white cells, and large mononuclears and transitionals about 10%. The presence of eosinophils is slightly above normal, with basophils present in normal proportion.

In the chronic cases, a leukocytosis was observed with counts ranging from 7,500-30,000, the average of all cases being 14,000 per c.mm., with 10,000 or thereabouts the usual count. The average for neutrophils was from 60% to 70%, with small mononuclears present in the proportion of 20% to 25%, and large mononuclears 10%. Eosinophils are found more commonly than in the acute cases, while basophils are rarely observed.

Total erythrocyte counts in acute cases could not be distinguished from a series of controls on normal individuals. In the chronic cases here reported, a secondary anemia was found to develop consistently, with counts below normal in almost every instance. Four cases showed counts of less than 4,000,000, the lowest being 3,200,000 per c.mm. The usual count was within the range of from 4,000,000-5,000,000. Hemoglobin estimation gave an average reading of 85%.

The presence of this secondary anemia may be attributed to the universal presence of an initial hemolytic streptococcus infection.

BACTERIAL CONTROL OF TREATMENT

In the treatment of suppurative pleuritis by irrigation with antiseptics, the variation of the treatment is directed to a large extent by the results attained in freeing the cavity of bacterial contamination. Routine weekly smears have been made during the course of treatment. The method employed is essentially that recommended in the Carrel-Dakin treatment of open wounds, but its application to empyema cavities presents some technical difficulties. At first smears were obtained by passing a platinum looped needle through the drainage tube, but this was soon discarded. It was realized that erroneous counts might well be obtained through growth of organisms within the rubber tube, and the collection of old pus, in cases where tubes were not removed and cleaned each day. Consequently the practice of first removing the tubes was adopted, and the needle was passed in through the external sinus. This likewise proved not altogether satisfactory, as it is difficult to prevent contamination of the needle around the opening and along the walls of the sinus, in entering the cavity. The making of the smear from the end of the drainage tube resting in the cavity was also tried, the smear being made immediately following its removal. Finally, a method suggested by the use of the West tube in meningococcus work, was developed. A long series of smears have been made simultaneously by the various methods outlined, and the bacterial counts compared. The following gives the most consistently satisfactory results:

The drainage tube is removed and is replaced by a sterile rubber tube much smaller in diameter than the tube removed. It is also shorter and should be about 5 cm. long, or just long enough to reach through the external sinus. A long looped needle is then introduced through this sterile tube into the cavity, the pus pocket is smeared, and the needle with its loop of pus, carefully withdrawn through the sterile tube. With this technic one eliminates all error due to old pus collected within the drainage tube, or along the walls of the sinus. A representative specimen of the fluid inside the pleural cavity is obtained. Before determining finally the bacteriologic fitness of the wound for closure, smears must be made from the sinus as well as the cavity.

Smears of the fluid were made on glass slides, stained with carbol-thionin, and examined. Large numbers of leukocytes are invariably present. They show signs of necrosis as a rule, and appear in various stages of degeneration. In smears from chronic cases there is rarely evidence of phagocytosis.

Counts of the bacteria present are made under the microscope, using the immersion lens.

The value of the bacteriologic control rests on a standardization of technic. A standard sized looped needle should be used, and the system of lenses, and tube length of the microscope must always be the same. This is necessary to obtain true comparative results, and a comparison of results is the basis on which this method rests, a comparative increase or decrease of bacteria in a standard field. It is believed that the method just outlined for obtaining the material for smears tends more nearly to standardize that part of the procedure. The rest of the technic is a matter of mechanical detail, leaving the personal equation in the actual counting as the variable factor.

TECHNIC OF CULTURE

Material for culture was obtained from the pleural cavity in the manner outlined for obtaining exudate for bacterial counts. Streak inoculations were made on plates in the manner recommended for meningococcus work.[11] The medium used was a beef infusion agar titrated to a P_H of 7.4-7.6, to which was added aseptically 5% of sterile horse blood. Direct smears were made at the time of culture, and the microscopic examination checked by the cultural results.

In all cases in which thoracotomy or rib resection was done from time to time, previous to operation 10 c c of fluid was withdrawn aseptically from the

[11] Standard Methods for the Detection of Meningococcus Carriers, U. S. Army, 1918.

pus pocket with a sterile syringe. The fluid thus obtained was examined culturally and microscopically in the same way as exudate obtained from the open cavity.

BACTERIOLOGY OF PLEURAL EXUDATES

A systematic program of culturing every case at weekly intervals was instituted, and has been followed through a period of 3 months.

Only one case of the series (11) gave a history of the pneumococcus as the etiologic factor. At the time of the first culturing in the present study, no cultural evidence of the pneumococcus could be found in that case, nor was it subsequently obtained in culture. In fact the pneumococcus has not been obtained in culture in any of the present work.

In the remaining 24 cases, hemolytic streptococci were the primary invaders causing the suppurative condition of the pleural cavity. The examination of the fluid at the time of the first aspiration demonstrated streptococci as the primary agents in the case of all those patients who were admitted from this command. In those cases transferred from overseas, or from other hospitals, the organism still persisted in the cavity at the time of admittance. However, as brought out later, with the persistence of the condition, it appears that the original flora is displaced in many instances by secondary invaders. At the time this investigation was undertaken, the hemolytic streptococcus could be demonstrated in only 11 cases of 24 of known streptococcal etiology.

Green-producing streptococci have been cultivated in something over half of the cases during the series of cultures taken, but have been found with no regularity, and in but one case do they seem to be the predominating organism. This type of streptococcus is among the most common secondary invaders. Their presence, in the small numbers in which they have been found, is probably of little significance.

By far the most interesting result is the finding in a large percentage of these old chronic cases of some member of a broad proteolytic group of bacilli. Nineteen of 25 show the presence of these organisms in culture and in smear.

Staphylococci in varying numbers have been found in practically all of the cases, and the majority of the cultures as they are taken from week to week will show a few colonies of the aureus or albus varieties.

Diphtheroids, usually of the solid staining, but occasionally of the barred type, are encountered from time to time, but never in large numbers, or predominating in a culture. Occasional colonies of chromogenic air bacteria have been found, as would be expected.

Such is the varied flora encountered.

The most significant results have been obtained in cultures derived from pus of secondarily encysted areas at the time of operation. Frequent fluoroscopy has denoted from time to time walled off areas of infection which had developed subsequent to the primary operation, often some months following it. A second thoracotomy was made to allow drainage of these pockets. In 10 of 11 fluids obtained at the time of operation, a proteolytic bacillus was found to be the predominating organism. Oftentimes it was obtained in pure culture, sometimes with an accompanying staphylococcus, and in two instances with a Streptococcus viridans as well as staphylococci. In all specimens, however, it was the predominating organism. Neither hemolytic streptococci nor pneumococci have been isolated from any of these fluids.

SEROLOGIC STUDY OF PATIENT'S BLOOD

The interesting results which were attained in the bacteriologic study of these empyemic lesions suggested that a more definite idea of the history and course of the infection might be deduced from a study of the blood.

A representative strain of hemolytic streptococcus was selected from a number isolated from cultures of chest fluids. It corresponded to Streptococcus pyogenes of the Holman classification. Macroscopic agglutination tests, using this strain, were made with the serum of patients. The results were most interesting. Twenty serums were tested, and all showed positive agglutination for this streptococcus. Four serums showed agglutination at a dilution of 1 : 400, in 10 cases the titer proved to be 1 : 800, and in 5 cases, 1 : 1,600. For one serum a titer of 1 : 3,200 was demonstrated. All of these serums were from cases of initial streptococcic empyema. At the time of making the tests, streptococci were absent from cavity culture in all but one case. The general absence in culture, and the uniform high titer for the organism, would indicate that the body had established a well fixed immunity for that organism.

As has been noted, streptococci of the green producing type have been obtained in culture in numerous instances, and in a number of the cases. Agglutination tests, employing a like technic, were made with the same serums, using this time as the agglutinogen, a strain of Streptococcus viridans isolated in the course of the work. No antibodies, even in a dilution of 1 : 10, could be demonstrated in any serum.

A slight antibody content for one or the other of the two types of proteolytic bacilli to be described later, was found present in seven serums, all from cases in which the organism had been demonstrated in culture from the cavity. In only one case did agglutination occur in a higher serum dilution than 1 : 20. A positive reaction at a dilution of 1 : 40 was obtained in that instance.

As controls on these four sets of agglutinations, like tests were made with serum from 15 normal individuals. No agglutinins for the same strain of streptococcus employed in the first experiment were demonstrable. Neither were agglutinins for Streptococcus viridans or either group of proteolytic bacilli present.

The relative frequency of tuberculous complications in protracted empyemas has been emphasized. To determine the possibility of tuberculous empyema being the cause of some of these chronic cases, complement fixation tests for the tubercle bacillus were made with negative results in all cases. Sputum examinations likewise failed to demonstrate the presence of B. tuberculosis.

Routine Wassermann tests also proved negative in every instance.

HEMOLYTIC STREPTOCOCCI IN CHRONIC EMPYEMA

The importance of hemolytic streptococcus in primary pleural infections has been thoroughly demonstrated by the reports of its presence in the majority of cases throughout the country. The cases here reported have all shown it in the first culture with one exception. The importance of the streptococcus in the development of the chronic state is open to question. It will be remembered that only 11 of the 25 cases here reported have at any time during this investigation given positive cultures of the organism. Of these 11 cases which gave positive findings at the beginning of the study, only 1 (22) continued to show the organism 3 months later. Eight cases (2, 6, 10, 16, 19, 20, 23 and 25) continued free drainage at that time, with discharge of fetid pus, although hemolytic streptococci had not been demonstrated in culture for a minimum of 4 weeks, and in some instances longer. Two patients (3 and 12) have been discharged to duty as recovered, streptococci having been present in only the early cultures. In but 1 case can the persisting condition be attributed to the streptococcus.

In this entire study the persistence of hemolytic streptococci has been of shorter duration, under daily irrigations of antiseptic solution, than that of the group of proteolytic bacilli already mentioned. Taken in general, the flora of these wounds seemed to follow, under treatment with antiseptic irrigations, a course much as follows: The first cultures showed hemolytic streptococci in pure culture. Under treatment following operation this organism was gradually replaced by a varying flora, usually staphylococci first being found with the streptococci, and occasionally a few diphtheroids. Soon some member of the proteolytic group became the predominating organism in culture. It continued so under treatment until gradually eliminated by the action

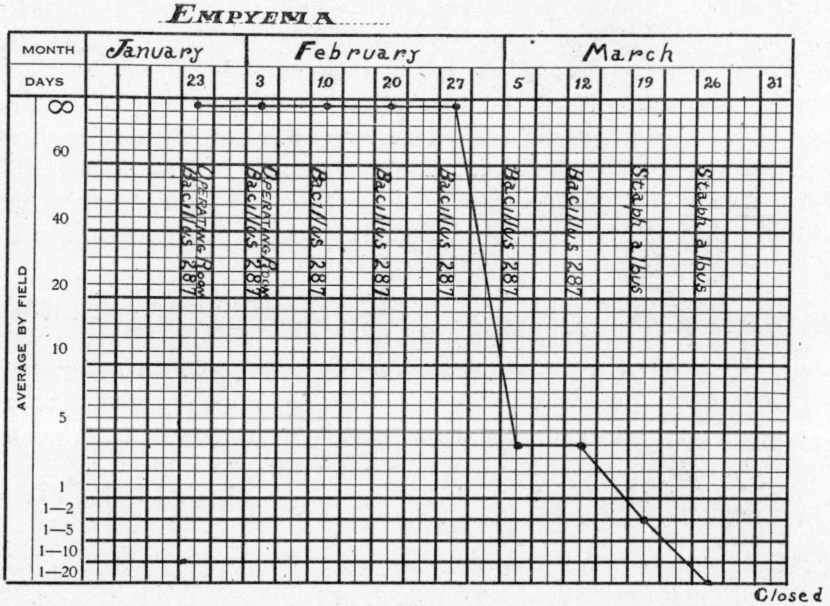

Fig. 1.—Typical bacterial count and flora in chronic empyema.

of the antiseptic. With the disappearance of the later organisms, the discharge decreased in amount. The end result was a small amount of secretion, viscid and translucent, and serous in nature. Culture showed only an occasional staphylococcus colony, with a very low bacterial smear count. Closure of the wound followed.

These results are at variance with the findings of the empyema commission working at Camp Lee. The members of the commission state that hemolytic streptococci are by no means the first organisms to disappear under antiseptic treatment in mixed infection of cavities neglected after operation, and likewise that putrefactive organisms and B. pyocyaneus disappear much earlier than hemolytic streptococci, as indicated by plate cultures. The results which I have attained from weekly cultures of wounds, and from the culture of secondarily walled off pockets, at the time of operation, would seem to ascribe a greater importance to the heterologous group of proteolytic bacilli, especially a predominating organism of the Friedländer group, than to streptococci as the bacterial factor in protracted empyema.

No detailed study of the streptococci isolated from these cases has been undertaken, but in connection with some other work on streptococci, sugar reactions were determined on strains picked from plate cultures, all of the hemolytic type.

Inoculations were made on a beef infusion broth to which 5% of horse serum and 1% of Andrade indicator had been added. Twenty per cent. solutions of the sugars were sterilized at 100 C. for three successive days, and added in sufficient amount to give a final 1% sugar medium. Holman's classification was employed in grouping the strains. Nine of 13 tested were found to be Streptococcus pyogenes, 2, S. hemolyticus III, and 3, S. infrequens.

Serum against strains of S. hemolyticus III, and against S. pyogenes, were used in agglutination tests. No differential characteristics could be observed. Positive agglutinations were obtained in a serum dilution of 1:2,500 irrespective of heterogeneous or homogeneous serum. The results bear out the accepted conclusions that agglutination reactions are of little value in the differentiation of streptococci.

PUTREFACTIVE BACTERIA

The consistent finding in successive cavity cultures, from 19 of 25 cases, and the universal observation in operative fluids, of these proteolytic bacilli, seemed to warrant a closer and more exact study of their biologic nature.

BACILLUS PROTEUS

In 5 of these cases I have isolated a proteus bacillus. It was also obtained late in the course of 2 other cases in which the organism to be described later predominated. It agrees culturally with the usual B. proteus vulgaris, fermenting glucose and saccharose with gas production, but showing no action on lactose. Morphologically, it is a typical proteus bacillus, and shows motility. It seems to be a variant of the common type of B. proteus, for it is wholly inagglutinable by an immune serum produced with a known strain as antigen. Furthermore, it shows a well developed tendency to retain the Gram stain.

Still, agglutination reactions among various strains of the proteus group are always variable, and lack of agglutinative power was rather to be expected. All of the strains isolated from empyema are, however, agglutinated in at least a dilution of 1 : 1,000 by an immune serum produced by one of the strains (192). Results indicate that these 7 strains encountered in the course of the work represent a single type of the large and varying proteus group.

BACILLUS OF FRIEDLÄNDER GROUP

A small gram-negative bacillus has been obtained in 14 cases by wound culture, and in 10 cases from fluids drawn from cavities just prior to operation.

Morphology.—The bacillus is a rather broad, rod-shaped organism, the length not exceeding 1-2 mikrons. Sometimes, in old cultures especially, besides the coccobacillary forms, longer and even filamentous bacilli are observed. The organism is nonmotile and spores are never found. Capsule formation is irregularly observed, but can usually be demonstrated in growths from animal fluids, rarely from artificial culture. The bacillus stains readily with all of the basic anilin dyes, and is negative to Gram's stain.

Cultural Characteristics.—The organism is a facultative anaerobe, and grows very luxuriantly on all culture mediums. Blood agar was used in all primary cultures, but equally good growths are obtained on beef extract agar, and on plain broth. Colonies on agar plates develop in a few hours. The growth appears in the form of grayish white, mucous-like colonies, having a characteristic slimy and semifluid appearance. Colonies have a marked tendency to become confluent, so that the surface of plates even at the end of 24 hours has the appearance of being covered with a glistening sticky exudate. The odor given off by cultures is decidedly penetrating and disagreeable, and of that distinctive quality characteristic of the Friedländer group. Cultures on agar remain viable over long periods. Gelatin is liquefied, as is Loeffler's blood serum. Evidence of hemolytic action on blood medium is present, but may be due to the marked proteolytic enzymic action, rather than to any distinct hemolytic power. Milk is an excellent medium for the growth of the bacillus. It is rendered alkaline with no coagulation. Proteolysis at the end of 5 days is practically complete, and partial reduction of the litmus is present.

Fermentation Reactions.—The various strains isolated were found by sugar reactions, and later by serologic tests, to be differentiated into one main group, and a smaller sub-group or variant. Strains from 12 cases fermented glucose without gas production. Lactose was not affected. Saccharose was fermented but without the production of gas. Acid production in inulin was always present. Strain 287, isolated from a secondary pus pocket at operation, is representative of the organism described.

Strains consistently present in 2 cases differed from the usual organism found in that gas as well as acid production followed in glucose and saccharose mediums, with lactose remaining unaffected as usual. Inulin was unaffected by these strains. Like strains were isolated in 4 other instances from cases in which the usual nongas-producing bacillus was consistently present. Culturally, the organisms were otherwise identical. Strain 086 of table 2, likewise isolated at operation, is typical of this variant.

Serologic Reactions.—An immune rabbit serum was developed against strain 287. The serum gave a titer of 1:6,000 against the homologous organism. All strains isolated were tested by agglutination against this serum, and in each instance reacted positively. All strains culturally the same, in that sugar reactions showed absence of gas production, were agglutinated by the serum in at least a dilution of 1:1,000. Those strains producing acid and gas in glucose and saccharose, and seemingly denoted as being a variant of the bacillus, were found to show agglutination at 1:20 and 1:40 dilution only. Aserum developed against strain 086, a gas producing type, agglutinated all of that variety in a serum dilution of at least 1:1,000, with low cross agglutination for the nongas-producing type.

The sugar and serologic reactions of these gas-producing strains are sufficient to distinguish them from the nonfermenting type. The morphology and growth characteristics are otherwise identical. It would seem that this smaller group was a variant of the main group. That it is closely allied is denoted by its cross agglutination, serum 287 agglutinating strain 086, and vice versa, serum 086 showing cross agglutination with strain 287. Cross agglutination with B. proteus vulgaris, B. mucosus capsulatus, and B. rhinoscleromatis was entirely absent.

Virulence.—White mice are killed by 0.001 c c of a 24-hour old broth culture of the bacillus, when injected intraperitoneally. One cubic centimeter of a like culture proves fatal for guinea-pigs of about 300 gm. weight. It is less virulent for rabbits.

Distribution.—In addition to being commonly found in these cases of chronic empyema, the organism has also been observed in 2 cases of pneumonia, typed pneumococcus I, and in a case of influenza; all encountered in the course of routine cultural work.

TABLE 2

CULTURAL CHARACTERISTICS

Organism	Glucose		Lactose		Saccharose		Maltose		Galactose		Mannite		Inulin	Litmus Milk	Gelatin
	Gas	Acid	Gas	Acid	Gas	Acid	Gas	Acid	Gas	Acid	Gas	Acid			
B. proteus vulgaris	+	+	—	—	+	+	+	+	+	+	—	—	—	Acid Coagulation Proteolysis	+
B. mucosus	+	+	—	—	+	+	+	+	+	+	—	—	—	Acid Coagulation Proteolysis	—
B. rhinoscleromatis	—	+	—	—	—	+	—	+	—	+	—	—	—	Alkaline No coagulation No proteolysis	—
B. proteus 192	+	+	—	—	+	+	+	+	+	+	—	—	—	Acid Coagulation Proteolysis	+
Bacillus 086	+	+	—	—	+	+	+	+	+	+	—	—	—	Alkaline Reduction litmus Proteolysis	+
Bacillus 287	—	+	—	—	—	+	—	+	—	+	—	—	+	Alkaline Reduction litmus Proteolysis	+

Table 2 shows the cultural reactions of this organism, its variant 086, as well as those of the proteus bacillus isolated in this study. Comparison is afforded with the cultural characteristics of known strains of B. proteus vulgaris, B. mucosus capsulatus of Friedländer, and B. rhinoscleromatis.

The exact classification of this organism is undetermined. The main group is clearly differentiated from the proteus group by its lack of gas production in any of the sugar mediums. It is related to that general group of bacilli of which B. mucosus is the dominating member. The close relationship of B. mucosus, B. rhinoscleromatis and the ozena bacillus serves to place them in a general group, the Friedländer or capsulated group. As indicated in the table, this bacillus resembles most closely B. rhinoscleromatis and the ozena bacillus, but differs from either by its rapid liquefaction of gelatin. The gas producing type is a variant in the direction of B. mucosus capsulatus itself. Biologically, the bacillus would seem to fall into the general Friedländer group. Its biochemical and cultural reactions, however, serve to differentiate it as a distinct species.

SUMMARY AND CONCLUSIONS

The blood picture in chronic empyema, in contradistinction to that of acute cases where the leukocytosis is high with a high percentage of polymorphonuclears, gives a low grade leukocytosis of about 10,000 white cells per c.mm. and a neutrophilia of 60-70%. A secondary anemia is invariably present in old and protracted cases.

A new technic for obtaining smears for bacterial counts from the pleural cavity is described. The use of a sterile protective tube in entering the cavity through the external sinus gives more uniform and consistent results in bacterial counts for the control of treatment.

Hemolytic streptococci are the usual causative agent in the series of cases here reported. These findings are in accordance with general observations in military practice of the past two years.

Study of the cases at Camp Gordon would seem to indicate that hemolytic streptococci play a minor part in empyemas which have developed into the chronic state. Fetid, purulent discharges continue to be given off, and closure of the wound is impossible, long after the hemolytic streptococcus is absent in culture or smear from wound or secondary operative fluid. A high degree of immunity to hemolytic streptococci has been demonstrated in these cases.

A heterologous group of proteolytic bacilli, of which one group predominates, has been observed in a large percentage of cases.

The typical bacterial picture in the present cases seems to be (1) hemolytic streptococci in pure culture, (2) gradual supplanting of the streptococci by a flora of secondary invaders, and (3) freeing of the wound of these organisms under treatment, followed by closure.

A variety of the proteus group has been isolated from this secondary flora of the cavity, and group classification established.

The predominating organism among secondary invaders has in these cases been a gram-negative bacillus, broadly belonging to the Friedländer group. The reactions and cultural characteristics have been described.

PHENOL RED-CHINA BLUE AS AN INDICATOR IN FERMENTATION TESTS OF BACTERIAL CULTURES

Kan-ichiro Morishima

From the Department of Pathology, U. S. Army Medical School, Washington, D. C.

A special medium for the differentiation of members of the typhoid-coli group of bacteria was devised by me[1] in 1916; it contained decolorized china blue as an indicator. The use of this stain in combination with malachite green had been recommended in 1911 by Bitter[2] in a special medium for the isolation of typhoid bacilli from stools. Harding and Ostenberg[3] employed decolorized "soluble blue," a stain related to china blue, as an indicator for acid formation in broth cultures. Bronfenbrenner[4] recommended the use of a combination of china blue and rosolic acid as an indicator for both acid and alkali in fluid mediums for fermentation tests of growing bacterial cultures. He did not decolorize the china blue before adding it to the medium; but if the medium was sufficiently alkaline, the china blue was decolorized during the sterilization. Bronfenbrenner, Davis, and Morishima[5] described the action of this indicator in milk mediums. The fact that rosolic acid is insoluble in water appeared to me to be a disadvantage.

The indicator which I herewith recommend is composed of phenol red and decolorized china blue. A 1% solution of china blue in distilled water is prepared and, while the solution is kept hot on a water bath, normal sodium hydroxid solution is added slowly until the blue color disappears and the solution becomes brown. This is the decolorized china blue solution. It should be kept in a flask with a rubber stopper. About 3.5 c c of normal sodium hydroxid are required to decolorize 100 c c of the 1% china blue solution. To the peptone solution, sugar-free broth or other fluid medium to be used, are added 5 c c of 0.02% solution of phenol red per 100 c c of medium, and the reaction is adjusted to the desired P_H. For the typhoid-coli group I have used $P_H = 7.0$ to 7.2. Then 1.2 c c of the decolorized china blue solution is added to every 100 c c of medium, and sterilization is carried out in the autoclave. The sugar solution can be sterilized separately and then added to the sterilized medium containing the

Received for publication Aug. 28, 1919.

[1] Jour. Bacteriol., 1916, 3, p. 19.
[2] München. med. Wchnschr., 1911, 58, p. 709.
[3] Jour. Infect. Dis., 1906, 2, p. 109.
[4] Jour. Med. Research, 1919, 39, p. 25.
[5] Ibid., p. 345.

indicators, when the tubing must, of course, be performed under aseptic conditions; or, the sugar can be added to the previously sterilized medium, and after being tubed, this can be heated a second time in the autoclave—this time, however, for only 10 minutes and at 10 lbs. pressure. If properly prepared, the medium is almost colorless; if, however, after sterilization, it is tinged with color, it can still be satisfactorily employed by carrying a control uninoculated tube with every set of fermentation tests. The control tube should in any case never be omitted as the mediums during incubation, for longer periods of time may absorb carbon dioxid and become more acid. After inoculation and incubation of the medium the production of alkali during bacterial growth is indicated by a pink color due to the phenol red, the china blue remaining colorless. The production of acid causes first a bright green color, due to the yellow of the phenol red plus the blue of the china blue; later, when much acid is formed, the green color changes to a deep blue. The color changes are much sharper, and consequently more easily and accurately read than those due to litmus.

I have also employed the decolorized china blue as an indicator in agar instead of the decolorized fuchsin of Endo. The nutrient agar is adjusted to the neutral point of litmus or to $P_H = 7.0$ to 7.2, the sugar is added, and 1.2 c c of the decolorized china blue per 100 c c of agar.

On plates of this medium colonies fermenting the contained sugar take on a deep blue color, while the nonfermenters remain white or pale blue. The decolorized china blue plates possess a distinct advantage over the endo-plates, in that they do not change color on exposure to light as do the latter.

Both the fluid and solid mediums described above have been used with very satisfactory results by Dr. Teague and myself in a large series of tests in connection with some experimental work on typhoid and paratyphoid bacilli.

THE METABOLISM OF VIRULENT HUMAN TUBERCLE BACILLI

STUDIES IN ACID-FAST BACTERIA. XI.

Arthur I. Kendall, Alexander A. Day
and
Arthur W. Walker

From the Patten Research Foundation, Northwestern University Medical School, Chicago

A study of the nitrogenous metabolism of certain rapidly growing acid-fast bacteria,[1] so-called saprophytic human tubercle bacilli, in plain, glucose, mannitol and glycerol broths, revealed the fact that the organisms produced moderate amounts of ammonia, comparable quantitatively with that of the colon group, or approximately 30 mg. per 100 c c of culture medium.[2]

The maximum production of ammonia was reached about the third week in the plain, glucose and mannitol cultures, the reaction becoming progressively alkaline during this period. In glycerol medium, on the other hand, the increase in ammonia was progressive to the fourth week, although the rate of production was slower and the reaction became acid, contrasting sharply in this respect with the alkalinity of the other cultures.

The ammonia curve gradually diminished from the maximum, particularly in plain glucose and mannitol mediums, until scarcely half the amount remained in solution at the end of the sixth week. The rise in ammonia coincides chronologically with the luxuriance of growth of the bacteria; the decline in ammonia is accompanied by recessive changes in the organisms, shown by a loss of staining intensity and the appearance of beaded forms.

A definite explanation for this phenomenon of waxing and waning of ammonia production is not apparent, but available evidence points to a coincidence between luxuriance of growth and ammonia increase (deamination) followed by autolysis of the organisms and a decrease in ammonia. Evidence in favor of this view is furnished by the rise

Received for publication Sept. 16, 1919.

[1] Kendall, Day and Walker: Jour. Infect. Dis., 1914, 15, p. 417.
[2] Kendall, Day and Walker: Jour. Am. Chem. Soc., 1913, 35, p. 1201.

and fall of esterase and lipase activity of the bacteria-free filtrates of these cultures as well as the esterase and lipase content of the bacteria themselves.[3]

Furthermore, total nitrogen determinations of the bacteria-free cultures show a small but unmistakable decrease at the height of bacterial development, indicating the incorporation of this element in the bacterial bodies, followed later by an increase in nitrogen, suggesting a gradual autolysis of the organisms with the liberation of some of the nitrogen in soluble form.[4]

The saprophytic human tubercle bacilli mentioned differ sharply from virulent human strains not only in their relative rapidity and luxuriance of growth in all ordinary mediums, but they fail to produce potent tuberculin even on prolonged cultivation.[5]

An important question, therefore, presents itself: In what way do virulent tubercle bacilli differ from avirulent types, and are there gradations in virulence among acid-fast organisms of the tubercle bacillus group?

In answering this question, it is of course necessary to keep constantly in view the probable difference in rates of chemical change which may result from difference in rate of development. A mere variation in the accumulation rate of the products of metabolism, coincident with corresponding relative luxuriance of growth of virulent and avirulent organisms, would be of far less significance than well defined differences in the types of reactions induced in parallel mediums.

A study was made of the nitrogenous metabolism of two virulent human tubercle bacilli, A and B, each of which would kill a full-grown guinea-pig in from 3-4 weeks following the subcutaneous injection of 1 mg. of culture. Rabbits were unaffected by 10 mg. of culture. Each organism was inoculated into a sufficient number of 250 c c Erlenmeyer flasks (each containing 100 c c of 3% glycerol broth) so that 5 flasks could be studied in parallel at weekly intervals for a period of 8 weeks. The slow development of these two organisms make this plurality of parallel cultures desirable.

Evaporation is of necessity an important factor to control in prolonged cultivations because the free surface exposed, even in a moist incubator, will permit the loss of water, with a resulting confusion of results. Each flask, therefore, was incubated 24 hours prior to inoculation to insure sterility, and then weighed. Before analysis, the loss due to evaporation was compensated for by the addition of distilled water. By so doing, errors due to evaporation

[3] Kendall, Day and Walker: Jour. Infect. Dis., 1914, 15, p. 443.
[4] Kendall, Day and Walker: Ibid., 1914, 15, p. 433.
[5] Unpublished experiments by Arthur I. Kendall.

were reduced to a minimum. Naturally, slight variations in the amount of evaporation between the different flasks occurred, but, on the whole, the results were surprisingly constant. The average replacement of water per flask at the end of the second week was 7.5 c c; the fourth week, 13.6 c c; the sixth week, 19 c c, and the eighth week, 24 c c.

The cultures in the various flasks grew at parallel rates. At the end of 2 weeks about 12% of the surface was covered with growth; 3 weeks, about 70%, and at the 4th week the bacilli formed a wrinkled, complete pellicle. The organisms were found to be completely acid-fast at the end of the 2nd week. By the 4th week, however, beaded forms began to appear, suggesting the beginning of recessive changes in the organisms.

The analyses comprised the determination of changes in the titratable reaction, using both neutral red and phenolphthalein, as indicators, the measurement of the ammonia, the total nitrogen and the amino-acid content of the bacteria-free medium.

A control was made from an uninoculated flask each week, and a composite sample, prepared from equal portions of each of the five flasks, was analyzed as well as the regular samples. The analyses of the individual flasks ran so closely parallel, the composite sample really added nothing to the definiteness of the data, and the results from it are omitted from the analytic data and the discussion.

The significance of a change in reaction, as a means for differentiating between human and bovine tubercle bacilli, has been studied by Theobald Smith[6] and Marie Grund.[7] Generally speaking, the human type of culture in glycerol broth becomes acid; the bovine type, on the contrary, becomes progressively alkaline. Occasional variants intermediate between the two have been reported by Lewis[8] and Grund.[7]

The significance of ammonia formation (deamination) as an index of the intracellular utilization of protein and protein derivatives has been emphasized in previous communications.[2]

The titration of amino-acids by the method of Sörenson is the only new analytic process introduced. The method followed was to add to 10 c c of culture medium, exactly neutral to phenolphthalein, 5 c c of exactly neutral liquor formaldehydi (using phenolphthalein as an indicator), and titrate with N/50 NaOH. The determinations were made in duplicate and a variation of 0.1 c c N/50 reagent was allowed as the greatest permissible deviation between two determinations from the same sample. Agreement within this limit was readily obtained.

Inasmuch as ammonia in the sample reacts with liquor formaldehydi, it is desirable to distinguish between total amino nitrogen and that portion which remains after ammonia is subtracted. The results in the following table are expressed as milligrams of amino nitrogen minus ammonia per 100 c c of sample.

Esterase and lipase determinations were made by the same methods as those previously described.[8]

The accompanying table contains the essential analytic data. The analyses of uninoculated control flasks, run in parallel with the inoculated flasks, are included to indicate the precision of the method used. It will be seen that the

[6] Jour. Med. Research, 1904-1905, 13, p. 405.

[7] Studies from the Research Laboratory, Department of Health, New York City, 1911, 6, p. 116.

[8] Jour. Exper. Med., 1910, 12, p. 82.

TABLE 1

Metabolism of Virulent Human Tubercle Bacilli

B. Tuberculosis A

Weeks	Flask A: Neutral Red	Flask A: Phenolphthalein	Flask A: Ammonia, mg. per 100 c c	Flask A: $\frac{NH_3}{N}$ %	Flask A: Amino Nitrogen, mg. per 100 c c	Flask A: Lipase	Flask B: Neutral Red	Flask B: Phenolphthalein	Flask B: Ammonia, mg. per 100 c c	Flask B: $\frac{NH_3}{N}$ %	Flask B: Amino Nitrogen, mg. per 100 c c	Flask B: Lipase	Flask C: Neutral Red	Flask C: Phenolphthalein	Flask C: Ammonia, mg. per 100 c c	Flask C: $\frac{NH_3}{N}$ %	Flask C: Amino Nitrogen, mg. per 100 c c	Flask C: Lipase
2	—0.30	+0.10	—0.7	—0.29	+0.5	—	—0.30	+0.10	—0.7	—0.29	+2.1	—	—0.30	+0.10	—0.7	—0.29	+1.4	—
3	+0.10	—0.10	—0.7	—0.29	—1.4	00	+0.10	000	—0.7	—0.29	+0.7	00	+0.10	000	00	00	+0.7	00
4	+0.10	000	—1.4	—0.59	—4.9	0.20	+0.10	000	—2.1	—0.88	—4.9	+0.05	+0.10	000	—2.8	—1.17	—1.4	+0.05
5	+0.30	000	—2.1	—0.88	—6.3	—	+0.30	000	—2.1	—0.88	—7.7	—	+0.30	000	—2.8	—1.17	—1.4	—
6	+0.10	+0.10	—1.4	—0.59	—0.7	00	+0.10	+0.10	—1.4	—0.59	00	00	000	+0.10	—0.7	—0.29	+2.1	00
7	000	+0.10	00	00	+4.9	00	000	+0.10	—2.1	—0.88	+5.6	00	000	+0.10	—0.7	—0.29	+2.1	00
8	+0.20	000	+1.4	+0.59	+9.1	00	+0.20	000	+1.4	+0.59	+7.7	00	+0.20	+0.10	+2.1	+0.88	+2.1	00

Weeks	Flask D: Neutral Red	Flask D: Phenolphthalein	Flask D: Ammonia, mg. per 100 c c	Flask D: $\frac{NH_3}{N}$ %	Flask D: Amino Nitrogen, mg. per 100 c c	Flask D: Lipase	Flask E: Neutral Red	Flask E: Phenolphthalein	Flask E: Ammonia, mg. per 100 c c	Flask E: $\frac{NH_3}{N}$ %	Flask E: Amino Nitrogen, mg. per 100 c c	Flask E: Lipase	Control Flask: Neutral Red	Control Flask: Phenolphthalein	Control Flask: Ammonia, mg. per c c	Control Flask: Amino Nitrogen, mg. per 100 c c	Control Flask: Lipase
2	—0.30	+0.10	—0.7	—0.29	+1.4	—	—0.30	+0.10	—1.4	—0.59	+2.1	—	+0.10	+0.30	4.9	23.8	0.25
3	+0.10	000	00	00	00	00	+0.10	000	00	00	00	00	+0.10	+0.40	3.5	23.8	0.20
4	+0.10	000	—2.1	—0.88	—1.4	—0.05	+0.10	000	—2.1	—0.88	—1.4	0.05	—0.20	+0.40	4.2	23.8	0.20
5	+0.30	000	—2.1	—0.88	—7.0	—	+0.30	000	—2.1	—0.88	—7.0	—	—0.20	+0.40	4.2	23.8	—
6	+0.10	+0.10	—2.1	—0.88	+0.7	00	+0.10	+0.10	—2.1	—0.88	—0.7	00	—0.20	+0.40	4.2	23.1	0.20
7	000	+0.10	00	00	+3.5	00	000	+0.10	—0.7	—0.29	+4.2	00	—0.20	+0.30	4.9	25.2	0.20
8	+0.20	000	+0.7	+0.29	+9.1	00	+0.20	+0.10	+1.4	+0.59	+10.5	00	—0.10	+0.40	4.9	24.5	0.20

B. Tuberculosis B

Weeks	Flask A: Neutral Red	Flask A: Phenolphthalein	Flask A: Ammonia, mg. per 100 c c	Flask A: $\frac{NH_3}{N}$ %	Flask A: Amino Nitrogen, mg. per 100 c c	Flask A: Lipase	Flask B: Neutral Red	Flask B: Phenolphthalein	Flask B: Ammonia, mg. per 100 c c	Flask B: $\frac{NH_3}{N}$ %	Flask B: Amino Nitrogen, mg. per 100 c c	Flask B: Lipase	Flask C: Neutral Red	Flask C: Phenolphthalein	Flask C: Ammonia, mg. per 100 c c	Flask C: $\frac{NH_3}{N}$ %	Flask C: Amino Nitrogen, mg. per 100 c c	Flask C: Lipase
2	+0.10	000	—0.7	—0.29	—1.4	—0.05	+0.10	000	—0.7	—0.29	+2.1	—0.05	+0.10	000	—0.7	—0.29	+1.4	—0.05
3	000	000	+0.7	+0.29	—0.7	+0.05	000	000	+0.7	+0.29	00	00	000	000	00	00	00	00
4	000	000	—2.8	—1.17	—2.8	—	000	000	—2.1	—0.88	—2.8	—	000	000	00	00	+0.7	—
5	+0.10	+0.10	—2.8	—1.17	—0.7	+0.05	+0.10	+0.10	—2.1	—0.88	—7.0	+0.05	+0.10	+0.10	—2.8	—1.17	—2.8	+0.05
6	+0.10	000	—0.7	—0.29	—2.1	00	+0.10	000	—2.1	—0.88	00	00	+0.20	000	—2.1	—0.88	00	00
7	—0.10	000	+2.8	+1.17	—0.7	00	+0.10	000	+0.7	+0.29	—2.8	00	+0.10	000	—0.7	+0.29	—2.8	00
8	+0.10	000	00	00	00	00	+0.40	000	—1.4	—0.59	—2.8	00	+0.30	000	—1.4	—0.59	—5.6	00

Weeks	Flask D: Neutral Red	Flask D: Phenolphthalein	Flask D: Ammonia, mg. per 100 c c	Flask D: $\frac{NH_3}{N}$ %	Flask D: Amino Nitrogen, mg. per 100 c c	Flask D: Lipase	Flask E: Neutral Red	Flask E: Phenolphthalein	Flask E: Ammonia, mg. per 100 c c	Flask E: $\frac{NH_3}{N}$ %	Flask E: Amino Nitrogen, mg. per 100 c c	Flask E: Lipase	Control Flask: Neutral Red	Control Flask: Phenolphthalein	Control Flask: Ammonia, mg. per c c	Control Flask: Amino Nitrogen, mg. per 100 c c	Control Flask: Lipase
2	+0.10	000	00	00	+1.4	—0.05	+0.10	000	00	00	+1.4	—0.05	+0.10	+0.40	4.9	23.8	0.25
3	000	000	+0.7	+0.29	00	00	000	000	00	00	+1.4	+0.05	+0.10	+0.40	3.5	22.4	0.20
4	000	000	—3.5	—1.47	—2.1	—	000	000	—2.1	—0.88	—3.5	—	—0.10	+0.40	4.2	22.4	—
5	+0.10	+0.10	—2.8	—1.17	—4.9	+0.05	+0.10	+0.10	—2.8	—1.17	—4.9	+0.05	000	+0.40	4.2	23.8	0.20
6	+0.10	000	—1.4	—0.59	—1.4	00	+0.10	000	—1.4	—0.59	—2.1	00	000	+0.40	4.2	21.7	0.15
7	+0.10	000	+2.1	+0.88	—2.8	00	+0.20	000	00	00	—2.8	00	000	+0.40	4.9	22.4	0.20
8	+0.10	000	+0.7	+0.29	00	00	+0.10	000	00	00	+5.6	00	000	+0.40	7.0	22.4	0.20

slight differences between parallel control flasks for each week, and variations from week to week, are within the limits of error of the analytic procedures employed in this study.

DISCUSSION

Reaction.—Neutral red: The change in reaction is slight, but there is an unmistakable increase in titratable acidity from the first week of analysis.

Phenolphthalein: The change in reaction to phenolphthalein is less than that observed with neutral red, but it is toward the acid side.

The change in reaction from neutrality to acid is in accord with the general results of Theobald Smith and Marie Grund, and it is quite possible that the acidity is due in the last analysis to the utilization of glycerol for energy by the human types of tubercle bacilli.

Ammonia.—The ammonia curves for both strains are quantitatively very similar. There is a progressive decrease in the amount up to the end of the fourth week, then a gradual increase which reaches or even surpasses that found in the controls. Inasmuch as the decrease in ammonia parallels chronologically the period of increasing luxuriance of growth of the bacteria, it may be inferred that the two phenomena are inter-related. Conversely, the period of increasing soluble ammonia coincides in point of time with the recessive changes in the bacillary bodies, shown by the appearance in ever increasing numbers of beaded and feebly staining organisms. In other words, autolytic changes in the bacilli are accompanied by an increase in soluble ammonia.

Amino Nitrogen.—In general, the amino nitrogen curve follows the ammonia curve quite closely, but the excursion is somewhat greater, as might be expected. There is no evidence of proteolytic or enzymic action, however; otherwise, the amino nitrogen would tend to increase rather than diminish during the period of luxuriance of growth. Available evidence suggests that the decrease in ammonia and amino nitrogen is associated with the growth of the bacilli, and the gradual increase of these substances in solution, as the degenerative processes in the organisms become prominent, would be in harmony with this view.

Inasmuch as the final amount of amino nitrogen exceeds somewhat both that of the controls and of uninoculated broth at the start of the experiment, it would appear that the autolytic processes result in a liberation of amino-acids or polypeptids from the bacillary substance.

Total Nitrogen.—A study of the total nitrogen in solution shows a gradual decrease which reaches a maximum at the height of vegetative activity of the organism, thus coinciding approximately with the corresponding period of greatest decrease both in ammonia and in amino nitrogen. The amount of decrease in total nitrogen is greater than the sums of the ammonia and amino nitrogen at this time, which is in harmony with the obvious incorporation of this element in the substance of the bacilli. The gradual increase in soluble total nitrogen, as autolysis proceeds, is in accord with the observations recorded above.

Esterase and Lipase.—A study of the esterase and lipase content of the mediums was made, using the methods described in previous communications.[8] Both the esterase and lipase content of the culture medium was practically nil, contrasting sharply in this respect with corresponding observations in cultures of rapidly growing "saprophytic" tubercle bacilli, previously studied. This observation is in harmony with that of Wells and Corper,[9] who found that the lipase activity of tubercle bacilli was decidedly less pronounced than that of staphylococci and Bacillus pyocyaneus. In this respect, the virulent human tubercle bacilli studied differ sharply from so-called avirulent types.

SUMMARY

Parallel cultures of virulent human tubercle bacilli, grown under the same conditions in glycerol broth, develop with remarkably uniform luxuriance, and the chemical changes associated with this development are quantitatively and qualitatively very similar.

The noteworthy chemical features are the production of a feebly acid reaction, together with a gradual decrease in ammonia, amino nitrogen and total nitrogen in solution up to the point of maximum development of the culture. As the recessive changes, resulting presumably in autolysis of the bacilli, become dominant, a resolution of nitrogeneous constituents becomes manifest. This proceeds until a very considerable return to conditions in the original quantitative nitrogenous composition of the culture medium is attained. The amino nitrogen, however, is somewhat greater than the original content, suggesting that the autolytic process yields considerable amounts of nitrogenous substance, which can be measured by the Sörenson method of formol titration.

[9] Jour. Infect. Dis., 1912, 11, p. 388.

The contrast between the development of an acid reaction, on the one hand, and the minimal evidence of deamination (shown by the ammonia curve) and of action on the protein constituents of the medium (amino nitrogen production), on the other hand, suggests that glycerol may be utilized largely for the energy requirements of the bacilli, thus shielding the protein constituents from extensive breakdown. In other words, the glycerol appears to exert a sparing action for the protein constituents of the medium. This is in harmony with the generally accepted view that glycerol is a desirable, if not essential, constituent of medium suitable for the cultivation of the human types of the tubercle bacillus.

It is in sharp contrast to the bovine types of tubercle bacilli, which do not appear to require the addition of glycerol as a constituent of mediums adapted to their cultivation.

THE ACTION OF B. TYPHOSUS ON XYLOSE AND SOME OF THE OTHER LESS FREQUENTLY USED SUGARS

With One Plate

Oscar Teague and Kan-ichiro Morishima

From the Department of Pathology, U. S. Army Medical School, Washington, D. C.

The bacillus of typhoid fever was discovered early in the course of the development of the science of bacteriology and has been subjected to intensive study by a great number of workers. It has come to be generally regarded as being possessed of greater stability and uniformity with regard to most of its properties than many other pathogenic bacteria, some of which have been subdivided into varieties by means of immunity reactions, fermentation tests, or morphologic differences; the typhoid bacillus is still described in our textbooks as being homogeneous or of a single type.

In 1917, Weiss[1] found that 6 of 31 typhoid strains investigated by him did not produce acid in xylose broth; 4 of these appeared to be also atypical antigenically in that they did not absorb out agglutinins for the xylose-fermenting typhoid strains. The "Rawlings" strain, which has been used so extensively in the preparation of typhoid vaccine, was one of those that did not ferment xylose. This fact appeared to render the question as to whether there are two distinct groups of typhoid bacilli one of practical significance, for, if such is the case, our army was being vaccinated with a strain of the minority type. Shortly after the publication of Weiss' work, Teague and McWilliams[2] showed that by plating and selecting different colonies of a single culture of B. typhosus, similar differences with regard to the absorption of agglutinins could be observed at times with these subcultures as were obtained by Weiss when using his xylose-fermenting and nonfermenting strains. It was suggested that differences in physical aggregation in cultures with varying tendencies toward spontaneous agglutination might, perhaps, cause differences in the absorption of agglutinins in the complete absence of specific antigenic differences in the strains tested. The fact that only four of the six

Received for publication Aug. 28, 1919.

[1] Jour. Med. Research, 1917, 31, p. 135.
[2] Jour. Immunol. 1917, 2, p. 383.

nonfermenting strains of Weiss were observed to behave atypically with regard to the absorption of agglutinins made it appear doubtful that these strains really differed immunologically from other typhoid strains; the evidence offered did not lead to the addition of other strains of B. typhosus to the vaccine prepared at the Army Medical School.

In 1918, strains of typhoid that did not ferment xylose were encountered in blood and stool cultures of certain typhoid patients among the American soldiers in France and the interesting observation was made that patients infected with the nonfermenting type of B. typhosus sometimes occurred in definite small groups. An investigation of these cultures, particularly with regard to their immunologic relationship to the xylose fermenting typhoids, is being carried out at the Army Medical School by the officers who collected the cultures in France. The question as to whether additional strains of B. typhosus should be used along with the "Rawlings" strain in the preparation of vaccine thus again arose, and Col. F. F. Russell directed us to investigate a larger number of cultures than had been used by Weiss with regard to their ability to ferment xylose. It was thought advisable to study at the same time the action of B. typhosus on some of the other less frequently used sugars. We decided to study the action of the growing bacilli both in fluid medium and when inoculated on the surface of agar plates containing the sugar and a suitable indicator for acid-production.

We shall first present the results of our experiments and will then try to point out in what respects they are confirmatory of results previously obtained by other workers and in what respects they supplement those previous observations.

The cultures of B. typhosus used in this investigation may be considered in three groups:

1. The collection of the Army Medical School, consisting of 116 strains. The sources of these cultures were as follows:

Blood cultures	40 strains
Stool cultures	11 strains
Urine cultures	11 strains
Bile cultures	1 strain
Source not recorded	53 strains

The cultures had been carried on artificial mediums for the following lengths of time:

More than two years	5 strains
Between one and two years	25 strains
Between six months and one year	36 strains
Less than six months	32 strains
Isolated during this investigation	11 strains
Age not recorded	7 strains

Of the 116 strains, 94 were obtained from army camps in the United States, 9 from camps in France, and the majority of the remaining 12 from civilian hospitals in the United States.

Two of the strains, namely, Pierce and Lelito, were recovered from chronic typhoid carriers. Numbers 25 and 33 are duplicate cultures obtained from Lelito at different times and 34 is a duplicate culture obtained from Pierce.

One of the strains is the well-known "Rawlings" strain, which has been used for many years in England and the United States for the preparation of typhoid vaccine. It was obtained for this collection from the Royal Army Medical School, England, in March, 1908.

2. A group of older cultures, consisting of 10 strains. Three of these had been obtained from Dr. J. C. Torrey of the Cornell University Medical School, New York, more than 5 years ago; 5 were isolated by one of us (Teague) about 3 years ago at the Quarantine Laboratory, Port of New York; and 2 came from Boston. Four of the 5 cultures from the Quarantine Laboratory were from blood cultures, the other from a stool culture; the 2 cultures from Boston were obtained from blood cultures.

3. A group of 12 cultures obtained from R. C. Colwell, 1st Lieut. Sanitary Corps, U. S. Army, through the courtesy of Lieut.-Col. H. J. Nichols. It was stated that these cultures did not ferment xylose and that they had been selected by Lieut. Colwell, precisely on account of this property, from a large number of cultures of B. typhosus obtained from American army camps in France. The 12 strains were derived from 9 patients, cultures from both blood and stools of 3 patients having been included. The duplicate strains were the following:

C-175	Blood culture
C-176	Stool culture
C-48	Blood culture
C-59	Stool culture
C-188	Blood culture
C-189	Stool culture

Six of these 12 cultures were isolated between Nov. 22, 1918, and Feb. 6, 1919.

RESULTS OF EXPERIMENTS

Xylose.—We shall consider first the results of the inoculation of the cultures of groups 1 and 2 into xylose broth. These cultures came from widely separated districts and varied greatly as to the length of time they had been carried on artificial culture mediums. The proportion of strains that do not ferment xylose found among them should represent, therefore, approximately the proportion in which such strains actually occur.

April 19, 1919, in the first tests; 115 cultures were included. The medium consisted of 1% peptone, 1% nutrose, 1% xylose and 0.5% sodium chlorid with litmus as an indicator. Two c c amounts were placed in small test tubes and sterilized in the autoclave at 10 lbs. pressure for 10 minutes. Peptone-water tubes were inoculated with the cultures and, after they had been incubated over night, one loopful of the peptone water growth was transferred to each xylose broth tube; the latter were then kept in the incubator until the close of the experiment. Endo plates were inoculated from the xylose broth cultures in the hope of detecting any accidental contaminations that may have taken place during the inoculation of the tubes. The result of these first tests was as follows—"positive" indicated that the medium became unmistakably acid, "negative" that the medium remained neutral or became alkaline:

Positive in 24 hours	106 cultures
Positive on the 5th day (57 and 156)	2 cultures
Positive on the 6th day (Rawlings and Wright)	2 cultures
Positive on the 7th day (K-9)	1 culture
Positive on the 8th day (77)	1 culture
Negative on the 27th day (49, 75 and Jones)	3 cultures

Thus, 9 of the 115 cultures did not ferment the xylose or fermented it very slowly; however, when transplants of these 9 cultures were made from the xylose broth tubes on the eleventh day to new xylose-broth tubes, all of them with the exception of Wright showed acid production in 24 hours.

April 25, 1919, in the second tests, the same cultures as in the preceding tests were employed, and the xylose broth was prepared in the same way. The results were as follows:

Positive in 24 hours.. 107 cultures
Positive on the 5th day (57)................................ 1 culture
Positive on the 8th day (49, 77, Rawling)................... 3 cultures
Positive on the 10th day (Wright)........................... 1 culture
Positive on the 11th day (75 and Jones)..................... 2 cultures
Positive on the 21st day (K-9).............................. 1 culture

Culture 156, a slow fermenter of the previous tests, was found to be contaminated in this series and is not included; with this exception, the negative cultures and slow fermenters of the first series correspond exactly to the slow fermenters of the second series of tests. Two other cultures, 10 and 163-D, showed only questionable acidity in 24 hours, but were strongly acid, the one in 48 hours and the other on the third day.

May 17, 1919, in the third tests, the same cultures were again used, but the medium was prepared from meat infusion rendered sugar-free by inoculation with B. coli, to which was added 1% peptone, 1% xylose and 0.5% sodium chlorid. Litmus was the indicator. The results were as follows:

Positive in 24 hours.. 107 cultures
Positive on the 7th day (57)................................ 1 culture
Negative on the 16th day (49, 75, 77, 156, Jones, Wright, Rawlings and K-9) .... 8 cultures

The negative and slowly fermenting cultures correspond to the negative and slowly fermenting cultures of the two preceding series of tests.

June 26, 1919, in the fourth tests, freshly isolated cultures of B. typhosus, which were not included in the preceding tests, were employed. The medium contained 0.25% nutrose, 1% peptone, 0.5% sodium chlorid and 1% xylose. Phenol red and decolorized china blue (Morishima[3]) were used as indicators. The results were as follows:

Positive in 24 hours.. 9 cultures
Negative on the 32nd day (Brockney)......................... 1 culture

A total of 126 cultures of B. typhosus were examined with regard to their ability to ferment xylose; 92% of them fermented the xylose promptly, the other 8% produced an acid reaction in the xylose-broth not at all, or only after a number of days' incubation.

The histories of the negative cultures, so far as they are available, are in table 1.

TABLE 1

HISTORIES OF CULTURES THAT DO NOT FERMENT XYLOSE OR FERMENT IT VERY SLOWLY

Number of Culture	Date Received at the Army Medical School	Source	Material Cultured	Approximate Age of Culture
49	Aug. 23, 1918	Columbus Barracks, O.	Blood	8 months
57	Aug. 3, 1918	Camp Logan, Texas	Blood	9 months
75	Aug. 29, 1918	Camp Travis, Texas	......	8 months
77	Aug. 30, 1918	Camp Dodge, Ia.	Blood	8 months
156	Feb. 20, 1919	Camp Eustis, Va.	Blood	2 months
Jones	1915	....	......	4 years
Wright	1909	From Sir A. E. Wright, London, England	......	10 years
Rawlings	1908	From the Royal Army Medical College, England	......	11 years
Brockney	June 6, 1919	Port of Embarkation, Hoboken, N. J.	Blood	a few days
K-9	....	From Dr. J. C. Torrey, Cornell University Medical School, New York	......	6 years

[3] Morishima, this journal, preceding article.

It is seen that the failure to ferment xylose promptly is not due to long continued cultivation of the B. typhosus on artificial mediums. No evidence is afforded in favor of the view that infections with the atypical typhoid bacillus are particularly frequent in certain districts.

June 26, 1919, in the fifth series of tests cultures of group 3 were used, which were selected on account of not fermenting xylose from a large number of cultures obtained in France. The medium contained 0.25% nutrose, 1% peptone, 0.5% sodium chlorid and 1% xylose. Phenol red and decolorized china blue served as the indicator.

Positive in 24 hours	0 cultures
Positive on the 6th day (C-51)	1 culture
Positive on the 8th day (C-49 and C-175)	2 cultures
Positive on the 14th day (C-60, C-176 and C-195)	3 cultures
Positive on the 18th day (C-50 and C-189)	2 cultures
Negative on the 32nd day (C-48, C-59, C-183 and C-188)	4 cultures

It is seen that the statement that these cultures do not ferment xylose is not, strictly speaking, correct. Only 4 of the cultures failed to call forth an acid reaction in the xylose broth and one of them produced acid as early as the sixth day.

July 4, 1919, in the sixth series of tests, the same cultures were used as in the preceding tests. The medium consisted of meat infusion rendered free from sugar by inoculation with B. coli, to which were added 1% peptone, 0.5% sodium chlorid and 1% xylose. Phenol red and decolorized china blue served as the indicator.

Positive in 24 hours	0 cultures
Negative on the 25th day	12 cultures

Xylose-agar plates.—In the preceding experiments the phenol red and decolorized china blue in combination served as a very satisfactory indicator in the xylose-broth. The phenol red was added to the broth and the reaction was adjusted to $P_H = 7.1$; then the decolorized china blue was added. The medium was usually almost colorless, but if the reaction had been improperly adjusted it had a greenish or pinkish tinge; even then it was quite satisfactory if a control uninoculated tube was used for comparison. A small amount of acid turned the medium bright green, a larger amount made it deep blue; alkali made the medium pink. The slowly fermenting typhoid bacilli almost invariably called forth an alkaline reaction in the medium during the first few days of incubation, and consequently the contrast between the pink color of the negative cultures and the green or blue color of the positive ones was most striking. It was decided to use the decolorized china blue as an indicator in the xylose agar also, the nutrient agar having been first adjusted to approximately $P_H = 7.1$ by the use of phenol red. We also employed the methylene blue-eosin medium of Holt-Harris and Teague.[4] Both of these plates remain unaffected by light and hence offered a distinct advantage over the Endo plate in these experiments, where the period

[4] Jour. Infect. Dis., 1916, 18, pp. 596-600.

of observation was often one or two weeks and sometimes three weeks. The nutrient agar employed contained 1% peptone, 0.33% Liebig's beef extract and 0.5% sodium chlorid; xylose to the amount of 1% and an appropriate amount of the indicators were added to the sterile melted agar, which was heated in the autoclave for 10 minutes at 10 lbs. pressure and then poured into petri dishes.

When typhoid cultures that ferment xylose rapidly are inoculated on the xylose-china-blue plate, large blue colonies develop in 24 hours; these colonies increase in size and intensity of color during the succeeding days but show no changes of interest when observed for 10 days or 2 weeks. Usually the isolated colonies are all of the same color, but occasionally some are paler during the first day or two of incubation. The color diffuses into the medium around the colonies, and the whole plate soon becomes blue. When the rapidly fermenting cultures are inoculataed on methylene blue-eosin xylose plates, the isolated colonies show black centers by transmitted light after 24 hours' incubation; on the succeeding days the black centers become larger, but the colonies offer no developments of interest over long periods of observation. Occasionally some of the isolated colonies did not have black centers after 24 hours' incubation, but when such colonies were fished and inoculated into xylose broth, they invariably caused good acid production in 24 hours; this was also true of the paler colonies on the china plates. It seemed possible that some of the cultures, which fermented xylose in broth rapidly, might contain slowly fermenting typhoid bacilli together with the rapidly fermenting ones. Consequently 38 different strains of B. typhosus which had been found to ferment xylose rapidly in broth were inoculated on the china blue-xylose plate, on the methylene blue-eosin-xylose plate, or on both. Not a single colony that was fished from the plate, yielded a slowly fermenting culture when transplanted to xylose broth. Hence the conclusion seems warranted that the rapidly fermenting strains of B. typhosus are homogeneous; i. e., they consist solely of rapidly fermenting individuals even though the culture may have been carried on agar slants for long periods of time.

If typhoid cultures that ferment xylose slowly are inoculated on xylose-china-blue plates, colorless colonies develop, which after 24 hours' incubation are somewhat thinner and consequently more transparent than colonies on control plates without xylose. On the second day, or somewhat later according to the culture used, many very small daughter colonies appear within the isolated colonies on the plate. The daughter colonies rapidly become much more opaque than the colony in which they are developing and project above the surface of the main colony as papillae. Each isolated colony on the plate may contain a dozen or more of the daughter colonies. If such a plate is viewed by transmitted light on the fifth or sixth day, the rather delicate typhoid colonies speckled with round opaque daughter colonies present an appearance entirely foreign to that of the usual typhoid colonies. A few days later deep blue areas appear in a few of the colonies; these are obviously daughter colonies that are producing acid from the xylose in the culture medium. The blue daughter colonies frequently grow with surprising rapidity and become much larger than the colony in which they originated. They yield a heaped up growth, which is quite different in appearance from the usual flat typhoid colony. In the succeeding days other colonies may show blue daughter colonies, which in turn soon develop into the large heaped up growths; later the china blue in some of the large colonies may become reduced giving the growth a brownish yellow color. Any one unfamiliar with the phenomenon under consideration would regard such a typhoid plate with large daughter colonies as being surely contaminated with other bacteria. The number of large blue colonies that develop on the plate varies greatly according to the strain of B. typhosus employed; sometimes only 1, 2 or 3 appear, in other instances 50, or 100 or more may develop. It is our custom to inoculate one edge of the plate with a loopful of a 24 hour peptone water culture of B. typhosus and then gradually spread the material over the rest of the plate; the developing colonies give a confluent growth over about one-third of the plate and yield well isolated colonies over about half the plate. The confluent growth becomes spotted with opaque colonies which jut above the surface of the growth, and some of these become blue and exhibit the same rapidity of growth shown by the blue daughter colonies of the isolated colonies.

If the methylene blue-eosin-xylose plate is inoculated with the slowly fermenting B. typhosus, the same phenomenon is observed. The colonies are all pink after 24 hours' incubation; a day or so later daughter colonies develop which appear by transmitted light as white dots within the pink colonies. Some of the daughter colonies soon become black. The small round black dots within the pink colony give a beautiful picture and show quite plainly that the acid production begins within the daughter colony. Some of the black daughter colonies exhibit the same rapidity of growth in the succeeding days that was described in the case of the blue daughter colonies of the china blue plate.

If one of the large, opaque, blue colonies of the china blue-xylose plate or one of the large, black colonies of the methylene blue-eosin xylose plate is fished and inoculated into xylose broth, the latter may show acid production in 24 hours, whereas the culture inoculated on the plate may have required 6, 8, or more days to produce acid in xylose broth; if at the same time one of the small colonies or pink colonies is fished from the xylose plate into xylose broth, as much time may be required for acid production as in the case of the original culture or even more.

All of the slowly fermenting cultures examined by us have produced daughter colonies on the xylose agar plates. The number of blue colonies found on a series of china blue-xylose plates on the eighth day after inoculation with slowly fermenting cultures was:

TABLE 2

NUMBER OF BLUE COLONIES ON THE EIGHTH DAY

Culture	
Jones	2
Wright	25
59	25
75	5
156	12
Rawlings	5
K-9	0
49	4

The cultures were inoculated at the same time on plates poured from the same batch of culture medium.

That different slowly fermenting cultures require varying lengths of time for the development of blue colonies on xylose-china blue plates is shown also by the following results:

TABLE 3

LENGTH OF TIME REQUIRED BY THE VARIOUS CULTURES FOR DEVELOPMENT OF BLUE COLONIES

Culture	Day of Reading	Number of Blue Colonies
C-49	2	4
C-50	13	0
C-51	3	0
C-51	5	8
C-59	3	9
C-60	6	2
C-60	9	8
C-175	6	2
C-183	5	1
C-188	13	0
C-189	5	1
C-48	9	11

Since the slowly fermenting strains of B. typhosus usually produce more and more blue colonies on the china blue-xylose plate as the period of incubation becomes longer, it was thought probable that the proportion of typhoid bacilli capable of fermenting xylose rapidly would increase in xylose broth cultures with increased time of incubation. In order to study the changes occurring in the xylose-broth culture with regard to the behavior of the contained bacilli toward xylose, it was decided to inoculate, at intervals of one or two days, one loopful of the xylose-broth culture on a xylose-china blue plate and to record the behavior of the colonies developing on these plates. Four cultures, known to ferment xylose-broth slowly, were selected for this experiment. To insure the absence of all contaminating bacteria, each culture was plated on the surface of a plain nutrient agar plate; one colony was fished from this plate, emulsified in sterile salt solution and plated on a second plain agar plate; a colony from the second plate was inoculated in like manner on a third plate; finally, a colony from the third plate was fished and inoculated on an agar slant. These agar slant cultures were used for the experiment, a xylose-broth tube being inoculated from each culture. A loopful of each of these xylose-broth cultures was inoculated at intervals on china blue-xylose plates with the results recorded in tables 4, 5, 6 and 7.

TABLE 4

CULTURE 57; THE XYLOSE-BROTH BECAME ACID IN FORTY-EIGHT HOURS

Age of Xylose Broth Culture in Days	Days after Inoculation of the China-Blue-Xylose Plates						
	1	2	3	4	5	7	9
At once	All white	All white*	5 blue*	7 blue	10 blue	22 blue	32 blue
1	All white	⅕ blue					
2	All pale blue	All blue					
3	Two white others blue	4 pale blue others blue					
6	All blue						

* White = white colonies. * Blue = blue colonies.

Culture 57 of table 4 fermented xylose more quickly than the other cultures, producing acid in xylose in 48 hours. On the control china blue plate of the first day only 10 blue colonies had developed on

TABLE 5

CULTURE K-9. THE XYLOSE BROTH CULTURE BECAME ACID ON THE EIGHTH DAY

Age of Xylose Broth Culture in Days	Days after Inoculation of the China-Blue-Xylose Plates					
	2	3	4	5	8	11
At once	All white	All white	All white	All white	All white	3 blue
3					1 blue	
6		3 blue		7 blue		
8	½ white ½ blue	⅓ white ⅔ blue	All blue			
10	All blue					

TABLE 6

CULTURE JONES; THE XYLOSE-BROTH BECAME ACID ON THE 11TH DAY

Age of Xylose Broth Culture in Days	Days after Inoculation of the China-Blue-Xylose Plates							
	2	3	4	5	6	8	10	11
At once	All white	All white	All white	All white	All white	All white	All white	4 blue
1					1 blue	3 blue	7 blue	
3					1 blue	3 blue		
6		45 blue		⅔ blue				
8		6 blue	40 blue					
9	Few white, others blue							
12			1 white, others blue					

TABLE 7

CULTURE RAWLINGS; THE XYLOSE BROTH BECAME ACID ON THE 8TH DAY

Age of Xylose Broth Culture in Days	Days after Inoculation of the China-Blue-Xylose Plates							
	2	3	5	6	7	8	9	10
At once	All white	All white	All white	All white	3 blue		7 blue	
1						3 blue		12 blue
3				2 blue		6 blue	7 blue	
4		2 blue	6 blue		18 blue	25 blue		
6		¾ blue		All blue				
8	Few pale blue, many blue	All blue						
10	All blue							

the fifth day. After the bacteria had grown for only 24 hours in the xylose broth, they had undergone a marked change; for, when inoculated on a china blue xylose plate, about one-fifth of all the colonies on the plate were blue on the second day. Culture K-9 of table 2 had developed on the control plate only 3 blue colonies on the eleventh day. After 7 days' growth in the xylose broth the bacteria had changed only slightly in their behavior toward xylose, but during the next 2 days they underwent a profound change, most of the bacteria producing blue colonies on the xylose plate quite promptly. Cultures Jones and Rawlings behaved similarly to K-9 but the change in the bacteria apparently took place somewhat more gradually.

To prove that the development of the daughter colonies in the preceding experiments was in no wise due to the stains contained in the agar, slowly fermenting cultures were inoculated on plain nutrient agar containing 1% xylose; on these plates daughter colonies developed in the same manner as on the china blue-xylose plates and the methylene blue-eosin xylose plates. The great majority of the cultures tested showed no daughter colonies on the control agar plates without xylose; the others showed very small daughter colonies which developed very late—usually after the tenth day of incubation. Cultures that fermented xylose rapidly, as well as those that fermented this sugar slowly, were represented among the cultures showing the late development of small daughter colonies on the control plates; among these a rapidly fermenting culture, obtained through the kindness of Dr. A. F. Coca from the New York Hospital soon after isolation from a blood culture, revealed the best developed daughter colonies on the control plate. Since the daughter colonies due to the presence in the medium of xylose appeared between the second and fifth days of incubation, the late daughter colonies, probably called forth by some unknown substance in the nutrient agar, caused no confusion. We gained the impression that daughter colonies were less likely to appear on the control plates if the cultures had been carried for a long time on nutrient agar than if they had been isolated from patients comparatively recently.

A systematic attempt was made to obtain from each of the cultures that fermented xylose slowly a subculture which would ferment this sugar in 24 hours. Two methods were employed to accomplish this purpose: First, transplants were made from the xylose broth cultures after a number of days' incubation to fresh xylose broth tubes; and second, the cultures were inoculated on china blue-xylose plates and large blue colonies, which developed on the plates, were fished and inoculated into xylose broth. Rapidly fermenting subcultures were readily obtained from many of the cultures by both of these methods. Some of the cultures, however, were quite refractory and positive results were obtained in these instances only after repeated attempts. Rapidly fermenting subcultures have been obtained from all of the slowly fermenting strains with the single exception of culture C-188. These subcultures were plated to demonstrate their purity and were agglutinated with a typhoid immune serum and found to agglutinate to the same limits as the original cultures. Since cultures C-188 and C-189 were from the same patient, the former from a blood culture, the latter from a stool, they may be regarded as the same strain; we succeeded in obtaining from C-189 a subculture that fermented xylose in 24 hours.

Arabinose Broth.—It is generally stated that B. typhosus does not ferment arabinose. Nevertheless, we carried out a series of experiments with this sugar similar to those described above for xylose. It will suffice for the present to indicate briefly the results obtained, the discussion of these results being reserved for a later section of this articles.

June 2, 1919, in the first series of tests, 114 cultures of groups 1 and 2 were employed. The medium consisted of meat infusion rendered sugar-free by inoculation with B. coli, to which was added 1% peptone, 0.5% sodium chlorid and 1% arabinose. Litmus was the indicator. Sterilization was carried out in the autoclave at 10 lbs.' pressure for 10 minutes.

Positive on the 2nd day (1)	1 culture
Positive on the 7th day (9, 34, 134 and 138)	4 cultures
Positive on the 9th day (63)	1 culture
Positive on the 11th day (16)	1 culture
Positive on the 28th day (3)	1 culture
Negative on the 28th day	107 cultures

Only 7% of the cultures showed acid production in the arabinose broth tubes of this series.

June 22, 1919, in the second series of tests, 117 cultures of groups 1 and 2 were employed. The medium contained 1% peptone, 0.25% nutrose and 1% arabinose. Phenol red and decolorized china blue served as indicators.

Positive on the 3rd day (75)	1 culture
Positive on the 4th day (100 and 161)	2 cultures
Positive on the 10th day (63)	1 culture
Positive on the 14th day (31)	1 culture
Positive on the 23rd day (162)	1 culture
Positive on the 24th day (28)	1 culture
Negative on the 30th day	110 cultures

Only 6% of the cultures showed acid production in the arabinose broth. Although there is a fairly good agreement in the percentage of positives in the two sets of tests, yet the positives of the first series were with one exception, culture 63, negative in the second series.

June 26, 1919, in the third series of tests, the 12 cultures from France that fermented xylose slowly and 9 recently isolated cultures were used. The medium was the same as in the second series.

Positive on the 6th day (C-188)..........................	1 culture
Negative on the 32nd day..................................	20 cultures

July 4, 1919, in the fourth series of tests, the cultures that had given positive results in either of the first two series of tests and the 12 cultures from France that fermented xylose slowly were plated on plain nutrient agar, and a single colony from each plate was fished and inoculated on an agar slant. The latter cultures were employed in this experiment. The medium was meat infusion rendered sugar-free by inoculation with B. coli, to which was added 1% peptone, 0.5% sodium chlorid and 1% arabinose. Phenol red and decolorized china blue served as indicators.

Positive on the 2nd day (98)............................	1 culture
Positive on the 6th day (C-51, C-59, C-175, 191 and 134).....	5 cultures
Positive on the 10th day (C-176)........................	1 culture
Negative on the 25th day................................	20 cultures

Arabinose Plates.—All of the typhoid cultures inoculated by us on arabinose-china blue plates have without exception produced daughter colonies similar to those described above. In the case of xylose we have seen that only about 10% of the cultures, namely, those that fermented xylose in broth very slowly, gave rise to daughter colonies. On the arabinose china-blue plates each isolated colony usually contains many small daughter colonies; between the second and tenth days, one or two or more blue colonies may appear. A number of the latter, when fished into arabinose broth, caused acid production in 24 hours. The blue colonies grow with great rapidity, but, instead of yielding a heaped up growth as in the case of xylose, they usually give a flat spreading growth which may form an opaque, round colony having several times the diameter of the original colony from which it started. Furthermore, the large blue colonies on the arabinose plate do not usually increase in number on further incubation to the same extent as is the case with the slowly fermenting typhoid cultures on xylose plates.

We have made no systematic attempt to obtain from each typhoid culture of our collection a subculture that would ferment arabinose in 24 hours, but we have obtained a number of such subcultures and have proved them to be typhoid bacilli by means of the agglutination test. These subcultures when inoculated on arabinose-china blue plates yield colonies, uniform in type, which do not develop daughter colonies. Our records show that we have inoculated on china blue-arabinose plates 33 different typhoid cultures, 11 of which were of the type that ferments xylose rapidly and 22 of the type that ferments xylose slowly; 5 of the former group and 8 of the latter group gave rise to one or more large blue colonies. In the arabinose-broth tests also positive cultures were found among the strains that fermented xylose slowly, as well as among those that fermented xylose rapidly. There thus appears to be no relation between the development of ferments for xylose and for arabinose by different strains of B. typhosus, although these two sugars are closely related chemically.

When subcultures that fermented xylose rapidly were obtained from slow fermenters, these subcultures remained rapid fermenters when kept on agar slants containing no xylose. By fishing both blue and white colonies from xylose-china blue plates on agar slants and at the same time into xylose broth, we obtained rapid and slow fermenters from the same cultures. Twenty-five of these subcultures, which gave a good acid reaction in xylose broth in from 24 to 48 hours, yielded the same result when inoculated into xylose broth from 1 to 3 months later, though they had not been in contact with xylose during the interval. Eighteen subcultures that produced acid not at all or after the eighth day on the first test reacted in the same way after from 1 to 3 months on plain agar. One subculture, 57-C-ii, which produced acid only after 20 days on the first test, gave an acid reaction on the 7th day in the second test. Two subcultures, C-189-1 and Lewis B-2, which were positive on the third and fifth day, respectively, in the first test, were negative on the sixteenth day of the second test.

Similarly, 19 subcultures that fermented arabinose in from 24 to 48 hours on the first test still fermented arabinose after an interval of from 1 to 2 months on plain agar, in from 24 to 48 hours. Since most of the typhoid cultures gave negative results in arabinose broth, only a few of the white colonies were fished from arabinose-china blue plates; five of these were negative in both tests, one was negative in the first test and gave acid reaction in arabinose broth on the fourth day in the second test.

All of these subcultures from the arabinose and xylose plates were shown to be typhoid bacilli by agglutination with a typhoid serum.

Dulcite Broth.—It will be seen below that none of the cultures tested produced acid in dulcite broth before the fourth day. A large percentage of the cultures — in the first series, 37 — fermented the xylose if the tubes were observed for a period of 30 days. The positive cultures of one series of tests did not at all correspond with the positives of other series; a culture might ferment the dulcite comparatively early in one test and not produce an acid reaction at all in two or three succeeding tests. We have seen in the foregoing that many typhoid cultures behaved in a similar way with regard to arabinose broth, but that the two groups of cultures were quite constant in their behavior in xylose broth in that the rapid fermenters always fermented rapidly and the slow fermenters never fermented rapidly, though the time required by the latter in different tests varied considerably.

June 2, 1919, in the first series of tests, 115 typhoid cultures of groups 1 and 2 were used. The medium consisted of meat infusion, rendered free from sugar by inoculation with B. coli, to which were added 1% peptone, 0.5% sodium chlorid and 1% dulcite. Litmus was the indicator.

Positive on the 4th day	1 culture
Positive on the 7th day	15 cultures
Positive on the 9th day	8 cultures
Positive on the 11th day	7 cultures
Positive on the 13th day	9 cultures
Positive on the 16th day	2 cultures
Positive on the 19th day	1 culture
Negative on the 40th day	72 cultures

Forty-three of the cultures, or 37%, were positive.

June 22, 1919, in the second series of tests, 57 cultures of group 1 were used. The dulcite broth was prepared as in the preceding tests.

Positive on the 10th day	1 culture
Positive on the 14th day	5 cultures
Positive on the 23rd day	12 cultures
Positive on the 30th day	9 cultures
Negative on the 30th day	30 cultures

Twenty-seven of the cultures, or 47%, were positive.

June 26, 1919, in the third series, 9 recently isolated cultures, all except one of which fermented xylose rapidly, and 12 cultures from France, which fermented xylose slowly. The medium contained 0.25% nutrose, 0.5% sodium chlorid, 1% peptone and 1% dulcite. Phenol red and decolorized china blue served as indicators.

Positive on the 14th day	6 cultures
Positive on the 16th day	1 culture
Negative on the 32nd day	14 cultures

Four of the strains that ferment xylose rapidly were positive and only 3 of the 12 cultures that ferment xylose slowly were positive.

July 4, 1919, in the fourth series, 12 cultures from France which ferment xylose slowly and 17 selected cultures, which in at least one test had fermented arabinose in broth, were used. The medium consisted of meat infusion, rendered sugar-free by inoculation with B. coli, to which were added 1% peptone, 0.5% sodium chlorid and 1% dulcite. The cultures were plated on nutrient agar and single colonies were fished and inoculated on agar slants; the latter cultures were used in the experiment.

Positive on the 10th day	1 culture
Positive on the 15th day	2 cultures
Positive on the 31st day	1 culture
Negative on the 31st day	25 cultures

Only 14% of the cultures were positive; the smaller percentage of positives in this test than in the preceding tests may have been due to the fact that cultures freshly started from a single colony were used.

A fifth series, including all of our 139 cultures, gave 74 positives on or before the twenty-sixth day; that is, 54% of positives.

In all of the above dulcite-broth tests there was a greater tendency for the indicator (litmus or china blue) to become reduced than in the tests with xylose broth or arabinose broth; it is highly probable that some of the tubes that were recorded as negative were, in fact, positive, and that the percentage of positives, as given, is consequently too low.

Dulcite plates.—When typhoid cultures are inoculated on dulcite-china blue plates, daughter colonies appear on from the second to fifth day. They appear at first in comparatively few of the colonies on the plate and each of these colonies usually contains only one or two daughter colonies; in both of these respects the dulcite plate is different from the xylose or arabinose plates. Another difference consists in the fact that almost all the daughter colonies on the dulcite plate increase rapidly in size, while on the xylose or arabinose only an extremely small percentage of the daughter colonies, which are usually crowded together within a colony, exhibit this rapid growth. It is quite characteristic for the confluent growth on the dulcite plate to become studded with large opaque colonies and large opaque daughter colonies appear also in scattered isolated colonies. Such daughter colonies, almost without exception, grow very rapidly, yielding a heaped up growth, and some of them become blue or have blue centers, though there is a tendency for the china blue to become reduced as the growth further increases. It is the rule rather than the exception for the dulcite plate to have 25 or 50 or more of the large opaque colonies between the fifth and tenth day of incubation. When the large blue colonies are fished and inoculated into dulcite broth, some produce acid in 48 hours, others produce acid more slowly, still others call forth an alkaline reaction, and many cause reduction of the indicator.

No culture that we have tested has failed to produce the large opaque colonies on the dulcite agar and we have tested both cultures that ferment xylose slowly and cultures that ferment xylose rapidly—in all 40 cultures.

These experiments have furnished some evidence that ferments for xylose, arabinose and dulcite appear quite independently of each other in typhoid cultures. It was planned to secure by artificial means strains or subcultures showing maximum and minimum activity respectively for each of the sugars and then to test strains against all three of the sugars. The method pursued was to plate a culture on a china blue plate containing the sugar and to fish from the plate, after a suitable period of incubation, a blue and a white colony. The blue colony was inoculated into broth containing the sugar in question and was transplanted in such broth at intervals, if necessary, until a strongly acid reaction was produced in 24 hours. The slowly fermenting strains were kept on agar slants until time for the experiment. The results of this experiment are recorded in table 8.

Both the subcultures that fermented xylose slowly and those that fermented xylose rapidly failed to ferment arabinose; one of the rapid xylose fermenters and one of the slow xylose fermenters produced acid in dulcite.

Three of the rapid arabinose fermenters and four of the slow (or negative) arabinose fermenters produced acid in dulcite. The subculture A-K-9-1, which was trained to ferment arabinose in 24 hours, continued to ferment xylose slowly like the culture from which it was derived. The same is true of the culture D-K-9-1, which was trained to ferment dulcite in 48 hours. The two subcultures from the culture Jones, which fermented dulcite rapidly and slowly respectively, both fermented xylose slowly, though the rapid dulcite fermenter did produce acid in xylose earlier than the slow dulcite fermenter. Two of the rapid dulcite fermenters produced acid in arabinose, while none of the slow dulcite fermenters did so.

TABLE 8

RESULT IN XYLOSE, ARABINOSE AND DULCITE BROTH

Culture	Type	Xylose Broth 1 Day	3 Days	4 Days	6 Days	9 Days	21 Days	35 Days	Arabinose Broth 1 Day	4 Days	21 Days	35 Days	Dulcite Broth 1 Day	2 Days	3 Days	4 Days	6 Days	9 Days	17 Days	27 Days	35 Days
Rawling I	Rapid in xylose	++	..	..	..	..	..	++	±	..	..	—	±	..	..	..	..	..	..	..	—
Rawlings II	Slow in xylose	±	..	..	..	..	..	—	±	..	..	—	±	..	..	..	..	++	..	..	++
Jones M I	Rapid in xylose	++	..	..	..	..	..	++	±	..	..	—	±	..	..	..	..	..	..	..	—
Jones M II	Slow in xylose	±	..	..	..	..	..	—	±	..	..	—	±	..	..	..	..	..	..	..	—
156 I	Rapid in xylose	++	..	..	..	..	..	++	±	..	..	—	±	..	..	..	..	..	..	..	—
156 II a	Slow in xylose	±	..	..	..	..	..	—	±	..	..	—	±	..	..	..	..	..	..	..	—
57 C I	Rapid in xylose	++	..	..	..	..	..	++	±	..	..	—	±	..	..	..	..	..	..	..	—
57 C II	Slow in xylose	±	++	..	..	..	..	++	±	..	..	—	±	..	..	..	..	..	..	..	—
K-9 II C II	Rapid in xylose	++	..	..	..	..	..	++	±	..	..	—	±	..	++	..	..	..	..	..	++
K-9 II C I	Slow in xylose	±	..	..	..	..	..	—	±	..	..	—	±	..	..	..	..	..	..	..	—
Wright P II	Rapid in xylose	++	..	..	..	..	..	++	±	..	..	—	±	..	..	..	..	..	..	..	—
Wright C II a	Slow in xylose	±	..	..	..	++	..	++	±	..	..	—	±	..	..	..	..	..	..	..	—
A 18 I	Rapid in arabinose	++	..	..	..	..	..	++	++	..	..	++	±	..	..	..	..	..	..	..	—
A K-9 I	Rapid in arabinose	±	..	..	++	..	..	++	++	..	..	++	±	..	..	..	..	++	..	..	++
A 9	Rapid in arabinose	++	..	..	..	..	..	++	++	..	..	++	±	..	..	..	++	..	..	..	..
A 32	Rapid in arabinose	++	..	..	..	..	..	++	++	..	..	++	±	..	..	..	..	..	..	..	—
A 34	Rapid in arabinose	++	..	..	..	..	..	++	++	..	..	++	±	..	..	..	..	..	..	..	—
A 51	Rapid in arabinose	++	..	..	..	..	..	++	++	..	..	++	±	..	..	..	..	..	++	..	++
A 134	Rapid in arabinose	++	..	..	..	..	..	++	++	..	..	++	±	..	..	..	..	..	..	..	—
a 2	Slow in arabinose	++	..	..	..	..	..	++	±	..	..	—	±	..	..	..	..	..	..	..	—
a 25	Slow in arabinose	++	..	..	..	..	..	++	±	..	..	—	±	..	..	..	..	..	..	..	—
a 78	Slow in arabinose	++	..	..	..	..	..	++	±	..	..	—	±	..	..	..	..	++	..	..	++
a 91	Slow in arabinose	++	..	..	..	..	..	++	±	..	..	—	±	..	..	..	..	++	..	..	++
a 105	Slow in arabinose	++	..	..	..	..	..	++	±	..	..	—	±	..	..	..	..	..	++	..	++
a 163 D	Slow in arabinose	++	..	..	..	..	..	++	±	..	..	—	±	..	..	++	..	..	..	..	++
D Jones II	Rapid in dulcite	±	..	++	..	..	..	..	±	..	..	—	++	..	..	..	..	..	..	..	++
D K-9 I	Rapid in dulcite	±	..	..	..	..	++	++	±	..	..	—	..	++	..	..	..	..	..	..	++
D 2-I	Rapid in dulcite	++	..	..	..	..	..	++	±	..	..	—	++	..	..	..	..	..	..	..	++
D K31-I	Rapid in dulcite	++	..	..	..	..	..	++	±	..	..	—	++	..	..	..	..	..	..	..	++
D 163 D I	Rapid in dulcite	++	..	..	..	..	..	++	±	..	..	—	++	..	..	..	..	..	..	..	++
D 126	Rapid in dulcite	++	..	..	..	..	..	++	±	..	++	++	++	..	..	..	..	..	..	..	++
D 129	Rapid in dulcite	++	..	..	..	..	..	++	±	..	..	—	++	..	..	..	..	..	..	..	—
D 136	Rapid in dulcite	++	..	..	..	..	..	++	±	++	..	++	++	..	..	..	..	..	..	..	++
D 163 I	Rapid in dulcite	++	..	..	..	..	..	++	±	..	..	—	++	..	..	..	..	..	..	..	++
d 163 II	Slow in dulcite	++	..	..	..	..	..	++	±	..	..	—	±	..	..	..	..	..	..	..	—
d 3	Slow in dulcite	++	..	..	..	..	..	++	±	..	..	—	±	..	..	..	..	..	..	..	—
d 106	Slow in dulcite	++	..	..	..	..	..	++	±	..	..	—	±	..	..	..	..	..	..	..	++
d 127	Slow in dulcite	++	..	..	..	..	..	++	±	..	..	—	±	..	..	..	..	..	..	..	—
d 136	Slow in dulcite	++	..	..	..	..	..	++	±	..	..	—	±	..	..	..	..	..	..	..	—
d Rawling	Slow in dulcite	±	..	..	++	..	..	++	±	..	..	—	±	..	..	..	..	..	..	++	++
d Jones	Slow in dulcite	±	..	..	++	..	..	++	±	..	..	—	±	..	..	..	..	..	..	..	—

All in all, this experiment offers strong evidence that an increased or decreased production of the ferment for one of the three sugars — xylose, arabinose, or dulcite — induced by experimental means in a typhoid culture, does not affect the production by the culture of ferments for the other sugars.

Three subcultures that fermented xylose rapidly were transplanted every 3 days in xylose broth for 2 weeks; 3 rapid arabinose cultures were similarly transplanted in arabinose broth, and 3 rapid dulcite fermenters in dulcite broth. These 9 cultures were also transplanted every 3 days for 2 weeks in sugar-free broth. At the end of the time both sets of cultures were inoculated into xylose broth, arabinose broth and dulcite broth, as were also 9 slowly fermenting cultures. The results of this experiment are recorded in tables 9, 10 and 11.

TABLE 9

RAPIDLY FERMENTING CULTURES TRANSPLANTED EVERY THREE DAYS FOR TWO WEEKS IN BROTH CONTAINING THE SUGAR THAT IS FERMENTED

Culture	Transplanted in	Xylose Broth			Arabinose Broth			Dulcite Broth				
		1 Day	6 Days	28 Days	1 Day	4 Days	28 Days	1 Day	4 Days	11 Days	19 aDys	28 Days
X Rawling I	Xylose broth	++	..	++	±	..	—	..	..	++	..	..
X Jones M I	Xylose broth	++	..	++	±	..	—	..	++	..	..	++
X K 9 II C II	Xylose broth	++	..	++	±	..	—	..	++	..	..	..
A K 9-1	Arabinose broth	±	..	—	++	..	++	..	..	..	++	++
A 9 M	Arabinose broth	++	..	++	++	..	++	±	..	..	..	—
A 32 M	Arabinose broth	++	..	++	++	..	++	±	..	..	..	—
D Jones I	Dulcite broth	..	++	++	±	..	—	++	..	..	..	++
D 163 I	Dulcite broth	++	..	++	..	++	..	++	..	..	..	++
D 126	Dulcite broth	++	..	++	±	..	—	++	..	..	..	++

TABLE 10

THE SAME RAPIDLY FERMENTING CULTURES TRANSPLANTED EVERY THREE DAYS FOR TWO WEEKS IN SUGAR-FREE BROTH

Culture	Transplanted in	Xylose Broth		Arabinose Broth		Dulcite Broth			
		1 Day	28 Days	1 Day	28 Days	1 Day	3 Days	9 Days	28 Days
X Rawling I	Xylose broth	++	++	±	—	..	++	..	..
X Jones M I	Xylose broth	++	++	±	—	..	++	..	..
X K 9-II C II	Xylose broth	++	++	±	—	±	..	..	—
A K 9-1	Arabinose broth	±	—	++	++	..	..	++	..
A 9 M	Arabinose broth	++	++	++	++	±	..	..	—
A 32 M	Arabinose broth	++	++	++	++	±	..	..	—
D Jones I	Dulcite broth	±	—	±	—	++	..	..	++
D 163 I	Dulcite broth	++	++	±	—	++	..	..	++
D 126	Dulcite broth	++	++	±	—	++	..	..	++

TABLE 11

SLOWLY FERMENTING CULTURES

Culture	Type	Xylose Broth			Arabinose Broth			Dulcite Broth					
		1 Day	19 Days	28 Days	1 Day	6 Days	28 Days	2 Days	6 Days	9 Days	11 Days	12 Days	28 Days
x K 9-11 C I	Slow in xylose	±	..	—	±	..	—	—	++	..	..	..	++
x Jones M II	Slow in xylose	..	++	++	±	..	—	++	++	..	..	..	++
x Rawlings II a	Slow in xylose	±	..	—	±	..	—	..	..	++	..	..	..
a 105	Slow in arabinose	++	..	++	±	++	++	..	..	++	..	..	..
a 91	Slow in arabinose	++	..	++	..	..	..	±	..	..	..	..	—
a 78	Slow in arabinose	++	..	++	±	++	++	..	++	..	..	..	++
d 3	Slow in dulcite	++	..	++	±	..	—	..	..	..	..	++	..
d 163 II	Slow in dulcite	++	..	++	±	++	..	±	..	..	..	..	—
d Jones	Slow in dulcite	±	..	—	±	..	—	±	..	..	++	..	..

It is seen that the further cultivation of a rapidly fermenting strain in broth containing the sugar that it fermented rapidly did not influence the production of ferments for the other two sugars. It is seen also that the removal of the rapid fermenters from contact with the sugars for a period of two weeks, during which time they were transplanted every three days, leads to no apparent diminution in the rapidity with which they fermented their respecttive sugars.

Inoculation on china blue agar containing a given sugar often affords a more accurate idea of the behavior of a culture toward this sugar than does inoculation into broth containing the sugar. Consequently, 3 rapid fermenters and 1 slow fermenter of each of the 3 sugars were inoculated on a series of china blue plates containing 1% of xylose, arabinose, dulcite and rhamnose. Rhamnose was also employed because all the typhoid cultures inoculated on rhamnose agar had been found by us to yield many daughter colonies. Cultures which fermented rapidly the sugar contained in the agar produced blue colonies and no daughter colonies appeared on these plates. All of the cultures — the rapid fermenters of xylose, arabinose and dulcite as well as the slow fermenters — produced daughter colonies on the rhamnose plates. Subcultures of slow xylose fermenters, which had been trained to ferment arabinose or dulcite rapidly, behaved on the xylose plates like the original slow xylose fermenters from which they were derived. Rapid arabinose fermenters and rapid xylose fermenters produced the usual daughter colonies and large opaque colonies on dulcite plates. Thus additional evidence was obtained in favor of the view that the production of the ferment for one of these sugars may be increased without affecting the ferments for the other two sugars.

It was decided to inoculate typhoid cultures on a number of sugars and on salicin and glycerol to see if other sugars besides those investigated above gave rise to daughter colonies. Six cultures that were known to ferment xylose slowly and two that fermented xylose rapidly were selected for the experiment; one of the rapid fermenters had been recently isolated from the blood of a typhoid patient and showed many daughter colonies on the control plate on the fourteenth day. All of the sugars and salicin were used in 1% amounts, but 3% glycerol was employed. None of the sugars except xylose, arabinose and dulcite gave rise to daughter colonies, but the types of colonies that developed on the other plates after a few days' incubation were interesting. On the dextrose, mannite, maltose and galactose plates the colonies were small, round, flat and opaque, and apparently increased but little in size after the first 48 hours' incubation. On the salicin, lactose, saccharose and raffinose plates the colonies were like those of the control plates, while on dextrin they appeared to be somewhat larger and thicker than on the control plates. On the glycerol plates the colonies soon became very much larger and thicker than the colonies of the control plates, and after five or six or more days of incubation they were quite different from the colonies on all the other plates, so that the glycerol plates could be picked from the others at a glance; still later, the colonies on the glycerol plates became quite brown. Rhamnose was not available to us at the time this experiment was performed.

The colonies in which daughter colonies develop on the xylose, arabinose and rhamnose plates are transparent in type, being usually somewhat thinner and more delicate than the typhoid colonies on the control plate.

With regard to the smallest amounts of the sugars that give rise to daughter colonies, we have found that cultures giving good daughter colonies on 1% xylose agar on the second or third day require from 10 to 12 days on 0.2% xylose agar, and produce very few daughter colonies on 0.04% of xylose. On 0.25% and 0.1% arabinose the daughter colonies are smaller and appear later than on 1% arabinose agar. Rhamnose yields well developed daughter colonies in much greater dilution than xylose and arabinose, 0.02% of rhamnose giving good daughter colonies on the 4th day, and 0.01% many small daughter colonies on the 10th day. One one hundreth per cent. of dulcite also gives rise to daughter colonies.

One fourth per cent. dextrose added to 1% xylose agar did not interfere with the production of daughter colonies. No daughter colonies were observed on plates containing 1% xylose and 0.5 or 2% glycerin.

Raffinose.—None of our typhoid cultures produced acid in raffinose broth; after 30 days' incubation all of the tubes showed an alkaline reaction. No daughter colonies appeared on raffinose agar plates. Three per cent. and 2% raffinose agar gave rise to typhoid colonies that were larger and more opaque than the colonies of the control plate, thus indicating that B. typhosus is able to utilize this sugar as a food.

Inosite.—None of our typhoid cultures produced acid in inosite broth. No daughter colonies were seen on the inosite plates. Three per cent. inosite does not inhibit the growth of B. typhosus.

Discussion

Having presented the results of our experiments in some detail, we shall next consider the results of similar experiments that have been carried out by other workers. Daughter colonies have been observed and studied in connection with cultures of B. anthracis, V. cholerae, B. coli, B. dysenteriae and some other organisms, but they were either caused by sugars not considered in this paper or were not due to sugars at all. Twort,[5] after growing a strain of B. typhosus for two years in lactose medium, succeeded in producing a strain that fermented lactose. This experience is unique; Penfold,[6] working with 20 strains and having carried many of them for more than a year in lactose medium, obtained only negative results; he showed that the Twort lactose fermenting strain produced daughter colonies on lactose agar. This Twort culture fermented sorbite in broth only after a number of days, and Penfold found that it also gave rise to daughter colonies on sorbite agar.

Reiner Mueller[7] showed that B. typhosus produces daughter colonies on rhamnose agar. He examined a large number of cultures in this regard and found that they all gave rise to daughter colonies. He did not see acid production in rhamnose by any of his typhoid cultures. He noticed that the colonies on the rhamnose plates remain small and delicate and found that 5% rhamnose produced no more inhibition than 0.5% in the agar. He showed further that other bacteria of the typhoid-coli group are not inhibited by rhamnose and that B. typhosus gives rise to daughter colonies in 8 days on agar containing as little as 0.025% of rhamnose and in 14 days on agar containing only 0.01%. He endeavors to bring the inhibition into causal connection with the production of daughter colonies by assuming that certain bacteria within the typhoid colony overcome the inhibition, grow rapidly and give rise to daughter colonies. Penfold found that the 20 strains of B. typhosus investigated by him all gave daughter colonies on rhamnose neutral red agar and he noticed acid production in none of the daughter colonies. He did observe with some of his cultures late acid production in rhamnose broth and, on transplanting from rhamnose broth to rhamnose broth after several weeks of incubation, he was able to obtain subcultures which fermented in 1, 2 or 3 days. Such a rapid fermenter no longer produced daughter colonies on rhamnose agar and, even when it was passed through 13 generations of peptone water and plated on rhamnose agar, it still did not give rise to

[5] Proc. Roy. Soc., London, 1907, 79, p. 329.

[6] Jour. of Hyg., 1911, 11, p. 30.

[7] Centralbl. f. Bakteriol., I., O., 1911, 58, p. 97.

daughter colonies. He found that the Twort lactose-fermenting B. typhosus and a typhoid culture which had been trained to ferment dulcite rapidly both produced daughter colonies on rhamnose agar.

Reiner Mueller suggests that the development of daughter colonies on rhamnose agar might be utilized in the identification of B. typhosus; the results obtained by Penfold and by us, as far as they go, indicate that he was right in concluding that all typhoid cultures exhibit the phenomenon. Mueller found that some other bacteria besides B. typhosus also give rise to daughter colonies on rhamnose agar.

Typhoid bacilli inoculated on litmus agar containing arabinose, dulcite or raffinose produced no change in the medium according to Reiner Mueller. This is difficult to understand in view of Penfold's results with dulcite and our results with arabinose and dulcite. Penfold made a very careful study of the behavior of B. typhosus in dulcite broth and on neutral red dulcite agar. In one of his experiments in which 14 strains were inoculated into dulcite broth, the first signs of acidity occurred in from 5 to 15 days. If, after one month, subcultures were made in new dulcite broth, an acid reaction was produced in from 1 to 4 days. Three strains inoculated on neutral red dulcite agar yielded daughter colonies as early as the 3rd day and some of the latter were acid by the 5th day. Some plates showed as low as 2% of colonies with daughter colonies, some as high as 50%. Different plates inoculated with the same culture also showed variations within these limits. Subcultures, which had been trained to ferment dulcite rapidly, showed great permanency; one such culture, transplanted 25 times in peptone water during a period of 5 months and then plated on neutral red dulcite agar, yielded only fermenting colonies. Twenty colonies from a MacConkey plate of pure typhoid were inoculated into dulcite broth; the time required for acidity to appear varied from 11 to 32 days. This observation is in harmony with our findings with regard to the varying results yielded by typhoid cultures on successive tests in dulcite broth.

Krumwiede, Kohn and Valentine[8] inoculated 37 strains of B. typhosus into xylose broth and found that 29 produced acid in 24 hours while 8 of the strains required from 5 to 13 days for the production of acid.

Mandelbaum[9] obtained in Munich from the blood or feces of more than 50 patients with clinical typhoid fever a bacillus which he called Bacterium metatyphi. This bacillus resembled B. typhosus in all respects except that it produced alkali instead of acid in mediums containing glycerol. He showed that these cases were infected, in all probability, from a typhoid carrier, a woman who served as a milker in a dairy near Munich. The interesting observation was made that this carrier had both the typical B. typhosus and the B. metatyphi in her stools. The B. metatyphi had retained the property of producing alkali in glycerol mediums for 5½ years when transplanted on plain nutrient agar.

Some of the strains of B. metatyphi produced daughter colonies on glycerol agar, and from the daughter colonies cultures were obtained which behaved in all respects like B. typhosus. Since B. metatyphi would be overlooked in the usual technic for the isolation of B. typhosus, little is known at present concerning its prevalence. Russowici[10] reported having found one strain, and

[8] Jour. Med. Res., 1918, 38, p. 89.

[9] Centralbl. f. Bakteriol., I., O., 1912, 63, p. 46.

[10] München. med. Wchnschr., 1908, 55, p. 2507.

[11] Centralbl. f. Bakteriol., I., O., 1911, 58, p. 97.

Ditthorn and Luerssen[11] two strains. All of our 138 cultures produced acid in glycerol broth.

From a small epidemic of clinical typhoid fever in an insane asylum in Denmark Jacobsen[12] obtained a bacillus which he described as Bacterium typhi mutabile. The bacillus resembled B. typhosus in all respects except the following: (1) Its growth was strongly retarded on Konradi-Drigalski agar or plain nutrient agar, which had been sterilized in the autoclave, and (2) it did not agglutinate in typhoid immune serum. On the plates showing retarded growth, a few large colonies appeared on the 5th or 6th day, which when fished on agar slants gave typical agglutination with typhoid immune serum and resembled B. typhosus also in all other respects. B. typhi mutabile itself gave good agglutination three months after its isolation. Although there was an inhibited growth on Conradi-Drigalski plates, yet the organism exhibited good growth on Endo plates. Jacobsen showed that it was the sodium sulphite of the Endo plates which abolished the inhibition. Fromme[13] studied a bacillus the growth of which was retarded on nutrient agar but good on nutrient agar to which sodium sulphite was added. His bacillus differed from Jacobsen's in that it agglutinated with typhoid immune serum from the start and in that no large colonies developed on the plates showing the retarded growth.

It has been shown that the so-called nonfermenters of Weiss are in reality slow fermenters and can be made to revert to the typical rapidly fermenting type of B. typhosus. There are the following variants of B. typhosus:

1. Bacterium metatyphi (Mendelbaum), a nonfermenter of glycerol; in contact with glycerol it reverts to the typical B. typhosus.

2. Bacterium typhi mutabile (Jacobsen), the growth of which is inhibited on autoclaved nutrient agar; it reverts to the typical B. typhosus.

3. Nonfermenter of xylose (Weiss), really slow fermenters of xylose, which, growing in contact with xylose, revert to the typical B. typhosus.

4. Artificially produced variants (rapid arabinose fermenters, rapid dulcite fermenters and others).

Two other variants may be mentioned in passing: (a) freshly isolated strains which do not agglutinate with typhoid immune serum; they usually agglutinate typically after having been transplanted a number of times on artificial mediums, and (b) the so-called "blue typhoids" which produce a deep blue color in litmus milk early (from the third to sixth day); they retain this property indefinitely when propagated on nutrient agar.

[12] Centralbl. f. Bakteriol., I., O., 1910, 56, p. 208.

[13] Centralbl. f. Bakteriol., I., O., 1911, 58, p. 445.

It is obvious from the discussion that B. typhosus should not be divided into different types or groups or varieties. The variants described are very interesting and may at times, as suggested by Lieut. R. C. Colwell, be of epidemiologic value in tracing the source of infections, but since they revert to the typical B. typhosus under certain conditions, and since they have not been shown to be constantly and permanently different from B. typhosus serologically, they cannot be allowed to alter the conception of B. typhosus as a homogeneous organism.

SUMMARY

The so-called nonfermenters of xylose among typhoid strains were shown to be slow fermenters; rapidly fermenting subcultures were obtained from them.

The slowly fermenting strains produce daughter colonies on 1% xylose agar plates; some of these daughter colonies increase greatly in size and produce acid on further incubation.

Only a small percentage of the typhoid cultures investigated produced acid in arabinose broth, and these cultures did not do so constantly. Rapidly fermenting subcultures were obtained from a number of strains by plating on arabinose-china blue agar.

Typhoid cultures inoculated on 1% arabinose agar gave rise to daughter colonies; a few of the daughter colonies may increase greatly in size and produce acid on further incubation.

Subcultures that ferment arabinose rapidly still retain this characteristic after having been kept on plain nutrient agar for one or two months; the same is true of the subcultures that ferment xylose rapidly, which were obtained from slowly fermenting strains.

The amount of ferment for one of the sugars, xylose, arabinose or dulcite produced by a strain of B. typhosus may be greatly increased without affecting the production of ferments for the other two sugars.

The evidence at hand, it is thought, does not justify the division of typhoid bacilli into separate groups.

EXPLANATION OF PLATE

Fig. 1.—Colonies of B. typhosus "Rawlings" on nutrient agar containing 1% xylose after 13 days' incubation.

Fig. 2.—Colonies of B. typhosus "Rawlings" on a control plate of the same nutrient agar without xylose.

Fig. 3.—Colonies of B. typhosus 156 on nutrient agar containing 1% arabinose after 13 days' incubation.

Fig. 4.—Colonies of B. typhosus 156 on nutrient agar containing 1% dulcite after 13 days' incubation.

Plate I

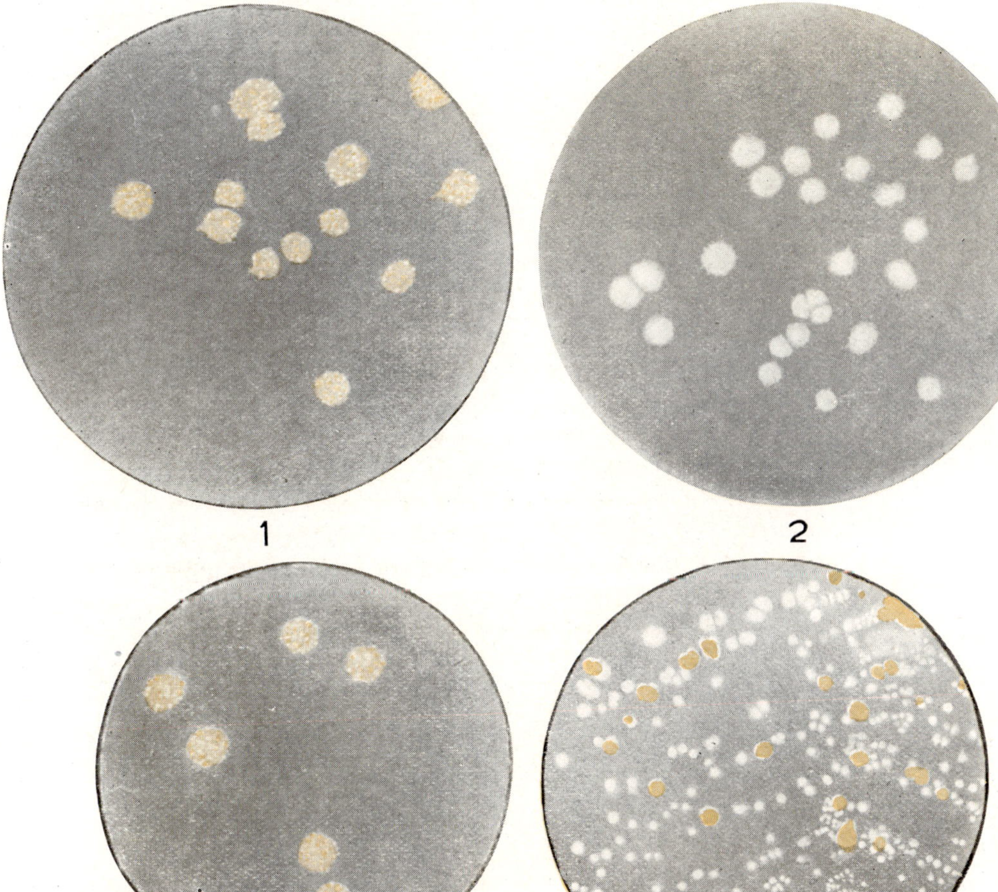

Teague and Morishima
Action of B. Typhosus on Xylose and Other Sugars

THE METABOLISM OF BOVINE TUBERCLE BACILLI

STUDIES IN ACID-FAST BACTERIA. XII

Arthur I. Kendall, Alexander A. Day
and
Arthur W. Walker

From the Patten Research Foundation, Northwestern University Medical School, Chicago

Studies of the nitrogenous metabolism of bovine tubercle bacilli do not appear to have been recorded, although certain peculiar and characteristic progressive changes in the reaction of broth mediums, in which bovine tubercle bacilli have grown, are reported by Theobald Smith[1] and others.

The comprehensive study of Marie Grund[2] on 173 acid-fast viruses, chiefly human and bovine strains of tubercle bacilli, has done much toward explaining the occasional variant which has been reported since Smith's important contribution to this subject.

Bovine tubercle bacilli, generally speaking, differ from human tubercle bacilli in two important particulars. Bovine strains, even in minute doses, are virulent for rabbits, and they produce progressive, titratable alkalinity in bouillon cultures, with or without the addition of glycerol.

Human tubercle bacilli, on the contrary, are practically avirulent for rabbits, and they tend to produce a permanent acid reaction in glycerol broth. There are, however, a few strains of acid-fast bacilli of the tubercle group which appear to be intermediate between the human and bovine types so far as the reaction curve is concerned, and Grund's conclusion that "the glycerin reaction curve is undoubtedly a valuable corroborative evidence of a division of tubercle bacilli into two types, but that its value is lessened by the number of irregular and atypical reactions" may be regarded as expressing the status of the relationship between the reaction curve and the type of tubercle bacillus at the present time.

Received for publication Sept. 16, 1919.

[1] Jour. Med. Research, 1904-1905, 13, p. 405.

[2] Studies from the Research Laboratory, Department of Health, New York City, 1911, 6, p. 116.

In a preceding communication[3] on the nitrogenous metabolism of virulent human tubercle bacilli in glycerol broth, it was shown that the reaction curve and the nitrogenous changes in the medium were so related that the conclusion could be drawn that glycerol is an available source of energy for human tubercle bacilli, and as such it spares the nitrogenous constituents of the medium to a considerable degree from bacterial breakdown. The increase in acidity of the medium, together with the practical absence of indications of deamination or proteolysis, are the principal factors on which this assumption was based.

The present investigation is a study of the metabolism of bovine tubercle bacilli. The primary objective is the acquisition of data explanatory of the difference in reaction curves exhibited by human and bovine tubercle bacilli, respectively. That such a distinction exists has long been known. An adequate exposition of the cause has apparently never been made.

The cultures studied were 4—P and M, very virulent for rabbits; G and D, slightly virulent for rabbits. Approximately 1 mg. of P or M inoculated subcutaneously would produce death. Several milligrams of G or D would be required to induce a fatal ending.

The procedure followed was precisely that reported in the study on the metabolism of virulent human tubercle bacilli.[3]

Culture P was inoculated into enough flasks to provide 5 parallel growths for each analysis. Culture M was inoculated in duplicate. Culture D was run in a series of 6 flasks, but only the composite sample, prepared from equal amounts of each flask in the series, is recorded. Culture G was run in a series of 4 flasks. The analyses of the individual flasks, together with the composite, are recorded.

Cultures D and G grew more rapidly and luxuriantly than P and M. This suggests that rapidity of growth is more or less inversely proportional to virulence, an observation which also held true for the human types, studied previously.

The tables show the analytical results.

DISCUSSION

Reaction.—Neutral red: The reaction curves, both of the virulent and avirulent cultures, follow those generally characteristic of bovine types of tubercle bacilli, namely, progressive increases in the titratable alkalinity of the mediums. The maximum degree of the reaction is reached about the sixth week. This is somewhat later than the time of greatest luxuriance in growth, which occurs on or about the fourth week.

[3] Jour. Infect. Dis., 1919, 26, p. 45.

TABLE 1

VIRULENT BOVINE TUBERCLE BACILLUS CULTURE P

Weeks	Flask A					Flask B					Flask C					Flask D					Flask E					Control				
	Neutral Red	Phenolphthalein	Ammonia, mg. per 100 c c	Amino Nitrogen, mg. per 100 c c	Lipase	Neutral Red	Phenolphthalein	Ammonia, mg. per 100 c c	Amino Nitrogen, mg. per 100 c c	Lipase	Neutral Red	Phenolphthalein	Ammonia, mg. per 100 c c	Amino Nitrogen, mg. per 100 c c	Lipase	Neutral Red	Phenolphthalein	Ammonia, mg. per 100 c c	Amino Nitrogen, mg. per 100 c c	Lipase	Neutral Red	Phenolphthalein	Ammonia, mg. per 100 c c	Amino Nitrogen, mg. per 100 c c	Lipase	Neutral Red	Phenolphthalein	Ammonia, mg. per 100 c c	Amino Nitrogen, mg. per 100 c c	Lipase
2	+0.30	000	—2.8	+0.7	—0.05	+0.30	000	—2.8	00	—0.05	+0.30	000	—2.8	00	—0.05	+0.30	000	—2.1	—1.4	—0.05	+0.30	000	—2.8	00	—0.05	—0.10	+0.20	4.9	22.4	0.25
3	000	—0.10	00	+2.1	00	000	—0.10	00	+1.4	00	000	—0.10	00	+2.1	00	000	—0.10	00	+1.4	00	000	—0.10	00	+2.1	00	+0.20	+0.30	4.2	19.6	0.20
4	000	—0.10	+0.7	+0.7	—	000	—0.10	+0.7	+1.4	—	000	—0.10	+0.7	+2.1	—	000	—0.10	00	+1.4	—	000	—0.10	+0.7	+1.4	—	+0.20	+0.30	5.6	19.6	—
5	000	000	00	+0.7	00	—0.10	000	00	00	00	—0.10	000	00	00	00	—0.10	000	00	00	00	—0.10	000	—0.7	+0.7	00	+0.20	+0.30	4.2	21.0	0.15
6	—0.40	000	+0.7	+2.1	00	—0.40	000	+1.4	+2.8	00	—0.40	000	+2.1	+4.9	00	—0.40	000	+1.4	00	00	—0.40	—0.10	+1.4	+2.8	00	+0.10	+0.30	4.9	19.6	0.15
7	—0.50	000	—1.4	+1.4	00	—0.40	—0.10	—1.4	—1.4	00	—0.50	—0.10	—1.4	00	00	—0.50	—0.10	—1.4	00	00	—0.60	—0.10	—2.1	—0.7	00	+0.20	+0.40	4.9	21.0	0.15
8	000	000	+3.5	+1.4	00	000	000	+3.5	+5.6	00	—	—	—	—	—	000	000	+3.5	+5.6	00	—0.10	000	+1.4	+5.6	00	—0.30	+0.30	4.2	22.4	0.20

Phenolphthalein: The increase in titratable alkalinity is less marked, although the change toward the basic side is unmistakable at the height of the development of the cultures. The same relationship between the maximum reaction change and greatest development was also observed in cultures of human tubercle bacilli.[3]

Ammonia.—The ammonia curve of culture P shows an increase from the beginning of the analyses, and this is true, but with greater intensity, for the relatively avirulent cultures G and D. Culture M, on the other hand, is characterized by a minimal increase in ammonia, scarcely greater than can be accounted for by the limits of accuracy of the method. The growth was fairly luxuriant, however, although less rapid than the other strains, indicating that the explanation of the chemical inertness of the organism is to be sought for in some undetermined factor.

TABLE 2

VIRULENT BOVINE TUBERCLE BACILLUS CULTURE M

Weeks	Flask A						Flask B					
	Neutral Red	Phenolphthalein	Ammonia mg. per 100 c c	NH_3 / N %	Amino Nitrogen, mg. per 100 c c	Lipase	Neutral Red	Phenolphthalein	Am. monia mg. per 100 c c	NH_3 / N %	Amino Nitrogen, mg. per 100 c c	Lipase
Control	+0.30	+0.40	4.9		12.6	0.15	+0.30	+0.40	4.9		12.6	0.15
2	—0.10	—0.10	00	00	—1.4	00	—0.10	—0.10	00	00	—1.4	00
3	—0.10	—0.10	+0.7	—0.29	00	00	—0.10	—0.10	00	00	+1.4	00
4	—0.20	—0.10	—1.4	—0.59	+0.7	00	—0.20	—0.10	—1.4	—0.59	00	00
5	—0.30	—0.20	—1.4	—0.59	—0.7	00	—0.30	—0.20	—0.7	—0.29	00	00
6	—0.50	000	—0.7	—0.29	00	—	—0.50	000	—0.7	—0.29	00	—
7	—0.50	+0.10	—2.1	—0.88	+0.7	00	—0.50	+0.10	—1.4	—0.59	00	00
8	—0.50	—0.10	—1.4	—0.59	00	00	—0.40	—0.10	—1.4	—0.59	00	00
9	—0.60	—0.10	—1.4	—0.59	00	00	—0.20	—0.10	—1.4	—0.59	00	00

Amino Nitrogen.—The amino nitrogen curves, contrary to the human tubercle bacillus amino nitrogen curves, show a slight but unmistakable increase up to the point of maximum development of the culture. After this time, the changes are somewhat irregular, possibly due to unequal rates of autolysis of the bacteria. The general picture is one in which a moderate degree of proteolysis is taking place, contrasting sharply in this respect with human strains, which in glycerol mediums are practically devoid of proteolytic powers.

Total Nitrogen.—A study of the total nitrogen in two of the strains showed a progressive decrease in the amount of this element in the bacteria-free medium. This indicates its incorporation in the bacillary substance. Recessive changes in the bacteria, leading to partial resolution of nitrogen in the underlying medium, as the autolytic processes became dominant in the cultures, were clearly shown by a gradual increase in soluble nitrogen.

Esterase and Lipase.—The esterase and lipase content of the germ-free broth was practically nil in the virulent strains, but it was distinctly increased in the two avirulent strains. A similar observation was made in the virulent and avirulent human strains.[3]

TABLE 3

AVIRULENT BOVINE TUBERCLE BACILLUS CULTURE D

Weeks	Control				Composite			
	Neutral Red	Am. monia, mg. per 100 c c	Total Nitrogen, mg. per 100 c c	Lipase	Neutral Red	Am. monia, mg. per 100 c c	Total Nitrogen, mg. per 100 c c	Lipase
4	+0.46	13.3	266	0.20	—0.90	+18.2	252	+1.00
5	+0.40	15.7	266	0.20	—1.00	+20.7	259	+1.00
6	+0.40	14.0	273	0.20	—1.20	+21.7	252	+1.10
7	+0.40	14.0	273	0.20	—1.20	+22.4	259	+1.15
8	+0.20	14.0	280	0.20	—1.00	+23.8	252	+1.10
9	+0.20	14.0	287	0.20	—1.10	+23.8	259	+1.15

The composite sample is a mixture of equal portions of the bacillus-free filtrate from six parallel cultures.

The studies on both virulent human and bovine types of tubercle bacilli have shown that these organisms are not very reactive chemically. The lipase and esterase activities also are virtually negative. Less virulent strains grow more rapidly, their chemical activities are greater, and lipase and esterase production becomes a distinct feature of the germ-free filtrates from broth cultures. This difference between virulent and avirulent, or less virulent strains, is of considerable theoretical interest, although nitrogenous metabolic changes fail to reveal the underlying cause. The possibility that tuberculin, a reaction product of growth, may vary somewhat in potency with luxuriance of development suggests itself as a distinct concomitant phenomenon, which may furnish additional information. A communication on this point will be made in the near future.

SUMMARY AND CONCLUSIONS

The neutral red reaction curves of virulent and slightly virulent bovine tubercle bacilli show a small but definite increase in titratable alkalinity, which is progressive. This observation agrees with the typical curves said to be characteristic of the bovine type. The phenol-

TABLE 4

AVIRULENT BOVINE TUBERCLE BACILLUS CULTURE G

Weeks	Control				Flask A			Flask B			Flask C			Flask D			Flask E			Composite Sample				
	Neutral Red	Ammonia, mg. per 100 c c	Total Nitrogen, mg. per 100 c c	Lipase	Neutral Red	Ammonia, mg. per 100 c c	$\frac{NH_3}{N}$ %	Neutral Red	Ammonia, mg. per 100 c c	$\frac{NH_3}{N}$ %	Neutral Red	Ammonia, mg. per 100 c c	$\frac{NH_3}{N}$ %	Neutral Red	Ammonia, mg. per 100 c c	$\frac{NH_3}{N}$ %	Neutral Red	Ammonia, mg. per 100 c c	$\frac{NH_3}{N}$ %	Neutral Red	Ammonia, mg. per 100 c c	Total Nitrogen, mg. per 100 c c	$\frac{NH_3}{N}$ %	Lipase
1	+0.20	19.6	350	0.00	—0.90	+2.1	+0.06	—0.80	+6.3	+1.80	—0.80	+8.4	+2.40	—0.80	+7.7	+2.20	—	—	—	—0.80	+6.3	350	1.80	+0.05
2	+0.25	19.6	350	0.00	—0.60	+13.3	+3.80	—0.60	+11.2	+3.20	—0.70	+16.8	+4.80	—0.70	+19.6	+5.50	—0.70	+16.8	+4.8	—0.70	+15.4	308	5.00	+1.10
3	+0.20	19.6	357	0.05	—0.60	+19.6	+5.49	—0.60	+19.6	+5.49	—0.40	+12.6	+3.53	—0.60	+25.9	+7.25	—0.60	+24.5	+6.86	—0.60	+21.7	315	6.90	+1.15
4	+0.25	21.0	364	0.00	—0.90	+16.1	+2.43	—0.90	+7.0	+1.92	—1.00	+9.8	+2.69	—1.00	+15.4	+4.23	—0.90	+14.0	+3.85	—0.90	+14.0	301	1.80	+1.15
5	+0.25	21.0	371	0.00	—1.00	+19.6	+5.28	—1.10	+30.1	+8.11	—1.10	+14.7	+3.97	—1.10	+31.5	+8.50	—1.10	+22.4	+6.04	—1.10	+24.5	315	7.78	+1.55
6	+0.20	20.3	364	0.00	—1.40	+27.3	+7.50	—1.90	+32.9	+9.04	—2.10	+30.1	+8.28	—1.70	+29.4	+8.08	—1.70	+30.8	+8.46	—1.80	+31.5	294	10.70	+1.50

The composite sample is an analysis of a mixture of equal parts of the bacillus-free filtrates from flasks A, B, C, D and E, inclusive.

phthalein reaction curve is less pronounced in this respect, but the period of greatest luxuriance in growth is accompanied by a slight increase in alkalinity. The ammonia curves are suggestive of increased deamination as the culture develops, but unlike the human tubercle bacillus curve, the trend is constantly toward an increase. Presumably the latter part of the ammonia rise is associated rather with autolysis of the bacteria than with an increase in protein utilization when the culture is decadent. There is also an increase in soluble nitrogen during the autolytic period, which in a measure supports this view.

Culture M is characterized by a minimal change in the ammonia curve, but evidence drawn from the amino nitrogen curve leads to the conclusion that this variation from the other strains is merely one of degree, not of type.

Generally speaking, the ammonia curves and curves of deamination of the bovine tubercle are the reverse of this characteristic of virulent human tubercle bacilli. The former increase with luxuriance of development in the culture, the latter decrease under the same conditions.

Increased ammonia production suggests increased action on the proteolytic constituents of the medium, and decreased ammonia indicates the virtual absence of proteolysis.

The amino-acid curves are in harmony with this view. In bovine strains the amount of soluble amino-acid increases with the development of the bacteria, and the maximum of amino-acid and of growth practically coincide in point of time. The exact reverse is true for those strains of virulent human tubercle bacilli which have been studied.

The three noteworthy features in the metabolism of the bovine tubercle bacilli herein studied — progressively alkaline reaction in glycerol mediums, increase in ammonia (or deamination), and parallel increase of amino-acids — point definitely to two significant facts: First, that the character of the metabolism of these organisms, both virulent and avirulent, is distinctly proteolytic in glycerol broth, and, secondly, that glycerol does not appear to spare the protein constituents of the broth from bacterial breakdown. Glycerol, in other words, is not a source of energy for bovine tubercle bacilli. On the contrary, glycerol appears to be an important source of energy for human tubercle bacilli, and the marked differences between the metabolism curves of the human and bovine types, including the Smith reaction curves, appear to depend on this very definite and simple fact.

The limited number of observations herein recorded do not, of course, permit of too great generalization on this point, but the chemical evidence, so far as it goes, taken into consideration with the reaction curves characteristc of the human and bovine types, are absolutely in harmony and appear to justify the conclusion that glycerol is a source of energy to human tubercle bacilli, but it is not a source of energy to bovine tubercle bacilli.

The development of an acid reaction in glycerol cultures of human tubercle bacilli and the absence of chemical evidence of proteolysis indicate that the human type can ferment glycerol. The development of an alkaline reaction in glycerol cultures of bovine tubercle bacilli, together with the unmistakable increase of deamination and cleavage of protein to amino-acids, indicates equally strongly that bovine tubercle bacilli cannot or do not ferment glycerol. This appears to be the true explanation for the observed differences in reaction curves of the two types of organisms.

COMPLEMENT FIXATION IN DIAGNOSIS OF TUBERCULOSIS

W. H. Moursund

From the Department Laboratory, Fort Sam Houston, Texas

Since there have been good reviews of the literature on this subject published recently,[1] it does not seem advisable at this time to review it again. Further, no effort will be made to give a detailed classification of the cases, as it is felt that in the hands of different clinicians the same set of cases would receive different classifications. Cases considered as incipient by some observers would be considered as moderately advanced by others and vice versa. Varying degrees of importance are placed on certain symptoms or physical signs by different observers, and the enthusiastic observer might find what he considers evidence of tuberculosis in a case which on more thorough and more extended observation proves to be nontuberculous. The cases reported in this article have been grouped as follows: active cases, inactive cases and nontuberculous cases. It is realized that in some cases the differentiation between activity and inactivity might be impossible. However, the clinical examinations of these cases were made by well qualified, competent and conservative clinicians, and it is felt that the classification is as near correct as can be obtained.

The complement fixation tests were made independently of the clinical examinations and no reference was made to the clinical records until the series of fixation tests had been completed.

TECHNIC

Serum.—The serum was removed from the clot as soon as possible and inactivated at 56 C. for 30 minutes; 0.1 c c of the undiluted serum was used in the test and the same amount was used as a control for anticomplementary action.

Antigen.—Petroff's Antigen[2] 2 was used, 250 mgm. of dried, pulverized tubercle bacilli were extracted with 50 c c of methyl alcohol at 38 C. for from 5-10 days, when it was well corked and set aside in a dark place at room temperature. After several weeks the supernatant fluid was pipetted off and was ready for use. The container should be sealed or well corked. When used it is diluted with the necessary amount of salt solution as determined by titration.

Received for publication Sept. 16, 1919.

[1] Stoll, H. F., and Newman L.: Jour. Am. Med. Assn. 1919, 72, p. 1403; Von Wedel, H. J.: Jour. of Immunology, 1918, 3, p. 351; Moon, V. H.: Jour. Am. Med. Assn., 1918, 71, p. 1127; Stivelman, B.: Am. Rev. Tuberc., 1918, 546, p. 550.

[2] Am. Rev. Tuberc., 1917, 1, p. 35.

Using 0.1 c c positive serum, 0.01 c c antigen gives partial fixation; 0.05 c c gives fairly complete fixation; 0.1 c c gives complete fixation. With negative serum it is not anticomplementary until 0.5 c c of the antigen is used. The tests were made by using 0.1 c c of antigen. Before setting up tests, the antigen was titrated each day to determine fixing power with positive serum, and anticomplementary limit.

Complement.—The pooled serum from 4 to 6 guinea-pigs was used in a 1:10 dilution. The complement was titrated, using 3 units of amboceptor and 0.1 c c of 5% sheep cell suspension, 0.05 c c of pooled negative serums (10 serums containing no natural amboceptor) with 0.1 c c of antigen in the front row of tubes. The amount of complement to be used in the tests is indicated by the smallest amount necessary for complete hemolysis.

Hemolytic System.—One-tenth c c of 5% washed sheep corpuscles is used with 0.2 c c of diluted amboceptor containing 3 standard units.

Controls.—Known positive and negative serums were used as controls each day.

The titrations of complement and amboceptor are incubated in water bath at 37.5 for 1 hour and the fixation tests in icebox for 2 hours. Then in water bath for 30 minutes and after addition of sheep cells and amboceptor for 1 hour in the water bath. The tests are read immediately after last incubation.

In a certain number of cases both water bath fixation at 37 C. and icebox fixation at about 10 C. were used with the same serums. The results obtained would indicate that the icebox method gives better results in that more positives were obtained and the fixation in doubtful water bath reactions became more complete in the icebox method.

Tests were made on the serums of 186 patients, 103 being active cases and 51 inactive cases of pulmonary tuberculosis; one was a case of tuberculosis of the epididymis (test made some time after operation) and 31 were nontuberculous cases.

Of the 103 active cases, 15 gave + + reactions, 1 gave a + reaction, 5 gave ± reactions, and 83 gave negative reactions. Considering the + + and + reactions as positive, only 16, or 15.53%, of the total number of active cases gave positive complement fixation tests.

Of the inactive cases, 50 gave negative reactions and one gave a + + fixation test for tuberculosis and also a + + Wassermann reaction.

Of the nontuberculous cases, 29 gave negative reactions and one gave a + + fixation test for tuberculosis and also a + + Wassermann reaction.

Sputum examinations were made in all cases. The antiformin concentration method was used. From one to eight sputum examinations were made in each case. Of the 103 active cases, 10 gave positive sputum and positive complement fixation tests, 6 gave negative sputum and positive fixation tests, 41 gave positive sputum and negative fixation tests, and 46 gave negative sputum and negative fixation tests.

DISCUSSION

A laboratory test to be of value to the clinician must be either of diagnostic or prognostic aid. The degree of activity in the 103 cases varied considerably, and in the 16 cases giving positive complement fixation tests the degree of activity varied so markedly that the fixation test cannot be considered of any prognostic value.

The test is of very little, if any, value as a diagnostic aid, at least in the type of cases examined. Of the 16 cases which gave positive complement fixation tests, 10 gave positive sputum at the time of or before the fixation test was made. So in only 6 cases of the entire series of active and inactive cases can the complement fixation test be said to have been of any diagnostic aid. Also without the laboratory tests the diagnosis could be easily made in all these cases by the clinician with the aid of the roentgen-ray laboratory. It will be noted that approximately 50% of the active cases had tubercle bacilli in the sputum, and no doubt further sputum examinations in the other cases would increase this percentage.

Since the inactive cases, except the one which gave a positive Wassermann test, gave negative fixation tests for tuberculosis, it might be considered that the test is of some importance in distinguishing active from inactive cases. However, when one stops to consider the large number of active cases that gave negative reactions it does not seem that the test can be considered of any practical value in differentiating active from inactive cases. The same thing can be said relative to the value of a negative reaction in excluding the presence of tuberculosis in a patient.

Of course it is realized that the system of the fixation test used in the examination of these cases might not be the ideal one for this kind of work, and also the antigen used may not be the best.

Another question to be decided in connection with this test is whether or not it is a specfic reaction. In all cases in this article a Wassermann test was made at the same time as the fixation test for tuberculosis. Of the cases giving positive fixation for tuberculosis 3 cases also gave positive Wassermann tests. In 2 of the 3 cases the patients denied all history of syphilitic infection and there was nothing to indicate the presence of such infection.

In two of the active cases giving negative fixation for tuberculosis, positive Wassermann reactions were obtained. In neither case was there any history nor evidence of any syphilitic infection.

TABLE 1

WASSERMANN AND COMPLEMENT FIXATION TESTS

Serum	Syphilis Showing Strength of Reaction						Tuberculosis, 0.1 c c	Gonococcus, 0.1 c c	Glanders, 0.1 c c	Streptococcus, 0.1 c c
	0.05 c c	0.025 c c	0.0126 c c	0.0062 c c	0.0031 c c	0.0015 c c				
1	++	0	0	0	0	0		0	0	0
2	++	0	0	0	0	0		0	0	0
3	++	0	0	0	0	0		0	0	0
4	++	0	0	0	0	0		0	0	0
5	++	0	0	0	0	0		0	0	0
6	++	++	++	++	++	±	++	0	0	0
7	++	0	0	0	0	0		0	0	0
8	++	0	0	0	0	0		0	0	0
9	++	0	0	0	0	0		0	0	0
10	++	0	0	0	0	0		0	0	0
11	++	0	0	0	0	0		0	0	0
12	++	0	0	0	0	0		0	0	0
13	++	0	0	0	0	0		0	0	0
14	++	0	0	0	0	0		0	0	0
15	++	0	0	0	0	0		0	0	0
16	++	++	++	++	++	±	++	0		
17	++	++	++	++	+			0	0	0
18	++	++						0	0	0
19	++	++	++	++			++	0	0	0
20	++	++	++	++	++				0	0
21	++								0	0
22	++									
23	++	++	++	++					0	0
24	++	++							0	0
25	++	++	++	±					0	0
26	++	++	++	++				0	0	0
27	++						+	++		0
28	++	++	++	++	+			++	0	0
29	++	±						++		0
30	++	++	++	+				+	0	0
31	++	++	+							
32	++	+								
33	++						++			
34	++	++	++	++	±		++	+		0
35	++	++	+							0
36	++	++	±				++	++		
37	++								0	0
38	++	++	+						0	0
39	++	++						0	0	0
40	++	++						++	0	0
41	++	++					+		0	0
42	++	+						±	0	0
43	++	++	+						0	0
44	++	++	+	±				++		
45	++	++					++	++		
46	++	++	++	+				+		
47	++	++	++	++					0	0
48	++	++	++	+				+		
49	++	++						++		
50	++	++	±					0		
51	++	++	+	±				0		
52	++	++	++	+	±			0		
53	++	++	++	++	±			0		
54	++	++	++	++	+		+	0		
55	++	++	±					0		
56	++	++	+				+	0		
57	++	++	++	+			++	0		
58	++	++	++	±			++	0		
59	++	++	++	++			++	0		
60	++	++	++	±				0		
61	++	++	+				+	0		
62	++	++	++	+	±			0		
63	++	++	++	+			++	0		
64	++	++	++	++	±		++	0	+	
65	++	++	++	+			++	0		
66	++	+	±				+	0	0	0
67	++	++	++	+	±		+	0		
68	++	+					++	0		
69	++	++	++				+	0		

TABLE 1—*Continued*

WASSERMANN AND COMPLEMENT FIXATION TESTS

Serum	Syphilis Showing Strength of Reaction						Tuberculosis, 0.1 c c	Gonococcus, 0.1 c c	Glanders, 0.1 c c	Streptococcus, 0.1 c c
	0.05 c c	0.025 c c	0.0126 c c	0.0062 c c	0.0031 c c	0.0015 c c				
70	++	++	++	++	+	±	++	0		
71	++	++	+				+	0		
72	++	+					++	0		
73	++	++	++	+	±		++	0		
74	++	++	++	±				0		
75	++	++						0		
76	++						+	0		
77	++	++	++	++	++	++	++	0		
78	++	++	++	+	±		++	0		
79	++	+	±				+	0	0	0
80	++	++	±				+	0		
81	++	+						0	0	0
82	++	++	++	++	+	±	+	0		
83	++	++	++	+			++	0	0	0
84	++	++					++	0		
85	++	++	++				+	0	+	
86	++	++	++	++	++	++	++	0		
87	++	++	++	+				0	0	0
88	++	++	+	±				0		
89	++	++	++	++	++	+	++	0		
90	++	++	++	++	+	+	++	0	0	0
91	++	++	++	++	+	+	+	0	0	0
92	++	++	++	++	+	±		0		
93	++	++	++	++	++	+	++	0		
94	++	++	++					0		
95	++	+						0		
96	++	++	++	++	+		++	0		
97	++	+					+	0		
98	++	++	±				+	0		
99	++	++	++	++	++	++	++	0		
100	++	++	++	++	++	+	+	0		

Of the inactive cases, one gave + + reactions in both tests. This patient gave a history of syphilitic infection, but nothing to indicate the presence of tuberculosis. That a patient might have tuberculosis and syphilis at the same time must be recognized, but that all these cases giving both positive fixation for tuberculosis and syphilis had both tuberculosis and syphilis seems very questionable.

It is still believed by some workers that a few cases of tuberculosis give a positive Wassermann reaction without any evidence or history of syphilitic infection. That the Wassermann test is not specific is recognized by serologists. While it is generally supposed that bacterial complement fixation tests are specific, this work suggests the possibility that they are nonspecific. An attempt was therefore made to determine whether serum that gave a positive complement fixation for syphilis would also produce a positive complement fixation with various bacterial antigens. The table presents the results obtained.

Complement fixation tests for tuberculosis (as described) were made in 100 patients who gave a + + complement fixation for syphilis; 45 gave positive fixation tests for tuberculosis. Fixation tests using gonococcus antigen were made in 28 with positive results in 12. Fifty-nine were tested with glanders antigen with weak + reactions in 3; 55 were tested with streptococcus antigen with no positive reactions. In 86 the serum was titrated to determine the strength of complement fixation for syphilis, and from these titrations the following summary is compiled.

TABLE 2

COMPLEMENT FIXATION FOR SYPILIS

Dilution of Serum	0.05 c c	0.025 c c	0.0125 c c	0.0062 c c	0.0031 c c	0.0015 c c
Positive tubercle fixation........	3	11	6	10	6	8
Negative tubercle fixation.......	4	13	10	12	3	0
Per cent. positive................	42.8	45.8	37.5	45.4	66.6	100

In the cases giving positive fixation for syphilis in serum dilution from 0.05 c c to 0.0062 c c there is no marked difference in the percentage of positive cross fixation with tubercle antigen in each dilution, but the percentage of positives increases in the cases giving positive fixation for syphilis in dilutions higher than 0.0062 c c, even giving 100% positive in the dilution of 0.0015 c.c. This would indicate that the greater the fixing properties of the serum with syphilitic antigen, the greater the possibility of cross fixation with tubercle antigen. To determine whether or not only syphilitic serum would give cross fixation with tubercle antigen, 100 serums giving negative fixation for syphilis were tested for fixation with tubercle antigen. Of this number, 17 gave positive complement fixation for tuberculosis, none of which gave any history or evidence of tuberculosis, and in only two was there a history of syphilis (two old treated cases). Naturally the question would arise as to the possibility of double infections explaining the cross fixation of syphilitic serums with tubercle and gonococcus antigens.

In 15 of the cases giving cross fixation with tubercle antigen and in 4 giving cross fixation with gonococcus antigen there was no history obtainable. In only 2 of the cases was there a history of tuberculosis, both being cases of active chronic pulmonary tuberculosis. Of the 8 cases giving cross fixation with gonococcus antigen, and in which the history obtained is dependable, none gave a history of recent gonococcus infection, and only two gave a history of such infection, one in 1910, the other in 1917.

It can hardly be conceived that approximately 45% of all syphilitic individuals also have tuberculosis without any signs or indications of the latter disease.

It is recognized that a large number of individuals at some time during life become infected with tubercle bacilli, but the disease is arrested in some and cured in the majority. Granting that all patients giving cross fixation have had tuberculosis at some time during life, it does not seem possible that complement fixing bodies would remain for any length of time after such cases are arrested or cured. The positive Wassermann in a syphilitic is considered indicative of activity of the disease and that such a case should receive more treatment. From the work done, it is not believed this rule can be applied to complement fixation tests with bacterial antigens.

Apparently, the serums of a large number of syphilitics and of some normal individuals contain complement fixing bodies in the presence of tubercle and gonococcus antigens. What these fixing bodies are is not known. Possibly they are of a protein nature, and when in sufficient quantity combine with lipoids in the antigen to produce fixation of complement.

An idea is advanced that the greater the amount of lipoidal substances contained in an antigen, the less specific such an antigen is, since in the series of tests reported in this article it is noted that cross fixations are more numerous with tubercle and gonococcus antigens than with glanders and streptococcus antigens, the tubercle bacilli and gonococci containing more lipoidal substances than either the glanders bacilli or streptococci.

CONCLUSIONS

The complement fixation test for tuberculosis as described in this article is of no value as a diagnostic or prognostic aid.

The complement fixation test for tuberculosis with alcoholic extract of tubercle bacilli as antigen, is not specific.

Not all complement fixation tests with bacterial antigens are specific.

A large percentage of serums giving a positive Wassermann give fixation with tubercle and gonococcus antigens.

A certain number of individuals not infected with tuberculosis or gonorrhea will give positive fixation tests with one or both of the corresponding antigens.

VARIETIES OF STREPTOCOCCI WITH SPECIAL REFERENCE TO CONSTANCY

Benjamin Junior Clawson

From the Department of Hygiene and Bacteriology, University of Chicago

The work reported in the following pages deals with the characteristics of strains of streptococci isolated from various sources. Particular attention is given to the constancy of the special characteristics of streptococci such as peculiarities in morphology, the action on the blood-agar plate, the fermentation of the various carbohydrates, and the immune reactions such as agglutination and complement fixation. An attempt has been made to discover whether the various classes adopted by different workers have sufficient relationship to source, habits, pathogenesis, or any other particular characteristic to justify such grouping. A review of the literature is not given, since the literature on the work which has been done on streptococci has been well summarized by such recent workers as Holman,[1] Blake,[2] Aschner,[3] and Brown.[4]

Methods

Mediums Used.—Meat infusion agar with a reaction of from 0.3-0.5% acid was used in all the work; 1.5% of agar was used. This gave a soft agar in which a considerable quantity of water of condensation was always present. Sodium chlorid, 0.85%, was added to all mediums. The broth for sugar mediums was made sugar free by incubating the filtered meat infusion inoculated with B. coli for about twelve hours. The broth was adjusted to from 0.1-0.5% acid to phenolphthalein, P_H 7.9-7.4. All of the broth contained 1% of Armour's peptone. The sugar broths were prepared by adding 1% of the sugar to the sugar-free broth, and enough litmus was added to give the broth a faint blue color. The broth was then sterilized in the autoclave at 10 lbs. of pressure for ten minutes. The inulin was placed in a mixture of 1 part serum and 3 parts water. Blood agar was prepared by adding 10% of defibrinated sheep blood to salt meat infusion agar. Ascitic fluid agar was prepared by adding 10% of ascitic fluid to the agar. Certified milk was used.

Method of Isolation and Cultivation.—Material was plated on blood agar or glucose litmus agar, and the plates were incubated at 37 C. for from 15-24 hours. The dilution method was used in all cases. Well isolated colonies were picked and transferred to blood agar slants or glucose broth. In all cases

Received for publication Oct. 4, 1919.

[1] Jour. Med. Research, 1916, 34, p. 377.

[2] Ibid., 1917, 36, p. 99.

[3] Jour. Infect. Dis., 1917, 21, p. 409.

[4] Monograph of Rockefeller Institute for Medical Research, No. 9, January, 1919.

these blood agar or glucose broth cultures were replated on blood agar and repicked to the blood agar slants. Pneumococci and streptococci were differentiated on the basis of morphology, the inulin fermentation, and the bile solubility test. All sugar mediums were inoculated from a 15-24 hour glucose-broth culture with one standard loopful of the culture. The glucose-broth culture from which the sugars were inoculated was tested by smear preparation for growth and purity of culture. The cultures in sugar mediums were grown at 37 C. for 5 days and then examined for acidity. All tubes which did not show an evident change in color were reported negative. These negative cultures were checked by using Andrade's indicator. All cultures were kept in storage on blood-agar slants at icebox temperature and transferred each month. Fifteen strains were kept at 37 C. for 10 months on blood-agar slants and ascitic-fluid-agar slants and transferred every week.

Agglutination.—Suspensions for agglutination were prepared by growing the organisms in salt broth for about twenty-four hours. A homogeneous suspension was obtained by shaking the salt-broth tube. Immune serum was prepared by injecting from 2-10 c c of a 24-hour broth culture intravenously into a rabbit. These injections were continued for from 5-7 injections at intervals of from 5-8 days. The blood was taken from the heart, centrifugalized, and preserved in 0.5% phenol. Twelve rabbits were immunized respectively to 12 different hemolytic strains, and 5 rabbits were immunized to 5 different nonhemolytic strains. Controls were made with normal rabbit serum and with salt solution. The serum was also controlled with sterile salt broth to see that precipitation was not produced.

Complement Fixation.—The same serum was used as in the work with agglutination. The antigen was prepared according to Kinsella and Swift's[5] method. The organisms to be used in the antigens were grown in large tubes of glucose-broth for 24 hours. The broth was centrifugalized and the sediment was washed twice with salt solution. The sediment was then dried and 10 mg. were dissolved in 5 c c of a 2% antiformin solution in a water bath at 56 C. This solution was then neutralized to phenolphthalein with N/20 H_2SO_4 and made up to 10 c c. The chlorin was removed by adding a few drops of a 5% solution of sodium thiosulphate. The antigens were preserved with 0.5% phenol. In the complement fixation test 0.1 c c of antigen was used with 3 different amounts of serum (0.1 c c, 0.05 c c, and 0.025 c c) and 2 units of complement. After incubation for one hour at 37 C., 2 units of hemolytic amboceptor and 0.5 c c of washed sheep red blood cells were added, and the tubes were incubated for another hour. The usual controls were made.

Sources of Material

The sources from which the organisms used in this series were isolated may be grouped as follows: necropsies, respiratory passages and accessory openings, feces and urine, local suppurative processes, milk and milk products.

Classification

Morphology.—The early workers differentiated the strains of streptococci on the basis of morphology. It was thought at first that pathogenic strains of streptococci produced long chains and saprophytic strains short chains. Lingelsheim[6] in 1899 first differentiated the pathogenic streptococci from those

[5] Jour. Exper. Med., 1918, 28, p. 181.
[6] Beitr. z. exper. Therap., 1899, 1, —.

TABLE 1

Strain	
	NECROPSIES
2, 7, 45	Pyemia following puerperal sepsis
17	Peritonitis following rupture of diverticulum of urinary bladder
18	Spinal fluid, Little's disease
23, 34, 63, 106	Lobar pneumonia
24	Spinal fluid, death after nephrectomy
25	Pericardial fluid, death after nephrectomy
30, 109	Hemorrhagic infarcts of lung, general septicemia
31	Carcinoma of liver and pelvic abscess
32	Pus from pelvic abscess
38	Carcinoma of larynx and bronchopneumonia
40	Carcinoma of larynx and lobar pneumonia
41	Primary carcinoma of mediastinum
46	Unresolved pneumonia
59	Pus from stomach in phlegmonous gastritis
60	Tuberculous bronchopneumonia
64, 66	Tuberculous peritonitis
113	Carcinoma of stomach, generalized septicemia
114	Nodular tuberculosis of lung
5	Pus from lung abscess of cow
10	Septicemia of cow
	RESPIRATORY PASSAGES
8	Sputum in cold
21	Infected mouth of meningitis child
36	Pus from frontal sinus
47–55, 57, 61, 62, 68–71, 74, 75, 78, 80, 81, 83, 86–89, 91–94, 97–99, 107, 108, 111	Removed tonsils
103–105	Sputum in pneumonia
112	Acute pharyngitis
116–118, 120–133, 135, 137–140, 142–150, 152, 153, 155, 155B, 157–159, 162, 164, 166, 168, 170, 171, 174–186, 188, 189, 191–198, 200, 203–209, 307, 313, 317, 318, 329, 330, 326, 333–335, 342, 343, 345, 353, 354, 359, 366–368, 370–372, 375, 379, 382, 383, 386–388, 390, 395, 397, 399, 400	Normal throat
411	Sputum in pneumonia following influenza
412-415, 422, 423, 436, 437, 453, 454	Sputum in influenza patients
448	Tonsillitis
	URINE AND FECES
19	Urine of meningitis child
20	Urine of normal child
140, 199, 202, 211, 213, 401-410, 425-429, 431-434, 440-447, 459, 461-467	Normal horse feces
416-421, 438, 439, 449-452, 460, 493-496	Normal human feces
	LOCAL SUPPURATIVE PROCESSES
4	Suppurative infection on face
6	Ulcer on abdomen of dog
22	Pus from mastoid infection
67	Pus at root of tooth
173	Ulcer of stomach from a dog
	MILK AND MILK PRODUCTS
163, 455, 456	Buttermilk tablet
115, 457, 458, 468-492	Milk

less pathogenic by means of the length of the chains produced. Those strains which formed chains of 8 or more cells he classified as Streptococcus longus, and those strains forming less than 8 cells in a chain he classified as Streptococcus brevis. The former was considered to be more pathogenic and more common in suppurative processes, while the latter was characteristic of the more saprophytic forms. I have found considerable variation in the length of chains depending on the medium whether solid or liquid and on the amount of water of condensation on the solid medium, but I have not found any direct relation between the length of chains and pathogenesis. Many strains which were isolated from the blood of septicemia patients at first produced short chains on blood agar slants, but after growing for several months developed longer chains. When strains having long chains were grown on sterile tissue in salt solution there was a tendency to produce shorter chains. In general, streptococci isolated from the throat were found to be more segmented into pairs in the chain than the strains isolated from the blood of patients dying with septicemia. The shape of the cells seems to have some significance. Those strains isolated from the blood in general septicemia have cells which retain the spherical shape while those isolated from saprophytic conditions show elongation in the long axis of the chain. Several strains of pleomorphic streptococci were isolated from various sources, strain 17 from a case of peritonitis, strain 34 from the blood of a case of lobar pneumonia, strains 54 and 55 from removed tonsils, and strain 155 from the normal throat. All of these strains have changed to the segmented slightly elongated cells which form in chains.

The morphology of those strains grown at 37 C. for 10 months corresponds in general with the morphology of the same strains kept at icebox temperature and transferred once a month.

The question of the production of capsules in the streptococcus pneumococcus group has stimulated considerable discussion. Hiss,[7] working with the various types of capsules produced by the pneumococci and the streptococci, decided that the capsule formation was not sufficient to separate the streptococci from the pneumococci. Holman[1] in his scheme of classification represents the streptococci as noncapsule producers. In my series it has been found that the capsule-producing property varies somewhat. Of the 134 strains of hemolyzers, 20 produced capsules at one or more times. The intervals between the tests ranged from 1-11 months in duration. The strains which produce capsules seem to vary from time to time. Of the 20 strains of hemolyzers which produced capsules 15 varied from time to time. Sixty hours incubation proved to be the best time for determining capsular formation in milk. Most of the capsule producers among the hemolyzers were strains associated with acute pathologic processes such as pyemia, septicemia, and removed tonsils.

Capsule production among the nonhemolytic strains is more common than among the hemolyzers. Of the 150 strains of nonhemolyzers, 47 produced capsules at one or more determinations. Of these 47 strains, 27 showed the presence of capsules at every determination. Ten of these capsule producers were isolated from the pulp of removed tonsils, 5 from blood at necropsies, 2 from spinal fluid, one from a suppurative infection on the face, 24 from the normal throat, one from urine, one from a buttermilk tablet, 2 from milk, and one from the sputum of an influenza patient. As among the hemolytic

[7] Jour. Exper. Med., 1905, 6, p. 317.

capsule producers the nonhemolytic-capsule-producing strains of this series are among the strains which tend to be parasitic in their habits.

Blood-Agar Plate.—Recent workers agree concerning the value of the blood-agar plate for the separation of streptococci into two main groups, the hemolyzers and the nonhemolyzers. Different investigators have recommended various amounts of defibrinated blood for use in the agar plate. Shottmüller,[8] who first used the blood-agar plate, recommended the use of 40% of defibrinated blood. Holman used 5%; Blake found 10% satisfactory. Becker[9] emphasizes the necessity of a standard blood agar, and favors as the standard the medium recommended by the committee on standard methods in water analysis. He recommends that 1 c c of defibrinated blood be added to 6 c c of agar. Brown[4] considers 5% sufficient. Approximately 10% has been found satisfactory in this work. I agree with Blake that it is necessary to have the blood well mixed. A smaller amount than 10% may lead to confusion in recording the presence of green producing streptococci since after more than 24 hours these organisms may show a slight zone of hemolysis. This is particularly true if part of the plate contains a small amount of blood. This zone of slight hemolysis about a colony with a greenish zone at the periphery of the hemolytic zone, which is produced by many of the green-producing organisms when the plate is read at longer periods than 24 hours, corresponds closely with that described as the alpha type by Smith and Brown.[10] It is important to take into consideration the temperature of the agar at the time when the blood is added. If the blood and agar remain above 40 C. for any considerable length of time, the mixture becomes brown. The green organisms are then slow in producing methemoglobin and may be mistaken for hemolyzers when after more than 24 hours some slight hemolysis is shown without any methemoglobin around the periphery of the zone of hemolysis or around the colony.

Hopkins and Lang[11] point out that hemolysis depends on the depth of the medium at which the colony is grown. I have found that using approximately 10 c c of agar and 1 c c of blood in plating the depth of the medium in the ordinary petri dish has no noticeable effect on hemolysis if the agar and the blood are well mixed and not allowed to remain above 40 C. Hopkins and Lang state that they found all gradations of action on the blood-agar plate between complete hemolysis and no action at all. Their conflicting results as pointed out by Blake probably were due to making observations at variable times, from 1-3 days after plating.

The zone of hemolysis in this series of 134 strains of hemolytic streptococci was found to vary but little in size. The average diameter was about 2 mm. This corresponds to the beta type of some writers. In one case in which at the time of swabbing the patient complained of a sore throat and showed an inflamed pharynx hemolytic streptococci were found which produced a very small zone of hemolysis. Hemolytic streptococci that produced a similar zone of hemolysis were isolated from the canal of an extracted tooth. Both of these strains, 14 and 155B, grew poorly on blood agar and in all other mediums. Strain 14 required at least 48 hours to produce any visible growth on any mediums. It has been under observation for more than a year and has not shown any variation in its method of growth. In carbo-

[8] München. med. Wchnschr., 1903, 50, pp. 849, 909.
[9] Jour. Infect. Dis., 1916, 19, p. 754.
[10] Jour. Med. Research, 1915, 31, p. 455.
[11] Jour. Infect. Dis., 1914, 15, p. 63.

hydrate mediums these strains are regular in their fermentation reactions. Floyd and Wolbach[12] state that the zone of hemolysis varied greatly in their series and that most of their cultures retained the hemolytic property for several weeks. A number lost this property after being cultivated for several months on blood serum medium. They decided that in general hemolysis among the streptococci is characteristic of pathogenic types. In no case in their series did nonhemolytic strains acquire the hemolytic property while under cultivation. No mention is made of the kind of blood used.

All of my 134 hemolytic strains, several of which are more than a year old, have remained constant in the production of hemolysis. Of the 15 strains which were grown at 37 C. on blood agar and ascitic fluid agar for 10 months, 7 were hemolyzers. At the end of 10 months when plated on blood agar hemolysis was produced as readily as at first. This is true of the strains grown on ascitic fluid agar as well as those grown on blood agar. Six of these strains at the end of 10 months were kept at icebox temperature for 5 months without being transferred. When plated out all of those strains which had been kept on blood were alive and produced hemolysis on the blood-agar plate. Four of these strains which had been kept on ascitic fluid agar were alive and produced hemolysis on the blood-agar plate.

Ruediger[13] has shown that hemolysis does not readily take place if glucose is present in the agar. Shigeki Shikiguchi[14] has found that this power of glucose to retard hemolysis bears no relation to the amount of acid that is produced by the action of the streptococci on the glucose in the medium. Although little hemolysis takes place when 2% of glucose is present in the medium, the organism itself is not changed in its power to hemolyze. Strain 345 was grown on 2% glucose blood agar at 37 C. for 11 weeks. This strain was then plated on ordinary blood agar, and hemolysis occurred as readily as at first.

Two types of nonhemolytic streptococci, the methemoglobin producers and those indifferent on blood, are recognized by Lyall,[15] Holman, Blake, Brown, and others. Lyall states that this division is sufficiently constant to justify grouping on this basis. He groups the fecal streptococci among the organisms inactive on the blood-agar plate. Brown[4] calls these inactive strains the gamma type. Aschner[3] found that streptococci which would not produce methemoglobin on human blood would produce methemoglobin on ox blood. Strain 6, isolated from an ulcer on the abdomen of a dog, and strains 455 and 456, isolated from different commercial buttermilk tablets, are the only strains in the series of the 150 nonhemolytic strains which were inactive on blood when isolated. These 3 strains became active in producing methemoglobin after being grown on blood agar for from one to two generations. All the nonhemolytic strains isolated from human feces (17), all those isolated from milk (27), and all those isolated from horse feces (30) produced green colonies on the blood-agar plate and have continued to from time to time. The green about the colonies of some of these strains was faint, but after one or two transfers the green zone became typical.

Four strains of nonhemolyzers which had been grown on blood agar and on ascitic fluid agar for 10 months were then left in the icebox for 5 months without being transferred. The following results were obtained when these strains were plated out:

[12] Jour. Med. Research, 1914, 29, p. 493.
[13] Jour. Infect. Dis., 1906, 3, p. 663.
[14] Jour. Infect. Dis., 1917, 21, p. 475.
[15] Jour. Med. Research, 1914, 30, pp. 487, 515.

Strains 4, 5, 18,	grown on blood agar	green colonies
Strain 21	grown on ascitic fluid agar	dead
	grown on blood agar	indifferent
	grown on ascitic fluid agar	indifferent

Strain 21 was transferred but once when the colonies on the blood-agar plate showed the typical green zone again. The evidence is that all non-hemolytic strains of streptococci when grown on suitable mediums are methemoglobin producers.

DISTRIBUTION OF HEMOLYTIC STREPTOCOCCI

Although hemolytic streptococci are found in different places under apparently normal conditions as in the normal throat, milk, horse feces, and occasionally human feces, yet the fact still remains that acute processes such as septicemia and pyemia are generally caused by hemolytic streptococci. To what extent hemolytic organisms are pathogenic is still a question of considerable doubt. Some clinicians have accepted hemolysis as an indication of virulence. My 134 strains were collected from the following sources:

TABLE 2

SOURCES OF STRAINS

Normal throats	69
Removed tonsils	18
Canal of tooth	1
Acute mastoiditis	1
Blood at necropsy	18
Horse feces	10
Throats of influenza patients	9
Acute pharyngitis	2
Sputum of pneumonia patients	3
Frontal sinusitis	1
Milk	1
Tonsillitis	1

Of these 134 strains, 79 were found in the normal throat and from horse feces. Several of those found in horse feces were tested and found to be pathogenic to rabbits. Several of the hemolyzers from the normal throat were tested for pathogenesis in rabbits, but death was not produced.

It is interesting to note the relative frequency of hemolytic streptococci in the normal throat. During the winter of 1917-1918 respiratory diseases, due apparently to hemolytic streptococci, were frequent in the army camps.

An epidemic of empyema following bronchopneumonia was reported by the Empyema Commission[16] at Camp Lee; hemolytic streptococci were isolated in pure cultures from the aspirated fluid. Irons[17] found at Camp Custer in cases of empyema following measles that the exciting organism was Streptococcus hemolyticus. In a streptococcus epidemic at Camp Zachary Taylor, in which there were evidences of septicemia, an investigation was made by Fox and Hamburger[18] to determine the portal of entry. Fifteen per cent. of the men of one contingent were found to be harboring hemolytic streptococci in the pharynx when they entered the camp. In one company which had been at the camp for 6 months the percentage of those carrying hemolytic streptococci in the pharynx was 85. In the base hospital at Fort Riley 28.2% of the sputum of 428 cases of pneumonia contained hemolytic streptococci. Of the 155 cases of empyema, 68.4% were found to be produced by hemolytic

[16] Jour. Am. Med. Assn., 1918, 71, p. 443.

[17] Ibid., 1918, 70, p. 687.

[18] Ibid., p. 1758.

streptococci. Small[19] found that nearly 25% of the sputum from the pneumonia patients examined between September, 1917, and April, 1918, at Camp Pike showed the presence of hemolytic streptococci. At Camp Dodge, Miller[20] reported an epidemic of pneumonia and empyema due to streptococci. The exudates in 95 of these cases were examined bacteriologically, and 88 pure cultures of hemolytic streptococci were found. Smillie[21] reported in 1907 that of 100 normal throats examined the beta type of hemolytic streptococci, according to Smith and Brown, was found in only one of the 100 throats.

The fact that some of these workers have found apparently normal individuals harboring the hemolytic streptococci in the pharynx, and the fact that these organisms were found in such a large number of individuals at the time and at the place of these epidemics, has led me to make observations on the relative frequency of hemolytic streptococci in the normal nasopharynx and on the normal tonsil.

The throats of 100 students at the University of Chicago were examined during the summer quarter of 1918. During the autumn quarter of 1918, another 100 throats were examined. Most of these students were medical students from the classes of bacteriology and pathology. Those who had lived in Chicago before the beginning of the quarter in which their throats were examined were classified as residents of Chicago; of these there were 117. The remaining 83 were from various states. The work was started shortly after June 16, 1918. One hundred and sixty of the students examined were males; ages ran from 20-40.

The nasopharynx was swabbed with a curved wire swab as recommended in the Standard Technique of Meningococcus Carrier Detection.[22] Each tonsil was swabbed with a separate straight swab. Both tonsillar swabs were immediately put into about 3 c c of sterile salt solution; the nasopharyngeal swab was put into a separate tube of salt solution. The content of these swabs was well mixed in the salt solution by stirring the swabs in the solution. The swabs were removed and the mixture of organisms was at once plated. Often only a few hemolytic colonies appeared, and these had to be replated to obtain them in pure culture.

Comparisons were made between the streak method on cooled and hardened blood-agar plates and dilutions. It was found that if hemolyzers were few they could be detected by the dilution method where they would be missed by the streaking method.

In every case where positive hemolyzers are reported the colony was picked from the plate and replated. The organism was then isolated and confirmed as a streptococcus morphologically and by Gram staining. Morphologic and staining confirmation seems to be necessary, as in many of the plates examined an organism was present at 24 hours' incubation which produced a slight hemolysis somewhat similar to that of some of the colonies of hemolytic streptococci. After about 48 hours these colonies become pyramidal in shape and show a milk-white color. Morphologically, the organism is biscuit-shaped diplococci. In staining by the Gram method the stain is not retained.

Thirty-seven per cent. of the students examined in the summer quarter and 36% of those examined in the fall quarter showed hemolytic streptococci in the nasopharynx or on the tonsil. Of the number examined, 34 had had tonsils removed; of these 8 contained hemolyzers. Of the 200 throats examined, 14 had somewhat enlarged tonsils; 7 of these showed hemolyzers. It is interesting to compare this with a series of 25 pairs of tonsils which were removed in the dispensary of Rush Medical School. These tonsils were collected under as aseptic conditions as possible and brought to the laboratory. The posterior portion of the tonsil was seared with a hot iron, and the tonsil was opened in the seared portion with a sterile scalpel. Part of the tonsillar pulp was removed and placed in a sterile petri dish. This material was macerated and later plated. Of these 25 pairs of tonsils, 17 pairs showed the presence of

[19] Ibid., 1918, 71, p. 700.

[20] Ibid., p. 702.

[21] Jour. Infect. Dis., 1917, 20, p. 45.

[22] Standard Technique of Meningococcus Carrier Detection, U. S. Army, 1918.

hemolytic streptococci. It seems that the fact that the tonsils are enlarged does not indicate that the owner is surely harboring the hemolytic streptococci, and conversely the fact that the tonsils are removed does not indicate that the individual is free from hemolytic streptococci.

To determine in what manner the hemolytic flora varies from time to time 6 laboratory workers were selected. Swabs were made from once to twice a week for 12 weeks. Of these 6 persons, 3 were always free from hemolyzers, in 2 hemolyzers were always found, in one they were found every time except on one examination. It has been suggested that persons working or mingling with those who harbor the hemolyzers are apt to become carriers. Two of the 3 who never showed the presence of hemolyzers were present continually as instructors in the laboratory and in fairly close daily contact with individuals known to be harboring hemolytic streptococci.

The results obtained in this series of 200 throats justify the conclusion that a considerable number of healthy people are sometimes carriers of hemolytic streptococci.

Sherman[23] examined the throats of 32 dogs. Typical hemolytic streptococci were found in 39%. Poppins, working in this laboratory on the frequency of hemolytic streptococci in horse feces, found them present in 25% of the samples examined (personal communication). The hemolytic streptococci which are reported by me in the present series as being isolated from horse feces were isolated by him. Davis has frequently found hemolytic streptococci in milk. Out of 15 samples of pasteurized milk examined, I found 2 samples containing hemolytic streptococci.

DISTRIBUTION OF NONHEMOLYTIC STREPTOCOCCI

Nonhemolytic streptococci are found in almost any place where bacteria are present. These streptococci are normally present on the mucous membranes of the respiratory passages and in the intestinal canal. They were found in all the 200 throats and the 25 pairs of tonsils. They were present in the feces of the cow, horse and man in practically all determinations. Urine often contains these strains of nonhemolytic streptococci even when collected under aseptic conditions. Str. lacticus is present in commercial starters and in milk even when it is pasteurized. Heinemann found Str. lacticus on the skin of cows. He was able to raise the virulence of these organisms so that rabbits were killed when injected with doses of 0.1 c c of a broth culture. These streptococci isolated from milk and commercial starters produce the typical green colony on the blood-agar plate.

FERMENTATION REACTIONS

Attempts to classify the streptococci by their power to ferment various carbohydrates were first made by Gordon[24] in 1903 and Hiss[7] in 1905. Hiss indicated a classification which divided the streptococci into groups. One group fermented only the monosaccharids, another fermented the disaccharids, and another fermented the polysaccharids as starch, dextrin and glycogen. Gordon's work, 1905, in which he used 9 different tests, has led to much investigation in regard to classification in relation to the distribution of streptococci.

[23] Jour. Infect. Dis., 1919, 25, p. 259.
[24] Lancet, 1905, 2, p. 1400.

Andrewes and Horder,[25] using Gordon's tests, tabulated 1,200 strains isolated from various sources. These strains of streptococci, including the pneumococci, were placed in 7 groups, Str. equinus, Str. mitis, Str. pyogenes, Str. salivarius, Str. anginosus, Str. fecalis, and the pneumococcus.

Beattie and Yates[26] tested 42 strains of streptococci according to Gordon's tests and found these tests unreliable in their hands. The work of Floyd and Wolbach[12] is unique in that they reported a large number of organisms which failed to ferment any of the carbohydrates. The number which failed to ferment lactose is especially large. They state that their fermentation groups were supported by immune reactions, agglutination, and complement fixation.

Lyall,[15] working with 263 strains and using the fermentation tests as suggested by Gordon in combination with the blood-agar plates, reported that it is possible to recognize all the groups proposed by Andrewes and Horder, and another group not reported by them, a group which is capable of fermenting salicin and raffinose. Lyall's hemolytic group presented the most constant carbohydrate reactions. Seventy-four and nine tenths per cent. of this group conformed to Str. pyogenes of Andrewes and Horder. Lyall states that the ability to ferment raffinose is characteristic of the methemoglobin-producing organisms. He separates the pneumococci from the other streptococci primarily on the basis of their ability to ferment inulin.

The conclusion was reached by Hopkins and Lang,[11] after working with 105 strains, that streptococci occurring in severe infections of man may be differentiated from the saprophytic types by the fermentation tests. One pathogenic and six saprophytic groups are recognized. The pathogenic group differs from the six saprophytic groups in being able to ferment salicin and failing to ferment raffinose and mannite. These workers used the blood-agar plate, but did not consider it a reliable basis for classification.

Holman, using strains of his own collection and the data of others, reported the action on blood-agar plates and the fermentation reactions of 2,463 different strains of streptococci. He states that the constancy of these reactions is essential to the method of classification advocated and that evidence of transmutation or examples of inherent alteration of character have been insufficient to invalidate this method. He also concludes that the confusion in the results of the tests and the examples of so-called alteration are explained by the relative difficulty of growth and the morphologic similarity among different types. Holman makes 16 groups of streptococci on the basis of the reaction on the blood-agar plate and the various carbohydrates.

Blake's contribution to the classification of the streptococci, like Holman's, is based on observations with the blood-agar plate and the various fermentation reactions. He reduced the number of groups to four. He considers that the slight variation among the hemolytic organisms is not sufficient to demand separate classification. He divided the methemoglobin producers and those indifferent on the blood-agar plate into three groups, depending on their action on lactose and mannit.

Holman differs from Lyall and Blake in classifying hemolyzers, in that he separates them into eight groups mainly on the basis of the fermentation of the different carbohydrates. He at first divided them into two main groups on the basis of their lactose fermentation. This raises the question of the reliability of lactose fermentation.

Lactose Fermentation of Hemolytic Streptococci.—One hundred and fourteen of the 134 strains of hemolyzers always fermented lactose. Many of these strains have been tested from 2-6 times at intervals varying in duration from 3-15 months. Seven of these strains were grown on blood agar and ascitic fluid agar at 37 C. for 10 months. Twenty strains have at one or more times failed to ferment lactose. Only 4 of these 20 strains (32, 137, 345, 386) have always failed to ferment lactose at the end of the regular fermentation period of 5 days. Three of these strains (137, 345, 386) were isolated from the normal throat and one (32) from the blood of a patient dying of carcinoma of the liver and pelvic abscess. Only two strains (2, 7), both of which were isolated from the blood at necropsy from different cases of pyemia, varied more than once in their lactose fermentation (table 1, strains 2, 7).

[25] Ibid., 1906, 2, pp. 708, 775, 852.
[26] Jour. Path. and Bacteriol., 1911, 26, p. 247.

It is interesting to consider strain 31 in relation to strain 32. Both of these strains were isolated from the same individual at necropsy. Strain 31 was isolated from the blood, and strain 32 was isolated from the pus of a pelvis abscess. Strain 31 fermented lactose on only one occasion after it had been grown on ascitic fluid agar for 10 months; strain 32 never fermented lactose at the end of the regular fermentation period of 5 days. To determine whether a continuous growth in lactose broth and a longer period of incubation would have any effect on the fermentation of lactose negative hemolytic streptococci strains 32, 137 and 386 were grown in lactose broth for eight weeks with weekly transfers. Seventeen days after the sixth weekly transfer these strains fermented lactose when litmus was used as an indicator. When Andrade was used as an indicator slight fermentation occurred at the end of seven days.

TABLE 3

FERMENTATION REACTIONS

Strain	Lactose	Mannit	Salicin	Date	
2	—	—		11/22/17	
	+	—		12/12/17	
	+	—	+	1/ 2/18	
	—	—	+	11/20/18	
	+	—	+	12/10/18	
	—	—	+	1/ 7/18	Blood agar at 37 C.
	—	—	+	10/ 8/18	Blood agar at 37 C.
	—	—	+	1/ 7/18	Ascitic agar at 37 C.
	—	—	+	10/ 7/18	Ascitic agar at 37 C.
7	+	—		12/12/17	
	+	—		12/18/17	
	—	—	+	1/ 2/18	
	—	—	+	3/12/18	
	—	—	+	11/20/18	
	—	—	+	12/10/18	
	—	—	+	1/ 7/18	Blood agar at 37 C.
	—	—	+	10/ 7/18	Blood agar at 37 C.
	+	—	+	10/ 7/18	Ascitic agar at 37 C.
	—	—	+	10/ 7/18	Ascitic agar at 37 C.
80	+	—	+	3/ 4/18	
	+	+	+	4/28/18	
	+	—	+	11/25/18	
	+	+	+	11/26/18	
	+	+	+	1/ 9/18	

Strain 406 was irregular in its lactose fermentation. To determine to what extent the variation continued, this strain was plated out on blood agar. Ten colonies were picked off and put into separate lactose broth tubes. All of these tubes were fermented in 24 hours except two (1 and 10), which were but slightly fermented in 48 hours. Number 1 was then plated out and 20 separate colonies were picked off and inoculated into lactose broth tubes. All of these tubes of lactose were fermented but number 10. This one remained lactose negative for 5 days. Tube number 10 was then plated out and 10 colonies were picked and inoculated into 10 lactose broth tubes. All of these tubes of lactose broth were acidified in 24 hours except number 5, which fermented lactose in 48 hours. Tube 10 in the first plating was plated in blood agar. Four colonies were picked and inoculated into lactose broth tubes. All of these were fermented in 5 days except tube 3. Tube 3 was then plated and 10 colonies were picked off and inoculated into lactose broth. All of these 10 tubes were fermented except tube 6. This tube was plated in blood agar and 3 colonies picked. Of these 3 tubes, number one fermented lactose in 3 days, number two in 1 day, and number three in 2 days. Tube number one was plated out on blood agar and 10 colonies were picked off and put into lactose broth. All of these tubes fermented lactose except number 6, which failed to ferment lactose at all, and number 10, which fermented lactose after 3 days. In each negative tube growth was determined by plating. In all, 67 tubes of the same lot of lactose broth were tested in this experiment, and in 4 of these fermentation failed to occur in 5 days. On this test alone the organism might have been placed in either of 2 groups.

Mannite Fermentation of Hemolytic Streptococci.—The lactose positive and the lactose negative organisms are divided further by Holman on the basis of their ability to ferment mannite. Of the 134 hemolyzers in my series, 10 fermented mannite at least on one titration. Of these 10, only 2 strains (67, 371) fermented mannite on each titration. One of these was isolated from a removed tonsil, and the other from the normal throat. Both of these organisms would be classified as Str. infrequens according to Holman's classification. Only one strain (80) varied in its mannite fermentation more than once (table 1, strain 80).

Salicin Fermentation of Hemolytic Streptococci.—Holman divides the mannite fermenters and the mannite nonfermenters into separate groups on the basis of ability to ferment salicin. This brings up the reliability and constancy of the fermentation of salicin as a basis for classification. Of the 134 strains of hemolyzers tested by me, 5 strains (32, 40, 137, 174, 345) failed to ferment salicin at one or more titrations. Three of these (137, 174, 345) failed to ferment salicin at every titration. Comparison between lactose and salicin fermentation shows that all those strains which are irregular or fail to ferment salicin are either weak in their ability to ferment lactose or fail altogether to ferment it. Strains 32, 137 and 345, which always failed to ferment salicin, also failed to ferment lactose during the regular fermentation period. Strain 40 fermented lactose once out of 5 determinations. Strain 174 fermented lactose once out of 4 determinations. In all these determinations growth in the tube from which the test sugars were inoculated was confirmed by the fact that good growth occurred in the saccharose tube and the milk. Strain 32 was isolated from a pelvic abscess; strain 40 was isolated from the blood of a patient dying with carcinoma of the pharynx; strains 137, 174, 345 were isolated from the normal throat. In noting this it must be taken into consideration that 67 other strains which were isolated from the normal throat did ferment salicin.

Grouping of Hemolytic Streptococci.—According to Holman's nomenclature, 30 strains of the 134 hemolyzers could not be classified as Str. pyogenes at every titration. All of the 30 strains except 7 (61, 137, 345, 371, 386, 32, 174), however, did fall into the group Str. pyogenes at one or more determinations.

The class Str. infrequens is characterized by being a positive fermenter of lactose, mannite and salicin. It differs from the ordinary pyogenes only in being able to ferment mannite. Ruediger[27] has found this type associated with scarlatinal angina. He also found this type in normal throats, in throats of tonsillitis patients, in middle-ear infections, erysipelas and cellulitis, in the pericardial cavity, in blood in puerperal sepsis, in conjunctivitis, sinusitis, and in the throats of patients having measles. Of the 9 strains (61, 78, 80, 81, 91, 104, 112, 155B, 371) falling into Str. infrequens all except two (61, 371) on one or more titrations would fall back into the pyogenes class. Strain 61 is the only one of 19 strains isolated from removed tonsils which would always be

[27] Amer. Jour. Pub. Health, 1912, 2, p. 107.

placed in the class of Str. infrequens. Strain 371 is the only one of 69 strains isolated from the normal throat which would always fall into the infrequens group.

None of my strains would fall permanently into Str. hemolyticus I, II, or III, according to Holman's nomenclature. Strain 36 isolated from the pus of a frontal sinusitis would be grouped as Str. hemolyticus II once out of its 5 titrations. In the other 4 titrations it would be grouped as Str. pyogenes once and as Str. equi three times. One strain (83) isolated from a removed tonsil would fall into Str. hemolyticus II once out of 4 of its determinations. In the other 3 titrations it would be grouped as Str. pyogenes.

One strain (174) isolated from the swab from a cryptic tonsil where there had never been a history of sore throat would fall into Str. anginosus once out of three of its titrations. In the other 2 titrations it would be classified as Str. subacidus.

Sixteen strains would fall into group Str. equi. Of these, 14 during one or more titrations could be grouped as pyogenes, one (36) as hemolyticus II, and 2 (32, 40) as subacidus. One strain (386) remained true on each titration as Str. equi. It is interesting to note the source of these organisms which at one time or another could be grouped as Str. equi. This group has been considered as representing those strains which in one way or another are associated with the horse. The one strain remaining true to this group in all determinations was isolated from the normal throat. Two of the 16 strains which would be grouped as Str. equi, strains 403 and 406, were isolated from horse feces. Strain 403 fermented lactose two times out of 3 titrations, and 406 fermented lactose once out of 2 titrations. It is interesting to note that of the 10 hemolytic strains isolated from horse feces these two strains are the only two which at any time failed to ferment lactose. All other strains falling into the group Str. equi are from septicemia, removed tonsils, or normal throats. The source of these strains would not seem to suggest that they should be classified with those organisms obtained from horse feces. The strains isolated from horse feces were tested on rabbits and found to be pathogenic, killing in 4 days when $\frac{1}{10}$ c c of a 24-hour broth culture was injected intravenously.

Strains 137 and 345 always were grouped as Str. subacidus. Three strains (32, 40, 174) fell into this group in one or more determinations. This group was called subacidus by Holman because it failed to ferment any of the sugars except glucose and saccharose. Floyd and Wolbach have reported a large number of strains belonging to this group. The sources such as broncho-pneumonia and scarlet fever from which Floyd and Wolbach isolated their organisms would place them in as pathogenic a group as Str. pyogenes. Strains 137 and 345 were isolated from the normal throat.

Of the 134 hemolytic strains which cover a variety of sources, only 6 strains in all tests failed to group themselves as Str. pyogenes according to Holman's classification; that is, they failed to follow the usual order of fermentation to hemolytic streptococci in fermenting lactose and salicin but not fermenting mannite or raffinose. The sources of these 6 strains, 5 from the throat and 1 from septicemia, show no significance of relationship to their fermentation reactions. Thus it seems that Blake is justified in his decision that the slight variation among hemolytic organisms is not sufficient to demand a separate classification.

Lactose Fermentation of Nonhemolytic Streptococci.—As among the hemolyzers slight variation occurs among the nonhemolyzers in the fermentation of lactose. All except 16 of the 150 strains of nonhemolyzers reported in this series fermented lactose at every determination. Five of these 16 strains (189, 211, 213, 440, 466) never fermented lactose in any of their determinations. The sources of these strains which always failed to ferment lactose are as follows: strain 189 from the normal throat, strains 211, 213, 440, 446 from horse feces. Only two strains (86, 87) varied in their lactose fermentation more than once (table 4, strains 86, 87).

TABLE 4

Fermentation Reactions

Strain	Lactose	Mannite	Raffinose	Salicin	Date	
4	+	–	+		10/21/17	
	+	–	+		12/18/17	
	+	–	+		1/ 2/18	
	+	–	–	–	5/11/18	
	+	–	–	–	11/20/18	
10	+	+	–		12/12/17	
	+	+	–		12/18/17	
	+	–	–	+	1/ 2/18	
	+	+	–	+	11/20/18	
	+	–	–		1/ 7/18	Blood agar 37 C.
	+	+	–	+	10/ 7/18	Blood agar 37 C.
	+	–	–		1/ 7/18	Ascitic agar 37 C.
	+	+	–	+	10/ 7/18	Ascitic agar 37 C.
20	+	+	–		12/31/17	
	+	+	–		3/11/18	
	+	+	–	+	1/20/18	
	+	+	–		1/ 7/18	Blood agar 37 C.
	+	–	–	+	10/ 7/18	Blood agar 37 C.
	+	+	–		1/ 7/18	Ascitic agar 37 C.
	+	–	–	+	10/ 7/18	Ascitic agar 37 C.
86	+	+	–		3/ 6/18	
	+	–	–	–	4/28/18	
	–	–	–	+	11/22/18	
	–	–	–	–	12/19/18	
87	+	–	+		3/ 7/18	
	+	–	+		4/28/18	
	–	–	–	+	11/25/18	
	–	–	–	+	12/19/18	
88	+	–	–		3/ 6/18	
	+	+	–	+	4/28/18	
	+	–	+	–	11/25/18	
			+	–	12/ 9/18	

Mannite Fermentation of Nonhemolytic Streptococci.—Forty-two strains of the 150 nonhemolyzers fermented mannite one or more times during the various determinations; 36 of the 42 fermented it at each titration. Only two strains (10, 20) varied in their ability to ferment mannite more than once (table 4, strains 10, 20).

Salicin Fermentation of Nonhemolytic Streptococci.—Eighty-seven of the 150 nonhemolyzers fermented salicin; 12 of the 87 were irregular in their fermentation of salicin, but at no time did any of the strains vary more than once. Lyall states that all streptococci which are indifferent on blood agar are salicin fermenters. In his indifferent group he places the strains isolated from fecal sources. It has not been found that all of the strains of fecal origin in this series of 150 nonhemolyzers ferment salicin. Of the 24 strains isolated from horse feces, 14 strains fermented salicin. All of the 16 strains isolated from human feces did ferment salicin. The 27 strains isolated from milk — a material which might easily be contaminated with fecal matter — fermented salicin. Of the 67 strains of fecal origin, 57 were positive salicin fermenters.

Raffinose Fermentation of Nonhemolytic Streptococci.—Lyall[15] states that all the methemoglobin producers are raffinose fermenters. Blake considers the fermentation of raffinose unimportant since it so nearly coincides with the fermentation of inulin. All of the methemoglobin producers among the 150 strains are not raffinose fermenters. Only 50 strains at one or more times fermented raffinose. Eight of these positive raffinose fermenters showed a variation in their raffinose fermenting ability, but only three of these variable strains (4, 87, 88) varied more than once (table 2, strains 4, 87, 88). One of these raffinose fermenters was isolated from an infection on the face, 1 from a lung abscess of a cow, 1 from the blood of a patient dying with peritonitis, 1 from a pus pocket at the root of a tooth, 4 from removed tonsils, 5 from the normal throat, 17 from horse feces, 3 from human feces, and 1 from a buttermilk tablet. A greater proportion of those isolated from horse feces fermented raffinose than those isolated from any other source. Andrewes and Horder have two classes, Str. salivarius and Str. anginosus, which are reported as raffinose fermenters. Of the 60 strains isolated from the normal throat or removed tonsils, 19 fermented raffinose. This is a somewhat lower percentage of raffinose fermenters than is found among those strains isolated from horse feces. Twenty of the 40 strains isolated from feces (horse and human) fermented raffinose. There does not seem to be any direct relationship between the source of organism and their fermentation of raffinose unless it is that streptococci of fecal origin are often stronger raffinose fermenters than those strains isolated from other sources.

Grouping of Nonhemolytic Streptococci.—Thirty-one strains of the 150 nonhemolytic strains on every determination fell into the group Str. fecalis according to Holman since they were positive fermenters of lactose, mannite, and salicin. Eight of these 31 strains were from human feces, but these 8 were only one half of the strains isolated from human feces. Depending on their salicin fermentation, the other 8 strains from human feces would be classified either as Str. mitis or Str. salivarius. Eight of the 24 strains isolated from horse feces fell into group Str. fecalis on every determination. Depending on their salicin fermentation, 13 other strains from horse feces would be classified either as Str. mitis or salivarius. The remaining 3 strains from horse feces could be grouped as follows: Strain 441 varied in its lactose fermentation and could be placed in the salivarius group twice and the ignavus group once; strain 440 being lactose, mannite, and salicin negative could be grouped as ignavus, and strain 433 was lactose and mannite positive and salicin negative, and would fall into group Str. nonhemolyticus I.

Thirteen of the 31 strain isolated from milk or milk products always fell into the fecalis group. The remaining 17 milk strains could be placed in the mitis or salivarius group. Three strains (6, 24, 109) from pathologic processes were always grouped as fecalis. Nine other strains were irregular in their fermentation reactions and fell into Str. fecalis one or more times. Only one (434) was of fecal origin. The remaining 8 were mostly from pathologic processes. These irregular strains could be classified in other groups according to Holman as follows: strain 10 as Str. mitis 3, of 8 determinations; strain 18 as mitis, 5 of 7 determinations; strain 20 as mitis, 5 of 7 determinations; strain 60 as mitis, 2 of 3 determinations. Strain 86 on account of its irregularity in lactose, mannite and salicin fell one or more times into all of Holman's

8 groups of nonhemolyzers; strain 88 could be placed in the groups fecalis, nonhemolyticus I, mitis, and salivarius; strain 3 fell into mitis once in two determinations, and strains 121 and 434 could be grouped as mitis in 2 of 3 of their determinations.

Blake states that it has been thoroughly established that the majority of streptococci from the intestinal tract of man are characterized by the fermentation of mannite. This statement is not entirely borne out by the findings of workers who have studied the fecal streptococci. Houston[28] studied 300 strains isolated from human feces and found 73 of them capable of fermenting mannite. Holman reported in all 39 strains isolated from feces. Twenty-four of these fermented mannite. Buerger reported 5 strains from the stools of patients having diarrhea. Three fermented mannite. The results of these workers agree with my findings in showing that a high percentage of nonhemolytic streptococci isolated from human feces do not ferment mannite.

It is interesting to consider the source of the strains reported by various workers as grouping as Str. fecalis. Andrewes and Horder[25] reported that 21% of their strains isolated from pathologic sources fermented mannite. Holman, combining his findings with those of Andrewes and Horder, Hopkins and Lang, Kligler, Hartzell and Henrici, and Broadhurst, reported 298 strains of nonhemolyzers which grouped as Str. fecalis. Of these 298 strains, 24 were from human feces, 1 from horse feces, 2 from the intestinal canal of the guinea-pig, 13 from the intestines of the dog, 19 from the feces of the dog, 15 from the intestines of the cat. This shows that of the 298 strains reported by these workers as fermenting mannite, only 74, or less than 25%, were from fecal sources. The remaining 244 strains were isolated from such sources as milk, urine, blood, peritoneal cavity, throat (human, dog and cat), water, abdominal wall, abscesses and ulcers, osteomyelitis, pleural cavity, ear, pyorrhea, infarct of spleen, stump of leg, compound fracture, burn, pus, cellulitis, gallbladder, uterus and vagina of guinea-pig, esophagus and stomach of the dog and cat, and subcutaneous tissue of the frog.

A group of organisms could not well have a greater variety of sources. Broadhurst[29] reported 120 strains which were isolated from the alimentary tract of dog and cat which fermented mannite. Seventy-three of these strains were isolated from the throat, esophagus and stomach. Blake reported only four strains belonging to this group, all of which were from pathologic processes. Considering the low percentage of fecal streptococci grouping in this group and the wide limits from which organisms grouping as Str. fecalis may be isolated, it seems that such grouping carries little significance in respect to indicating the source of the organisms falling into this group.

One strain (433) grouped permanently as Str. nonhemolyticus I. This strain was isolated from horse feces. Strains 86 and 88 fell into this group on one titration. No strains could be grouped permanently as Str. nonhemolyticus II or III.

Three strains (211, 213, 466) were always negative in their lactose and mannite fermentation and positive in salicin fermentation, which placed them as Str. equinus according to Holman. They were isolated from horse feces. These are the only strains of the 24 isolated from horse feces which grouped as equinus. Strains 86, 92 and 173, which are irregular, fell into this group at times. Blake agrees with Holman in thinking that the relationship between

[28] Supplement Annual Report Local Government Board, 1904-5, p. 327.
[29] Jour. Infect. Dis., 1915, 17, p. 277.

grouping and specific fermentation of lactose and mannite is sufficient to justify calling nonhemolytic strains of streptococci which have a close association with the horse Str. equinus.

Andrewes and Horder reported 95 noninulin fermenting strains conforming to what they called class Str. equinus. Seventeen of these 95 strains were isolated from saliva, 23 from human feces, and 1 from urine. The remaining 54 strains were obtained mainly from air, dust, and horse dung. Buerger's[30] results agree in general with the other workers on the fermentation reactions of streptococci. His group, which only fails to ferment inulin and lactose, corresponds with Andrewes and Horder's class Str. equinus. Of his 33 strains isolated from different sources, he reported 2 strains which could be grouped as equinus. These strains represent 2 of 5 isolated from the stools of patients suffering from diarrhea. Holman, including his own series and those of other workers, reported 42 strains grouping as equinus. None of these were isolated from horse feces. He states that the sources often suggest air contamination. These 42 strains were isolated from such sources as normal throat, pyorrhea, human feces, urine and urethra, heart valves, blood, infected foot, hay, tonsils, milk, appendix, fractured clavicle, peritoneum of guinea-pig, and guinea-pig blood. Blake has reported but one strain, which was isolated from the tonsil of a diphtheria patient. Considering the few strains grouping as Str. equinus, the possibility of variation in lactose fermentation, the wide variation of sources of strains grouping as equinus, and the low percentage of strains from horse feces in this class, it is doubtful whether such nomenclature is very fortunate.

Two strains (189, 440) failed to ferment lactose, mannite, and salicin in all their determinations, and according to Holman, would be grouped as Str. ignavus. Ten other strains grouped as ignavus in one or more of their titrations, but fell back into mitis or salivarius. These strains in Str. ignavus, as in Holman's other small groups, show no relationship between source and fermentation.

Of the 150 nonhemolytic strains, 112 always grouped as Str. mitis or salivarius. Eighteen of the 38 nonhemolyzers which did not always group as mitis or salivarius fell into one or the other of these groups on one or more determinations. On the basis of salicin fermentation there are 11 strains which may be placed in either of these groups.

Blake differs from Holman in not considering salicin of significance. By this he eliminates all of Holman's lactose negative groups except Str. equinus. From the standpoint of the fermentation of mannite and salicin, according to my series, Blake is not justified in omitting salicin. From the standpoint of the relationship of source and fermentation reactions, he is not only justified in omitting salicin, but he may just as fairly omit the mannite and lactose and consider the few strains which will not ferment lactose as strains which show a variation from the main type. It has been observed that those strains failing to ferment lactose are feeble in their growth in other mediums. By omitting salicin fermentation, as Blake does, he places the two large groups, mitis and salivarius, in one group, Str. buccalis. This seems reasonable, since the relationship between source, pathogenesis and fermentation reactions of these throat organisms cannot be established in my series. If we eliminate the significance of the occasional failure to ferment lactose and the significance of salicin fermentation, the only two groups of the nonhemolytic streptococci remaining would be Str. buccalis and fecalis. This division is made on the basis of

[30] Jour. Exper. Med., 1907, 9, p. 428.

mannite fermentation. While the relationship between source and the fermentation of mannite seems to be noticeable in the group classified as Str. fecalis by Holman and Blake, yet it is a question whether this relationship is sufficient to make a separate group.

IMMUNE REACTION

Agglutination.—In the work on streptococci, Floyd and Wolbach[12] report that they found the 6 groups of streptococci, which they established on the basis of fermentations, were borne out by agglutination as well as by complement fixation. Kligler's[31] results differ from Floyd and Wolbach's. He reported agglutination tests with 60 strains isolated mostly from pathologic processes. He concluded that agglutination did not separate streptococci into large groups; that classification on the basis of hemolysis was not confirmed by agglutination; that classification on the basis of fermentation reactions seemed to coincide more nearly with agglutination tests. For the agglutination tests which are reported in this paper the serum was titrated and found to produce complete agglutination at dilutions of 1:360 in 4 hours. Two hours of incubation in the water bath at 37 C. followed by 2 hours at room temperature was the period of incubation adopted. Low dilutions (1:50) were used. Controls were made with normal serum and with uninoculated broth to guard against spontaneous agglutination which is common among streptococci and against any possible precipitation which might be produced as a result of inoculating the animals with broth cultures. Thirteen serums were used in the various agglutination tests. Nine of these (2, 372, 368, 399, 367, 411, 371, 345, 174) were produced with hemolytic streptococci and five with nonhemolytic (425, 158, 416, 4, 115).

Twenty-seven hemolytic organisms were tested with the 9 hemolytic serums. Twenty-seven other hemolytic organisms were tested with 4 hemolytic serums (372, 368, 399, 367). This represents in all 351 agglutination tests between suspensions and serums of hemolytic organisms. Of these 351 tests, 64, or 18%, failed to agglutinate. The same 27 hemolytic organisms were also tested with 5 serums of nonhemolytic origin. Of the 135 tests represented in agglutinating the hemolytic serums with the nonhemolytic suspensions, 126, or 93%, failed to agglutinate.

Twenty-five nonhemolytic organisms were tested with the five nonhemolytic serums. Of the 125 tests represented in this series of nonhemolytic serums with nonhemolytic suspensions, 111, or about 89%, failed to give positive agglutinations. These 25 nonhemolytic suspensions were further tested with the 9 hemolytic serums, and in the 225 tests, 145, or 64%, failed to bring about agglutination.

The relative frequency of agglutination in the hemolytic and nonhemolytic groups in these series may be summarized as follows:

Hemolytic serum plus hemolytic streptococci.........	18% failure
Hemolytic serum plus nonhemolytic streptococci......	64% failure
Nonhemolytic serum plus nonhemolytic streptococci...	89% failure
Nonhemolytic serum plus hemolytic streptococci......	93% failure

These results seem to show that agglutination between hemolytic serum and hemolytic streptococci is relatively constant, that less than one half of the tests with hemolytic serum, and nonhemolytic streptococci show agglutination, that with nonhemolytic serum and other strain of hemolytic streptococci agglutination is infrequent, and that with nonhemolytic serum and hemolytic organ-

[31] Jour. Infect. Dis., 1915, 16, p. 327.

isms the agglutination is less frequent. Each serum whether hemolytic or non-hemolytic when tested with its homologous suspension gave typical agglutination.

Complement Fixation.—Floyd and Wolbach[12] tested antigens prepared from six groups of streptococci with the serum of each group. They found in general that complement was fixed when each group was tested with its specific serum, but no fixation occurred when the serum of the other groups were used. Katharine Howell[32] tested 65 strains (28 hemolyzers and 37 nonhemolyzers) with 28 antiserums. She prepared the antigens by washing the cells in salt solution and heating them at 56 C. for 30 minutes. She decided that no correlation existed between complement fixation and groups based on disease; that nonhemolytic antiserums gave less specific complement fixation reactions than hemolytic serums; that the organisms giving positive fixation could not be grouped in any way that would justify a classification of streptococci based on complement fixation. Kinsella and Swift,[5] found a difference between hemolytic and nonhemolytic groups in their complement fixing properties. They considered that the first group was homogeneous, since nearly all these strains reacted in almost an identical way with hemolytic antiserums in their fixation reactions. They regarded the nonhemolytic streptococci as a heterogeneous group and represented it as possessing a right-handed element which would not fix complement with hemolytic serums and a left-handed element which would fix complement with hemolytic serums.

In my work the technic of Kinsella and Swift was followed except that 0.1 c c instead of 0.05 c c of antigen was used. Controls were made with broth as antigen to guard against complement fixation resulting from the possible presence in the antigen of protein from the broth. Such complement fixation might occur if antibodies against the protein in the broth were present in the serum as a result of injecting broth cultures in immunizing the animals. Seventeen animals were immunized against 17 different strains, respectively. Twelve strains (367, 372, 368, 389, 381, 345, 174, 386, 2, 32, 14, 411) were hemolyzers, five (416, 158, 4, 115, 425) nonhemolyzers.

The 12 hemolytic serums were tested against 15 antigens prepared from hemolytic organisms (367, 174, 345, 386, 371, 352, 177, 166, 159, 411, 14, 2, 30, 32, 38) (table 5). All of the 180 tests showed complete inhibition of hemolysis in 0.1 c c of the serum except in 4, or 2% of the tests. Three of these failures were with serum 32. This organism was isolated from the blood of a case of septicemia. One of the antigens (2), with which serum 32 failed to fix, was also from a case of septicemia. The other two antigens which failed to fix complement with serum 32 were from organisms from the normal throat, but 7 of the 9 antigens from organisms from the normal throat fixed complement with serum 32. Three antigens from septicemia other than strain 2 fixed complement with antiserum 32. The fourth failure between hemolytic serum and hemolytic antigens to fix was antiserum 371 with antigen 367, both from organisms from the normal throat. Thirty, or 16%, of the tests with hemolytic antiserums and antigens failed to fix complement with 0.05 c c of serum. Sixteen of these failures were with antigens of mouth origin and serum developed with organisms isolated from cases of septicemia or with organisms from the mouth and antigens of septicemia origin. When it is taken into consideration that in all these tests with hemolytic antiserum and antigens, there were only two serums and four antigens of septicemia origin, it is seen that failure to fix complement is much greater between the throat group and the septicemia group than it is in these groups themselves.

32 Ibid., 1918, 22, p. 230.

TABLE 5

COMPLEMENT FIXATION

Antiserum (hemolytic)	Dilution of Serum in c c	Hemolytic Antigens														
		367	38	32	30	2	174	345	411	386	371	152	14	177	166	159
367	.1	+	+	+	+	+	+	+	+	+	+	+	+	+	+	+
	.05	+	+	+	−	+	+	+	+	+	+	+	+	+	+	+
	.025	+	+	+	−	−	+	+	+	+	+	−	+	+	−	+
372	.1	+	+	+	+	+	+	+	+	+	+	+	+	+	+	+
	.05	+	+	−	+	−	+	+	+	+	+	+	+	+	+	+
	.025	+	−	−	−	−	+	+	+	+	+	−	−	+	−	+
399	.1	+	+	+	+	+	+	+	+	+	+	+	+	+	+	+
	.05	+	+	+	+	+	+	+	+	+	+	+	+	+	+	+
	.025	+	+	+	−	−	+	+	−	+	+	−	−	−	−	+
2	.1	+	+	+	+	+	+	+	+	+	+	+	+	+	+	+
	.05	−	+	+	+	+	+	+	+	+	+	−	+	−	+	+
	.025	−	+	+	+	+	−	−	+	+	+	−	+	−	−	+
32	.1	−	+	+	+	−	+	+	+	+	+	−	+	+	+	+
	.05	−	−	+	−	−	−	−	+	+	+	−	+	+	+	+
	025	−	−	+	−	−	−	−	−	+	−	−	−	−	−	−
411	.1	+	+	+	+	+	+	+	+	+	+	+	+	+	+	+
	.05	−	+	+	+	+	+	+	+	+	+	+	+	+	+	+
	.025	−	+	+	+	+	+	+	+	+	+	+	+	+	+	+
371	.1	−	+	+	+	+	+	+	+	+	+	+	+	+	+	+
	.05	−	+	+	+	+	+	−	+	+	+	+	+	+	+	+
	.025	−	+	+	+	+	+	−	−	−	+	+	+	+	+	+
345	.1	+	+	+	+	+	+	+	+	+	+	+	+	+	+	+
	.05	−	+	+	+	+	+	+	+	+	+	+	+	+	+	+
	.025	−	+	+	+	−	+	+	−	−	+	+	+	+	+	+
174	.1	+	+	+	+	+	+	+	+	+	+	+	+	+	+	+
	05	−	+	+	+	−	+	+	+	+	+	+	+	+	−	+
	.025	−	−	+	+	−	+	+	−	+	+	+	+	+	+	+
386	.1	+	+	+	+	+	+	+	+	+	+	+	+	+	+	+
	.05	−	+	−	+	−	+	−	+	+	+	+	+	+	+	+
	.025	−	−	−	−	−	+	−	−	−	−	−	−	−	−	−
14	.1	+	+	+	+	+	+	+	+	+	+	+	+	+	+	+
	.05	+	+	−	+	−	+	+	+	+	+	−	+	+	+	+
	.025	+	−	−	−	−	+	+	−	−	+	−	+	−	−	−
368	.1	+	+	+	+	+	+	+	+	+	+	+	+	+	+	+
	.05	+	+	−	+	+	+	−	+	+	+	−	+	+	+	+
	.025	−	−	−	−	−	−	−	−	+	+	−	−	−	−	−

The same 12 hemolytic serums used in testing the hemolytic antigens were used in tests in the same way with 18 nonhemolytic antigens (18, 115, 416, 425, 158, 4, 170, 474, 73, 357, 466, 132, 119, 483, 211, 148, 15, 420) (table 6). Deducting the number which were not tested with serums 32 and 386, 193 tests were made. In these 193 tests, 47, or 25%, failed to fix complement with 0.1 c c of serum. With 0.05 c c of serum, 71, or 36%, of the tests failed to fix complement. Antigens 115 and 175 showed a larger number of failures to fix than any of the other antigens. Both of these antigens fixed in all dilutions with their specific serum.

The five nonhemolytic antiserum were tested with the 18 nonhemolytic antigens (table 7). Of the 90 tests represented, 18, or 20%, failed to fix complement with 0.1 c c of serum. Forty-nine, or 53%, failed to fix complement with 0.05 c c of serum. The failure to fix complement occurred mainly with the same antigens as in the tests with hemolytic serum. The five nonhemolytic

TABLE 6

COMPLEMENT FIXATION

Antiserum (hemolytic)	Dilution of Serum in c c	Nonhemolytic Antigens																	
		18	115	416	425	158	4	170	474	73	457	466	132	119	483	211	148	415	420
367	.1	+	—	+	+	+	—	—	+	+	+	—	+	+	+	+	—	+	+
	.05	+	—	+	+	+	—	—	+	+	+	—	+	+	+	+	—	+	+
	.025	+	—	+	+	+	—	—	—	—	+	+	+	—	+	—	—	—	—
372	.1	+	—	+	+	+	—	—	+	+	+	+	+	+	+	+	+	+	+
	.05	—	—	+	+	+	—	—	+	+	+	+	+	+	+	+	+	+	+
	.025	—	—	+	+	+	—	—	—	+	+	—	+	+	+	+	—	+	—
368	.1	+	—	+	+	—	+	—	+	+	+	—	+	+	+	+	+	+	+
	0.5	+	—	+	+	—	—	—	+	+	+	—	+	+	—	—	+	+	+
	.025	—	—	—	—	—	—	—	—	—	+	—	—	—	—	—	—	—	—
399	.1	+	—	+	+	+	+	—	+	+	+	+	+	+	+	+	—	+	—
	.05	+	—	+	+	+	—	—	+	+	+	+	+	+	+	+	—	+	—
	.025	+	—	+	+	—	—	—	—	+	+	+	+	—	+	—	—	—	—
2	.1	+	—	+	+	—	+	—	+	+	+	—	+	+	+	+	—	+	+
	.05	+	—	—	+	—	—	—	—	—	+	—	—	+	+	+	—	+	+
	.025	—	—	—	+	—	—	—	—	—	—	—	—	—	—	—	—	—	—
32	.1	—	—	+	—	—	—												
	.05	—	—	—	—	—	—												
	.025	—	—	—	—	—	—												
411	.1	+	+	+	+	—	+	—	+	+	+	+	+	+	+	+	+	+	+
	.05	+	+	+	+	—	—	—	—	—	+	—	—	+	—	+	—	+	—
	.025	+	+	+	+	—	—	—	—	—	—	—	—	—	—	+	—	—	—
371	.1	+	—	+	+	—	—	—	+	+	+	—	+	+	+	—	—	+	+
	.05	+	—	+	+	—	—	—	+	+	+	—	+	+	+	—	—	—	+
	.025	+	—	—	+	—	—	—	+	—	+	—	—	+	—	—	—	—	—
345	.1	+	+	+	+	+	+	—	+	+	+	+	+	+	+	+	+	+	+
	.05	+	+	+	+	+	+	—	+	+	+	+	+	+	+	+	—	+	+
	.025	+	—	—	+	—	—	—	—	+	+	—	+	+	—	+	—	—	—
174	.1	+	+	+	+	—	—	+	+	+	+	+	+	+	+	—	+	+	+
	.05	+	—	+	+	—	—	—	+	—	+	—	—	+	+	—	—	—	+
	.025	+	—	—	—	—	—	—	+	—	—	—	—	+	+	—	—	—	+
386	.1	+	+	+	+	—	—	—											
	.05	—	—	+	+	—	—	—											
	.025	—	—	—	—	—	—	—											
14	.1		+	+	+	—	—	—	+	+	+	+	+	+	+	+	—	+	+
	0.5		—	+	+	—	—	—	—	+	+	+	—	+	+	—	—	+	—
	.025		—	—	+	—	—	—	—	—	+	—	—	+	—	—	—	—	—

serums were further tested with the 15 hemolytic antigens (table 8). This represents 75 tests, of which 7, or 9%, failed to fix complement with 0.1 c c of serum, and 35, or 47%, failed to fix with 0.05 c c of serum. The percentages of failure to fix complement may be summarized as follows:

Hemolytic serum (0.1 c c) plus hemolytic antigen....	2% failure
Hemolytic serum (0.05 c c) plus hemolytic antigen....	16% failure
Nonhemolytic serum (0.1 c c) plus nonhemolytic antigen	20% failure
Nonhemolytic serum (0.05 c c) plus nonhemolytic antigen	53% failure
Hemolytic serum (0.1 c c) plus nonhemolytic antigen.	25% failure
Hemolytic serum (0.05 c c) plus nonhemolytic antigen	36% failure
Nonhemolytic serum (0.1 c c) plus hemolytic antigen.	9% failure
Nonhemolytic serum (0.05 c c) plus hemolytic antigen	47% failure

As shown by these tests, it seems that there is a greater constancy among hemolyzers than there is between hemolyzers and nonhemolyzers or among nonhemolyzers themselves.

In general, the results obtained in agglutination and complement fixation seem to agree with the findings of Kinsella and Swift, who, by fixation tests, decided that the hemolytic organisms represented a homogeneous group, and the nonhemolytic organisms represented a heterogeneous group, having a left-handed element more closely related to the hemolytic group than the right-handed element. A relationship between a grouping based on agglutination or complement fixation and a grouping based on fermentation reactions or source does not seem to be evident.

TABLE 7

COMPLEMENT FIXATION

Antiserum (nonhemolytic)	Dilution of Serum in c c	Nonhemolytic Antigens																	
		18	115	416	425	158	4	170	474	73	457	466	132	119	483	211	148	415	420
416	.1	+	+	+	+	−	+	−	+	+	+	+	+	+	+	+	+	+	+
	.05	+	+	+	+	−	−	−	−	−	+	−	−	−	−	+	−	+	−
	.025	+	+	+	+	−	−	−	−	−	−	−	−	−	−	+	−	−	−
158	.1	+	−	+	+	+	+	−	−	+	+	+	+	+	+	+	−	+	+
	.05	+	−	+	−	+	−	−	−	+	+	+	+	−	−	−	−	+	−
	.025	+	−	−	−	+	−	−	−	+	−	−	+	−	−	−	−	−	−
425	.1	+	+	+	+	−	−	−	+	−	+	+	+	+	+	+	+	+	+
	.05	+	−	+	+	−	−	−	+	−	+	+	+	−	+	+	+	+	−
	.025	+	−	+	+	−	−	−	−	−	+	−	−	−	+	+	+	−	−
4	.1	+	+	+	+	+	+	+	−	+	+	−	+	+	+	−	+	+	+
	.05	−	+	+	−	−	+	−	−	+	−	−	−	−	−	−	−	−	−
	.025	−	−	−	−	−	+	−	−	+	−	−	−	−	−	−	−	−	−
115	.1	+	+	+	+	+	−	−	+	+	+	+	+	+	+	+	−	+	+
	.05	+	+	+	+	−	−	−	+	+	+	+	−	+	+	−	+	+	−
	.025	+	+	+	+	−	−	−	−	−	+	−	−	+	−	−	−	−	−

TABLE 8

COMPLEMENT FIXATION

Antiserum (nonhemolytic)	Dilution of Serum in c c	Hemolytic Antigens														
		367	38	32	30	2	174	345	411	386	371	152	14	177	166	159
416	.1	+	+	+	+	+	+	+	+	+	+	+	+	+	+	+
	.05	−	−	+	+	+	+	+	−	−	−	−	+	+	+	+
	.025	−	−	−	−	−	−	−	−	−	−	−		+	+	+
158	.1	+	+	−	+	+	+	−	+	+	+	+	+	−	+	+
	.05	−	−	−	+	−	−	−	+	−	+	−	−	−	+	+
	.025	−	−	−	−	−	−	−	+	−	+	−	−	−	+	+
425	.1	+	+	+	+	+	+	+	+	+	+	+	+	+	+	+
	.05	+	+	+	+	−	+	−	−	−	+	+	+	+	+	+
	.025	−	−	+	+	−	+	−	−	−	+	−	+	−	+	+
4	.1	−	+	−	+	+	+	−	+	+	+	+	+	−	+	+
	.05	−	−	−	−	−	+	−	−	−	+	−	−	−	+	+
	.025	−	−	−	−	−	−	−	−	−	−	−	−	−	−	−
115	.1	+	+	+	+	+	+	+	+	+	+	+	+	+	+	+
	.05	+	−	+	+	+	+	+	−	−	+	−	+	+	+	+
	.025	−	−	+	+	+	+	+	−	−	+	−	−	−	−	+

SUMMARY AND CONCLUSIONS

There seems to be no direct relationship between the length of chains and pathogenesis in streptococci.

Pleomorphic strains may change to segmented chains with slightly elongated cells.

Capsules are less commonly found among hemolyzers than among nonhemolyzers.

Hemolysis as shown in this series of 134 strains is constant even after nearly two years of artificial cultivation.

Evidence points to the fact that all nonhemolytic strains are methemoglobin producers when grown on suitable mediums.

Thirty-seven per cent. of 200 normal throats examined contained hemolytic streptococci. Hemolytic streptococci may be present in horse feces, crypts of tonsils, milk, throats of dogs, and occasionally in human feces.

Of the 134 hemolytic strains, only four regularly failed to ferment lactose. Lactose was fermented by these four strains at a longer period of incubation than five days. Only two of the hemolytic strains always fermented mannite; and only three always failed to ferment salicin.

There seems to be more uniformity of fermentation among the hemolytic streptococci than among the nonhemolytic.

None of the minor groups of hemolytic streptococci show sufficient relation to source, habits or pathogenesis to warrant a separate classification.

The term Str. hemolyticus is to be preferred to Str. pyogenes.

Of the 150 strains of nonhemolyzers, only five always failed to ferment lactose; 36 always fermented mannite, and 75 always fermented salicin.

The regular type of fermentation places most of the nonhemolyzers in the class Str. mitis and salivarius according to Holman, or Str. buccalis according to Blake.

Considering the lack of relationship between fermentation reactions and source or pathogenesis, and the wide distribution of organisms falling into nonhemolytic groups, it is doubtful whether any of the smaller groups of the nonhemolytic streptococci deserve a place in classification.

The term Str. viridans seems to be preferable to Str. buccalis.

Agglutination reactions between hemolytic organisms and homologous serum in the series examined show a high degree of uniformity. The reactions of hemolytic serum with nonhemolytic organisms, nonhemolytic serum with hemolytic organisms, or nonhemolytic serum with nonhemolytic organisms, except with homologous strains, give a low percentage of positive results.

The reactions of hemolytic serum with hemolytic antigen yield a higher percentage of complement fixation than those of hemolytic serum with nonhemolytic antigen, nonhemolytic serum with nonhemolytic antigen, or nonhemolytic serum with hemolytic antigen.

The results of both agglutination and complement fixation tests strengthen the belief that the hemolytic group is a homogeneous group in which there is a relatively high degree of constancy and that the nonhemolytic group is heterogeneous or at all events less homogeneous than the hemolytic group.

THE HUMAN FECAL STREPTOCOCCI

C. J. Oppenheim

From the Department of Hygiene and Bacteriology, University of Chicago

Ever since the discovery of the typhoid bacillus by Eberth in 1880, gastro-intestinal bacteriology has concerned itself largely with the study of various organisms that have been thought to have a possible bearing on the etiology of specific diseases. It is not surprising, therefore, that among the large number of organisms isolated from the intestinal tract and studied, the streptococcus has come in for its share of attention as a possible inciter of certain of the diarrheal diseases as well as local gastro-intestinal disturbances in infants and adults.

As early as 1890, Kruse and Pasquale[1] in an investigation on dysentery and tropical abscess, found streptococci to be the predominant organism in dysentery stools, and though they observed that streptococci also seemed to predominate in the diarrheal stools of nondysenteric origin, they nevertheless felt the possibility of etiologic relationship between this disease and streptococci. Beck[2] reported a case of cholera nostras in which he was able to isolate "almost pure cultures" from the stools on the third day of the disease. Streptococci isolated from the organs of the case were found to be highly pathogenic for mice. He concludes that the streptococci isolated were the causative organisms.

Metschnikoff[3] mentions Drasch's report of a streptococcus which, after isolation from a case, was found to be able to produce diarrheas resembling in all respects those provoked by the cholera vibrio. Askanazy[4] reports a case of phlegmonous enteritis with fatal termination in which streptococci seemed to have had some provocative significance. A series of small epidemics of severe gastro-enteritis, apparently due to the consumption of raw milk in Christiania, were studied by Axel Holst[5] in 1895 and the blame placed on a cow found to harbor streptococci in a subacute udder infection. The streptococci isolated were able to produce a rather intense hyperemia of the intestinal vessels of mice and dogs to which cultures were fed, and provoked diarrheal attacks when cultures were swallowed by Holst and his colleagues. Holst remarks on the variance in virulence of these organisms, which seemed to be morphologically and culturally identical with the streptococci ordinarily found in the Christiania market milk.

Received for publication Oct. 4, 1919.

[1] Ztschr. f. Hyg. u. Infektionskr., 1891, 16, p. 1.
[2] Centralbl. f. Bakteriol., 1892, 12, p. 632.
[3] Ann. de l'Inst. Pasteur, 8, p. 258.
[4] Centralbl. f. allg. Path. u. path. Anat., 1895, 6, p. 313.
[5] Baumgartens Jahresbericht, 1896, 52, p. 545.

Tavel, Cérenville, Eguet, and Krumbein[6] noted a series of cases of severe gastro-enteritis of a somewhat typhoidal clinical course, in which a peculiarly varying streptococcus was found. Cérenville believed this organism differed perceptibly in morphology from the normal intestinal streptococci and termed the clinical cases "streptococcus enteritis."

Lameris and Harrevelt[7] record an epidemic in a hospital in which boiled milk, previously heavily polluted from the milk of a cow recovering from a subacute mastitis, was being used; and attributed the epidemic to toxic material produced by the organisms in the milk, though live cultures were found to be nonpathogenic for laboratory animals. Baermann and Eckersdorff[8] studied a series of cases of dysenterial appearance occurring in a Sumatra hospital in which only hemolytic streptococci were to be found in the stools. These organisms failed to have sharply defined agglutinative powers with the patients' serum, and produced no changes in macacus monkeys to which broth cultures were fed.

Ungermann,[9] in a bacteriologic investigation of appendicitis, found streptococci in 47% of 38 cases of acute and chronic appendicitis. He found, however, that staphylococci occurred in about 75% of the cultures from the same series. In 1916, Rosenow and Dunlap[10] reported an outbreak of appendicitis at Culver Military Academy, which they attributed to streptococci probably disseminated in dairy products. These streptococci, in a number of cases, produced in animals lesions resembling appendicitis.

As early as 1886, streptococci were recognized as normal inhabitants of the bowel of infants by Escherisch,[11] who described their morphology in detail. Czerny and Moser[12] described their appearance in blood cultures from cases of infantile gastro-enteritis. Fischl[13] studied 22 cases of septic gastro-intestinal conditions in sucklings, and found streptococci to be the predominating organisms.

In 1895, Booker[14] made a thorough study of over 100 cases of summer diarrhea, covering a period of 5 years' observations, in which bacteriologic and anatomic findings were correlated. He concluded that summer diarrhea, though not attributable to any single micro-organism, may be induced by the activity of several varieties of ordinary occurrence and wide distribution, the principal ones being B. proteus and the streptococcus.

Several cases of so-called "streptococcus enteritis" in sucklings were reported by Hirsch,[15] Libman,[16] and Spiegelberg[17] from the clinic at Graz, and were reviewed by Escherisch.[18] The interesting feature of these cases is the fact that practically all occurred in infants reared on cow's milk, and that streptococci predominated in the blood cultures and were found in large numbers in bacteriologic examinations of the stools.

[6] Ann. Suisses des Sc. Méd., Ser. H, 2, 11.
[7] Ztschr. f. Fleisch u. Milch Hyg., 1901, 11, p. 114.
[8] München. med. Wchnschr., 1909, 56, p. 1169.
[9] Centralbl. f. Bakteriol., I, O., 1909, 1, p. 513.
[10] J. Infect. Dis., 1916, 18, p. 383.
[11] Die Darmbakterien des Saüglings, 1886.
[12] Jahr. f. Kinderh., 1894, 38, p. 430.
[13] Ztschr. f. Heilk., 1894, 15.
[14] Johns Hopkins Hosp. Repts., 1897, 6, p. 159.
[15] Centralbl. f. Bakteriol., 1897, 22, p. 369.
[16] Ibid., p. 376.
[17] Ibid., 1898, 24, p. 401.
[18] Jahrb. f. Kinderh., 49, p. 1898.

Jehle[19] presented a study of 49 cases of enteritis in sucklings and concluded that the evidence points to a milk-borne streptococcus infection. The impression seems to be general that cow's milk offers more opportunity for infection with streptococci than human milk, and the tendency is rather to underestimate other factors incident to artificial feeding which might profoundly influence the opportunity for, and the unfavorable outcome of, infection. In this connection, it is interesting to find that Cohn and Neumann[20] have found that human milk commonly contains pyogenic cocci, including streptococci.

The difficulty of evaluating the literature of streptococcal alimentary infection is at once apparent, since the allusions are rather fragmentary and for the most part based on the report of single or small series of cases, in which the bacteriologic investigations have usually been carried out under older methods or with insufficient detail. These frequent allusions have also, as Nobécourt[21] has observed, tended rather to complicate than to simplify matters, since the streptococcus has long received recognition as a normal inhabitant of the skin and mucous membranes; and since morphologic, biologic and pathogenic characteristics have not assisted materially in bringing about a differentiation of the pathogenic from the nonpathogenic strains. Newer methods of classification based on a combination of observations on growth on blood mediums, as originally proposed by Schottmüller.[22] and fermentative groupings originating with Gordon,[23] have perhaps given a little more hopeful aspect to the possibility of identifying certain types as normal flora, and in addition have brought about the necessity of restudying these organisms under more modern methods.

The first exhaustive studies on the human fecal streptococci were made by Houston[24] in 1904, who examined 300 strains taken from 19 stools, and classified them on the basis of the Gordon fermentations. Houston found that the organisms fall into about 40 groups in their fermentative characteristics, and proposed 10 large classes into which the majority of his strains fell. In a later work, Houston reported on an additional 100 strains.[25]

Winslow and Palmer[26] reported on the fermentative characteristics of 116 strains of streptococci isolated from 15 samples taken from 10 persons, the majority of which were obtained from diarrheal stools. Fuller and Armstrong[27] made further studies on fecal streptococci, and reported on 123 strains, using methods of study similar to those employed by Winslow and Palmer.

19 Jahrb. f. Kinderh., 1907, 65, p. 40.
20 Virchow's Arch., 1891, 126, p. 391.
21 Presse méd., 1903, 2, p. 677.
22 München. med. Wchnschr., 1903, 1, p. 849.
23 Report of the Medical Officer, Local Gov't Board, 1903-4.
24 Ibid., Supplement, 1904-5.
25 Fifth Research Report, Metropolitan Water Board, 1910.
26 J. Infect. Dis., 1910, 7, p. 1.
27 Ibid., 1913, 13, p. 442.

Aside from these observations, there exist practically no studies on the streptococci of normal feces with the exception of strains which Broadhurst[28] has included in her studies, and 53 strains reported by Holman.[29] With the exception of the last two, no account has been taken of the characteristics on blood mediums. One thing, and practically the only one on which all observers seem to agree, is the rather constant presence of mannite-fermenting organisms in human feces, thus giving some justification to the name "fecalis" which has been used in all of the later classifications from that of Andrewes and Horder[30] up through the more recent groupings suggested by Blake[31] and by Holman.[29] Numerical estimations of the preponderance of mannite-fermenters in human feces are, however, at great variance. Thus Houston reports 24%, Winslow and Palmer 28%, Broadhurst 45%, Holman 50%, and Fuller and Armstrong 65%.

On closer examination, it is apparent, however, that the dissimilarity is not so pronounced as one would be led to believe by a mere casual survey of the percentage tabulations. The number of persons examined has been variable, and is not mentioned by some of the observers. The number of strains from each sample also varied greatly; and the methods of study were so different that it would scarcely be expected to find much greater accord in the results. Certain of these points will be taken into consideration later in this paper in more detail.

A conservative point of view is highly desirable in the interpretation of any infection along the basis of streptococcal specificity; and though the limitations of present methods of study of the streptococcus group are perhaps great, there nevertheless exists the desirability of establishing a norm in accord with the recent methods of classification, deviations from which may aid us in more firmly establishing future implications of streptococcal specificity. Up to the present, most observers have rather casually taken "streptococcus enteritis" and other "streptococcal" alimentary infections for granted. The case against the streptococcus rests, however, on a very insecure footing and will remain so until more comprehensive and precise studies of the normal streptococcal flora of the alimentary tract have been made.

The present study represents the examination of 55 stools from 15 persons, from which 323 strains were isolated. All the subjects were healthy adults, and care was taken to avoid any material which was of diarrheal character. The distribution of the samples and strains was:

[28] Ibid., 1915, 17, p. 277.
[29] J. Med. Research, 1916, 34, p. 377.
[30] Lancet, 1906, 2, p. 708.
[31] J. Med. Research, 1917, 36, p. 99.

TABLE 1

DISTRIBUTION OF SAMPLES AND STRAINS FROM PERSONS EXAMINED

Subject	Samples	No. of Strains
1	5	49
2	5	33
3	2	16
4	2	14
5	4	20
6	4	20
7	4	17
8	4	21
9	4	20
10	4	20
11	4	21
12	4	20
13	4	21
14	4	20
15	1	11

METHODS

Material.—Fecal material was collected in sterile paraffined pasteboard containers. The stools were inspected to eliminate loose, watery stools which occasionally were found incident to slight transient diarrheas in the subjects under observation. Material was plated as quickly as it could be obtained, and in no case did more than four hours elapse between deposition of the stool and plating. Plates were always made immediately before use, as it was found that the organisms grew more readily on fresh, moist blood agar.

A few loops of feces taken from the center of the stool were placed in tubes containing sterile salt solution, and after shaking until a uniform, slightly turbid suspension was obtained, two or three loops of the suspension were placed on the edge of a fresh plate. The loop, after being resterilized in the flame, was used to spread the suspension across the plate in radial streaks, "fan-wise" with cross streaks at the spread ends.

Plates were incubated for 18-24 hours at 37 C., at the end of which time, colonies appearing to be streptococci were fished into glucose broth and re-incubated. Replatings were then made from broth, and after the usual incubation, a single colony was picked and streaked on a fresh blood-agar slant. Such slants were used as stock slants, and all morphologic study and transfers to carbohydrate mediums were made from them.

Morphologic study included a Gram stain, and examination for capsule by means of the Welch capsule stain and hanging drop with darkened field.

The appearance of colonies was noted from the replating; transfers to carbohydrate mediums were made from slants, and readings made at the end of 5 days' incubation. All negative fermentations were controlled by three methods: (1) Morphology, (2) re-inoculation into glucose broth to demonstrate viability, (3) retesting in the carbohydrate which failed to show signs of fermentation. Fermentations were in this way controlled to assure the presence of growing organisms in the mediums. Practically all negative fermentations have been repeated twice, and in every case at least once, before recording.

Mediums.—Meat infusion has been used entirely for the base of carbohydrate mediums in which fermentative characteristics were studied, and also in the preparation of agar. The broth has been rendered "sugar-free" by incubating for about eight hours at 37 C. with heavy inoculations of B. coli. Two per cent. of peptone (Armour's) and ½% of salt have been used. The various carbohydrates were added to the quantity of 1% (except in the case of salicin, when ½% was employed) and were added directly to the broth. All broths were titrated to approximate neutrality to phenolphthalein (hot). Determination of the hydrogen-ion concentration of several lots of broth showed a quite uniform P_H value of 7.5 or slightly higher (more alkaline).

One and a half per cent. agar prepared from the meat infusion was found satisfactory for both blood-plates and stock slants. Greater amounts of agar tend to decrease the moisture of the plates and slants, and thereby impair both the growth and longevity of the organisms. Green formation was found to occur most readily on a 10% blood-agar made from sterile defibrinated sheep blood. The formation of green pigment seems to vary greatly and be favored by the alkalinity of the plate. It was found that a P_H value of about 7.5 forms an excellent base for the demonstration of methemoglobin on the blood-plate.

Sterilization.—All mediums have been sterilized by autoclaving for 10 minutes at 10 lbs. of pressure. This was found fully satisfactory after comparison with fermentations in carbohydrate mediums sterilized by the fractional method.

Indicator.—In recent years, biometric studies with titration methods have frequently been used in the study of fermentations. Such methods are not without certain disadvantages: 1. They are more cumbersome and time-consuming. 2. They allow for an element of personal error which perhaps exceeds methods in which a sharply defining two-color indicator is employed. 3. They tend to give a fictitious security in quantitative values, which are by no means uniform, especially where different mediums are employed. This has been thoroughly studied, with regard to nutrient qualities, by Broadhurst;[32] and by Bronfenbrenner and Schlesinger[33] with reference to peptone, buffer and carbohydrate content. 4. Even in biometric studies, an arbitrary point has to be agreed on as the criterion of fermentation, so that the method does not therefore excel the use of any well chosen indicator. I have, therefore, used an indicator without titration in the routine study of my cultures. In the selection of an indicator, it is necessary to consider the initial reaction of the mediums, the range of acidities characteristically produced by the species of organism being studied, and the range at which the indicator employed customarily undergoes its color change.

"Bromcresol purple" (dibromo-ortho-cresol-sulphone-phthalein) was used, as suggested by Clark and Lubs[34] for milk, except that only half the quantity was found necessary to use in broth (5 c c to the liter of broth). These authors[35] denote the useful range of this indicator as lying between P_H values of 5.2 and 6.8, which is perhaps preferable for the demonstration of acidity in a medium of as distinct alkalinity as that which I have employed, and fully coincides with the amount of change in hydrogen-ion concentration which I have been able to demonstrate in 5-day incubations of several of my strains (vide infra).

In addition, this indicator has the advantage of sharp color contrast (from purple to bright yellow) on acidification, and is not reduced or impaired by autoclaving. (The "CR" indicator proposed by Bronfenbrenner[36] because it is much less expensive, would perhaps serve the purpose as well, since its range of usefulness about corresponds to that of bromcresol purple.)

[32] J. Infect. Dis., 1913, 13, p. 404.
[33] Proc. Soc. Exper. Biol. and Med., 1918, 16, p. 44.
[34] J. Agric. Research, 1917, 10, p. 105.
[35] J. Bacteriol., 1917, 2, p. 104.
[36] J. Med. Research, 1918-19, 49, p. 25.

OBSERVATIONS

Appearance of Colonies.—On blood-agar plates, the characteristic colony is the small, granularly opaque, varying from about one to two millimeters in diameter. With the plate on a white background, it is rather easy to differentiate the streptococcus colony by the slightly darkened zone about it; by transmitted light, a distinct green discoloration is readily noted about the colony in a medium of proper chemical reactivity.

I have been unable to distinguish the so-called "indifferent" variety of streptococcus among those isolated from feces. At times, colonies have failed to produce green on blood-agar, but no strain has persistently maintained indifference to the formation of green. It would seem highly suggestive that certain qualities in the medium are the principal determinants of methemoglobin formation. I have found agar of rather pronounced alkalinity (P_H of 7.5 or higher) to favor the production of green pigmentation.

Hemolytic streptococci in the feces of man are apparently the exception and not the rule. Davis[37] in an examination of 53 stools from a series of persons, several of whom were known to harbor hemolytic streptococci in their throats, failed to find a single hemolytic colony. On the other hand, Holman, in his studies reports the finding of 9 hemolytic strains out of a total of 53. Similarly, Broadhurst reports 9 hemolytics in her series of 31 fecal streptococci. I have been able to recover hemolytic streptococci from 5 persons in 15, twice from 2 and once from 3. They were apparently transient or accidental in occurrence, but their presence was nevertheless noted. As to constancy, the 12 strains isolated remained hemolytic over a period of months without exception. No attempt was made to estimate the percentage of hemolytics in stools where they were noted, but a rather general distribution usually occurred, though in no case did they predominate. In the two persons in whom they occurred twice, they appeared in the first and fifth, and first and third samples examined, the stools being collected at about weekly intervals.

General Morphology.—All organisms studied were gram-positive. The appearance of a capsule was rarely noted. One strain (239) maintained a capsule through several transfers. This strain also fermented inulin persistently. Insolubility in bile, however, caused me to disregard the possibility of its being a pneumococcus.

The typical morphology of young cultures in plain broth or from agar slants, was that of a short-chained, diplococcoid, rather lanceolate and coarsely beaded streptococcus. Earlier observers were inclined to confer a certain characteristic morphology on streptococci from various sources. A great number of bacteriologic studies on streptococci isolated from normal and pathologic fecal material from both infants and adults are given over to the description of the organisms. The value of such observations is perhaps quite slight, since it is possible to alter the appearance quite freely with conditions of growth. Thus, in glucose broth after 18 hours' incubation, the majority of fecal organisms tend to become diplococcoid, even in chain formation rather lanceolate and swollen. Addition of calcium carbonate to the glucose broth, which provides for a permanent alkalinity, allows the organisms to become smaller and rounder, and grow out in long strands. Morphology, therefore, would seem to vary with luxuriance of growth and reaction of the mediums.

[37] J. Am. Med. Assn., 1919, 72, p. 319.

Fecal streptococci are, in general, rapidly growing, active organisms. From this standpoint there might be some basis for characterizing them as occurring in short chains and with a tendency to diplococcoid appearance. Over 100 strains were tested for bile solubility. I was unable to find any bile soluble strain in my series.

Constancy of Fermentative Characteristics.—In general, there has been but slight, almost insignificant variation in the constancy of fermentative characteristics. Walker[38] believes that inconstancy is due to transient changes in the metabolic reactions of the organisms. Thro[39] has shown that repeated replatings give rise to single colonies which vary in their fermentative characters. Broadhurst[28] noted two varieties of inconstancy; one dependent on physical or chemical factors which tends to be rather inhibitory and temporary; the other due to marked environmental changes and tending to awaken more active, latent fermentative powers which remain more fixed and permanent.

Too much emphasis cannot be placed on carefully avoiding the acquisition of a mixed culture. In these studies, the progeny of a single colony from a subculture has been selected for study. Other factors that enter prominently into errors which may be interpreted as variability in reaction are the use of mediums which are not uniformly prepared. Thus Broadhurst[32] has found wide variation in acid production by identical strains in meat extract and meat infusion. Titration studies of 10 of my strains (314 to 323) made after 5 days' incubation at 37 C., of mannite and lactose-broth cultures in measured amounts of the extract and infusion, showed markedly higher acid production throughout the infusion cultures in spite of the fact that both extract and infusion cultures were proved to be viable at the end of that time (See table 3, p. 126).

The use of carefully controlled fermentations helps to eliminate the report of a negative fermentation where a failure to inoculate or to grow has accidently occurred. Variability after animal passage is always susceptible of the error inherent in the use of laboratory animals, namely, failure to recover the same organism that was introduced into the animal. This is particularly true of streptococci, which are commonly found as secondary and terminal invaders of the blood stream. Of especial interest in this connection are the observations of Richey and Goehring,[40] who were able to obtain positive postmortem blood cultures in about 33% of 206 cases within 10 minutes after death, and in a large number of antemortem results taken from the arm vein immediately before death; and who found cocci to be the most frequent invaders.

Nevertheless, it must be admitted that the nonhemolytic group of streptococci present a more heterogeneous complex than the hemolytic group, as is readily seen in the lack of specificity of complement fixation phenomena noted by Kinsella and Swift.[41] The general tendency, however, is for the large majority of streptococci under normal conditions of growth and preservation in vitro, to retain rather fixed fermentative characters. It is, then, unlikely that slight variations frequently observed will be sufficient to vitiate the value of fermentative differentiation.

[38] J. Path. and Bacteriol., 1912-13, 17, p. 140.
[39] J. Infect. Dis., 1914, 15, p. 234; 1915, 17, p. 227.
[40] J. Med. Research, 1918, 38, p. 421.
[41] J. Exper. Med., 1917, 65, p. 40.

Fermentations.—Early studies on the streptococci of normal human feces have usually embraced a grouping based on all or several of the Gordon test mediums. In recent years, the tendency has been to reduce the number of test substances, and in this way to avoid "species-mongering." In these studies, for the most part, all fermentative differentiation has been attempted on the basis of fermentations in glucose, lactose, mannite and salicin, so that together with the blood-plate findings, the organisms may readily be identified in the new groupings suggested by Blake[31] and Holman.[29]

All organisms fermented glucose. One strain (14) was markedly less vigorous in its fermentation of this carbohydrate than the others, which rapidly changed the color of the indicator. Of 323, but 8 failed to ferment lactose; 9 strains failed to ferment salicin; 84 failed to ferment mannite. All strains but 2 were negative in inulin broth. About 80 strains were tested in raffinose broth, and but 3 fermented this carbohydrate. A classification of the nonhemolytic streptococci found in human feces, based on a gross percentage from my studies, and classified according to the groupings of Blake and of Holman is:

Blake =	Str. fecalis	74.0%
	Str. buccalis	24.5%
	Str. equinus	1.5%
Holman =	Str. fecalis	73.0%
	Str. salivarius	1.0%
	Str. nonhemolyticus i	23.0%
	Str. equinus	1.5%
	Str. ignavus	1.5%

The result of these studies apparently would justify the assumption that the predominant fecal streptococcus is a nonhemolytic, mannite fermenting organism. That mannite fermenting organisms are characteristic of human fecal streptococci is a generally acknowledged fact, but their numerical frequency according to the results of various observers is somewhat in question.

In the following table are arranged the percentage fermentations in several carbohydrates, noted by various observers, together with my own observations:

TABLE 2

PERCENTAGE OF FERMENTATIONS IN VARIOUS CARBOHYDRATES

Observer	Glucose	Lactose	Salicin	Inulin	Mannite
Houston	..	76	93	5	24
Winslow and Palmer	89	62	..	..	28
Fuller and Armstrong	95	94	..	..	65
Broadhurst	..	87	96	16	45
Holman	..	100	99	2	50
Oppenheim	100	97	97	1	76

At once, it is apparent that there exist many points in common between the data of these observers; but it is equally true that there are many things on which the numerical evidence seems to be quite variable.

In considering the work, it is necessary to survey the several methods used by the workers in obtaining their results. Houston's fermentations were noted in meat extract broth after 48 hours' incubation, with litmus as an indicator.

Winslow and Palmer's fermentations were noted by titration methods in meat extract broth after 3 days' incubation; Fuller and Armstrong used practically the same methods as Winslow; Broadhurst used titration methods, but with meat infusion; Holman employed longer incubations in serum broth and used Andrade's indicator; while in my studies, 5-day incubations were read in meat infusion broth that had a distinct initial alkalinity, with bromcresol purple as an indicator.

Variations in mediums alone suffice to allow large differences to occur. Thus, 10 strains inoculated into 5 c c quantities of meat extract and meat infusion broths and titrated at the end of 5-days' incubation, gave these differences: All strains titrated were retransferred to glucose broth, in which they grew well, proving viability. It is obvious from the tabulations that meat infusion is a better medium for growth and for the demonstration of acidity production than is broth made from the extract.

TABLE 3

Differences in Results with Various Mediums

Strain	Lactose		Mannite	
	Extract	Infusion	Extract	Infusion
314	1.1	3.1	0.1	0.2
315	1.4	3.2	0.2	0.5
316	1.6	3.0	1.0	2.6
317	1.4	2.9	1.0	2.8
318	1.2	3.2	0.8	2.4
319	1.3	3.0	0.6	2.5
320	1.1	3.1	0.8	2.7
321	1.1	3.1	0.8	2.7
322	0.8	3.0	0.6	2.3
323	0.8	3.0	0.7	2.2

Initial p_H of infusion broths = 7.3; of extracts = 7.1.

The element of time also affects the readings greatly. It is therefore important in comparing fermentation readings, to ascertain whether readings were made on the second, third, fourth or fifth day. Frequently mannite fermentation was not complete until the fourth day, so that readings taken prior to this would have led to negative recordings. The choice of indicator and the range at which it best operates has been mentioned. Control of negative fermentations by repetition also helps in eliminating observational errors.

An examination of the changes in final hydrogen-ion concentration produced in 5 c c quantities of mannite and lactose broths, by several strains picked indiscriminately from my stock cultures and inoculated from newly incubated 24-hour blood-agar slants proves interesting (Table 4).

A noteworthy point illustrated by the tabulations is that, although lactose-broth changes are quite uniform, the changes in mannite are more variable and less sharply demarcated; and in several instances did not correspond with the classification of the strains as made by the routine methods with an indicator in these studies; this only by way of further suggesting the differences inherent to a fermentative classification.

It remains to be said, however, that mannite fermentation seems to be the crucial characterizing feature of a large part of fecal strains among the nonhemolytic streptococci; this has been accorded recognition by most workers on classification, and by the few who have studied the human fecal streptococci, and suggests the possibilities of an as yet unworked practical application.

TABLE 4

FINAL HYDROGEN-ION CONCENTRATION CHANGES IN MANNITE AND LACTOSE INFUSIONS

Strain		Type (Blake)	Change in p_H Concentration in Mannite	Change in p_H Concentration in Lactose
1	25	Fecalis	2.0	2.6
2	120	Buccalis	0.8	2.6
3	47	Fecalis	2.2	2.8
4	41	Buccalis	2.2	2.7
5	13	Buccalis	0.0	2.7
6	50	Buccalis	0.0	2.7
7	52	Buccalis	0.0	2.4
8	110	Buccalis	0.0	2.7
9	66	Buccalis	0.0	2.6
10	74	Buccalis	0.0	2.4
11	67	Buccalis	0.0	2.6
12	82	Buccalis	0.0	2.6
13	152	Fecalis	2.5	2.4
14	33	Fecalis	2.5	2.5
15	135	Fecalis	2.4	2.6
16	95	Buccalis	0.0	2.3
17	73	Buccalis	0.0	2.6
18	118	Fecalis	2.5	2.7
19	177	Fecalis	2.6	2.5
20	77	Buccalis	0.0	2.6
21	233	Buccalis	0.1	2.6
22	46	Buccalis	0.1	2.7
23	189	Fecalis	2.4	2.6
24	133	Fecalis	2.3	2.7
25	104	Fecalis	2.5	2.6
26	248	Buccalis	1.3	2.3
27	100	Buccalis	0.0	2.6
28	194	Fecalis	2.5	2.5
29	274	Fecalis	1.8	2.5
30	116	Fecalis	2.4	2.7
31	151	Fecalis	2.4	2.7
32	56	Fecalis	1.6	2.4
33	273	Buccalis	2.0	2.6
34	72	Buccalis	1.6	2.3
35	2	Fecalis	2.2	2.5

Average p_H of sterile incubated broths = 7.3.
These determinations were made with colorimetric methods proposed by Haskins.[42] I am indebted to Miss Helen Penn for valuable assistance in making the determinations.

In the studies of Winslow and Palmer, 85 of 116 strains of the organisms isolated were taken from diarrheal stools; and several strains (36) failed to produce acidity in lactose, a few (9) even proving negative in glucose. This has suggested the possibility that some variation may exist in the fermenting power of streptococci of diarrheal stools.

With this in mind, I have examined 4 stools from typhoid patients, of distinctly diarrheal character; 2 from persons suffering from diarrheas of non-specific origin; and 2 from a patient after free catharsis with a nonantiseptic purgative (elaterin). The organisms isolated were studied in the same manner as those from normal stools, and the same general appearance of colonies and morphology noted. A total of 84 strains was studied, no hemolytics occurring.

The tabulated results from carbohydrate fermentations among these strains are:

[42] J. Lab. and Clin. Med., 1919, 4, p. 6.

TABLE 5

RESULTS FROM CARBOHYDRATE FERMENTATIONS

Percentage Fermentations in	Typhoid Strains (48 Strains)	Strains from an Individual after Administration of Purgative (20 Strains)	Strains from Persons with Nonspecific Diarrheas (2 Subjects; 10 Strains from Each)
Glucose	100	90	100
Lactose	95	80	100
Salicin	90	90	90
Inulin	0	0	0
Mannite	25	50	25

The foregoing data are not strictly comparable to those of the studies made on the fecal streptococci of normal stools, since they represent a much smaller aggregate of observations. It is, however, highly suggestive. It was noted in all cases that fermentation of glucose was much slower than in the case of the streptococci from normal stools, usually requiring three times as long to be complete. In general, all fermentative activity seemed to be retarded or inhibited to some extent in this series. Whether this explains in part the fact that Fuller and Armstrong as well as myself obtained a higher percentage of fermentations than Winslow and Palmer, who used, for the most part, strains from diarrheal material for study, will require a more extensive series of observations to decide.

If further work were to reveal that fermentative characteristics of the fecal streptococci vary from the norm in diarrheal material, three questions will be raised, namely:

1. Are such variants, failing to ferment mannite, identical with the non-mannite fermenters normally found in the buccal cavity and nasopharynx, and not converted into more active fermentative forms due to unnatural conditions in the alimentary tract or unduly rapid transit through it?

2. Are these less active fermenters less resistant and less active forms normally found in the intestinal tract, but not hardly enough under normal conditions to remain viable in as great numbers until passed with the feces?

3. Or are they the characteristic mannite fermenting organism, active fermentatively, but rather permanently impaired in fermentative characters by marked environmental changes? These questions remain as interesting topics for further study, should the evidence furnished by these 84 strains prove true in the case of a larger number. A matter of some interest is the apparent preponderance of streptococci over other organisms on blood-agar plates from diarrheal stools. The proportionate number is perceptibly greater than in the case of nondiarrheal stools.

Eight stools from 3 healthy infants were examined, and streptococci recovered from 5 stools. The youngest subject was not quite 1 month old, and 3 examinations were necessary before suitable plates could be obtained. The next youngest was about 6 months of age, and plates from 2 out of 3 samples showed streptococci. The oldest subject was approximately 2 years of age, and yielded plates showing streptococci in the first 2 samples examined. It would appear from the number of streptococci found on the plates that their numerical frequency in infants is not so great as in the feces of adults.

Altogether, but 34 strains from infants were studied. They presented no striking differences from those found in the feces of adults with regard to morphology or appearance of colonies on the blood-plates. In fermentative reaction on carbohydrates, they presented the following gross percentages:

Glucose	100
Lactose	100
Salicin	97
Inulin	0
Mannite	82

The foregoing number is probably insufficient to use in comparison with the 323 strains reported from normal adult feces; it is, however, demonstrative of the fact that the fermentative types commonly found in adult feces are established at a very early age, and are found normally even in very young infants.

SUMMARY

Frequent allusions have been made in the literature to the streptococcus as an etiologic factor in the diseases of the alimentary tract. The lack of means of sharp demarcation between the streptococcus as a normal inhabitant of the bowel and as an incitor of specific disease, and the position of the streptococcus as a common secondary invader, make it difficult to confirm the clinical evidence offered.

Mannite fermenting nonhemolytic streptococci are the characteristic predominant types found in the feces of normal individuals.

Mannite fermentation is quantitatively less uniform, among the strains of human fecal streptococci, than that of other carbohydrates; it is, however, the most important fermentative characteristic, its numerical frequency depending to a great extent on the method of cultivation employed.

The "indifferent" variety of streptococcus in the feces of normal persons is inconstant in its indifference to the formation of green; green-formation would seem to be favorably influenced by the alkalinity of the mediums.

Hemolytic streptococci are but exceptional findings in the stools of normal, healthy people, and are inconstant in occurrence.

No apparent morphologic characteristics aside from those dependent on rapid, luxurious growth, characterize the human fecal streptococci.

Examination of the diarrheal stools from specific and nonspecific diarrheas as well as after catharsis, would suggest the presence of streptococci not so marked fermenters of mannite, and less active generally in the fermentation of carbohydrates.

Stools from infants contain streptococci, slightly less in numerical proportion than those of adults, but conforming in morphologic and fermentative types quite closely with those found in the feces of adults.

SOME FACTORS INFLUENCING THE POTENCY OF CONCENTRATED ANTITOXIC SERUM

CHARLES R. HIXSON

From the Laboratories of the United States Standard Serum Company, Woodworth, Wis.

The concentration of antidiphtheric serum has been carried on for a considerable period, but the process is still largely empirical as our knowledge of the chemistry of blood proteins is incomplete. The relation of antitoxic content to the blood protein is one of much interest both from a scientific and practical point of view, and any research which throws light on this question must be of value.

The first practical method of serum concentration was devised by Gibson[1] and consisted of precipitating the globulins of the blood serum or plasma by half saturation with ammonium sulphate solution and eliminating the albumin in the filtrate. The globulin precipitate, which is generally conceded to contain the bulk of antitoxin, was then dissolved in saturated sodium chlorid solution in order to further eliminate nonantitoxic protein, and the antitoxin globulins were precipitated from this solution with acetic acid. The precipitate was then gathered on hard filters, pressed and dialyzed against running water and the acid neutralized with sodium carbonate.

Banzhaf[2] modified the Gibson method as follows: The plasma was heated to 57 C. for from twelve to fifteen hours, cooled and diluted with half its volume of water and three parts saturated ammonium sulphate solution added to seven parts of diluted plasma. The precipitate was gathered on hard filters, pressed and dialyzed. By this method two serums were obtained, one of low and one of high potency.

In 1912 Banzhaf[3] published a further modification which consists of diluting the plasma with half its volume of water and adding enough saturated ammonium sulphate solution to make a 30% saturation. The mixture is heated to 60 C. in a water bath, and filtered while hot. The precipitate remaining on the filters is either washed with 33⅓% ammonium sulphate solution or is dissolved in water and ammonium sulphate solution added to bring the saturation to 33⅓%. The solution is filtered, the filtrate united with the first filtrate and the whole brought to 50% saturation with ammonium sulphate solution. The resulting precipitate is pressed and dialyzed as in the previous method. Later in 1915 Banzhaf[4] recommended holding the plasma ammonium sulphate mixture at 60 C. for 15 minutes. Banzhaf has since advocated the addition of 0.25 to 0.3% phenol to the plasma as a preservative. The added phenol tends to prevent clotting of the plasma and also gives a higher concentration of the finished product.

Received for publication Oct. 7, 1919.

[1] Jour. Biol. Chem., 1906, 1, p. 161.

[2] Collected Studies from the Research Laboratory, Dept. of Health, City of New York, 1908-9, 4, p. 230.

[3] Ibid., 1912-13, 7, p. 114.

[4] A report presented by the Committee on Standard Preparation of Diphtheria Antitoxin to the American Public Health Association in September, 1915.

Homer[5] advocated the following modifications of the Banzhaf methods:

"The serum or plasma, diluted with one-third or even with only one-fifth its volume of water, and made 1.5 to 2% with solid sodium chlorid, is heated to a temperature of 56-57 C. for 15 hours or to 57-58 C. for 8 hours, stage 1.

"The heated plasma is then made 30% of saturation with ammonium sulphate and the mixture is heated to a temperature of 61 C. and kept at that temperature for a few minutes only, stage 2.

"The mixture after cooling to 40-45 C. is filtered. The precipitate is washed with 33% of saturation with ammonium sulphate. The washings, after being filtered, are added to the main bulk of the filtrate which is then made 50% of saturation with ammonium sulphate.

"The resulting precipitate is filtered off, pressed and dialyzed. The pressed precipitate has a yellowish color and not the bluish green color of Banzhaf's product."

Homer[6] stated that before heating, the reaction of the plasma should be adjusted to about P_H 8 or that 0.25 and not more than 0.30% trikresol should be added.

The relation of antitoxin to the proteins of the blood is not fully understood. It has been demonstrated by Pick[7] and others that antitoxin is associated with the pseudoglobulin fraction of the blood proteins. However, little is known as to the nature of this association.

The experiments reported in this paper were designed to investigate the influence of heat on the antitoxic content of the globulin fraction, and are considered under two heads, namely:

(A). Determination of the effect of heat on antitoxic plasma, by the application of increasingly greater amounts of heat to the plasma ammonium sulphate mixture.

(B). Determination of the changes that have been produced in the dialyzed products by fractioning.

The blood proteins are usually divided into three more or less clearly defined fractions, according to their property of being precipitated by various salts.

Experience has shown that a variable portion of antitoxin is precipitated by 30-38% saturation with ammonium sulphate solution. It is therefore expedient for economic reasons to preserve the globulin precipitated with ammonium sulphate in saturation from 30 to 50%, otherwise the loss would be too great when antitoxin is concentrated for commercial purposes.

The precipitability of the different proteins in the plasma depends on the influence of several factors, namely, the presence of different salts, the degree of saturation with ammonium sulphate, the presence of phenol compounds, the amount of heat applied, the reaction

[5] Jour. Hyg., 1916, 15, p. 388.
[6] Jour. Hyg., 1918, 17, p. 51.
[7] Beitr. z. chem. physiol., 1901-2, 1, p. 351.

of the plasma, and possibly other factors. For example, trikresol or phenol when added to the plasma before concentration tends to alter the precipitating limits of the protein and gives a higher degree of concentration in the finished product. For this reason phenol compounds were purposely omitted from the experiments, although the final product gains in degree of concentration and in attractiveness. as has been shown by Heineman's[8] method of reconcentration.

The method used in concentrating the serums for the experimental work incorporated in this paper was the Banzhaf method modified by Heineman, excepting that different portions of the plasma were heated to 60, 64, 68 and 72 C., respectively. The first steps were the same as in the Banzhaf process except that the plasma ammonium sulphate mixture was heated for one and three quarter hours to reach the desired temperature, held at that temperature for one half hour, and filtered while hot. The resulting precipitate was stirred in water in order to separate the soluble from the insoluble globulins, and after the lapse of one hour, enough ammonium sulphate solution was added to equal one half of the amount of water used, thus making a 33⅓% saturation. The antitoxin globulins remain in solution while the fibrinoglobulin is precipitated and separated by filtration. The precipitate on the filters is washed twice with 33⅓% ammonium sulphate solution to recover the dissolved antitoxic globulins.

The resulting filtrate was added to the first filtrate and enough saturated ammonium sulphate solution added to make a 50% saturation. The precipitate was gathered on soft filters and stirred in a measured volume of water. After the solution was completed it was strained through cheese-cloth and the remaining paper pulp washed twice with water. To this solution a volume of saturated ammonium sulphate, equal to the total amount of water used for solution, was added and the precipitate gathered on soft filters. The process of redissolving and reprecipitating was repeated until the filtrate was colorless and clear. Usually two solutions were sufficient to accomplish this end so that finally the globulin precipitate could be gathered on hard filters. The precipitated globulins usually showed a greenish color. The precipitate was pressed and dialyzed in the usual manner.

(A) Determination of Effect of Heat on Antitoxic Plasma by the Application of Increasingly Greater Amounts of Heat to the Plasma Ammonium Sulphate Mixture

Forty liters of each diphtheria and tetanus plasma containing chloroform as a preservative were divided into 4 equal portions, each of which was heated to 60, 64, 68 and 72 C., respectively. The solids and potency[9] of each plasma were determined previous to heating.

The diphtheria plasma used had aged for three months. It was a mixture of several bleedings from two different horses, and was filtered through paper before further treatment was undertaken. Potency tests showed the mixture to contain 150 units per c c and 9.060% solids. One gram solids, therefore, contained 1,655 units diphtheria antitoxin.

[8] Jour. Infect. Dis., 1916, 19, p. 433.

[9] Potency tests were conducted in accordance with the rule laid down by the Hygienic Laboratory. No tests were taken as final unless the control guinea-pig died promptly in three days or somewhat less, and the final tests were based on the guinea-pig which survived 96 hours.

TABLE 1

RESULTS OF CONCENTRATING 10,000 c c QUANTITIES OF DIPHTHERIA PLASMA AT VARIOUS DEGREES OF TEMPERATURE

Degree of Heat Applied	Volume Obtained, c c	Total Number of Units Obtained	Percentage of Loss of Units	Percentage of Units Recovered	Percentage of Units Theoretically Lost but Recovered in the Soluble Globulin	Units per c c	Multiple of Concentration	Units per c c *	Multiple of Concentration*	Percentage of Solids	Solids Recovered, Gm.	Percentage of Solids Recovered	Percentage of Loss of Solids	Units in 1 gm. Solids	Percentage of Increase in Units per Gram Solids
60	1,200	1,260,000	16.0	84.0	39.6	1,050	7.0	625	4.1	33.54	402.480	44.4	55.6	3,130	89.12
64	840	1,134,000	24.4	75.6	46.1	1,350	9.0	850	5.6	31.74	266.616	29.5	70.5	4,253	156.98
68	570	712,500	52.5	47.5	32.0	1,250	8.3	1,017	6.7	24.58	140.106	15.5	84.5	5,085	207.25
72	230	241,500	83.9	16.1	10.0	1,050	7.0	930	6.2	22.60	51.980	6.1	93.9	4,646	206.46

* Reduced to a basis of 20% solids.

A study of table 1 brings out several important facts. The solids recovered decrease progressively as the temperature applied increases, but the potency per gram of solids increases as the temperature advances to 68 C. However, the potency of the solids obtained after heating to 72 C. is less than that of the solids heated to 68 degrees, although greater than that of the solids heated to 60 and 64 degrees. It is seen, therefore, that an increase in temperature for heating the plasma ammonium sulphate mixture eliminates a progressively greater amount of protein, while the potency of the dry globulins increases to

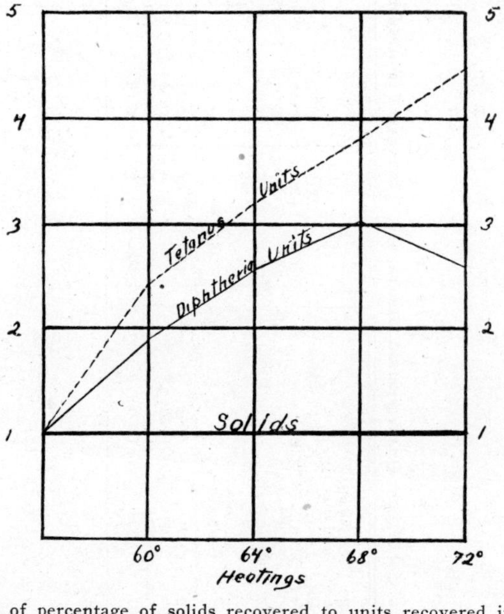

Chart 1.—Ratio of percentage of solids recovered to units recovered in both the tetanus and diphtheria concentrations.

a marked degree. The multiple of concentration is greatest at 68 C. Chart 1 shows the ratio of per cent. solids recovered to per cent. units recovered.

The total quantity of antitoxin lost by increase of temperature is so great as to render heating higher than 60 C. prohibitive from a commercial point of view. However, the interesting fact remains that with the elimination of protein a considerable amount of antitoxin is transferred from the globulin fraction which has been rendered insoluble by heat to the more soluble fraction. This principle holds throughout the heatings and is greatest at 64 C.

A preliminary series of experiments was conducted in which a portion of serum was heated to 76 C. The remaining antitoxin was so small that it seemed unprofitable to use a temperature higher than 72 C.

The relation of the loss of protein to the loss of antitoxin appears clearly from the following considerations: The loss of protein resulting from the heating to 64 C. is greater by 33.75% than the loss at 60 C., while the loss of antitoxin is only 10%. The loss of protein is 135.837 gm., representing a loss of 425,167 units if the antitoxin content of 3,130 units per gram solids of the 60 C. heating is taken as a basis for calculation. However, the actual loss in antitoxic units caused by heating to 64 degrees is greater by 126,000 units than the loss by heating to 60 C. The difference between the theoretical loss of 425,169 units and the actual loss of 126,000 units is 299,169 units, which were not lost in the precipitated protein but remained in the soluble portion.

Comparison of the results of the 68 C. heating with those of the 64 C. heating brings out similar relations. The globulin contained in the final product of the 68 C. heating is 126.510 gm. less than that contained in the 64 C. heating. This represents a loss of 538,047 units antitoxin if calculated on the value of the dialyzed product of the 64 C. heating, namely, 4,253 units per gram solids. The actual loss, however, was 421,500 units, leaving a difference of 116,547 units which were retained in the soluble portion of the globulin.

If the results of the 72 C. heating are compared with those of the 60 and 64 degree heatings, similar conditions present themselves, but when comparing the 72 C. heating with the 68 degree heating, it is found that there is no antitoxin transferred to the soluble globulin fraction.

(B) DETERMINATION OF CHANGES PRODUCED IN THE DIALYZED PRODUCTS BY FRACTIONING

To 200 c c of the diluted serum, which was equivalent to 100 c c of the original dialyzed product, was added enough distilled water to bring the solids to approximately 10%. This diluted serum was made to 38% saturation by the addition of saturated ammonium sulphate solution. After standing for about one hour it was placed on a hard filter, and the precipitate was washed twice with 38% ammonium sulphate solution and then pressed and dialyzed.

The filtrate was made to 50% saturation by adding saturated ammonium sulphate solution. This mixture stood for about an hour when it was placed on a hard filter. The gathered precipitate was pressed and dialyzed.

TABLE 2

RESULTS OF FRACTIONATING 100 C C OF THE DIALYZED PRODUCTS OF THE FOUR HEATINGS

Degree of Heat Applied	Units per 1 c c	Volume of Dialized Product	Fractionated 100 c c							Units Recovered	Units Lost
			Percentage of Solids	38%			50%				
				Solids	Entire Units	Units per Gram Solids	Solids	Entire Units	Units per Gram Solids		
60	1,050	1,200	33.540	29.206	93,500	3,201	1.890	8,250	4,365	101,750	3,250
64	1,350	840	31.740	25.380	85,500	3,368	3.680	18,750	5,095	104,250	30,750
68	1,250	570	24.580	19.123	84,500	4,418	3.744	19,500	5,208	104,000	21,000
68*	1,250	570	24.580	11.637	36,000	3,093	9.918	58,500	5,898	94,500	30,500
72	1.050	230	22.600	18.058	84,500	4,679	2.135	10,000	4,683	94,500	10,500

* Fractionated without the addition of trikresol or NaCl.

The percentage of solids in the dialyzed products of the various heatings vary to such an extent that, in order to compare the results of fractionating, the data of Table 2 were reduced to a basis of 20% solids and incorporated in Table 3.

TABLE 3

RESULTS OF FRACTIONATING REDUCED TO A BASIS OF 20% SOLIDS

Degree of Heat Applied	Fractionated 100 c c						
	38%		50%		Units Recovered	Units Lost	Solids Lost
	Solids	Units	Solids	Units			
60	17.415	55,745	1.127	4,919	60,664	1,836	1,458
64	15.992	53,861	2.318	11,810	65,671	19,330	1.690
68	15.543	68,669	3.046	15,864	84,533	17,127	1.411
68*	9,468	29,284	8.069	47,590	76,874	24,826	2.462
72	15.980	74,770	1.889	8,846	83,616	9,384	2.131

* Fractionated without the addition of trikresol or NaCl.

Table 3 shows a gradual increase of solids in the 50% fraction up to the 68 C. heating accompanied by an increase in units per gram solids. The unfractioned serums and their 38% fractions are lower in units per gram solids than their corresponding 50% fractions. After heating to 72 C. the solids of the 50% fraction decrease as do the units per gram solids.

The number of units lost in fractionating the serum prepared at 60 C. is small when compared with the units lost in fractionating serums prepared at higher temperature. The number of units lost in fractionating increases markedly as the temperature applied increases, while the amount of solids lost is not great.

The relation of the loss of protein to the loss of antitoxin is clearly shown by the following data: The solids lost in fractionating the serum of the 60 C. heating were 1.458 gm., which are equivalent to 4,564 units antitoxin if the potency of 1 gm. solids of the unfractionated product is taken as a basis of calculation. The actual loss of antitoxin was 1,836 units. The difference between the theoretical loss of 4,564 and the actual loss of 1,836 units is 2,728 units which were not lost with the protein but remained in the more soluble fraction. A small portion of the protein was lost during the manipulation, but since the proportionate amount of antitoxin was not lost an explanation must be looked for elsewhere. Possibly the added trikresol converted a sufficient quantity of nonantitoxic protein into an insoluble form so that loss of protein by precipitation and subsequent filtration and retention of antitoxin in solution resulted.

In fractionating the serums resulting from the 64, 68 and 72 degree heatings, the reverse was true. The number of units actually lost in fractionating exceeds the number of units represented by the solids lost. It is clear that in these cases the presence of trikresol is not the only factor that operates to increase the loss of both solids and antitoxin. Probably the higher degree of heat applied has so affected the antitoxic proteins that they are more readily precipitated by ammonium sulphate than the antitoxic proteins which are contained in the products resulting from the 60 degree heating. Therefore at degrees of temperature above 60 the actual loss of protein in fractionating is not materially different from the loss at 60 degrees, but the loss of antitoxin is decidedly greater. The protein rendered insoluble by heating to 60 C. of course is not contained in the dialyzed product used for fractionating as it was removed by filtration of the original heated plasma ammonium sulphate mixture.

In fractionating the 72 degree heating, the actual loss in units is represented by the solids lost in fractionating. This fact bears out the theory developed in the previous paragraph. Heating to 72 C. brings all the globulin so near the critical point of complete precipitation that but small quantities of both globulins and antitoxin remain.

The relation between the loss of solids and antitoxin in fractionating serums prepared at temperatures above 60 C. is shown by the fractionated 64 degree heating. The solids lost in fractionating were 1.690 gm., which are equivalent to 7,188 units if the units per gram solids of the unfractioned 64 degree heating are taken as a basis of calculation. The actual loss of antitoxin was 19,330 units. The difference between the theoretical loss of 7,188 units and the actual loss of 19,330 is 12,142 units.

The units per gram solids of the 38% fractions are lower than those of the corresponding unfractioned serums with the exception of the 60 and 72 degree heatings. In these the units per gram solids are practically the same as those in the unfractioned serum. The 50% fractions are considerably higher in units per gram protein than either those of the unfractioned serums or those of the 38% fractions, except in the 72 degree heating where the unfractioned and the 38 and 50% fractions each contain practically the same number of units per gram protein.

The tetanus plasma used had aged for two years and was prepared for concentration in the same manner as the diphtheria plasma. Potency tests showed the combined 40 liters of plasma to contain 45 units per c c and 8.570% solids. One gram of solids therefore contained 525 units tetanus antitoxin.

(A) Determination of the effect of heat on antitoxic plasma, by the application of increasingly greater amounts of heat to the plasma ammonium sulphate mixture.

TABLE 4

RESULTS OF CONCENTRATING 10,000 c c QUANTITIES OF TETANUS PLASMA AT VARIOUS DEGREES OF TEMPERATURE

Degree of Heat Applied	Volume Obtained, c c	Total Number of Units Obtained	Percentage of Loss of Units	Percentage of Units Recovered	Percentage of Units Theoretically Lost but Recovered in the Soluble Globulin	Units per c c	Multiple of Concentration	Units per c c*	Multiple of Concentration*	Percentage of Solids	Solids Recovered, Gm.	Percentage of Solids Recovered	Percentage of Loss of Solids	Units in 1 gm. Solids	Percentage of Increase in Units per Gram Solids
60	1,080	378,000	16.00	84.00	49.06	350	7.7	252	5.6	27.72	299.376	34.94	65.06	1,262	140.4
64	700	350,000	22.22	77.78	53.68	500	11.1	338	7.5	29.50	206.500	24.10	75.90	1,695	222.8
68	390	214,000	52.44	47.56	35.27	550	12.2	406	9.0	27.00	105.300	12.29	87.71	2,037	228.0
72	230	149,500	66.77	33.23	25.91	650	14.4	477	10.6	27.24	62.652	7.32	92.68	2,386	354.4

* Reduced to a basis of 20% solids.

A study of table 4 shows a similarity of results with those of the diphtheria concentrations. The progressive decrease in solids recovered, as the temperature applied increased, was somewhat greater than in the diphtheria concentrations with the exception of the 72 C. heating in which the solids recovered were proportionately greater than in the diphtheria heating. The potency per gram solids increased throughout the heatings, while in the diphtheria serums the highest unitage per gram protein was reached at 68 C. The multiple of concentration increased markedly as the temperature applied increased. The highest point was reached at 72 degrees, where the concentration of units per cubic centimeter was 14.4 times that of the plasma. The highest multiple of concentration in the diphtheria serums was at 68 degrees. See chart 1 for a comparative ratio of percentage of solids recovered to percentage of units recovered by both diphtheria and tetanus concentrations.

Throughout the heatings antitoxin was transferred from the globulin fraction, which was rendered insoluble by heat, to the more soluble fraction. The greatest percentage transfer of units occurred at 64 degrees, as was the case in the diphtheria concentrations. There was a greater percentage recovery of units and a decrease in percentage recovery of solids in the tetanus concentrations over the diphtheria concentrations.

The relation of the loss of protein to the loss of antitoxin was similar to that of the diphtheria heatings, except that the percentage transfer of units from the protein made insoluble by heat to the more soluble globulins was greater than in the diphtheria serums. This applies to all the heatings and to comparisons between the different heatings. There was no transfer of antitoxin to the soluble globulin fractions when comparing the loss of protein to the loss of antitoxin between the 72 and the 68 degree heatings of the diphtheria concentrations.

The percentage increase in units per gram solids increased markedly as the temperature applied increased and was much greater at 72 degrees than in the corresponding diphtheria heating.

DETERMINATION OF THE CHANGES THAT HAVE BEEN PRODUCED IN THE DIALYZED PRODUCTS BY FRACTIONATING

The same method was used in fractionating the tetanus serums as was used in fractionating the diphtheria serums.

TABLE 5

RESULTS OF FRACTIONATING 100 C C OF THE CONCENTRATED TETANUS SERUMS OF THE FOUR HEATINGS

Degree of Heat Applied	Units per 1 c c	Units per Gram Solids	Percentage of Solids	Fractionated 100 c c						Units Recovered	Units Lost
				38%			50%				
				Solids	Entire Units	Units per Gram Solids	Solids	Entire Units	Units per Gram Solids		
60	350	1,262	27.72	23.148	28,800	1,244	3.220	6,125	1,902	34,925	75
64	500	1,695	29.50	24.776	40,500	1,634	2.758	8,750	3,172	49,250	750
68	550	2,037	27.00	21.568	40,000	1,854	2.765	10,150	3,670	50,150	4,850
68*	550	2,037	27.00	16.969	......	.....	7.296	22,500	3,083		
72	650	2,386	27.24	20.143	52,500	2,606	3.780	12,250	3,240	64,750	250

* Fractionated without the addition of trikresol or NaCl.

The data of table 5 were reduced to a basis of 20% solids in order to compare better the results of fractioning, and were incorporated in table 6.

TABLE 6

Results of Fractionating Reduced to a Basis of 20% Solids

Degree of Heat Applied	Fractionated 100 c c						
	38%		50%		Units Recovered	Units Lost	Solids Lost
	Solids	Units	Solids	Units			
60	16.701	20,776	2.323	4,418	25,194	46	0.976
64	16.797	27,446	1.870	5,931	33,377	423	1.333
68	15.976	29,619	2.048	7,516	37,135	3,465	1.976
68	12.569	......	5.404	16,760	......	.....	2.027
72	14.789	38,540	2.738	8,871	47,411	289	2.473

* Fractionated without the addition of trikresol or NaCl.

There was no progressive rise or fall in the gram solids of the 50% fractions, but there was a decided increase in units per gram solids both of the 38 and 50% fractions, as the temperature applied increased. The 38% fractions corresponded closely in units per gram solids to the units in the unfractioned serums, while the potency of the 50% fractions showed a marked increase over that of the unfractioned serums and the 38% fractions. This difference became less marked in the 72 C. heating. It is possible that the aging of the plasma caused a change in the proteins so that on concentration a greater proportion of the less soluble or nonantitoxic protein was eliminated throughout all the heatings. Consequently, the end-products of the different heatings contained less of the less soluble globulins and a greater multiple of concentration resulted than in the diphtheria serums which were aged for three months only. In the fractionated diphtheria serums the 38% fractions of the 64 and 68 C. heatings were less in units per gram solids than the unfractioned serums.

In fractionating the serums resulting from the various heatings, the number of units actually lost is less than the number of units represented by the solids lost in fractionating. The reverse was true in the diphtheria heatings with the exception of the 60 degree heating. Perhaps the addition of trikresol to the globulin solutions of the tetanus heatings did not cause as marked a change in the proteins as was experienced with the diphtheria heatings, for the reason that the globulin of the tetanus heatings was more soluble than the corresponding diphtheria globulin. That so great a change was not experienced is seen by the results of fractionating both diphtheria and tetanus serums without trikresol and comparing them with the same serums fractionated with trikresol. In the diphtheria serums (see table 3) when fractionated without trikresol the ratio of the solids of the 38% and the 50% fractions is 1.18 to 1, while the same serum fractionated with trikresol is 5.1 to 1, indicating that the precipitating limits of the proteins have been so altered by the addition of trikresol that they are capable of precipitation at a lower saturation with ammonium sulphate. In the tetanus serums (see table 6) when fractionated without trikresol the ratio of solids in the 38 and 50% fractions is 2.3 to 1, while the same serum with trikresol added is 7.8 to 1. It is seen that the addition of trikresol to the tetanus serum did not cause as great a change in the protein as did the addition of trikresol to the diphtheria serums, for the reason that the diphtheria serums contained proportionately more of the less soluble globulins than did the tetanus serums.

The tendency of the 38 and 50% fractions of the 72 C. heatings of both diphtheria and tetanus serums to give a unitage per gram protein approaching that of the unfractioned serums, can be explained on the assumption that at this temperature the globulins have closely approached the point of complete precipitation, and that the remaining globulins are of the more soluble type. Therefore, when fractionated, the fractions will not be so materially different from the unfractioned serums both in solubility of globulins and in unitage per gram protein.

SUMMARY

The physical condition of refined serums is not at all constant, a fact which is disturbing and puzzling to those engaged in the production of antitoxins. Uniformity in color, clarity, viscosity, relative potency, and keeping qualities of different products, has so far not been successful. The desirability of obtaining uniform serums is obvious, and it was one of the problems underlying this research to attempt to locate the causes of this variability.

There are several factors which seem to be influential in determining the color of the finished product. Fresh plasma when concentrated has a decidedly greenish tint, but as the ripening process of plasma is lengthened the green color becomes less apparent. The diphtheria and tetanus plasmas used in these experiments had aged three months and two years, respectively, and were concentrated under otherwise identical conditions. The concentrated diphtheria serum had a decidedly greenish tint, while the concentrated tetanus serum was of a yellowish color, and no trace of green remained. Whether the addition of chloroform as a preservative has an influence on the color is problematical. It is certain, however, that when some kinds of trikresol are used in place of chloroform no green color appears.

Serums, concentrated by the method used in this work in which the precipitated globulins were dissolved and precipitated repeatedly, were greenish, while the aged products were light yellow. This change of green to yellow in most cases was not accompanied by a precipitate.

The degree of temperature applied to the plasma ammonium sulphate mixture seems to influence the color of the dialyzed product and also its clarity. As the temperature applied increased the color of the end-product was gradually obscured by the formation of a colloidal precipitate, as the critical point for complete precipitation of the globulins was approached. This precipitate was most marked at 72 C. After standing in the refrigerator for three months a marked precipitate settled in the serum prepared at the higher temperature, but none was perceptible in that of the lower heatings. The green color that was so marked in the diphtheria serums entirely disappeared after seven months.

An interesting point was observed in the color of the fractions of the different serums. The 38% fractions had the same color throughout the heatings as the unfractioned serums, while the 50% fractions were water clear and had a decidedly green tint. Even the tetanus serums showed a trace of green in the 50% fractions, but this color was lost after a few weeks' standing. The green color gradually changed to yellow after six month's standing in the refrigerator at a low temperature.

These facts indicate that the green color of serums is associated with the more soluble fractions of the globulins, and that it is not stable, but changes to a yellowish color on standing. The addition of either NaCl or trikresol to the plasma previous to concentration seems to produce a yellowish serum, and it is possible that NaCl or trikresol when added to a finished product with a greenish tint aids in the change from green to yellow.

Mention has been made of the fact that the degree of heat applied has some influence on the clarity of serums. This is true especially when the point of complete precipitation of the globulins is approached. It was found that by heating to as high a temperature as 72 C., a colloidal precipitate was formed that was not removed by filtration, but that after standing at a low temperature for several months it settled to a marked degree.

Some authors have stated that the addition of trikresol to the plasma before concentration gives a clear end-product with a high multiple of concentration. Different serums react differently in regard to the formation of an insoluble precipitate when trikresol is added to the dialyzed product and the kind of trikresol used has some bearing on this point. Serums that are concentrated with the addition of trikresol to the plasma, as well as those that are concentrated with trikresol, are able to form a precipitate after trikresol has been added to the final product. The end-products of the tetanus were of a clear, yellowish-brown color when removed from the dialyzing bags, but on the addition of trikresol a cloudiness formed which was not diminished after eight months' standing. The diphtheria serums did not react this way even though the same trikresol was used for both. Homer[10] states that the reaction of the plasma is of importance in gaining a clear end-product. The addition of trikresol to the plasma or the adjusting of the reaction seems to give a clear end-product in some but not in all cases.

Plasma from certain horses will usually give a cloudy end-product when the usual methods of concentration are used. If the concentration of ammonium sulphate is increased from 30 to 33%, a clear product can be obtained in most cases. This statement agrees with Homer's[11] findings.

The solubility of the globulins in different concentrated serums is not the same. Globulins precipitated between 30-38% tend to produce a cloudy serum and are less soluble than those precipitated between 38-50%, which usually yield a clear solution. The 38% fractions have the same clarity as the unfractioned serums. The addition of trikresol evidently so alters the precipitating limits of the globulins that the less soluble ones are precipitated at a lower saturation than they would be without trikresol. The more soluble globulins form a clearer solution when trikresol is added than without this addition.

[10] Biochem. Jour., 1917, 11, p. 21.
[11] Ibid., 1919, 13, p. 45.

In fractionating the concentrated serums without the addition of trikresol no precipitate was formed on making to 28% saturation with ammonium sulphate solution. However, after trikresol was added and the serums were aged for several days, a precipitate was formed on making to 28% saturation with ammonium sulphate. After dialysis this precipitate was but slightly soluble. The results obtained from serums containing trikresol were so at variance with those obtained from serums without trikresol that it was deemed best to reserve this subject for future study (see tables 3 and 4).

The viscosity of the various serums became less as the temperature applied increased and was not in direct proportion to the solid content of the various serums. In the concentrated diphtheria serums the percentage of solids decreased with a decrease in viscosity, but in the concentrated tetanus serums the percentage of solids did not vary to any great extent. However, the potency per gram solids of the viscous serums increased with a decrease in viscosity. As the temperature applied increased, an increasingly greater amount of protein was eliminated so that the globulins in the lower heatings contained more of the less soluble globulins than in higher heatings. The pressed globulin precipitates of the lower heatings, which gave viscous serums, were gummy. As the temperature applied increased, this property was gradually lost and the pressed precipitates became friable.

The 38% fractions were less soluble than the 50% fractions. The latter were friable and highly soluble. The potencies of the 38% fractions were lower than those of the 50% fractions per gram solids, and as the viscosity decreased the potency per gram solids of both fractions increased. Banzhaf and Gibson[12] also found that the more soluble portions of the "pseudoglobulin" are richest in antitoxin per gram protein.

As the temperature of the heatings increased, the percentage loss of protein and antitoxin increased, and after heating at 72 C. the protein rendered insoluble by heat and ammonium sulphate in the diphtheria plasma reached 94% with an accompanying loss of 84% of antitoxin, while in the tetanus plasma the percentage of loss of protein was 93 with 67% loss of antitoxin. In all of the heatings the percentage loss of protein was greater than the corresponding percentage loss of antitoxin. With an increase of temperature the multiple of concentration and units per gram solids were also increased, and at

[12] Jour. Biol. Chem., 1907, 3, p. 254.

the higher heatings the percentage increase in units per gram solids over the plasma used was around 207% in the diphtheria concentrations and 354% in the tetanus concentrations. The relative potency of the plasma is a factor in determining the final multiple of concentration. It was noted that in this experimental work, as well as in the routine concentration of serums, plasma of low potency yields a greater multiple of concentration than plasma of high potency.

In the fractioned serums of both diphtheria and tetanus, the 50% fractions contained more units per gram protein than the 38%, or the unfractioned serums, and as the temperature increased the units of the 50% fractions also increased. The 50% fractions of the tetanus serums showed a greater proportionate increase in units per gram protein over the unfractioned serums than did the 50% fractions of the diphtheria serums. The multiple of concentration was also greater than that in the diphtheria serums. This can be explained by the assumption that as the tetanus plasma had aged for a much longer period than the diphtheria plasma, a greater change had taken place in its proteins. In the aging of the plasma the proteins were so altered that on precipitation with 30% ammonium sulphate and heat a greater proportion of the less soluble globulins was removed than was the case with the diphtheria serum. This explanation is supported by the fact that the viscosity of the tetanus serums throughout all the heatings was less than the viscosity of the corresponding diphtheria serums. Furthermore, the units per gram protein of the 38% fraction of the tetanus serums approached closely the unitage of the unfractioned serums, while the unitage per gram protein of the 38% fraction of the diphtheria serums was smaller than the units per gram protein of the unfractioned serums with the exception of the 60 and 72 degree heatings.

Since the difference in unitage between the 38% fractions and the unfractioned serums of the tetanus serums is smaller than the difference between the 38% fraction and the unfractioned diphtheria serum, it seems probable that through prolonged aging the less soluble portion of globulin is so altered as to facilitate its removal by precipitation.

CONCLUSIONS

The color of concentrated serums is a factor determined by the age of the plasma previous to its concentration, by the method used in concentration, and by the presence of certain chemicals used as preservatives.

Serums concentrated by the method used in this work are green, but as the period of aging of the plasma is lengthened previous to concentration, the intensity of the green color gradually diminishes, and finally a product with a yellowish color remains.

The green color is associated chiefly with the more soluble portions of the pseudoglobulin.

The addition of trikresol to plasma previous to concentration causes the end-product to be of yellowish color with no trace of green.

When plasma is aged previous to concentration the proteins are so altered that a greater proportion of the nonantitoxic proteins is eliminated in concentrating than when plasma is not aged. The addition of trikresol to the fresh plasma previous to concentration seems to alter the proteins of the plasma in a similar way as does the process of aging.

The aging of the plasma or the addition of trikresol to the plasma previous to concentration lessens the viscosity of the finished product owing to the increased elimination of nonantitoxic proteins, which are of a less soluble nature, and a higher multiple of concentration is obtained.

The multiple of concentration depends in a measure on the potency of the plasma concentrated. It has been noted that the multiple of concentration is greater when low-unit plasma is concentrated than when high-unit plasma is concentrated.

The percentage precipitation of protein from heated plasma ammonium sulphate mixtures containing 30% ammonium sulphate solution is increased as the temperature applied is increased and is not complete at 76 C.

With the increased elimination of protein an increased percentage of antitoxin is also precipitated, but the percentage loss of antitoxin is less than the percentage loss of protein.

With the increased elimination of protein as the temperature applied is increased, there is a transfer of antitoxin from the protein rendered insoluble by heat and ammonium sulphate to the more soluble fraction. This principle is not lost even when the critical point for complete precipitation of the proteins is closely approached.

As the temperature is increased in concentrating, the potency of the end-products obtained becomes greater as also do the units per gram solids. However, heating higher than 60 C. for one half hour is not advisable owing to an appreciable loss of antitoxin.

The more soluble portion of the pseudoglobulin fraction is proportionately richer in antitoxin than the less soluble portion.

With the application of increasingly greater amounts of heat the ratio of solids of the more soluble to those of the less soluble fractions of the pseudoglobulin is not materially changed, but the potency of both fractions of the pseudoglobulins is increased.

As the temperature applied reaches a point near the complete precipitation of the globulins, the character of the end-product obtained is that of the more soluble fraction of the pseudoglobulin.

THE INFLUENCE OF NORMAL BEEF SERUM ON THE ANTHRAX BACILLUS

J. A. Kolmer; D. C. Wanner, and M. E. Koehler

From the Philadelphia Hospital for Contagious Diseases and the Dermatological Research Laboratories of Philadelphia

Our interest in this subject was aroused by the numerous reports of Penna, Cuenca and Kraus[1] on the favorable results in the treatment of the pustule and bacteremia of human anthrax with ordinary beef serum. These investigators injected normal beef serum, previously heated twice at 56 C. for 30 minutes for purposes of sterilization, in doses of 30 to 50 c c repeated in 12, 24 or 36 hours, as the case might require; the injections were made subcutaneously or intramuscularly except in very severe cases when the serum was given intravenously. According to their latest report on 200 cases, the mortality has been reduced to 0.5% as compared with 10% in 250 cases treated in the usual manner during the preceding 10 years. In an experimental study Kraus and his associates found normal beef serum just as effectual as horse anti-anthrax serum in the protection of rabbits against virulent anthrax bacilli.

Solari[2] has reported favorably on the treatment of 6 cases of anthrax with heated normal beef serum, and Langon[3] also has made a favorable report on 13 cases; Lignieres,[4] however, has reported unfavorably on the curative action of normal beef serum, stating that it is inferior to horse anti-anthrax serum and called attention to the prevalence of anthrax in cattle as evidence of the apparent lack of natural resistance to this disease and of defensive properties in their blood.

PURPOSE OF INVESTIGATION

Our studies were made with heated and unheated beef serum collected in abattoirs and under asceptic conditions from ordinary herd cattle; all of the animals were full grown and healthy at the time of

Received for publication Oct. 11, 1919.

[1] Prensa Medica Argentina, 1917, 3, 297; 1917, 4, 91 and 147; 1918, 4, 455.
[2] Semana méd., 1917, 24, 98.
[3] Ann d. l. Faculated d. Med., 1918, 3, 258.
[4] Prensa Medica Argentina, 1917, 4, 49, 370.

bleeding, but the histories were unknown in relation to previous attacks of anthrax.

The object was to study the protection and curative properties of beef serum in anthrax infections in rabbits and mice, and also to determine if beef serum contained bactericidins, agglutinins and complement fixing substances for anthrax bacilli.

Inasmuch as rabbits were found highly immune and white mice highly susceptible to the culture of anthrax bacilli employed in this investigation, the serum of these animals was included in the study for the purpose of comparison with beef serum and for study of the mechanism of the nature of natural immunity to anthrax.

TOXICITY OF BEEF SERUM FOR MICE

The majority of our protection tests were made with white mice inasmuch as rabbits were found too highly resistant to anthrax bacilli; accordingly, the toxicity of heated and unheated beef serum for mice was determined by intraperitoneal injection preliminary to the protection tests.

The general result of these tests was to show that fresh, unheated beef serum is but slightly toxic for white mice and that heated serum occasionally is somewhat less toxic. Mice receiving intraperitoneal injections of fresh, sterile beef serum in a dose of 0.2 c c per gram of body weight, equivalent to 5 c c undiluted serum for a 25 gm. mouse, occasionally died within 48 hours after injection, while similar doses of the same serum heated twice at 56 C. for 30 minutes rendered some of the mice toxic for from 24 to 48 hours followed by recovery. Mice receiving 0.1 c c of unheated or heated serum per gram of weight, or 2.5 c c for a 25 gm. mouse and equivalent to 100 c c per kilogram of weight usually survived for an indefinite period.

VIRULENCE OF ANTHRAX BACILLI FOR MICE AND RABBITS

All experiments were made with a single strain of the anthrax bacillus, kindly furnished by Dr. John Reichel, which was found to possess a high degree of virulence readily maintained by occasional passage through mice.

Twenty-four hour broth cultures of this strain thoroughly suspended by shaking with glass beads, regularly killed mice weighing from 14 to 18 gm. in 48 hours in a dose of 0.00002 c c injected intraperitoneally, the bacilli invariably being recovered from the blood of the heart; half this dose, or 0.00001 c c, killed mice of these weights occasionally within 48 hours, the survivors living at least 2 weeks or longer. In the protection tests with beef serum the minimal lethal dose of culture was taken as 0.00002 c c, equivalent to 0.2 c c of a 1:10,000 dilution or about 0.001 c c per kilogram of weight, and the virulence was readily maintained at this level for a period of several months.

The extremely high resistance of rabbits to the same culture is indicated by the fact that the minimal lethal dose was about 2,000 to 3,000 times greater than for mice, being about 3 c c of undiluted broth culture per kilogram of body weight injected intravenously; this dose usually killed in about 48 hours, 2 c c per kilogram in about 96 hours, while 1 c c per kilogram was usually without fatal effects over an indefinite period of time. Among the rabbits succumbing to these large doses within 96 hours after infection, anthrax bacilli were only occasionally recoverable from the blood of the heart.

TABLE 1

THE PROTECTIVE VALUE OF STERILE UNHEATED NORMAL BEEF SERUM FOR MICE INFECTED WITH B. ANTHRACIS

Weight in Grams	Administration of Serum	Duration of Life in Hours after Infection
26	12 hours before bacilli	72
24	12 hours before bacilli	44
25	6 hours before bacilli	28
21	6 hours before bacilli	26
21	2 hours before bacilli	122
23	2 hours before bacilli	28
26	Simultaneously with bacilli	36
29	Simultaneously with bacilli	60
24	2 hours after bacilli	36
26	2 hours after bacilli	Lived indefinitely
21	Culture control	48
23	Culture control	46
20	Serum control	Lived indefinitely

Mice infected by intraperitoneal injection of 2 M. L. D. (= 0.00004 c c culture).
Each mouse received 1 c c serum per 100 gm. of weight intraperitoneally.

Table 1 shows the results of an intraperitoneal injection of mice with 1 c c of fresh, unheated beef serum per 100 gm. of weight, equivalent to 10 c c per kilogram, at varying intervals before and after the intraperitoneal injection of 0.00004 c c of a broth culture of B. anthracis, equivalent to two minimal lethal doses; the culture controls died at the close of the second day after infection, and while the lives of two mice receiving serum were prolonged beyond this period, the results were irregular and failed to show protective or curative properties on the part of this serum. Anthrax bacilli were recovered from the blood of the heart of each dead mouse; the serum control lived indefinitely.

Table 2 shows the results of a similar experiment with a larger dose of serum, namely, 10 c c per 100 gm. of weight, equivalent to 100 c c per kilogram; each mouse was infected with two minimal lethal doses of culture, the culture controls succumbing in about 48 hours. The serum control lived indefinitely, and the general results of the experiment were that this serum failed appreciably to protect the mice.

TABLE 2

THE PROTECTIVE VALUE OF STERILE UNHEATED NORMAL BEEF SERUM WITH B. ANTHRACIS

Weight in Grams	Administration of Serum	Duration of Life in Hours after Infection
14	4 hours before bacilli	Lived indefinitely
18	4 hours before bacilli	34
22	2 hours before bacilli	40
18	2 hours before bacilli	24
22	Simultaneously with bacilli	36
18	Simultaneously with bacilli	24
14	2 hours after bacilli	36
27	2 hours after bacilli	34
26	4 hours after bacilli	24
16	4 hours after bacilli	36
18	6 hours after bacilli	Lived indefinitely
16	6 hours after bacilli	48
27	Culture control	48
16	Serum control	Lived indefinitely

Each mouse was infected by intraperitoneal injection of 2 M. L. D. of culture (= 0.00004 c c culture).
Each mouse received 10 c c serum per 100 gm. of weight intraperitoneally.

TABLE 3

THE PROTECTIVE VALUE OF STERILE UNHEATED NORMAL BEEF SERUM FOR MICE INFECTED WITH B. ANTHRACIS

Weight in Grams	Administration of Serum	Duration of Life in Hours after Infection
12	4 hours before bacilli	26
14	4 hours before bacilli	26
11	2 hours before bacilli	23
12	2 hours before bacilli	26
11	Simultaneously with bacilli	26
12	Simultaneously with bacilli	26
14	2 hours after bacilli	24
11	2 hours after bacilli	24
14	4 hours after bacilli	48
13	4 hours after bacilli	48
13	6 hours after bacilli	50
12	6 hours after bacilli	48
13	Culture control	24
14	Culture control	24
15	Serum control	Lived indefinitely

Each mouse was infected by intraperitoneal injection of 5 M. L. D. of culture (= 0.0001 c c).
Each mouse received 2 c c serum per 100 gm. of weight intraperitoneally.

Table 3 shows the results of the administration of 2 c c of fresh, unheated beef serum per 100 gm. of weight, equivalent to 20 c c per kilogram, at intervals before and after the injection of 5 minimal lethal doses of culture. As expected, the culture controls succumbed more quickly with the heavier infection; while the lives of 4 mice were prolonged 24 hours beyond the controls, the general results bearing on the protective value of the serum were negative.

Additional experiments were made with repeated injections of one minimal lethal dose of culture at intervals of 24 hours followed one hour after each injection of culture by intraperitoneal injection of 1 c c of fresh, unheated beef serum per 100 gm. of weight, equivalent to 10 c c per kilogram; the results of an experiment are shown in table 4 and indicate a lack of appreciable protective value on the part of normal beef serum.

TABLE 4

THE PROTECTIVE VALUE OF REPEATED DOSES OF STERILE UNHEATED NORMAL BEEF SERUM FOR MICE RECEIVING REPEATED INJECTIONS OF B. ANTHRACIS

Weight in Grams	Number of Injections of Culture	Number of Injections of Serum 2 Hours after Culture	Duration of Life in Hours
23	2	2	52
25	2	2	44
19	2	2	36
27	3	3	72
23	2	None	48
18	2	None	47
23	None	2	Lived indefinitely

By intraperitoneal injection; 1 M. L. D. (= 0.00002 c c culture) every 24 hours.
By intraperitoneal injection; 1 c c serum per 100 gm. of weight every 24 hours administered 1 hour after the culture.

TABLE 5

THE PROTECTIVE VALUE OF UNHEATED AND HEATED BEEF RABBIT SERUMS FOR MICE INFECTED WITH INCREASING AMOUNTS OF B. ANTHRACIS

Weight in Grams	Culture	Serum	Duration of Life in Hours
20	12 M. L. D. (control)	None	48
22	6 M. L. D. (control)	None	24
24	3 M. L. D. (control)	None	48
17	12 M. L. D.	Beef No. 1 unheated	48
26	6 M. L. D.	Beef No. 1 unheated	24
21	3 M. L. .D	Beef No. 1 unheated	24
17	12 M. L. D.	Beef No. 1 heated	24
14	6 M. L. D.	Beef No. 1 heated	24
17	3 M. L. D.	Beef No. 1 heated	24
14	12 M. L. D.	Beef No. 2 unheated	24
20	6 M. L. D.	Beef No. 2 unheated	48
17	3 M. L. D.	Beef No. 2 unheated	48
16	12 M. L. D.	Beef No. 2 heated	24
17	6 M. L. D.	Beef No. 2 heated	48
16	3 M. L. D.	Beef No. 2 heated	24
19	12 M. L. D.	Rabbit No. 1 unheated	24
16	6 M. L. D.	Rabbit No. 1 unheated	24
17	3 M. L. D.	Rabbit No. 1 unheated	24
15	12 M. L. D.	Rabbit No. 1 heated	24
14	6 M. L. D.	Rabbit No. 1 heated	48
16	3 M. L. D.	Rabbit No. 1 heated	48
18	None	Beef No. 1 unheated	Lived indefinitely
14	None	Beef No. 2 unheated	Lived indefinitely
17	None	Rabbit No. 1 unheated	Lived indefinitely
21	None	Rabbit No. 1 heated	Lived indefinitely

Injected intraperitoneally; 1 M. L. D. equaled 0.00002 c c 24-hour broth culture.
Injected intraperitoneally one hour after culture in dose of 1 c c per 100 gm.

The experiment in table 5 was made by infecting a series of mice with increasing doses of culture equivalent to 3, 6 and 12 minimal lethal doses followed in an hour by the intraperitoneal injection of a dose of unheated and heated normal beef and rabbit serums equivalent to 1 c c per 100 gm., or 10 c c per kilogram. The serums were heated twice at 56 C. for thirty minutes. Rabbit serum was included, by reason of the high resistance of rabbits to the anthrax bacillus, for the purpose of studying the possible protective value of this serum for mice. All of the serum controls lived indefinitely;

the culture controls succumbed in from 24 to 48 hours with anthrax bacteremia. Neither heated nor unheated normal beef or rabbit serum showed appreciable protective properties.

As previously stated, the natural resistance of rabbits to virulent anthrax bacilli was so high and variable as to render our experiments with these animals on the protective and curative properties of normal beef serum very uncertain and difficult of interpretation; the results of one experiment are shown in table 6.

In this experiment rabbits were injected intravenously with 1 c c of undiluted broth culture of B. anthracis per kilogram of weight every 24 hours followed in an hour by the intravenous injection of 2 c c of sterile normal beef serum (unheated) per kilogram of weight. The culture control died after 4 injections; the serum control received 6 injections and died on the eleventh day, or 5 days after the last injection of serum. The rabbits receiving culture and serum died in from 2 to 7 days and failed to show in this and similar experiments an undoubted protective value of normal beef serum for the culture employed.

TABLE 6

THE PROTECTIVE VALUE OF REPEATED DOSES OF STERILE UNHEATED NORMAL BEEF SERUM FOR RABBITS RECEIVING REPEATED INJECTIONS OF B. ANTHRACIS

Weight in Grams	Number of Injections of Culture	Number of Injections of Serum 2 Hours after Culture	Duration of Life
1326	4	4	7 days
1572	2	2	52 hours
1826	4	4	6 days
1246	4	None	6 days
1400	None	6	11 days

By intravenous injection; 1 c c of broth culture per kilogram of weight every 24 hours.
By intravenous innjection; 2 c c of serum per kilogram of weight every 24 hours one hour after the injection of culture.

TABLE 7

THE BACTERICIDAL ACTIVITY OF NORMAL BEEF AND RABBIT SERUMS FOR B. ANTHRACIS

Weight in Grams	Final Dilutions of Serum	Duration of Life in Hours
23	Beef No. 1 unheated 1:10	24
16	Beef No. 1 unheated 1:20	24
23	Beef No. 1 heated 1:10	48
20	Beef No. 1 heated 1:20	48
20	Beef No. 2 unheated 1:10	48
21	Beef No. 2 unheated 1:20	36
24	Beef No. 2 heated 1:10	24
18	Beef No. 2 heated 1:20	24
16	Rabbit unheated 1:10	48
14	Rabbit unheated 1:20	24
18	Rabbit heated 1:10	24
18	Rabbit heated 1:20	24
17	Sterile salt solution (Cult. Con.)	24
16	Sterile sale solution (Cult. Con.)	24

20 M. L. D. (= 0.0004 c c culture diluted with salt solution up to 1 c c exposed to 1 c c of serum dilutions for one hour at 38 C.).
1 c c of 1:5 and 1:10 dilutions mixed with 1 c c of culture giving final dilutions of 1:10 and 1:20.
After the intraperitoneal injection of 1 c c of each mixture.

Additional experiments were made with what may be designated as a combined in vitro-vivo method by mixing in sterile test tubes a constant dose of culture with varying amounts of serum and after a period in the water bath at 38 C., injecting a portion of the contents of each tube into the peritoneal cavities of mice to determine the bactericidal activity of the serum. The results of one experiment of this nature consisting in exposing 20 minimal lethal doses of culture to 1 c c of 1:5 and 1:10 dilutions of unheated and heated normal beef and rabbit serums are shown in table 7; while the lives of several mice were prolonged about 24 hours beyond the culture controls, these experiments showed an absence or at best but a feeble bactericidal activity of normal beef serum even when used in amounts of 1 c c of undiluted serum.

THE BACTERICIDAL ACTIVITY OF NORMAL BEEF, RABBIT AND MOUSE SERUM FOR THE ANTHRAX BACILLUS IN VITRO

Numerous experiments were made for the purpose of eliciting evidence of possible bactericidal activity of normal beef serum for anthrax bacilli in vitro. Inasmuch as rabbits are highly immune and mice highly susceptible to anthrax, the serum or whole blood of these animals was usually included in our experiments for the double purpose of serving as controls and for a study of the nature of natural immunity to anthrax infection.

The technic and results of these experiments may be summarized as follows:

1. Fresh, sterile normal beef or rabbit serum unheated and heated twice at 56 C. were mixed in amounts of 5 c c with 0.5 c c of a thoroughly emulsified 24-hour broth culture of anthrax bacilli (practically no spores) and kept in a water bath at 38 C.; at intervals varying from 15 minutes to 4 hours 0.1 c c of each mixture was plated in 10 c c of agar at 42 C. and the plates counted after 48 hours' incubation. Culture controls were included in which sterile salt solution was used instead of serum. Neither beef nor rabbit serum showed any demonstrable bactericidal activity in these experiments.

2. Fresh sterile normal beef or rabbit serum unheated and heated were placed in sterile test tubes in constant amounts of 1 c c and treated with increasing amounts of thoroughly emulsified 24-hour broth cultures of anthrax bacilli varying from 0.01 to 0.1 c c; culture controls were included in which physiological salt solution replaced serum. After mixing and incubation in a water bath at 38 C. for 2 hours, 0.1 c c of each tube was plated with 10 c c of agar at 42 C. The general result of these tests with this technic was to show that sterile normal beef serum possesses some bactericidal activity for the anthrax bacillus while rabbit serum is without any demonstrable effect.

3. Best results were secured with the Heist-Lacy technic;[5] in this test six capillary tubes were employed with varying dilutions of culture (table 8). The bacilli exposed to serum or whole blood were those adhering to the interior of capillary tubes measuring about 1 mm. in diameter after the culture had been allowed to flow in for a distance of about 20 mm. followed by expulsion and filling with serum or blood to the same distance. Culture controls were included in which sterile broth was used instead of blood or serum. Each tubule was sealed and incubated for 24 hours when smears were made

[5] Jour. Immunology, 1918, 3, 3261.

and stained for anthrax bacilli. The results of one experiment are shown in table 8; plates prepared with 0.1 c c of each dilution of culture at the close of the experiment showed an uncountable number of anthrax colonies in the undiluted, 1 : 10, 1 : 100 and 1 : 1,000 dilutions of culture; the 1 : 10,000 dilution showed 9,400 colonies and the 1 : 100,000 dilution 1,850 colonies per c c.

The results of several experiments with this technic were unusually clear and decisive; either the smear showed very large numbers of bacilli, or none at all. Mouse blood invariably showed growths even with the 1 : 100,000 dilutions of 24-hour broth cultures, and these animals were highly susceptible to the culture employed; rabbit blood usually inhibited or killed the bacilli even with undiluted culture, and these animals were highly immune to intravenous injections of the culture. Sterile normal beef serum showed a high degree of bactericidal activity in this test and fresh unheated serum was usually, but not always, more germicidal than after heating twice at 56 C. for 30 minutes.

TABLE 8

RESULTS OF BACTERICIDAL TESTS WITH THE HEIST-LACY METHOD

Animal	Serum	Dilutions of Culture					
		Undiluted	1:10	1:100	1:1,000	1:10,000	1:100,000
Mouse	Fresh whole blood	+	+	+	+	+	+
Mouse	Fresh whole blood	+	+	+	+	+	+
Mouse	Fresh whole blood	+	+	+	+	+	+
Mouse	Fresh whole blood	+	+	+	+	+	+
Rabbit	Fresh whole blood	—	—	—	—	—	—
Rabbit	Fresh whole blood	—	—	—	—	—	—
Beef No. 1	Unheated serum	+	—	—	—	—	—
Beef No. 2	Unheated serum	—	—	—	—	—	—
Beef No. 3	Unheated serum	—	—	—	—	—	—
Beef No. 1	Heated serum	+	—	—	—	—	—
Beef No. 2	Heated serum	—	—	—	—	—	—
Beef No. 3	Heated serum	+	—	—	—	—	—

THE AGGLUTINATION OF THE ANTHRAX BACILLUS BY NORMAL BEEF, RABBIT AND MOUSE SERUM

Since it is generally accepted that agglutinins may aid the protective and curative properties of a serum by aiding phagocytosis and bacteriolysis, normal beef serum has been examined for agglutinins for anthrax bacilli. The majority of the serums were secured from specimens of blood collected in abattoirs and a few from cattle on a neighboring farm; nothing could be learned of the previous histories of these animals, and it is unknown whether or not any of them had had anthrax.

Rabbit and mouse serum was also tested to study the rôle of agglutinins in natural immunity to anthrax.

For the macroscopic agglutination tests antigens were prepared by these two methods:

(1) Flasks containing 200 c c of plain neutral broth were inoculated and grown at 42 C. for several days yielding rich and almost sporeless cultures;

at the end of this time 2 c c of liquor formaldehydi were added to each flask and the contents shaken in a mechanical shaker with beads until microscopic examination showed the thorough breaking up of the chains of bacilli. The antigens were allowed to stand for a day in a refrigerator and either centrifuged briefly or filtered through sterile cotton to remove clumps. The resulting antigen was of proper density, showed no spontaneous agglutination and stood up well for at least 36 hours at 55 C.

(2) Agar slant cultures were cultivated for 48 hours at 42 C. and washed off with 0.5% of liquor formaldehydi in salt solution, thoroughly shaken and briefly centrifuged or filtered through cotton after standing 24 hours. The resulting antigen was then diluted with liquor formaldehydi salt solution to the proper density. These antigens were somewhat inferior to those prepared by the first method and yielded lower agglutination titers.

TABLE 9

THE AGGLUTINATION OF B. ANTHRACIS BY NORMAL BEEF AND RABBIT SERUMS BY MACROSCOPIC TECHNIC

Serum	Highest Titers of the Serum of Different Animals													
	1	2	3	4	5	6	7	8	9	10	11	12	13	14
Beef-unheated	1:96	1:160	1:144	1:192	1:192	1:224	1:120	1:18	1:48	1:56	1:32	1:24	1:40	1:48
Beef-heated	1:80	1:120	1:120	1:180	1:180	1:200	1:16	1:16	1:30	1:40	1:24	1:20	1:30	1:20
Rabbit-unheated	1:24	1:8	1:10	None	None	None	1:2	1:6	1:2	1:4	None	None	0	0
Rabbit-heated	1:6	1:2	None	None	None	None	None	1:4	None	None	None	None	0	0

TABLE 10

THE AGGLUTINATION OF B. ANTHRACIS BY NORMAL MOUSE AND RABBIT SERUMS BY MICROSCOPIC TECHNIC

Serum	Highest Titers of the Serum of Different Animals							
	1	2	3	4	5	6	7	8
Mouse—unheated	1:8	1:8	1:24	1:4	1:80	None	1:2	1:4
Rabbit—unheated	1:16	1:30	1:12	1:12	1:6	1:8	None	1:10

In the macroscopic tests each dilution of serum was used in a dose of 1 c c of anthrax antigen; the mixtures were kept at 55 C. for 16 to 18 hours and the results read. Salt solution controls were always included.

For the microscopic tests 24-hour broth cultures were thoroughly shaken in a mechanical shaker with beads and a loopful mixed on cover slides with a loopful of varying dilutions of serum. The results were read after one hour at room temperature. The controls occasionally showed some spontaneous agglutination requiring the frequent repetition of the tests.

The results of macroscopic agglutination tests with unheated and heated beef and rabbit serum are shown in table 9; all of these serums were tested within four days of the time of collection of the bloods.

As shown in table 9, normal beef serums contained agglutinin for our culture of anthrax but the amounts varied considerably in different animals as shown in a variation of titers ranging from 1:20 to 1:224; after heating once or twice at 56 C. for 30 minutes the titers were uniformly lower than those observed with fresh unheated serums.

While rabbits were highly immune to our culture of anthrax bacilli, their serum contained none or small amounts of agglutinin for this culture, the highest titer observed being 1:24.

The results of microscopic agglutination tests with unheated mouse and rabbit serums are shown in table 10; the highest titer observed with mouse serum was 1:80 while the majority were 1:8 or lower. With a macroscopic technic mouse serum yielded lower titers.

COMPLEMENT FIXATION WITH NORMAL BEEF, RABBIT AND MOUSE SERUMS AND ANTHRAX ANTIGENS

As a further study for anti-anthrax substances in normal beef serum, complement fixation tests were made; rabbit and mouse serums were included for purposes of comparison as representatives of animals possessing a high and low natural immunity to anthrax.

The antigens employed were those prepared after the methods described for the agglutination tests. Each antigen was used in a fresh state.

The tests were made with an antisheep hemolytic system, the antigen being titrated for anticomplementary activity just before the fixation tests and used in an amount equal to one-third the anticomplementary unit. All serums were freshly collected and tested unheated, and after heating at 56 C. for 30 minutes in graded doses varying from 0.01 to 0.2 c c. The usual serum antigen and hemolytic controls were included.

The primary incubation was conducted in a water bath at 38 C. for one hour; the secondary incubation was also in the water bath for about one hour depending on the hemolysis of the controls.

The results were entirely negative; 8 normal beef serums, 6 normal rabbit and 6 normal mouse serums yielded completely negative reactions with heated or unheated serum in the maximum dose of 0.2 c c. Occasionally a rabbit serum heated at 56 C. yielded a weakly positive reaction but all tests with active serum were negative and we ascribed these positive reactions with heated serums to the property of normal rabbit serums for fixing complement in a nonspecific manner with various lipoidal and bacterial antigens.

DISCUSSION

Normal beef serum may be said to possess some anti-anthrax properties by reason of its bactericidal properties in vitro demonstrated by the Heist-Lacy method, and to the presence of agglutinin for anthrax bacilli. The anti-anthrax properties of beef serum, however, are feeble, inasmuch as protection tests with mice in which the serum was injected intraperitoneally in doses varying from 10 to 100 c c per kilogram, and equivalent to 700 to 7,000 c c per 70 kilograms, or the weight of the average adult person, against one to five times the smallest amount of anthrax culture killing mice in a period of 48 hours, mainly yielded negative results. By reason of the virulence of the strain employed and the high susceptibility of the white mouse, these tests may not have been sufficiently delicate to elicit minor degrees of protective power of the serums tested; rabbits, however, which Kraus employed in his experiments, possessed such a high degree of natural immunity to our culture of anthrax as to render them unsuitable and the results too favorable to the serum being tested.

A favorable opinion based on the results of the treatment of anthrax of persons with any serum may readily be based on error in view of the clinical course generally pursued by this infection. As anthrax is encountered among persons in Philadelphia, the mortality is very low providing the blood is sterile; recovery is prompt and without complications if the pustule is excised. In the experience of one of us (J. A. K.) anthrax bacteremia is generally fatal despite the administration of horse anti-anthrax serum, although recently a man suffering with a pustule on the face and whose blood showed the presence of anthrax bacilli, on repeated cultures, recovered without the use of serum. At best it would appear on the basis of these experiments that normal beef serum, as secured from animals under ordinary conditions, is but feebly protective or curative for anthrax, and while its administration as described by Penna and his associates may favorably influence the pustule, it is doubtful if the serum is sufficiently powerful to influence anthrax bacteremia.

In so far as our experiments bear on the nature of the natural immunity of the rabbit to anthrax and the high susceptibility of the white mouse, it would appear that the bactericidal activity of the whole blood is important in this relation. The blood of the adult rabbit is highly bactericidal as shown by the Heist-Lacy method, whereas that of the mouse is practically without effect on the anthrax bacillus. The presence or absence of agglutinins in the serum of these animals is not nearly so definite in relation to the question of natural immunity; generally, however, the serum of rabbits contains more agglutinin for anthrax bacilli than the serum of white mice, and the former possesses the higher degree of natural immunity to this particular infection.

SUMMARY AND CONCLUSIONS

Fresh sterile, normal beef serum is but feebly toxic for white mice by intraperitoneal injection; doses equivalent to 10 c c per 100 gm. of weight are well borne. Serums heated twice at 56 C. for 30 minutes are slightly less toxic.

Protection tests consisting in the intraperitoneal injection of mice with heated and unheated normal beef serum in doses ranging from 1 to 10 c c per 100 gm. generally failed to protect mice against 1 to 5 minimal lethal doses of culture.

By reason of the high susceptibility of white mice to anthrax these tests may not have been sufficiently delicate; the high degree of natural immunity to anthrax possessed by rabbits, however, renders them unsuitable for protection tests.

Unheated normal beef serum is bactericidal for the anthrax bacillus in vitro; heated serum is somewhat less bactericidal.

Rabbit blood is highly bactericidal for anthrax bacilli in vitro while mouse blood is without appreciable effect. The natural immunity of rabbits to anthrax is probably due in part to the bactericidal activity of their blood.

Normal beef serum contains variable amounts of agglutinin for anthrax bacilli, the titers ranging from 1:16 to 1:224; rabbit and mouse serum also contains small amounts of agglutinin, the former somewhat more than the latter. Heated serums of the three animals contains less agglutinin.

Normal beef, rabbit and mouse serums do not contain complement fixing substances for antigens of anthrax bacilli.

While normal beef serum contains some anti-anthrax substances they were found without demonstrable protective and curative value in experimental anthrax infections of mice and rabbits.

SOME FACTORS INFLUENCING THE FINAL HYDROGEN-ION CONCENTRATION IN BACTERIAL CULTURES WITH SPECIAL REFERENCE TO STREPTOCOCCI

Horry Jones

From the Department of Pathology and Bacteriology, University of Illinois, College of Medicine, Chicago

It is a well known fact that a given organism in fermenting a utilizable carbohydrate, produces a gradual alteration in the reaction of the medium, and that this change in reaction eventually becomes so marked as to inhibit all further growth of the organism. The degree to which this alteration in reaction proceeds in a given culture is designated as the limiting or final hydrogen-ion concentration of that organism.

In some instances, accurate measurements of this final hydrogen-ion concentration have shown it to be one of the most remarkably constant characteristics, not only of a given organism, but of various strains of this organism. In fact, following the researches of Sorensen,[1] of Michaelis,[2] and later of Clark and Lubs,[3] the application of hydrogen-ion concentration determinations has come into quite prominent use in the differentiation of certain strains of bacteria from other strains more or less closely allied. For example, Clark and Lubs have shown that in the presumptive test for B. typhosus, an organism which, by the usual tests, is indistinguishable from B. coli of human fecal origin, is often encountered. They have shown, also, that this organism is not of human fecal origin, and that it may be differentiated from B. coli on the basis of differences in their final hydrogen-ion concentrations, when grown for five days in glucose broth.

In a similar way, Ayers[4] and others have shown that virulent hemolytic streptococci found in milk and other sources may be differentiated from nonvirulent hemolytic strains by differences in their final hydrogen-ion concentrations. Avery and Cullen[5] repeated this work with similar results.

Received for publication Oct. 13, 1919.

[1] Ergebn. Phisiol., 1912, 12, p. 303.
[2] Wasserstoffionenkonzentration, 1914.
[3] Jour. Infect. Dis., 1915, 17, p. 160; Jour. Bacteriol., 1917, 2, p. 1.
[4] Jour. Infect. Dis., 1918, 23, p. 290.
[5] Jour. Exper. Med., 1919, 29, p. 215.

The present work was undertaken for the purpose of determining if successive transfers of a given organism in the same medium, incubated under the same conditions, would develop identical concentrations of hydrogen-ion, and if so, to study the effect of some of the commoner factors, such as temperature, initial reaction, composition of medium, etc., in causing deviations from that final hydrogen-ion concentration.

METHODS

The hydrogen electrode described elsewhere[6] was used in making these determinations. The readings are accurate to half a millivolt, or about 0.01 of a P_H. Four day periods of incubation were used unless otherwise stated.

EXPERIMENTAL

To make valid any interpretations as to the effect of varying conditions on the final hydrogen-ion concentration, it was of course necessary, first of all, to determine whether a given organism could, under identical environment, reproduce identical concentrations of hydrogen-ion. The results of this experiment are recorded in table 1.

TABLE 1

HYDROGEN-ION CONCENTRATION PRODUCED BY SUCCESSIVE TRANSFER OF A HEMOLYTIC STREPTOCOCCUS OF VIRULENT TYPE

No. of Transfer	Reading in Millivolts	P_H	Variations
1	576.5	5.11	0
2	576.5	5.11	0
3	576.5	5.11	0
4	576.0	5.10	.01
5	576.5	5.11	0

Incubated at 37 C. for 4 days, in broth containing 1% peptone, 0.3% beef extract, 0.7% NaCl, and 1% glucose.

According to these results, a most surprising consistency is shown by Str. hemolyticus in its limit of hydrogen-ion tolerance, from one transfer to the next. Other strains of Str. hemolyticus and cultures of B. typhosus, B. paratyphosus, and B. proteus showed practically the same regularity through five successive transfers.

EFFECT OF VARYING THE PERCENTAGE OF GLUCOSE IN A GIVEN MEDIUM

Varying percentages of sugar were added to ordinary broth, beginning with 0.1% and increasing up to 1%. Some variation in ability to

[6] Jones, H. M., Jour. Infect. Dis., 1919, 25, p. 262.

completely remove glucose from the medium was observed in the various organisms studied. B. paratyphosus alpha and B. proteus removed all of the 0.2% of glucose and the reaction of the medium then turned back to alkalinity. With percentages above 0.2%, the final hydrogen-ion concentrations for a given organism were identical in the various sugar concentrations. The amount of glucose which a given organism can consume is influenced by the buffer content of the medium, i. e., by such constituents as phosphates, protein, etc., which aid in holding the concentration of hydrogen-ion from the toxic limit, thus permitting a larger amount of the sugar to be decomposed. An initial reaction with a P_H well over on the alkaline side has a similar effect. Streptococcus hemolyticus of virulent type did not remove all of the 0.2% glucose, while a Str. hemolyticus obtained from milk removed 0.2% and subsequently developed an alkalinity.

These two factors of buffer content of the medium and percentage of glucose deserve consideration. Berman and Rettger,[7] in studying the proteolytic activity and nitrogen metabolism of various organisms, erred in the interpretations of their results through lack of consideration of both of these factors.

EFFECT OF VARYING THE KIND OF UTILIZABLE CARBOHYDRATE

Str. hemolyticus, pneumococcus, and B. coli were inoculated into 1% glucose and 1% lactose broths, and incubated for 4 days at 37 C.

TABLE 2

RESULTS OF EXPERIMENT

Organism	P_H in Glucose	P_H in Lactose
Str. hemolyticus	5.11	6.0
Pneumococcus, type 1	5.43	6.2
Pneumococcus, type 3	5.6	6.02
B. coli	4.31	4.33

To extend the experiment to include other organisms and other sugars would doubtless show that the more vigorous organisms are affected more by the toxicity of the hydrogen-ion than by the nature of the sugar. These results, however, are sufficient to show that it is necessary to specify the kind of sugar used in the medium when referring to the limiting hydrogen-ion concentration of some organ-

[7] Jour. Bacteriol., 1918, 3, p. 389.

isms; they also show that a carbohydrate which is utilizable under certain conditions may not be utilizable under other slightly more adverse conditions.

EFFECT OF ADDITION OF HUMAN BODY TO GLUCOSE BROTH

Certain organisms are grown with difficulty in ordinary glucose broth, and for this reason blood, blood serum, or ascitic fluid are frequently added to the medium to favor growth. How ascitic fluid in varying amounts affects the final hydrogen-ion concentration is shown in the following table.

TABLE 3

FINAL HYDROGEN-ION CONCENTRATION OF STR. HEMOLYTICUS OF VIRULENT TYPE IN GLUCOSE BROTH CONTAINING VARYING AMOUNTS OF ASCITIC FLUID

Composition of Medium	Millivolts	P_H
10 c c glucose broth = 3 c c ascitic	548.5	4.63
10 c c glucose broth = 2 c c ascitic	548.5	4.63
10 c c glucose broth = 1 c c ascitic	548.5	4.63
10 c c glucose broth = ½ c c ascitic	548.5	4.63
10 c c glucose broth = 3 drops ascitic	548.5	4.63
10 c c glucose broth = no ascitic	576.5	5.11

From these results it is seen that, according to the work of Ayers and others referred to above, this organism when grown in 1% glucose broth would be classed as a streptococcus of virulent type because of its final hydrogen-ion concentration, but when grown in ascitic broth it would be classed as one of nonvirulent type, i. e., in ascitic broth its P_H is similar to that of a nonvirulent strain, while in plain broth its P_H is that of the virulent types. The final hydrogen-ion concentrations of different pneumococcus strains also show this same alteration when grown in ascitic broth. How the ascitic fluid brings about such a marked alteration in the tolerance of these organisms to the toxic hydrogen-ion is not clear. The phenomenon appears all the more puzzling when it is seen that the streptococci of nonvirulent types are not similarly affected by the presence of ascitic fluid in the medium. Furthermore, autoclaving the ascites broth reduces it to the condition of ordinary broth in this respect.

Delicately growing organisms, as Str. hemolyticus of virulent type and pneumococci of various type, showed wide variation even from one transfer to the next when subjected to conditions which tended to delay growth. For example, one strain of pneumococcus when inoculated into a medium whose initial reaction was P_H 7 grew poorly and developed a final concentration of only P_H 6.2, but in a medium with an initial reaction of P_H 7.6, the growth was abundant, and a final concentration of P_H 5.4 was reached.

Another strain required a heavy inoculum before abundant growth could be obtained, and its final concentration of hydrogen-ion varied from one transfer to another depending on the abundance of growth secured. Incubating at room temperature and also the age of the culture from which the transfer was made have a similar effect on growth, and, likewise, on the final hydrogen-ion concentration. The statement often made that the final hydrogen-ion concentration of a given organism is always the same regardless of the initial concentration, provided growth occurs, is therefore not true, at least, with certain delicately growing strains of bacteria.

CONCLUSION

From these results it is seen that, to obtain any accurate information regarding the final hydrogen-ion concentration of an organism, a number of factors should be taken into consideration. This characteristic, the limiting hydrogen-ion concentration of a given organism, to have any significance or subsequent application should be defined in terms of the composition of the medium, the initial reaction and any other conditions which favor or hinder abundant growth of that organism.

THE EFFECT OF PASTEURIZING TEMPERATURES ON THE PARATYPHOID GROUP

Edith M. Twiss

From the Department of Hygiene and Bacteriology, University of Chicago

Work on the thermal death point of micro-organisms in milk has been carefully reviewed, the difficulties of the problem stated, and the possible sources of error pointed out by M. J. Rosenau,[1] who investigated the thermal death point of a number of pathogenic micro-organisms. He concluded that milk heated to 60 C. and maintained there for 20 minutes may be considered safe so far as conveying infections with the micro-organisms tested is concerned. These results were later confirmed by Schorer and Rosenau,[2] using methods of actual pasteurization; the micro-organisms studied did not include B. paratyphosus A or B.

The first work on paratyphoid bacilli was by Bernhard Fischer in 1903.[3] It was mainly epidemiologic, but he makes the statement that he established by oft repeated experiment that the paratyphoid bacilli isolated in the epidemic studied were not killed by exposure to 60 C. for 30 minutes, that in two experiments bacilli were still living after exposure at 70 C. for from 10 to 25 minutes. Five minutes at 75 C. killed most of the organisms, but a few were living even then. The methods of experiment employed are not given in the report.

Friedel, Kutscher and Meinicke,[4] working in Koch's laboratory, reported all paratyphoid bacilli killed by 5 minutes' exposure to 58 C.

Exper. 1

The strains of bacilli used in this and in the following experiments are given in table 1. Their sources can be found in Jordan's article on the differentiation of this group.[5] Whole milk was used and sterilized in the autoclave for 10 minutes at 10 lbs. pressure. The milk used in Chicago was certified milk. In Topeka, where certified milk cannot be obtained, the milk came from a dairy where the milk count rarely exceeds 100,000 per c c.

The milk was sterilized in 100 c c lots in 150 c c Erlenmeyer flasks; 0.1 c c of a 24-hour broth culture of the strain to be tested was introduced with

Received for publication Sept. 17, 1919.

[1] Bull. 42, U. S. Public Health Service, 1908.
[2] Jour. Med. Research, 1912, 26, p. 127.
[3] Festschrift, R. Koch, 1903, p. 271.
[4] Klin. Jahrb., 1904-5, 13, p. 324.
[5] Jour. Infect. Dis., 1917, 29, p. 457.

a sterile pipet which was left in the flask and used for stirring and for withdrawing the milk for plating. Before pasteurization, the milk was thoroughly stirred and 1 c c portions withdrawn and plated in duplicate. The counts of these plates showed that the numbers of bacteria introduced in 0.1 c c of a 24-hour broth culture were consistently in the millions.

TABLE 1

STRAINS OF BACILLI USED IN EXPERIMENTS

B. paratyphosus B (26 strains)					B. paratyphosus A (15 strains)			B. typhosus (6 strains)	B. enteritidis (10 strains)		B. suipestifer (10 strains)	
5	115	161	185	224	3	48	215	Hopkins	50	205	63	162
8	149	169	202	240	4	138	219	189	51	206	66	163
12	150	175	211	245	9	158	229	190	52	207	116	167
47	151	179	222	250	40	188	230	197	53	226	136	173
62	152	180	223	251	42	198	231	247	204	228	166	227
								607				

Pasteurization was carried on in a water-bath set in a second bath so that the temperature could be carefully regulated. Thermometers were kept in the inner and outer bath and in the milk, and the temperature of the milk during the experiments did not vary more than 0.5 C. and usually less than 0.1 C. The flasks were set deep enough in the water so that the water came up on the outside of the flask to at least twice the depth of the milk inside. The greatest care was taken in moving the flasks, and in stirring and withdrawing the milk, to avoid getting any drops on the sides of the flask above the general level of the milk. At regular intervals, 1 c c portions were withdrawn and plated in duplicate. The plates were incubated at 37½ C. and counted after 24 hours, with a second count at 48 hours, when the colonies were very small and few.

The results of 12 strains of B. paratyphosus B tested in this way were: 3 strains showed no growth after the temperature reached 60 C., 2 strains showed no growth after 1 minute at 60 C., 4 strains showed no growth after 3 minutes at 60 C., 3 strains showed growth after 3 minutes at 60 C.

As has been noted by other investigators of the thermal death-point of micro-organisms in milk, the organisms decrease very rapidly as the temperature approaches 60 C. The test of one strain is given in table 2 as an illustration.

TABLE 2

B. PARATYPHOSUS B NO. 224

MILK AT 25 C. IMMERSED IN BATH AT 60 C.

Time after Immersion	Temperature, C.	Number of Colonies per c c
At start	25	0,900,000
4 minutes	55	1,600
8 minutes	59	154
12 minutes	60	9
13 minutes	1 minute at 60	2
14 minutes	2 minutes at 60	1
15 minutes	3 minutes at 60	0
16 minutes	4 minutes at 60	0

Different strains vary considerably in their resistance to heat. In most cases the milk reached 60 C. in from 10-12 minutes, but in two tests there was greater variation, and the results in these (table 3) seem to indicate that the difference in strains is, of the two, the factor of greater importance.

TABLE 3

RESULTS OF TESTS

Time to Reach 60 C.	Time at Which No More Growth Was Observed
7 minutes	1 minute at 60 C.
14 minutes	3 minutes at 60 C.

As the numbers are greatly reduced, it becomes more and more possible that the one or two surviving may not be included in the c c withdrawn to plate. For testing this possibility by allowing the few surviving to multiply to the point where their detection would be easy the following experiment was added:

At the close of the pasteurizing period, the flask was set first in cold water and then in the ice-box to duplicate the cooling of practical pasteurization. After cooling, it was incubated at 37½ for 24 hours, a loopful transferred to a tube of broth and this in turn incubated at 37½ C. From the broth a stab was made in a Russell double sugar slant. Typical growth on these slants showed survival at temperatures at which negative plates had been secured, and this method was accordingly used with a number of strains. To check results with those of investigators who used other methods, B. typhosus (Hopkins) was run in parallel experiments. Several strains of paratyphosus B were also tried in this way without repeating the plating. In these cases 0.1 c c of a 24-hour broth culture was introduced into 100 c c of milk. After stirring with a sterile pipet, a few drops were withdrawn into a broth tube and incubated. These served as checks on the presence of actively growing organisms at the beginning of pasteurization. The flask of milk was then put in the bath and treated like the others.

From one of these flasks B. typhosus was recovered after the milk had been held at 60 C. for 20 minutes. In order to be sure that this difference from the results obtained by Rosenau was not due to errors of technic in the method employed, I determined to test again the strains that had survived more than 3 minutes' exposure to 60 C., using Rosenau's method.

EXPER. 2

Accordingly, thin-walled tubes with approximately 10 c c of milk were substituted for 100 c c in flasks. Whole milk was used, sterilized as before, but the tube was always well shaken before the introduction of bacteria to break the cream layer. The tubes were open during pasteurization, but the plugs were flamed and replaced when the tubes were taken from the bath. The room temperature and the time taken to raise the temperature of the milk to 60 C. were always recorded. Neither varied much. The room temperature at Chicago (summer months) was from 26 C. to 31 C.; at Topeka (winter months), 22 C. or 23 C. The time taken to reach 60 C. was from 6 to 8 minutes.

Loopfuls were withdrawn into broth, in the greater number of cases at frequent intervals, but toward the end only twice—at from 58 C. to 60 C. and just at the close of pasteurization. Stabs from these broth tubes into Russell slants confirmed Rosenau's results. In approximately 35 tests of strains of B. paratyphosus B and 40 of parallel tests of B. typhosus (Hopkins) only one strain, of B. paratyphosus B, showed growth after exposure to 60 C. for 2 minutes.

These same tubes, from which loopfuls had been transferred to broth, were cooled and incubated at the close of pasteurization, and stabs made from them directly into Russell slants. Although the loopfuls removed to broth had failed, in every case except one, to indicate the presence of living bacilli after the temperature of the milk had been held at 60 C. for 2 minutes, after 24 hours' incubation of this same milk, the much smaller amount removed by a straight needle carried over into Russell slants bacilli which produced the effects of vigorous growth. Two strains of paratyphosus B were recovered from milk that had been held at 60 C. for 30 minutes. Their identity was confirmed by agglutination with immune serum. It is clear that results obtained by plating 1 c c of milk from 100, or transferring one loopful into broth, cannot be taken as proof of the death of all the organisms in the sample. It is possible that we have here, not only the difficulty of catching one or two organisms in a comparatively large sample, but also some such stunning of the organisms as occurs in the case of B. coli in chlorinated water,[6] though it is difficult to see why the organisms should not recover as well in broth and agar as in milk.

Tests were then made with a larger number of strains of B. paratyphosus B and B. typhosus and strains of B. paratyphosus A, B. enteritidis and B. suipestifer. The withdrawal of any portion of the milk to broth was omitted, but stabs were made into Russell slants before pasteurization, and strains in which these controls did not show active growth were discarded.

A summary of all results obtained from milk which was heated to 60 C., held at 60 C. for a definite time, cooled and incubated is contained in tables 4 and 5.

When one strain was tested a number of times, there appeared to be a time of exposure to 60 C. when the organisms sometimes died and in other experiments survived; a period just before the thermal death point. Such a period is seen in table 6 at from 15-20 minutes for B. typhosus Hopkins.

[6] H. E. Jordan cited by Race, Joseph, Chlorination of Water, 1918, p. 57.

TABLE 4

RESULTS OF TESTS

Temperature of Pasteurization, C.	Time of Exposure	Number of Strains Killed				
		Paratyphosus B	Paratyphosus A	B. typhosus	B. enteritidis	B. suipestifer
60	3 minutes	8	..	..	..	..
60	5 minutes	3	..	..	..	..
60	10 minutes	2	..	..	..	..
60	20 minutes	1	..	..	..	..
60	25 minutes	1	4	2	4	8
60	30 minutes	3	4	1	..	..
65	30 minutes	2	7	4	5	2
		20	15	7	9	10

TABLE 5

RESULTS OF TESTS

Organism	Number of Strains Tested	Number of Strains Surviving 30 Minutes at	
		60 C.	65 C.
Paratyphosus B	20	9	6*
Paratyphosus A	15	7	0
B. typhosus	7	4	0
B. enteritidis	9	5	0
B. suipestifer	10	2	0

* Confirmed by agglutination with immune serum.

TABLE 6

B. TYPHOSUS (HOPKINS)

Exposure to 60 C.	Russell Slants from Milk	
	+	—
5 minutes	3 times	once (from flask)
10 minutes	5 times	0 times
15 minutes	4 times	3 times
20 minutes	1 time	3 times
25 minutes	0 times	2 times
30 minutes	0 times	3 times

The same point was brought out by the work of three students (Edith Conard, Mary Holl, Edna Smith) at Washburn College, who used these methods for determining the thermal death point of four strains of B. paratyphosus A. They recovered them after 25 minutes' exposure to 60 C., had varying results after from 30-34 minutes' exposure, and failed in at least two tests of each strain to recover any organisms after 35 minutes at 60 C.

This is somewhat in line with the results of the investigation of the death of B. coli in pasteurized milk,[7] though the variation there

[7] Ayres and Johnson: Jour. Agric. Research, 1915, 3, p. 401.

seemed very irregular, and was noticed in tests of such organisms as had survived the higher temperatures. In my experiments, the broth culture used to inoculate the milk was always a 24-hour growth from the agar slant previously used.

SUMMARY

Negative tests of comparatively small amounts of milk removed during pasteurization, or just at its close, cannot be taken as proof of the death of all organisms. When infected milk which had been heated to 60 C., held there for a definite time and then cooled, was incubated at 37½ C., pathogenic organisms were recovered after exposures exceeding those of practical pasteurization. Of the strains of B. paratyphosus B tested, 6 were recovered from milk that had been held at 65 C. for 30 minutes, and 7 strains of B. paratyphosus A, 4 of B. typhosus, 5 of B. enteritidis, and 2 of B. suipestifer after 30 minutes at 60 C. It is possible that in a larger number of strains, some of even greater resistance might be found.

The greater number of organisms die out rapidly as the temperature approaches 60 C.

There is evidence that just before the exposure which kills all organisms, there is a period when survival is irregular, the few more resistant organisms sometimes living, in other tests dying.

THE FATE OF STREPTOCOCCUS HEMOLYTICUS IN THE GASTRO-INTESTINAL CANAL

DAVID J. DAVIS

From the Department of Pathology and Bacteriology, University of Illinois, College of Medicine, Chicago

Dangerous streptococci, especially Str. hemolyticus, are found very commonly in the throat. Our observations[1] show that in the crypts of the faucial tonsils hemolytic streptococci occur in nearly 100%. Often they occur in large numbers on the pharyngeal mucosa in normal persons, and especially in persons suffering with various respiratory infections, in which these organisms so often play an important rôle. Large numbers of streptococci are therefore constantly passing down the esophagus into the stomach in both normal and diseased persons. Furthermore, during milk-borne epidemics of streptococcus sore throat, milk from infected cows containing large numbers of streptococci is swallowed. The fate of these virulent hemolytic streptococci in the gastro-intestinal canal is the subject of this paper.

Three questions arise: First, the possibility of secondarily infecting the intestinal canal; second, the invasion of the body through the wall and third the possible danger of transmission of dangerous streptococci through sewage, etc.

As is well known, the gastric contents exercise a strong bactericidal effect on bacteria entering the stomach. Certain acidophils are able to live and develop in the stomach; spores and certain fungi, on account of their resisting properties, can do likewise. But the great mass of bacteria that enter the stomach through the act of swallowing are killed, and therefore the food passing into the duodenum contains relatively few organisms.

While these statements are generally true, there are exceptions due to several reasons; bacteria become enmeshed in particles of food and are thereby protected from acid until they enter the duodenum. This is especially true in cases of hypermotility. In achylia the bacteria pass through the stomach little affected by the feebly acid gastric contents.

Received for publication Oct. 24, 1919.

1 Pilot and Davis: Jour. Infect. Dis., 1919, 24, p. 386.

Consequently, under certain conditions many bacteria from the throat may pass through the stomach unharmed and invade the intestinal canal.

Little work has been done to determine specifically the effect of the intestinal juices on bacteria, and apparently nothing has been done to determine their effect on virulent streptococci.

The rabbit is especially susceptible to experimental infections with Str. hemolyticus; for this reason it was selected for certain experiments designed to test the action of the gastro-intestinal contents on this organism.

In the examination of material for hemolytic streptococci the following routine method was employed: Plain blood agar plates were made, using 0.5 c c of human blood to 5 c c of medium. This medium was inoculated usually with a small quantity of intestinal contents, which, whenever necessary, was properly macerated in sterile fluid. Several plates were made in order to obtain proper dilutions. The hemolyzing colonies were isolated and, when necessary, confirmatory tests were made. By hemolytic streptococci I mean streptococci having a wide, clear zone of complete hemolysis (type B or Theobald Smith) and not the imperfect hemolyzers (type A).

The intestinal contents from three normal rabbits living on a routine diet of carrots, hay and water were examined for hemolytic streptococci in the following manner: The animals were killed, the abdomen at once carefully opened, and several specimens of the contents were obtained from stomach, duodenum, ileum and colon, and plated on blood agar. In none of the specimens were hemolytic streptococci isolated; green streptococci of the fecalis type were common. Numerous other organisms, including hemolytic colon bacilli, appeared on the plates. Another normal rabbit was placed under observation for a period of nearly 3 weeks and each day one or more specimens of feces were cultured. Nineteen specimens thus collected were examined and all yielded negative results as to hemolytic streptococci. Many green producing streptococci appeared. This preliminary experiment was made primarily to determine the incidence of hemolytic streptococci in the intestinal canal of normal rabbits.

The following experiment was carried out to determine whether or not hemolytic streptococci fed to rabbits would live in the gastro-intestinal canal and cause symptoms: It was found that feeding was unsatisfactory and the streptococci were therefore introduced by means of a small catheter which serves as a satisfactory stomach tube for this animal.

Three healthy rabbits were carefully selected and their stools examined for hemolytic streptococci, with negative results. They were then given, by means of the rubber catheter, suspensions of streptococci. Three strains were given, one an old laboratory strain that appeared to be somewhat hardy and had lost most of its virulence (3 c c of a broth culture intravenously did not cause lesions) and two virulent strains recently isolated, one from a tonsillar abscess which killed a rabbit in doses of 1 c c given intravenously, and another isolated from the spinal fluid of a case of meningitis. Each day for ten days, from 10 to 20 c c of a 24-hour milk and broth culture of the relatively avirulent strain were given to the three rabbits, and each day the feces were collected and examined. In rabbit 1 on the ninth day a very considerable number of streptococcus colonies appeared on the plates which, on examination, were shown to be identical with those injected into the stomach. These cocci appeared suddenly, not being noted before in the feces. On the following day also a smaller number of the same streptococci were found, but on the third day none appeared. At the end of fourteen days, and for six days thereafter, the strain of streptococci from the tonsillar abscess was fed to the rabbit. No hemolytic streptococci were found in the feces in this time. Then for the next twelve days the freshly isolated strain of hemolytic streptococci from a fatal case of meningitis was given by mouth. During this time no hemolytic streptococci appeared in the feces. At no time did this rabbit show any evidence of infection or appear abnormal in any way. It was noted that on the two days when the hemolytic streptococci were found in the feces the latter were slightly more moist and softer than usual. Otherwise they remained throughout normally firm and well formed.

In rabbit 2 the streptococci were given as in 1. In this animal, on the fifth day after giving the meningitis streptococcus, there appeared in the feces numerous typical hemolytic streptococci like those given by stomach. They appeared suddenly, and the feces were slightly moist. On the following day they disappeared and were not recovered thereafter.

In rabbit 3 on the sixth day after feeding the avirulent streptococcus, streptococci appeared suddenly in the stools in large numbers. Two days later they were not found. Again six days after beginning the administration of the meningitis streptococcus about 25 colonies appeared on the plates, which proved to be identical with the original meningitis streptococcus. They did not reappear.

At the end of 31 days, during which these observations were being conducted, the three animals were killed and specimens for examination were obtained from various levels of the gastro-intestinal tract: 2 from the stomach, 8 from the small intestine and 4 from the cecum and large intestine. Cultures made from this material in the 3 rabbits in every case yielded no hemolytic streptococci. The stomach and intestinal mucosa appeared normal, as did all the other organs in the animals.

It appears from these experiments that when large numbers of streptococci are introduced they are usually killed promptly, presumably in the stomach, but that occasionally, as in each of the three animals, they may appear for a short interval in considerable numbers in the feces. They do not, however, permanently seed the intestinal canal with streptococci as evidenced by their absence in the examination made at necropsy. Nor is it possible, judging from these experiments, in this way to infect the rabbits or cause lesions of the intestinal tract.

In the light of these experiments it is difficult for me to understand the results of certain workers who report finding intestinal lesions and generalized infections followed by death after the administration by mouth of even small quantities of streptococci. Bail[2] states that he was able to so infect rabbits from 10 to 12 weeks old by injecting into the empty stomach far smaller quantities of streptococci than were used in my experiments. He believes that virulent pyogenic organisms may pass through the uninjured intestinal mucosa and cause a general infection. Holst[3] reports similar results with animals and with himself after feeding with cultures of streptococci. These results are not in accord with my own, nor are they in harmony with the general fact that in streptococcus pneumonia and other respiratory infections large numbers of streptococci are swallowed, but are not found, at least in large numbers, in the feces. The organisms may not have been hemolytic streptococci.

It was thought that perhaps the intestinal canal might become infected during a generalized infection with streptococci. Three rabbits were therefore inoculated with a virulent hemolytic strepto-

[2] Arch. f. klin. Chir., 1900, 62, p. 369.
[3] Baumgartens Jahresbericht, 1895, 11, p. 52.

coccus intravenously. Each developed severe multiple arthritis and had fever, loss of weight and other evidence of a generalized infection. Twelve days later the three animals were killed and cultures made from stomach, duodenum, ileum and cecum, as well as from heart blood and joint fluid. The various involved joints yielded streptococci in large numbers as did also the heart blood in one rabbit; but no hemolytic streptococci were found in the intestinal contents. In the duodenum very few bacteria of any kind were found in the intestinal contents; lower down the numbers were greatly increased. It appears therefore, that though the streptococci are in the blood and other tissues, the intestinal canal may remain free from these organisms.

HEMOLYTIC STREPTOCOCCI IN HUMAN FECES

There is little in the literature concerning the occurrence of hemolytic streptococci in human feces. Broadhurst[4] isolated strains from human feces, dog intestines and stomach, and various other sources, but does not clearly state whether they are the wide hemolyzers of the beta type.

A routine examination of 53 specimens of human feces was made. They were obtained from a variety of persons many of whom were patients in a large hospital and suffering with a variety of diseases, few of which were intestinal, however. Since we have shown that practically all tonsils contain hemolytic streptococci,[1] and since a large proportion of persons harbor many of these organisms at all times in their throats, we may be sure that many, if not all, of these patients were swallowing large numbers of them constantly in their foods. The feces were collected and cultured usually within a few hours after evacuation. Small particles were fished and stirred in a small quantity of broth or salt solution from which several blood-agar plate cultures were made. Suspicious colonies were fished and subjected to proper tests. In none of the 53 specimens were hemolytic streptococci demonstrated. In a number of the specimens broth was inoculated with a small particle of feces and incubated for from 12 to 18 hours, and from this material plates were made. These examinations also failed to reveal this organism in the specimens examined.

Since scarlet fever patients practically always have hemolytic streptococci in their throats and usually in very large numbers,[5] the feces from four cases were examined to determine if in this disease these

[4] Jour. Infect. Dis., 1915, 17, p. 277.
[5] Ruediger: Jour. Infect. Dis., 1906, 3, p. 755.

cocci passed through the canal. Examinations made in the usual way failed to reveal the hemolytic variety; many green streptococci were always present. Small particles of three of the specimens were suspended in salt solution and inoculated into the peritoneal cavity of three white mice. One white mouse was sick for two days, but recovered. On the fourth day examination revealed no streptococci in the peritoneal cavity. A second mouse died two days later. Small green streptococci were in the heart blood, but no hemolytic streptococci were found in the blood or peritoneal cavity. The third mouse died after four days. A few B. coli were in the peritoneal cavity and the heart blood was sterile; no hemolytic streptococci.

Thus, in none of the feces from normal or from the scarlet fever patients examined were hemolytic streptococci found. In this connection Kraft[6] working in this laboratory has examined 125 normal and pathologic appendices, cultivating the contents and also the scrapings of the mucosa. In 48 normal appendices he found only 2 in which hemolyzing streptococci occurred, and in these there were only a few. In 77 pathologic appendices examined he found 4 containing this organism and in decidedly larger numbers than in the normal ones.

The following experiment was made to determine how long hemolytic streptococci will live in feces: A specimen of fresh human feces was examined and no hemolytic streptococci found. A virulent freshly isolated throat hemolytic streptococcus was mixed with the feces, placed in the icebox, and at daily intervals cultures were made. At the end of seven days under these conditions the hemolytic streptococci seemed as numerous as in the first control. In a similar way, feces were mixed with hemolytic streptococci and kept at incubator temperature and cultivated from time to time. The results were different. While at the end of two hours numerous hemolytic streptococci were present, at the end of 24, 48 and 72 hours none were obtained in the feces. In the incubator the streptococci appear to be rapidly overgrown and destroyed by the normal fecal organisms. It should be pointed out that conditions in the test tube are not directly comparable to those in the intestinal canal where fresh alkaline intestinal secretions are being constantly poured, the reaction being thereby maintained normally not far from the neutral point. In the intestine also the mucosal surface might under certain conditions, especially pathologic, favor the development of hemolytic streptococci.

[6] Unpublished observations.

ACTION OF GASTRIC JUICE ON HEMOLYTIC STREPTOCOCCI

Strauss and Wurtz[7] showed that the destructive effect of stomach contents on bacteria, in vitro, runs parallel with the HCl content. Others have obtained evidence that in addition to the acid effect the pepsin may exert some germicidal action. This is probably slight, if it exists at all. The concentration of HCl in gastric contents varies according to Clark and Lubs,[8] from P_H 0.9 to P_H 1.6. This is far below the limiting H-ion concentration (5.2) at which hemolytic streptococci will develop, as determined by Jones[9] and others.

With concentrations of HCl in the stomach in ranges approaching normal we should, therefore, expect the hemolytic streptococci to be rapidly destroyed and the contents to become free from these organisms in a short time. This does occur.

In an examination of 15 stomach contents no hemolytic streptococci were found. In these the total acidity ranged from 14 to 85. In four no free acid was present when tested with the dimethyl test. In these cases of low acidity certain varieties of bacteria were far more numerous than in the other specimens, but hemolytic streptococci were not found.

In order to test the direct bactericidal action of the gastric juice on hemolytic streptococci pure suspensions of this organism were added to 5 c c of the stomach contents. Of 15 samples thus tested, 11 had free acid with total acidities ranging from 28 to 85, and in all the hemolytic streptococci were dead in five minutes, many of them in two minutes. Of the four samples with no free acid and with total acidities of from 14 to 19, the hemolytic streptococci lived from one to three hours, but were dead in twenty-four hours. Presumably in the stomach the action would go on somewhat more effectively than in the test tube owing to more favorable conditions. These results strikingly illustrate the effectiveness of proper acidity in the stomach in determining the character of the gastric flora.

In the older literature there are many references to work on streptococcal enteritis which seems to center largely around that of Escherich[10] and his school. The examinations made at that time do not permit one to classify the streptococci accurately, but there are reasons to believe that many, if not all, belong to the streptococcus fecalis

7 Quoted from Kolle and Wassermann, 1914, 1, p. 993.
8 Jour. Bacteriol., 1917, 2, p. 218.
9 Jour. Infect. Dis., 1919, 24, p. 386.
10 Die Darmbacterien des Säuglings, 1886.

group. Baermann and Eckersdorf[11] describe a series of cases of croupous enteritis simulating dysentery in which they say streptococci were found and cultured in large numbers from the stools and the intestinal exudate, and were strongly hemolytic on blood plates. Holst[12] describes a family epidemic of enteritis arising from the use of milk from a sick cow. These observations, together with several others of a similar character, suggest that streptococci of the hemolytic variety may at times play a rôle in gastro-intestinal infections, even as primary invaders. However, much of the literature is old and consequently the data are difficult to analyze in the light of more modern methods and conceptions. The problems involved, therefore, in the possible relation of hemolyzing streptococci to pathologic lesions (enteritis, diarrheas, dysenteries, etc.) in the intestinal canal require reinvestigation, and certain work along these lines has already been undertaken and will be reported shortly.

SUMMARY

Hemolytic streptococci do not occur normally in any appreciable numbers in the gastro-intestinal canal of rabbits. When introduced into the stomach of rabbits in large numbers, virulent hemolytic streptococci may occasionally pass through the canal and appear in the feces. Examination of the gastro-intestinal canal at various levels in rabbits thus fed indicates that the hemolytic streptococci do not develop appreciably in the intestines, nor do they readily gain a permanent foothold there. Rabbits with generalized streptococcus infection in joints, blood, etc., showed no hemolytic streptococci in the intestinal contents.

Gastric juice of normal acidity from man and from rabbits kills hemolytic streptococci in from two to five minutes. Gastric juice in achylia may not kill them in several hours.

In normal human feces hemolytic streptococci were not found in 53 cases.

Hemolytic streptococci when mixed with normal human feces will live in the icebox for at least several days. In the incubator they tend to die out rapidly.

[11] München. med. Wchnschr., 1909, 56, p. 1169.
[12] Baumgartens Jahresbericht, 1895, 11, p. 52.

THE INFLUENCE OF BRILLIANT GREEN ON THE DIPHTHERIA BACILLUS

J. A. Kolmer; S. S. Woody, and E. M. Yagle

From the Philadelphia Hospital for Contagious Diseases and the Dermatological Research Laboratories, Philadelphia.

Owing to the widespread distribution and prevalence of diphtheria and the tendency for the bacilli to persist for weeks and months in the tonsils and other tissues of the upper respiratory tract after an attack of the disease, any method promising a practical means for the disinfection of carriers is gratefully but somewhat skeptically received by those particularly interested in this problem.

Our interest in the use of solutions of brilliant green for the disinfection of diphtheria bacilli carriers was stimulated by Browning,[1] who states that the unpublished investigations of Mackie indicate that spraying 1:500-1:250 solutions of brilliant green over the fauces, tonsils and pharynx three times daily for a week, succeeded in eliminating diphtheria bacilli from the throats of chronic carriers whose infections had resisted various other forms of local treatment over periods of many months. Krumwiede and Pratt,[2] during the course of an extensive investigation on the influence of 40 dyes on 30 different pathogenic bacteria, found that dilutions of Grübler's and Bayer's brilliant green in agar as high as 1:500,000 restrained the growth of diphtheria and pseudodiphtheria (diphtheroid) bacilli, although the results were somewhat irregular, owing to the tendency for cultures to produce flakes and the failure of isolated bacilli to grow in plates. As shown by Krumwiede and his associates, brilliant green behaves in a somewhat similar manner as gentian violet toward gram-positive and gram-negative micro-organisms, being more highly bactericidal and antiseptic for the former. The dye has been used with considerable success in the isolation of typhoid bacilli from feces because it exerts an antiseptic influence on many bacteria of the fecal flora in dilutions that have no influence on the typhoid bacillus.

Received for publication Oct. 27, 1919.

[1] Applied Bacteriology, 1918, p. 87.

[2] Jour. Exper. Med., 1914, 19, p. 501.

We have studied the bactericidal activity of brilliant green in different culture mediums on one strain of the diphtheria bacillus (Park-Williams No. 8), with comparative tests employing B. typhosus, B. coli (communis) and Staph. aureus; also the influence of a 1:250 water solution of the dye applied three times daily to the fauces, noses and ears of a number of carriers of virulent and nonvirulent bacilli. The results are summarized in this paper.

THE BACTERICIDAL ACTIVITY OF BRILLIANT GREEN IN VITRO

Grübler's and Bayer's brilliant green were employed; the former occurred in greenish gold crystals readily soluble in water and permitting the preparation of solutions as concentrated as 1:10, the solution having a bright green color. Bayer's dye was of a bluish green color and not quite as soluble in water, 5% solution being near the limit of perfect solubility. The two dyes, however, were about equal in bactericidal activity; differences were slight and usually within the range of experimental error in disinfection tests.

The results of experiments shown in table 1 were conducted as follows: From a 10% stock solution of Grübler's dye in sterile distilled water, 1:100, 1:1000 and 1:10,000 dilutions were prepared with sterile water and distributed as follows in sterile test tubes:

1 c c brilliant green 1:100 + 8 c c glucose broth
1 c c brilliant green 1:1000 + 8 c c glucose broth
1 c c brilliant green 1:10,000 + 8 c c glucose broth
0.2 c c brilliant green 1:10,000 + 8.8 c c glucose broth
9 c c glucose broth (control)

To each tube was added 1 c c of a thoroughly emulsified 24-hour glucose broth culture of the diphtheria bacillus, the final dilutions of dye acting on the bacilli now being 1:1000, 1:10,000, 1:100,000 and 1:500,000. These mixtures were kept at 38 C. in a water bath and subcultured at intervals ranging from 5 minutes to 2 hours by planting several loopfuls on Loeffler's blood serum mediums and incubating for 48 hours.

The same tests were repeated with Hiss serum water glucose medium instead of glucose broth.

The controls always yielded luxuriant growths; the high diphthericidal activity of brilliant green in these tests is shown in table 1.

TABLE 1

THE DIPHTHERICIDAL ACTIVITY OF BRILLIANT GREEN (GRÜBLER)

Menstruum	Time Required for Complete Sterilization			
	1:1,000	1:10,000	1:100,000	1:500,000
Glucose broth..............	Less than 5 minutes	Less than 5 minutes	Less than 5 minutes	2 hours
Hiss serum water glucose...	....	10-20 minutes	More than 2 hours	More than 2 hours
Controls..................	....	Growth	Growth	Growth

The presence of serum in the Hiss medium evidently reduced the diphthericidal activity of the dye as compared with plain glucose broth; further evidence that protein reduces the bactericidal activity of brilliant green is shown in the results of the following experiments with citrated blood serum:

Five c c of human blood aspirated from a vein under aseptic conditions was added to 1 c c of a 10% solution of sodium citrate in salt solution; 1 c c of this citrated blood was mixed in small sterile test tubes with 1 c c of a 1:25,000 dilution of Grübler's dye and the mixture seeded with 0.1 c c of an emulsified 24-hour broth culture of the diphtheria bacillus. Similar mixtures were prepared with sterile unheated human serum and with sterile physiologic salt solution (control). These mixtures were kept at 38 C. in a water bath, and at intervals varying from 1 minute to 4 hours subcultures were made of each by transferring several loopfuls to Loeffler's medium.

Similar tests were conducted with 24-hour broth cultures of B. coli and Staph. aureus; the results are summarized in table 2.

TABLE 2

THE BACTERICIDAL ACTIVITY OF 1:50,000 SOLUTIONS OF BRILLIANT GREEN (GRÜBLER)

Organisms	Time Required for Sterilization		
	In 50% Citrated Blood	In 50% Serum	In Salt Solution
B. diphtheriae	Not in 4 hours	4 hours	15 minutes
B. coli	Not in 4 hours	Not in 4 hours	Not in 4 hours
Staphylococcus aureus	Not in 4 hours	Not in 4 hours	15 minutes
Controls	Growth	Growth	Growth

While the dye in final dilutions of 1:50,000 proved completely bactericidal in 15 minutes for diphtheria bacilli and staphylococci in a menstruum of salt solution, sterilization was incomplete after 4 hours in the menstruum of blood and serum. The relatively low bactericidal activity of brilliant green for a gram-negative bacillus (B. coli) was well shown in these experiments.

Additional experiments were made with cultures of B. diphtheriae, B. typhosus, B. coli and Staph. aureus as follows: dilutions of Grübler's brilliant green varying from 1:1000 to 1:100,000 were prepared with sterile water and distributed in amounts varying from 0.1 to 0.8 c c in sterile test tubes; to each tube was added sufficient culture medium to bring the total volume to exactly 5 c c. Two mediums were employed, namely, Hiss serum water glucose and plain glucose broth; before adding the medium to the tubes containing the dye, each 100 c c was seeded with 1 c c of a 24-hour broth culture of the test micro-organism. The final dilutions of dye acting on this number of each micro-organism was readily calculated and the ease of manipulation rendered the technic particularly serviceable. Controls were included in which sterile salt solution replaced the dye.

All tubes were observed daily for a period of 5 days and then subcultured by transferring several loopfuls to Loeffler's medium. When the mediums remained clear and the subcultures proved sterile, the results were recorded as showing the bactericidal activity of brilliant green for the various micro-organisms; when the mediums remained clear over the period of 5 days but the subcultures proved positive, the results were recorded as showing the restraining, antiseptic or bacteriostatic activity of the dye.

Table 3 shows the highest dilutions of each of these two dyes proving bactericidal for the 4 micro-organisms in the 2 culture mediums; table 4 shows the highest dilutions proving bacteriostatic at the end of 5 days.

TABLE 3

THE BACTERICIDAL ACTIVITY OF BRILLIANT GREEN

Organisms	Grúbler's Dye		Bayer's Dye	
	Hiss Serum Water	Glucose Broth	Hiss Serum Water	Glucose Broth
B. diphtheriae.............	1:125,000	1:625,000	1:125,000	1:500,000
B. typhosus................	Not in 1:6,250	1:6,250	Not in 1:6,250	1:6,250
B. coli......................	1:6,250	1:6,250	Not in 1:6,250	1:6,250
Staphylococcus aureus.....	1:50,000	1:250,000	1:16,000	1:125,000
Controls....................	Growth	Growth	Growth	Growth

TABLE 4

THE BABTERIOSTATIC ACTIVITY OF BRILLIANT GREEN

Organisms	Grúbler's Dye		Bayer's Dye	
	Hiss Serum Water	Glucose Broth	Hiss Serum Water	Glucose Broth
B. diphtheriae.............	1:160,000	1:820,000	1:160,000	1:820,000
B. typhosus................	Not in 1:6,250	1:160,000	Not in 1:6,250	1:125,000
B. coli......................	1:8,200	1:12,000	Not in 1:6,250	1:8,200
Staphylococcus aureus.....	1:60,000	1:300,000	1:25,000	1:160,000

As shown in these tables, both dyes exhibited high degrees of bactericidal and bacteriostatic activity for the two gram-positive micro-organisms, namely, B. diphtheria and Staph. aureus and particularly in plain glucose broth; bactericidal and bacteriostatic activity for the cultures of typhoid and colon bacilli were very much less, both dyes being, however, more bactericidal and antiseptic for colon than for typhoid bacilli.

Additional experiments were made with Grübler's brilliant green in agar prepared and standardized after the method described by Krumwiede, Kohn, Kuttner and Schumm.[3] A stock 0.1% of the dye in sterile distilled water was used in amounts of 0.2, 0.3 and 0.5 c c added to 10 c c of the agar medium at 40 C.; the four test micro-organisms were cultivated in broth for 24 hours, thoroughly shaken and filtered through sterile paper. Each culture was employed in doses of 0.05, 0.1, 0.2 and 0.5 c c of varying dilutions placed in sterile petri dishes and poured with the brilliant green agar. Controls of each micro-organism were included, and always showed heavy growths. Each plate was examined after 24 and 48 hours' incubation. The results observed with 0.1 c c of 1:50 dilutions of B. diphtheria and Staph. aureus, 1:200 dilution of B. coli and 1:500 of B. typhosus, are given in table 5.

[3] Jour. Infect. Dis., 1918, 23, p. 275.

TABLE 5

THE BACTERICIDAL ACTIVITY OF BRILLIANT GREEN (GRÜBLER'S) IN AGAR PLATES AFTER 48 HOURS INCUBATION

Culture	0.1 c c of Dilution of Culture Plate for Each	Number of Colonies in 1 c c of Diluted Culture			
		With 0.2 c c of 0.1 % Stock Solution of Dye	With 0.3 c c of 0.1 % Stock Solution of Dye	With 0.5 c c of 0.1 % Stock Solution of Dye	No Dye
B. diphtheriae..........	1:50	None	None	None	Uncountable
B. typhosus............	1:500	Uncountable	Uncountable	Uncountable	Uncountable
B. coli..................	1:200	Uncountable	Uncountable	720	Uncountable
Staphylococcus aureus	1:50	None	None	None	Uncountable

As shown in table 5, brilliant green proved highly bactericidal for B. diphtheriae and Staph. aureus and much less bactericidal for B. typhosus and B. coli, but more for the latter than the former.

THE TREATMENT OF DIPHTHERIA CARRIERS WITH BRILLIANT GREEN *

A 1:250 solution of Grübler's brilliant green in distilled water was sprayed three times daily over the fauces of 22 persons and into the noses of 17 persons carrying diphtheria bacilli for 2 weeks or longer after recovery from faucial and nasal diphtheria; the solution was also instilled into the ears of 10 persons with chronic or subacute otitis media showing the presence of diphtheroid bacilli in the discharges. The dye proved nonirritating and nontoxic.

Our plan was to take cultures from each person in the morning, followed by three treatments during the day.

The results may be said to have been negative; frequently and indeed usually, treatment of throat, nose and ear carriers for from 1-3 days resulted in the disappearance of diphtheria and pseudodiphtheria bacilli, but never permanently. By keeping persons under observation for from 1-2 weeks and stopping the treatments with dye after the first negative culture, it was found that the cultures may remain negative for varying periods up to 10 days, followed by the reappearance of the bacilli in the cultures. Very probably brilliant green in the concentration employed exerted some diphthericidal effect, but its potency was reduced by the presence of protein material in the discharges, failure to penetrate the follicles of the tonsils and the difficulty of applying the solution in a thorough manner to the nasal chambers,

* We are indebted to Dr. R. L. Works for aid in this part of the investigation.

nasopharynx and pharynx of children. Since brilliant green also possesses a high degree of bactericidal activity for gram-positive cocci, such as staphylococci, streptococci and pneumococci, its use for local application in diphtheria and tonsillitis due to the cocci mentioned above, may prove of value and is certainly worthy of clinical trial.

CONCLUSIONS

Brilliant green has been found highly bactericidal and antiseptic for a virulent diphtheria bacillus in vitro; the presence of blood and serum in the medium reduced the bactericidal activity.

The dye was found also highly bactericidal and antiseptic for staphylococci.

Brilliant green possesses much less bactericidal and antiseptic activity for B. typhosus and B. coli, particularly for the former.

The use of brilliant green in the treatment of carriers of diphtheria and pseudodiphtheria bacilli usually resulted in the temporary disappearance of these bacilli from the noses, throats and ears of the treated persons; permanent ridding of these tissues of the bacilli, however, was not observed.

Owing to the high bactericidal activity of brilliant green for B. diphtheriae and such pathogenic cocci as staphylococci, streptococci and pneumococci, it is probable that the clinical use of a 1:250 solution of the drug in water may prove of value in the local treatment of infections caused by these organisms.

STATISTICS OF THE 1918 EPIDEMIC OF INFLUENZA IN CONNECTICUT

WITH A CONSIDERATION OF THE FACTORS WHICH INFLUENCED THE PREVALENCE OF THIS DISEASE IN VARIOUS COMMUNITIES

C.-E. A. WINSLOW AND J. F. ROGERS

From the Department of Public Health, Yale School of Medicine, New Haven, Conn.

GENERAL HISTORY OF THE EPIDEMIC IN CONNECTICUT

According to the information courteously furnished to us by Dr. T. E. Reeks, epidemiologist of the State Department of Health:

"Influenza first appeared as an epidemic in Connecticut in New London, in the eastern part of the State, on or about September 1, 1918, when several cases of the disease were reported by the naval hospital at New London. These cases came primarily from the Experimental Station and Fort Trumbull where vessels from foreign ports had discharged patients. Within a day or two several cases were brought to the hospital from the submarine base located two miles above New London. About one hundred cases were sent to the New London naval hospital within the first ten days of September.

"On September 9, three cases were reported among the civilian population adjoining Fort Trumbull all of which were among employees in the Fort, and from September 12 on, a large number of cases were reported, particularly from the government station on the State pier where three hundred men from the Boston Navy Yard arrived on September 10. Nearly seven thousand of the naval men in the New London District were boarded in civilian homes, and the disease became generally prevalent among the civilians before the end of the month. The total number of cases (civilian) reported in New London for September was 901; in October, 936. No statistical data were furnished by the naval department after the first few cases.

"While the disease was primarily introduced into New London by ships arriving there from abroad and by men from the Boston Navy Yard, numerous foci developed in different parts of the State about the middle of September, the source of which was traced to other military establishments, principally Camp Devens, Mass.

"The towns early affected and in which a definite history was obtained of the disease developing two or three days following visits of soldiers from Camp Devens include Wallingford, Willimantic, Hartland, Rockville and Danbury. The wave of the infection in Connecticut was from east to west, reaching its peak in the eastern section about October 4, in the central section October 15, and in the western part of the State about October 24. These dates are based on morbidity and mortality reports from the various counties. The towns early infected by visitors from military establishments passed the climax sooner than the surrounding towns."

Received for publication Oct. 21, 1919.

The general story of the epidemic is clearly told in tables 1, 2 and 3, the data for which were obtained for us from the records of the State Department of Health through the courtesy of Mr. J. P. Balfe, Director of the Bureau of Vital Statistics of the Department. The rates, as calculated in table 2, have been presented in graphic form in figure 1. It will be noted that the increase in the death rate first became noticeable in the week ending September 21; that it rose to its height in the weeks ending October 19 and October 26, and then fell rapidly to a value only a little above normal in the week ending November 23. There were slight secondary rises in December and again in January, while by February the effects of the epidemic had entirely disappeared.

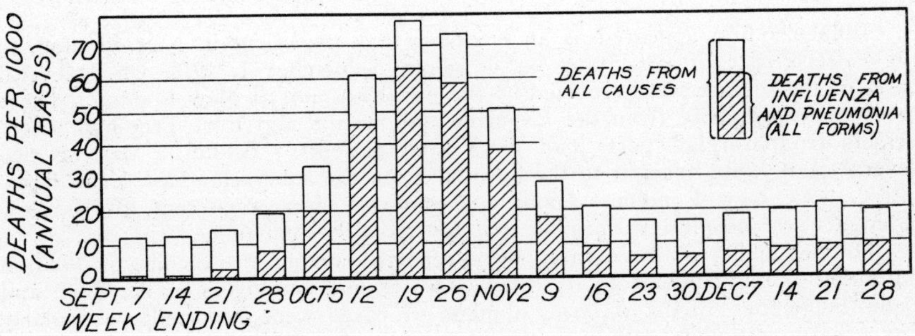

Fig. 1.—Weekly death rates in Connecticut, September to December, 1918.

EXTENT OF THE EPIDEMIC

The influenza epidemic of 1918 was by far the most serious outbreak of communicable disease from which the State of Connecticut has suffered since the beginning of its accurately recorded sanitary history. The annual death rate reported by the State Department of Health has reached 19 per 1,000 only four times since 1848. The two highest annual rates on record are both rates of 19.4 per 1,000, and these two rates are for the influenza epidemic years of 1892 and 1918.

The normal general death rate was, however, several points higher thirty years ago than today, so that the effect of the recent influenza epidemic was much more serious than was that of its predecessor during any single year.

The deaths actually reported as due to influenza and pneumonia (all forms) showed the following fluctuations during the winter months of 1918-1919.

TABLE 1

DEATHS FROM INFLUENZA AND PNEUMONIA

September, 1918	445
October, 1918	5,813
November, 1918	1,297
December, 1918	1,063
January, 1919	987
February, 1919	526

This table would indicate an excess of somewhat less than 7,000 deaths from influenza and pneumonia during the four epidemic months; although it is very difficult to make any estimate of this kind on account of the wide variations in pneumonia rates from year to year. Furthermore, the fact that statements of the cause of death are hastily entered during a severe epidemic makes an analysis based on such data necessarily incomplete.

TABLE 2

DEATHS FROM ALL CAUSES BY SEX AND WEEKS FROM SEPT. 1 TO DEC. 28, 1918, WITH DEATH RATE

Week Ending	Deaths from All Causes				Deaths from Influenza and Pneumonia			
	Male	Female	Total	Death Rate†	Male	Female	Total	Death Rate†
Sept. 7	178	154	332	12.2	10	5	15	0.5
14	181	162	343	12.6	12	6	18	0.6
21	221	171	392	14.4	42	20	62	2.2
28	310	222	532	19.6	149	79	228	8.4
Oct. 5	515	396	912*	33.6	324	223	547	20.1
12	914	742	1,656	61.0	709	544	1,253	46.1
19	1,176	929	2,105	77.5	979	735	1,714	63.1
26	1,075	915	1,990	73.3	858	746	1,604	59.1
Nov. 2	735	650	1,386*	51.0	557	489	1,046	38.5
9	410	363	774*	28.5	262	224	486	17.9
16	286	285	571	21.0	121	125	246	9.0
23	256	196	452	16.6	90	76	166	6.1
30	243	212	455	16.7	92	78	170	6.2
Dec. 7	258	239	497	18.3	82	110	192	7.0
14	280	252	532	19.6	122	102	224	8.2
21	332	260	592	21.8	137	119	256	9.4
28	290	247	537	19.7	142	119	261	9.6
	7,660	6,395	14,058	30.4	4,688	3,800	8,488	18.39

* 3 sex unknown.
† Death rates figured on annual basis.
1918—State population 1,410,665.

In an outbreak of such extraordinary proportions as this one, by far the safest measure of its actual extent is the death rate from all causes, compared with a reasonable norm, and for this purpose we have used the average of corresponding months for the five preceding years. Through the courtesy of Mr. J. P. Balfe, Chief of the Bureau of Vital

Statistics of the State Department of Health, we have obtained the complete data presented in table 3 for deaths and death rates from all causes by months from January, 1885, to February, 1919, inclusive. It will be noted from this table and from figure 2 that the monthly death rate for October, 1918, reached the enormous figure of 63.9 deaths per annum per 1,000 population, a figure more than double the highest figure recorded in the earlier epidemic, a rate of 30.6 for January, 1892. It should be noted, however, that there were rates of 27.2 for January, 1890, and of 27.6 for December, 1891, so that the total death rate from the 1890-1892 influenza was greater than that which has so far resulted from the present outbreak. For a single month, however, the death toll of last October was absolutely unprecedented.

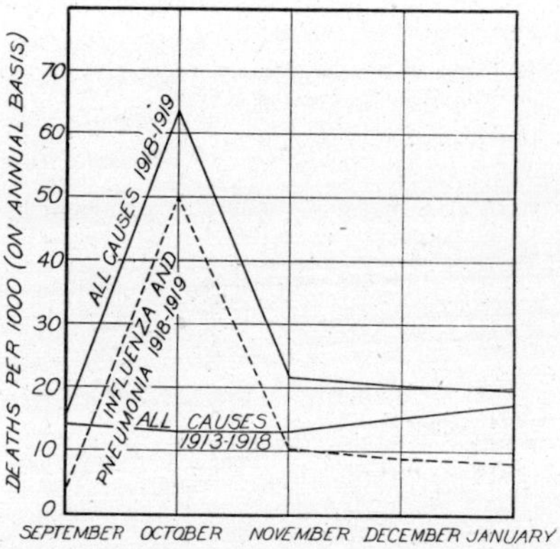

Fig. 3.—Monthly death rates in the state of Connecticut.

It will be noted from table 3 that the death rate for September, 1918, was a fairly normal one and that by February, 1919, the rate had again returned to a reasonably low figure. The death rate for October exceeded the October average for the five previous years by 51 points (see table 4), that for November exceeded its corresponding average by about 9 points, that for December exceeded its corresponding average by 5 points, and that for January its corresponding average by 2 points, a total of 67 points,—corresponding (since these are monthly death rates figured on an annual basis) to over 5.5 points for the year, indicating that the epidemic actually cost the state over 5.5 lives per 1,000 population, or over 7,700 lives.

TABLE 3

Deaths from All Causes by Months, and Monthly Death Rates from 1885 to 1919, Inclusive

Year	Estimated Population	January		February		March		April		May		June		July		August		September		October		November		December		Total Deaths	Yearly Death Rate
		Deaths	Rate	Deaths	Rate	Deaths	Rate	Deaths	Rate	Deaths	Rate	Deaths	Rate	Deaths	Rate	Deaths	Rate	Deaths	Rate	Deaths	Rate	Deaths	Rate	Deaths	Rate		
1885	684,478	945	16.6	988	17.3	1,222	21.4	1,173	20.6	998	17.5	833	14.6	1,276	22.4	1,156	20.3	887	15.5	847	14.8	842	14.7	841	14.7	12,008	17.5
1886	696,835	906	15.1	980	16.3	1.090	18.2	1,083	18.2	907	15.2	835	14.0	1,120	18.8	1,240	20.8	1,000	16.7	995	16.6	903	15.1	968	16.1	12,027	17.2
1887	709,192	942	15.5	880	14.4	1.067	17.6	1,036	17.1	930	15.3	920	15.2	1,688	27.8	1,386	22.8	1.094	18.0	933	15.2	844	13.8	966	15.9	12,686	17.9
1888	729,538	1,100	17.4	1,170	18.5	1,281	21.1	1,196	19.6	1,040	17.2	876	14.3	1,235	20.3	1,525	25.4	1,118	18.3	1,033	12.0	915	15.0	1,003	16.4	13,512	18.5
1889	733,906	912	14.9	956	15.6	1,076	17.5	1,101	18.0	957	15.6	946	15.4	1,367	22.3	1,204	19.6	1,074	17.5	1,053	17.2	917	14.9	965	15.7	12,529	17.1
1890	746,258	1,693	27.2	1,107	17.8	1,119	17.9	1,124	18.0	1,005	16.1	934	15.0	1,337	21.4	1,328	21.3	1,031	16.5	1,037	16.6	957	15.3	993	15.9	13,665	18.3
1891	762,468	1,005	15.8	975	15.3	1,147	18.0	1,285	20.2	1,196	18.8	1,000	15.7	1,335	21.0	1,296	20.3	1,131	17.8	1,143	17.9	1,118	17.5	1,754	27.6	14,385	18.8
1892	778,678	1.986	30.6	1,316	20.2	1,313	20.2	1,159	17.8	1,175	18.1	929	14.3	1,506	23.2	1,440	22.1	1,102	16.9	1,141	17.5	1,037	15.9	1,062	16.3	15,170	19.4
1893	794,888	1,298	19.5	1,149	17.3	1,333	20.1	1,418	21.4	1,245	18.7	1,005	15.1	1,396	21.0	1,468	22.1	1,081	16.3	1,098	16.5	1,054	15.9	1,353	20.4	14,901	18.7
1894	811,098	1,407	20.8	1,088	16.0	1,017	15.0	1,123	16.6	1,002	14.8	1,021	15.1	1,455	21.5	1,335	19.7	1,199	17.7	1,016	15.0	967	14.3	1,067	15.7	13,699	16.8
1895	827,308	1,059	15.3	1,380	20.0	1,443	20.9	1,220	17.6	1,122	16.2	986	14.3	1,320	19.1	1,387	20.1	1,251	18.1	1,192	17.2	1,053	15.2	1,131	16.4	14,546	17.5
1896	843,518	1,129	16.0	1,114	15.8	1,293	18.3.	1,230	17.4	1,121	15.9	1,642	23.3	1,642	23.3	1,675	23.8	1,225	17.4	1,121	16.0	1,015	14.4	1,159	16.4	15,025	17.8
1897	859,728	1,142	15.9	1,173	16.3	1,393	19.4	1,219	17.0	1,138	15.8	998	13.9	1,223	17.0	1,239	17.2	1,146	15.9	1,097	15.3	1.054	14.7	1.090	15.2	13,915	16.1
1898	875,938	1,159	15.8	1,035	14.1	1,280	17.5	1,197	16.4	1,139	15.6	983	13.4	1,230	16.8	1,407	19.2	1,355	18.4	1,123	15.3	1,029	14.0	1,231	16.8	14,170	16.1
1899	892,148	1,577	21.2	1,197	16.1	1,229	16.5	1,175	15.8	1,031	13.8	1.053	14.1	1,374	18.4	1,387	18.6	1,145	15.4	1,040	13.9	990	13.3	1,174	15.7	14.381	16.1
1900	908,355	1,367	18.2	1,265	16.7	1,698	22.4	1,684	22.2	1,231	16.2	1,126	14.8	1,587	20.9	1,652	21.8	1,291	17.0	1,210	15.9	1,100	14.5	1,140	13.0	16,368	18.0
1901	929,430	1,456	18.7	1,387	17.9	1,444	18.6	1,261	16.2	1,067	13.7	1,032	13.3	1,304	16.8	1,319	17.0	1,239	15.9	1,065	13.7	1,113	14.4	1,149	14.8	14,852	15.9
1902	950,506	1,182	14.9	1,128	14.2	1,251	15.7	1,195	15.0	1,100	13.8	1,065	13.4	1,407	17.7	1,349	17.0	1,165	14.7	1,138	14.3	1,089	13.7	1,301	16.4	14,386	15.1
1903	971,581	1,427	17.6	1,304	16.1	1,423	17.5	1,261	15.5	1,268	15.6	1,166	14.4	1,416	17.4	1,406	17.3	1,165	14.3	1,126	13.9	1,172	14.4	1,350	16.6	15,490	15.9
1904	992,657	1,445	17.4	1,387	16.7	1,524	18.4	1,377	16.6	1,317	15.9	1,127	13.6	1,407	17.0	1,365	16.5	1,163	14.0	1,165	14.0	1.162	14.0	1,262	15.2	15,711	15.8
1905	1,013,732	1,412	16.7	1,367	16.3	1,576	18.6	1,329	15.7	1,300	15.5	1,289	15.2	1,653	19.5	1,416	16.7	1,200	14.2	1,166	13.8	1,258	14.8	1,322	15.6	16,298	16.0
1906	1,034,808	1,344	15.5	1,236	14.3	1,489	17.2	1,430	16.5	1,403	16.2	1,248	14.4	1,538	17.8	1,649	19.1	1,341	15.5	1,288	14.9	1,296	15.0	1,486	17.2	16,766	16.2
1907	1,055,883	1,696	19.2	1,519	17.2	1,578	17.9	1,419	16.1	1,329	15.1	1,226	13.9	1,518	17.2	1,761	20.0	1,409	16.0	1,335	15.1	1,244	14.1	1,450	16.4	17,490	16.5
1908	1,076,959	1,557	17.3	1,515	16.8	1,456	16.2	1,330	14.8	1,204	13.4	1,146	12.7	1,496	16.6	1,410	15.7	1,240	13.8	1,215	13.5	1,144	12.7	1,280	14.2	16,000	14.8
1909	1,098,034	1,367	14.9	1,313	14.3	1,575	17.2	1,508	16.4	1,332	14.5	1,214	13.2	1,416	15.4	1,492	16.3	1,293	14.1	1,237	13.5	1,266	13.8	1,467	16.0	16,484	15.0
1910	1,119,110	1,498	16.0	1,421	15.2	1,632	17.4	1,505	16.1	1,421	15.2	1,266	13.5	1,735	18.6	1,426	15.2	1,387	14.8	1,381	14.8	1,252	13.4	1,575	16.8	17,500	15.6
1911	1,140,004	1,760	18.5	1,556	16.3	1,692	17.8	1,679	17.6	1,435	15.1	1,175	12.3	1,635	17.2	1,449	15.2	1,284	13.5	1,345	14.1	1,196	12.5	1,348	14.1	17,554	15.3
1912	1,160,898	1,600	16.5	1,567	16.1	1,681	17.8	1,428	14.7	1,406	14.5	1,213	12.5	1,454	15.0	1,433	14.8	1,391	14.3	1,397	14.4	1,256	12.9	1,489	15.3	17,315	14.9
1913	1,181,793	1,614	16.3	1,547	15.7	1,704	17.3	1,507	15.3	1,424	14.4	1,408	14.2	1,498	15.1	1,535	15.5	1,422	14.4	1,239	12.5	1,275	12.9	1,549	15.7	17,722	14.9
1914	1,202,688	1,671	16.6	1,623	16.1	1,845	18.4	1,650	16.4	1,509	15.0	1,233	12.3	1,440	14.3	1,596	15.9	1,526	15.2	1,323	13.1	1,321	13.1	1,474	14.7	18,211	15.1
1915	1,241,314	1,502	14.5	1,450	14.0	1,783	17.2	1,720	16.6	1,411	13.6	1,290	12.4	1,499	14.4	1,569	15.1	1,479	14.2	1,388	13.4	1,327	12.8	1,615	15.6	18,033	14.5
1916	1,291,989	2.170	20.1	1,769	16.4	1,773	16.4	1,765	16.3	1,664	15.4	1,473	13.6	1,555	14.4	1,685	15.6	1,507	13.9	1,409	13.0	1,534	14.2	1,839	17.0	20,142	15.5
1917	1,354,930	2,305	20.4	1,818	16.1	1,994	17.6	1,822	16.1	1,820	16.1	1,496	13.2	1,553	13.7	1,792	15.8	1,585	14.0	1,517	13.4	1,459	12.9	1,610	14.2	20,746	15.3
1918	1,410,665	1,877	15.9	1,717	14.6	2,010	17.0	1,834	15.6	1,489	12.6	1,273	10.8	1,418	12.0	1,431	12.1	1,818	15.4	7,516	63.9	2,566	21.8	2,421	20.5	27,378	19.4
1919	1,464,360	2,425	19.8	1,766	14.4																						

1885–1914 inclusive, population figured on U. S. census method.

1915–1919 inclusive, population figured on school population.

TABLE 4

DEATH RATES, 1913 TO 1918

	Average Death Rate from All Causes*		Excess for 1918-19	Death Rate from Influenza and Pneumonia* 1918-1919
	1913-1918	1918-1919		
September	14.3	15.4	1.1	3.7
October	13.1	63.9	50.8	50.0
November	13.2	21.8	8.6	10.4
December	15.4	20.5	5.1	9.0
January	17.5	19.8	2.3	8.4

* Death rates per 1,000 population on an annual basis.

These cold figures present but a faint picture of the actual extent of the tragedy. We must go back to records of bubonic plague to find a parallel for the conditions which existed in many Connecticut communities during the height of the epidemic. Emergency hospitals were improvised, 35 of them being established, supervised or assisted by the State Department of Health, and 100 nurses and 48 physicians, largely supplied by the U. S. Public Health Service, were sent to the places in greatest need. Yet as physicians and nurses were themselves stricken down by the epidemic, the lack of medical and nursing care was in many cases acute. Many persons died without any medical attention, and there were not a few instances of whole families being wiped out within a few days. In the cities most severely affected the great problem came to be the burial of the dead. At Waterbury and New Britain, for example, coffins remained for days on the ground, until in the latter case the mayor assigned the engineering force of the city to the task of digging graves.

MORBIDITY AND FATALITY RATES

Influenza was declared a reportable disease by the State Department of Health in New London on September 12 and throughout the State on September 18. The reporting was of course, however, exceedingly incomplete in face of the tremendous emergency faced by physicians during the epidemic. The actual number of cases of influenza and pneumonia (all forms) reported by months with the corresponding deaths and fatality rates are indicated in table 5.

The fatality figures are, of course, extravagantly high, due to incomplete case reports, particularly during the last three months.

A somewhat better idea of actual conditions may be gained from the excellent records of the Visiting Nurse Association of New Haven, courteously placed at our disposal by Miss Mary G. Hills, the superintendent of the Association, and analyzed by Mr. David Greenberg, instructor in the department of public health of the Yale School of Medicine. Seven hundred and thirty-six cases of influenza and pneumonia were cared for during the epidemic with 32 known deaths, giving a fatality rate of 4.3 deaths per 100 cases. Even this rate is certainly too high, since many light cases failed to receive nursing care.

TABLE 5

REPORTED MORBIDITY AND FATALITY, INFLUENZA AND PNEUMONIA, STATE OF CONNECTICUT

	Reported Cases	Deaths	Deaths per 100 Cases
September, 1918	7,864	432	5
October, 1918	92,698	5,895	6
November, 1918	6,244	1,297	21
December, 1918	8,043	1 063	13
January, 1919	6,804	987	15

The only way in which really complete data can be obtained in regard to morbidity and fatality from influenza is by detailed house to house canvasses, and a number of surveys of this sort were conducted by the State Department of Health. Dr. T. E. Reeks has supplied us with the following information in regard to one such study conducted in New Britain. Between December 3 and 6, 145 dwellings were visited in which there had been 2,757 persons. Of this number, 645 had had influenza and 25 had died. These figures would indicate a morbidity rate of 234 per 1,000 and a fatality rate of 3.9 deaths per 100 cases.

It seems probable that even in this instance the information obtained was incomplete in regard to light cases. Surveys conducted by the New York State Department of Health, reported by G. W. Baker,[1] and other studies made by the U. S. Public Health Service in selected districts of Maryland[2] indicate for a combined population of nearly 80,000 persons, a morbidity rate of 311 per 1,000, a mortality rate of 7.1 per 1,000, and a fatality rate of 2.3 deaths per 100 cases. We may perhaps safely conclude that the proportion of the population actually affected by the influenza epidemic varied between 200 and 400 per 1,000, and that the actual fatality rate was somewhere between 2 and 4 deaths per 100 cases, the higher morbidity rate and the lower fatality rate being more likely to be correct.

[1] Official Bulletin, New York State Department of Health, May 1, 1919, 4, V. S. No. 5.
[2] Public Health Reports, March 14, 1919.

EPIDEMIOLOGY

The first outstanding fact in regard to the epidemiology of the disease was the tremendous rapidity with which it spread throughout the state. Assuming that the epidemic was limited to the five months of September, 1918, to January, 1919, inclusive, we have calculated for each county the median day of the outbreak; that is, the day on which the first half of the total of reported deaths was reached. For New London County the median day was October 12; for Windham County, October 13; for Tolland County, October 21; for Middlesex and New Haven counties, October 22; for Hartford County, October 23, and for Fairfield and Litchfield counties, October 29 (Fig. 4).

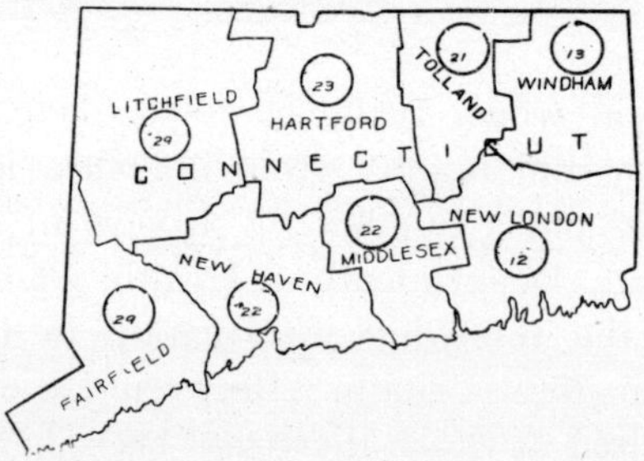

Fig. 4.—Median day of influenza epidemic in each county of Connecticut. Figures represent dates in October.

The outbreak, starting in the southeastern region of the state, passed north and then west, reaching its crest in New Haven and Hartford about ten days later than in New London, and in Fairfield County about a week later than in New Haven.

It seems very clear that a disease which spreads throughout a whole state within one month and ultimately affects from 20 to 40% of its population, must be a communicable disease of an exceedingly acute and readily transmissible type. One condition and one condition only temporarily checked the spread of the infection — complete institutional quarantine. There were many instances in Connecticut of schools, asylums, prisons and other institutions which maintained absolute quarantine and escaped infection, while it was raging all about them, — in every instance, so far as we are aware, to experience a normal incidence at a later date when the quarantine was lifted or accidentally broken.

One excellent illustration was furnished by an orphan asylum in New Haven, which completely escaped during the month of October when the epidemic was at its height in the city. One of the sisters and the priest in charge came down with influenza about December 15. On December 27, 127 cases occurred in the institution within 24 hours, and by January 7 there had been 424 cases with 7 deaths out of a total population of 464 persons. The most probable source of the sharp outbreak on December 27 seemed to be the sister first affected, who, on convalescence, resumed her duties in the kitchen, which included the inspection and handling of the milk served to the children.

This particular institutional outbreak might well have been due to food infection or transmission by eating utensils such as has been described in army camps by Drs. Lynch and Cumming.[3] In general, however, it seems clear that neither food nor insect transmission, under the general sanitary conditions of American life, can account for the spread of an epidemic on such a scale and at such a rate as that which characterized the influenza epidemic of October, 1918, as a whole. Direct contact transmission must certainly be looked on as the chief agent in such an outbreak.

The rapidity of the spread of the infection would also suggest an exceedingly short period of incubation, and we have ample evidence in individual cases that the incubation period for this disease is ordinarily close to 48 hours.

Further conclusions in regard to epidemiology can be formulated with much less certainty. In observing the spread of the disease through local population groups, we were at first inclined to believe that the usual source of infection was an early case, generally recognizable as suffering from some sort of respiratory infection. If this conclusion were justified, the problem, as in the case of measles, would be to isolate all contacts exhibiting any abnormal conditions; and control, though difficult, would not be impossible. Later experience has raised doubts as to the possible part played by convalescents and well carriers. In the case of the orphan asylum cited above, for example, the original infection appeared to come from a convalescent rather than an early case. Until we are certain as to the part played by well carriers, by incipient cases, by frank cases, and by convalescents, as sources, and until we can gauge the relative importance of mouth spray, hand contact, fomites, food and other possible vehicles of infection, it will be extremely difficult to formulate an intelligent policy of control. In any case, as we shall point out below in connection with the variations in the local incidence of the disease, there is no evidence that any method of control except absolute institutional quarantine had any influence upon its spread in the state of Connecticut.

[6] Amer. Jour. of Public Health, 1919, 9, p. 25.

AGE AND SEX AS PREDISPOSING FACTORS IN THE EPIDEMIC

One of the most striking features of the 1918 epidemic of influenza was the characteristic age incidence of the disease. All over the world, so far as we have seen reports of the outbreak, it displayed a marked predilection for the years of young adult life and passed lightly by the later age periods.

On account of the long period which has elapsed since the census of 1910, there are no accurate data available for the calculation of actual death rates on a large scale. The general age incidence of the epidemic can be easily brought out, however, by the calculation of ratios; and for this purpose we obtained from Mr. Balfe the number of deaths from all causes and from influenza and pneumonia classified by months for the four last months of 1918, and to furnish a basis of

TABLE 6

TOTAL NUMBER OF DEATHS FOR EACH MONTH

	Deaths from All Causes		Deaths from Influenza and Pneumonia
	1917	1918	1918
September	1,585	1,818	445
October	1,517	7,516	5,813
November	1,459	2,566	1,297
December	1,442	2,158	933

TABLE 7

PERCENTAGE OF DEATHS OCCURRING AT EACH AGE PERIOD

	Age											
	—1	1-4	5-9	10-14	15-19	20-24	25-29	-30-39	40-49	50-59	60-69	70+
All Causes 1917:												
September	23	9	2	1	2	3	3	8	8	10	13	18
October	18	6	2	2	2	3	2	9	10	11	15	20
November	15	5	2	1	1	4	4	7	11	13	14	23
December	16	7	3	1	2	3	4	7	9	11	14	23
Average	18	7	2	1	2	3	3	8	10	11	14	21
All Causes 1918:												
September	19	6	2	2	3	5	7	11	10	9	10	16
October	8	9	3	2	5	10	16	23	9	5	5	5
November	12	8	3	2	3	6	11	17	9	9	7	13
December	12	6	3	2	3	5	9	15	9	9	11	16
Average	11	8	3	2	4	8	13	19	9	7	6	10
Influenza and Pneumonia, 1918:												
September	6	6	2	2	5	12	19	26	10	5	4	3
October	5	10	3	2	5	12	19	27	9	4	2	1
November	7	12	3	3	4	10	18	25	8	5	3	3
December	8	7	3	3	5	8	15	24	9	6	5	6
Average	6	10	3	3	5	11	19	26	9	4	3	2

comparison, the deaths from all causes for the corresponding months of 1917. The total number of deaths for each month used in this analysis are presented in table 6, and the percentage distribution by age periods in table 7.

The four last months of 1917 show a normal age distribution, with one quarter of all deaths occurring under 5 years of age, one quarter between 5 and 40 years, and half over 40 years, the proportion of infant deaths decreasing and the proportion of deaths in old age increasing as one passes from the season of intestinal disturbances to the season of respiratory diseases.

In 1918 the distribution of deaths from all causes is strikingly different. Instead of less than a quarter of all deaths occurring between the ages of 5 and 40 years, this period included 49% of all deaths in 1918; and the two decades between 20 and 40 included 40% of all deaths (as against only 14% in 1917).

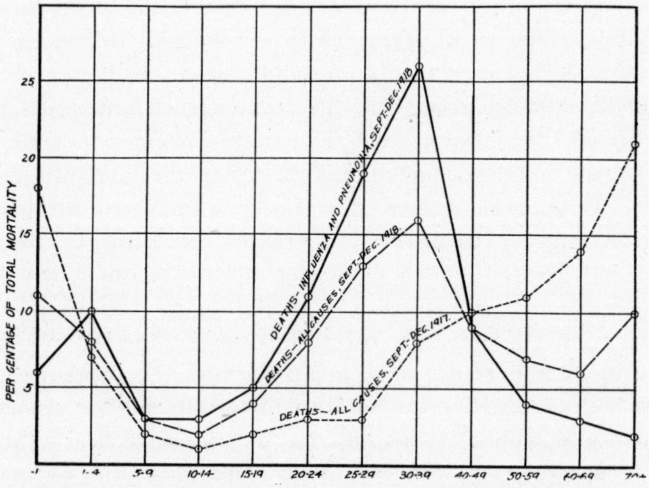

Fig. 5.—Age distribution of deaths from the influenza epidemic compared with normal.

Considering influenza and pneumonia alone, these two decades included 56% of the deaths, while only 9% occurred at ages over 49. The decade between 20 and 29 was most severely affected, including 30% of all deaths, while the decade between 30 and 39 was a close second with 26%.

An even higher incidence occurred at ages under 5 years, as has been brought out in other investigations,[4] since this age period con-

[4] Notably the summary presented by G. W. Baker, Official Bull., N. Y. State Depart. of Health, Vol. 4, V. S. No. 5.

tributed 16% of all the influenza-pneumonia deaths. The proportion of deaths from all causes in infancy did not rise even to normal, but with the enormous rise in total deaths the maintenance of a nearly normal ratio, of course, means a heavy influenza mortality.

Whether the high death rate under 5 years and between 20 and 40 years of age was due to an actually excessive incidence of influenza or merely to a higher fatality can only be determined by house to house surveys, since case reports during the outbreak were almost valueless. Frost[5] reports that a series of such intensive studies indicate that the actual case incidence of the disease was highest at ages 5-14 and uniformly decreased in later age periods.

It has been the tendency of some writers to assume that the relatively low mortality among those past middle life was due to artificial immunity acquired in the preceding epidemic of 1890-92. This seems to us somewhat doubtful. If such acquired immunity were the cause of the age distribution of influenza mortality, the drop should presumably have come at 30 years, while as a matter of fact the rate for the decade 30-40 was practically the same as that for the preceding one.

From the standpoint of sex, the Connecticut figures, as has been the case in other localities, show a distinctly heavier mortality among males. Of the influenza-pneumonia deaths in the last four months of 1918, 58% were among males. Two possible factors in producing such a condition suggest themselves, — greater exposure to the original infection and greater tendency to keep up and about when ill, which is one of the common factors in contributing to serious pneumonias. According to the Baker study referred to above, the latter would seem to be the more important, since in his surveys the incidence rate was alike for both sexes, but the fatality materially higher among males.

Frankel and Dublin[6] point out that an excessive death rate among males is characteristic of pneumonia and that the excess in the influenza-pneumonia of 1918 was rather less than the normal male excess for this disease.

RACE AS A PREDISPOSING FACTOR IN THE EPIDEMIC

The fundamental data presented in table 6 have been analyzed from the standpoint of the mother-nativity of the decedents, and the results are presented below in table 8 and in figure 6.

[5] Public Health Reports for Aug. 15, 1919.
[6] A. J. P. H., 1919 9, 731.

TABLE 8

DISTRIBUTION OF DEATHS BY MOTHER NATIVITY
PERCENTAGE IN EACH GROUP

	Birthplace of Mother											
	U. S.	Ireland	Italy	Russia	Austria	Germany	England	Canada	Poland	Russian Poland	Other Countries	Unknown
All Causes 1917:												
September	33	14	10	6	6	3	3	2	2	2	6	13
October	31	17	8	7	5	5	4	3	1	2	4	13
November	33	17	9	6	5	5	3	2	1	1	5	13
December	32	16	8	5	6	5	3	4	1	1	6	13
Average	32	16	9	6	6	5	3	3	1	1	5	13
All Causes 1918:												
September	32	13	9	8	6	3	3	4	2	2	5	13
October	24	11	18	10	7	3	2	4	2	3	5	11
November	30	13	14	6	7	4	3	2	1	2	6	12
December	36	14	8	6	6	4	3	3	1	1	7	11
Average	28	12	15	8	7	3	2	4	2	2	5	12
Influenza and Pneumonia, 1918												
September	24	9	12	10	7	2	3	7	4	1	7	14
October	21	10	21	11	7	3	2	4	2	3	5	10
November	26	9	20	8	9	3	3	2	2	2	7	9
December	39	12	10	5	8	4	3	3	1	1	8	8
Average	24	10	19	9	8	3	2	4	2	2	6	10

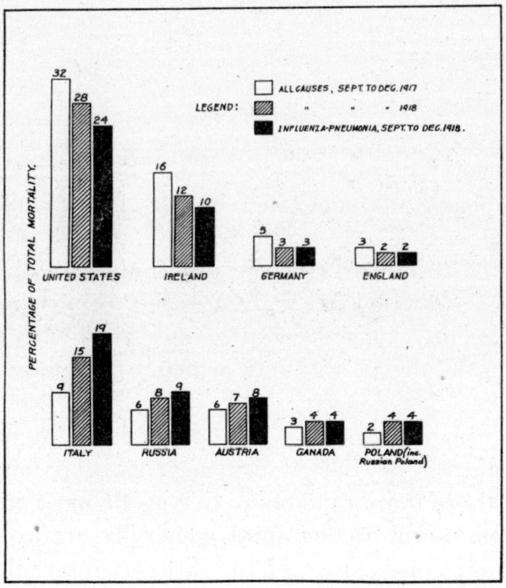

Fig. 6.—Distribution of deaths in Connecticut by mother nativity.

It appears evident that race (or some conditions associated with race) played a very large part in determining the incidence of mortality. The four months of 1917 and September, 1918, show closely concordant distributions by mother nativity; but with the onset of the epidemic marked divergences manifest themselves.

The proportion of influenza-pneumonia deaths is lower than would be expected among persons of native, Irish, English and German stock, higher than would be expected among Russian, Austrian, Canadian and Polish stock, and enormously high among Italians.

TABLE 9

DISTRIBUTION BY NATIVITY OF TOTAL CASES, TUBERCULOSIS CASES AND INFLUENZA CASES CARED FOR BY THE V. N. A. OF NEW HAVEN, SEPTEMBER-NOVEMBER, 1918

Race	Percentage of Total Cases Cared for by V. N. A.	Cases of Influenza		Cases of Tuberculosis	
		Number	Percentage	Number	Percentage
Native	24.3	160	21.8	102	29.6
Native, Austrian parentage	1.6	9	1.2	6	1.7
Native, English-Scotch parentage	0.9	8	1.1	1	1.7
Native, German parentage	0.9	10	1.4	1	0.3
Native, Irish parentage	4.7	20	2.7	48	13.9
Native, Italian parentage	23.3	183	24.9	46	13.3
Native, Russian parentage	12.2	83	11.3	17	4.9
Austrian	1.4	12	1.6	2	0.6
English	1.1	12	1.6	3	0.9
Irish	3.2	18	2.5	18	5.2
Italian	9.5	99	13.5	31	9.0
German	0.8	6	0.8	2	0.6
Russian	9.7	76	10.4	31	9.0
Swedish	0.7	6	0.8	5	1.5
Colored	....	6	0.8	...	....
Unknown	5.7	28	3.5	26	7.6
Total	100.0	736	100.0	345	100.0

It seems probable, as suggested by Dr. L. I. Dublin in personal discussions, that this marked difference in racial incidence is very largely due to the differences in age distribution of the various race-stocks, the races showing the highest ratios being those which have arrived more recently in the country and which are made up more largely of young adults at the ages which suffer most severely from influenza.

In part, too, this relation may be explained on the ground of differing economic status, the race-stocks disproportionately affected with influenza being those that are likely to live in the most crowded quarters of the community and under most generally unfavorable environmental conditions. The excess of the disease among the Italians is so enormous as to seem to call for some special explanation. Dr. D. B.

Armstrong[7] has pointed out an apparent inverse relation between racial susceptibility to chronic and acute respiratory disorders, the Irish suffering heavily from tuberculosis and lightly from influenza and pneumonia, while the reverse is true of the Italians. Our results for the state of Connecticut tend to confirm his conclusions in regard to the Italians, as do the figures presented in table 9 prepared by Mr. David Greenberg from the records of the Visiting Nurse Association of New Haven. It appears that Italy suffered very severely from the influenza epidemic in Europe, and Dublin has shown that the normal pneumonia rate of this race is a very high one.

GENERAL GEOGRAPHICAL VARIATIONS IN THE SEVERITY OF THE EPIDEMIC

In discussing variations in the severity of the epidemic in different parts of the state, we have thought it best to utilize the total death rate from all causes for the months from September to December, 1918,

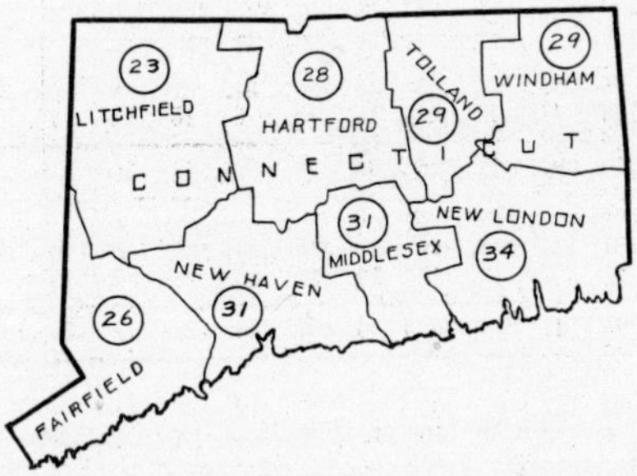

Fig. 7.—Severity of influenza epidemic by counties. Average death rate from all causes, September to December, 1918, on annual basis; deaths per 1,000.

inclusive. Actual variations in influenza-pneumonia are of course somewhat masked by the normal death rate from other causes, but in view of the errors in reporting causes of death we have felt this to be the safest course. Our figures are computed on an annual basis, the total number of deaths per 1,000 of population being multiplied by three (since the period included one third of a year). The rate for the entire state on this basis is 29.

The different counties of the state show slight but significant differences when computed in this manner. The figures are as follows: New London, 34; Middlesex, 31; New Haven, 31; Windham, 29; Tolland, 29; Hartford, 28; Fairfield, 26; Litchfield, 23.

[7] Boston Med. and Surg. Jour., 1919, 180, p. 65.

TABLE 10

DEATHS FROM ALL CAUSES, SEPTEMBER 1 TO DECEMBER 28, BY COUNTIES

	September				October				November					December					
	7	14	21	28	5	12	19	26	2	9	16	23	30	7	14	21	28	Total	Per 1.000
Middlesex:																			
Large towns..	14	9	11	13	22	49	60	46	26	24	20	18	10	15	18	24	15	394	39.4
Small towns..	6	5	5	12	7	13	24	21	9	10	10	2	8	6	9	7	13	167	18.6
Total.......	20	14	16	25	29	62	84	67	35	34	30	20	18	21	27	31	28	561	31.2
Tolland:																			
Large towns..	1	9	5	4	8	19	27	15	12	4	3	2	5	3	4	11	3	135	27.0
Small towns..	7	5	6	3	15	25	21	8	11	10	....	2	3	6	8	10	12	152	30.4
Total.......	8	14	11	7	23	44	48	23	23	14	3	4	8	9	12	21	15	287	28.7
Hartford:																			
Large towns..	66	79	79	105	177	368	502	429	269	132	93	86	93	102	110	109	107	2,906	29.7
Small towns..	8	12	11	12	20	38	46	43	32	22	12	15	8	16	17	13	12	337	19.6
Total.......	74	91	90	117	197	406	548	472	301	154	105	101	101	118	127	122	119	3,243	28.2
New Haven:																			
Large towns..	103	93	98	117	219	530	770	696	470	225	158	123	119	148	149	172	150	4,340	31.4
Small towns..	4	1	6	4	10	21	22	19	21	8	11	7	5	6	10	9	8	172	21.6
Total.......	107	94	104	121	229	551	792	715	491	233	169	130	124	154	159	181	158	4,512	30.8
New London:																			
Large towns..	21	24	47	95	159	157	85	46	26	31	32	28	30	31	26	42	35	915	35.2
Small towns..	14	7	16	24	41	55	41	18	13	8	15	11	11	5	12	8	13	312	31.2
Total.......	35	31	63	119	200	212	126	64	39	39	47	39	41	36	38	50	48	1,227	34.1
Fairfield:																			
Large towns..	62	61	67	84	135	206	316	481	390	234	165	110	116	120	109	124	112	2,892	26.4
Small towns..	6	4	5	11	7	12	17	19	13	10	8	7	10	7	7	5	10	158	17.6
Total.......	68	65	72	95	142	218	333	500	403	244	173	117	126	127	116	129	122	3,050	26.1
Windham:																			
Large towns..	2	7	16	29	57	92	65	33	25	12	13	14	9	5	13	14	16	422	32.4
Small towns..	4	4	2	4	2	13	10	12	7	4	4	4	8	5	6	6	5	100	20.0
Total.......	6	11	18	33	59	105	75	45	32	16	17	18	17	10	19	20	21	522	29.0
Litchfield:																			
Large towns..	9	13	7	9	19	31	77	73	45	28	17	18	12	16	20	22	16	432	25.4
Small towns..	5	10	11	6	14	27	22	31	17	12	10	5	8	6	14	16	10	224	20.4
Total.......	14	23	18	15	33	58	99	104	62	40	27	23	20	22	34	38	26	656	23.4

As indicated by figure 7 (which may be compared with figure 4), it is evident that the outbreak was most severe in the eastern counties where it broke out first, and that it decreased progressively in severity as it passed to the western and northwestern sections of the state.

It would seem probable that there was a gradual decrease either in the communicability of the disease or in its virulence after the great severity which characterized it at the time of its first invasion of New London.

TABLE 11

DEATHS, ALL CAUSES, BY LARGER TOWNS AND BY WEEKS, SEPTEMBER 1 TO DECEMBER 28

Towns	September				October				November					December				Total	Per 1,000
	7	14	21	28	5	12	19	26	2	9	16	28	30	7	14	21	28		
Ansonia	2	1	3	16	21	33	32	16	11	6	...	4	6	1	6	9	10	177	30.6
Berlin	2	1	...	3	...	3	4	5	6	1	1	2	1	1	1	2	2	35	18.4
Branford	2	...	1	1	2	2	6	5	11	10	7	3	2	1	1	1	2	57	23.7
Bridgeport	28	33	28	40	45	78	135	245	232	125	91	61	64	50	51	57	54	1,417	26.2
Bristol	4	4	2	3	7	36	38	33	11	7	4	2	5	4	7	4	2	173	26.2
Danbury	3	10	10	8	18	24	32	42	27	15	9	6	8	13	7	17	5	254	27.0
Darien	1	...	1	...	...	2	2	5	7	2	2	1	...	1	...	5	1	30	10.3
Derby	2	8	9	5	19	52	36	16	13	3	2	5	3	4	4	5	5	191	56.2
East Hartford	...	3	1	5	1	8	7	11	5	3	3	4	2	4	2	3	1	63	16.6
Enfield	2	2	4	3	3	9	20	15	19	6	3	1	4	3	3	6	1	104	25.4
Fairfield	...	1	4	3	2	5	6	10	14	17	5	3	5	3	3	6	1	88	21.4
Glastonbury	1	...	1	...	3	1	3	3	4	3	2	2	2	3	3	...	2	33	15.0
Greenwich	7	1	2	3	12	17	24	38	28	16	8	6	7	7	3	6	9	194	30.8
Groton	1	3	1	7	14	7	13	4	2	3	3	4	6	5	3	4	3	83	31.9
Hamden	1	1	...	3	4	7	9	12	8	6	2	2	2	3	1	2	2	65	19.7
Hartford	37	47	54	71	115	179	253	172	129	74	57	55	50	45	57	63	66	1,524	34.1
Killingly	...	...	3	6	9	15	6	4	4	1	2	5	1	1	1	3	2	63	24.2
Manchester	2	1	4	1	7	17	17	17	8	5	4	2	5	6	2	3	8	109	16.8
Meriden	13	9	10	9	30	100	81	44	26	10	13	14	10	11	10	12	13	415	38.0
Middletown	14	9	11	13	22	49	60	46	26	24	20	18	10	15	18	24	15	394	42.4
Milford	...	4	3	...	1	1	8	4	9	3	1	1	2	2	2	5	3	49	13.2
Naugatuck	6	1	2	2	18	29	37	34	12	1	6	1	3	2	3	1	6	164	35.7
New Britain	12	9	11	13	32	90	151	117	56	19	10	14	16	26	24	21	15	636	31.2
New Haven	37	42	44	44	67	129	204	243	218	127	81	62	55	81	69	83	60	1,646	29.4
New London	5	6	16	49	62	65	28	16	10	12	13	15	13	13	12	18	12	365	39.7
New Milford	1	...	2	1	...	1	5	7	6	3	1	1	...	...	...	...	1	29	17.1
Norwalk	6	5	6	4	12	30	42	43	32	20	19	10	7	15	11	9	10	281	29.0
Norwich	12	10	23	33	67	71	36	22	14	14	14	6	9	10	7	14	10	372	37.2
Orange	8	5	1	6	10	11	20	23	16	6	6	4	7	9	9	9	13	163	28.6
Plainfield	...	...	3	2	4	3	13	4	5	4	3	...	2	1	2	2	2	50	17.8
Plymouth	2	1	...	3	3	5	17	11	5	2	2	5	1	...	2	3	3	65	27.1
Putnam	...	4	1	6	8	12	20	9	11	6	6	6	4	3	5	3	5	109	37.6
Seymour	2	3	1	1	1	9	23	30	9	2	3	1	3	2	1	2	...	93	40.4
Shelton	3	5	2	8	12	12	8	5	2	4	5	2	2	6	4	3	6	89	26.7
Southington	3	4	...	1	3	7	2	21	13	5	4	3	2	5	6	6	4	89	28.9
Stafford	1	2	3	1	2	.....	3	3	4	3	...	2	1	1	2	5	1	34	16.2
Stamford	8	3	10	11	29	28	47	76	37	26	16	15	16	14	21	16	25	398	27.4
Stonington	3	5	7	6	16	14	8	4	.....	2	2	3	2	3	4	6	10	95	25.6
Stratford	4	3	2	2	5	5	10	11	7	8	8	5	1	3	6	3	1	84	17.5
Torrington	3	8	3	3	5	7	18	26	20	17	10	6	9	8	12	16	10	181	23.9
Vernon	...	7	2	3	6	19	24	12	8	1	3	...	4	2	2	6	2	101	33.7
Wallingford	1	3	2	8	12	20	12	6	3	...	1	2	1	2	2	2	2	79	19.7
Waterbury	29	16	22	22	34	137	302	263	134	51	36	24	25	30	41	41	34	1,241	34.8
Watertown	1	1	1	1	1	5	15	7	5	...	3	1	2	2	1	2	1	49	22.2
West Hartford	1	3	2	4	5	12	5	25	8	4	2	...	3	4	5	1	5	89	34.2
Westport	2	...	2	5	...	5	10	6	4	1	2	1	6	8	3	2	...	57	31.6
Winchester	2	3	1	1	10	13	22	22	9	6	1	5	...	6	5	1	1	108	32.7
Windham	2	3	9	15	36	62	26	16	5	1	2	3	2	...	5	6	7	200	42.6
Windsor	2	5	...	1	1	6	2	10	10	5	3	1	3	1	...	...	1	51	22.2
Towns under 5,000	54	48	62	76	116	204	203	171	123	84	70	53	61	57	83	74	83	1,622	22.3
Total	332	343	392	532	912	1,656	2,105	1,990	1,386	774	571	452	455	497	532	592	537	14,058	28.8
Unknown	2	...	...	...	1	....	....	....	....	...	...	...	...	1					

VARIATIONS IN URBAN AND RURAL INCIDENCE

A second relation, clearly brought out by an analysis of our figures is the greater incidence of influenza in large as compared with small communities. The respective rates for each county are shown in table 12.

With the single exception of Tolland County, in which the small towns were severely hit, the rates were in every case higher in the larger communities.

TABLE 12

DEATH RATE (TOTAL) PER 1,000 ON ANNUAL BASIS

County	Large Towns (over 5,000)	Small Towns (under 5,000)
New London	35	31
Middlesex	39	19
New Haven	31	22
Windham	32	20
Tolland	27	30
Hartford	30	20
Fairfiled	26	18
Litchfield	25	20

In certain counties we attempted a closer analysis of actual conditions by dividing some of the smaller towns into groups of a purely agricultural nature and groups in which manufacturing supplements agriculture to some extent.

In New Haven County, for example, the towns of Bethany, East Haven, Madison, Middlebury, North Branford, Oxford, Prospect, Wolcott and Woodbridge are purely agricultural. They had a combined death rate from influenza and pneumonia for the three months of September to November, inclusive, of 9.2 on an annual basis. The towns of Beacons Falls, Branford, Cheshire, Guilford, North Haven and Southbury, in which there are manufacturing plants, had a corresponding rate of 15.6.

In Litchfield County the purely agricultural towns of Bethlehem, Bridgewater, Canaan, Goshen, Harwinton, Kent, Morris, Roxbury, Sharon, Woodbury, Washington and Warren had a combined rate of 6.5. The partly manufacturing towns of Barkhamstead, Litchfield, New Hartford, New Milford, Norfolk, North Canaan, Plymouth, Salisbury, Thomaston, Watertown and Winchester had a rate of 18.3. Similar data for Fairfield County and for a group of towns in the state untouched by a railroad are presented in tables 13 and 14.

It will be noted that the data cited for these smaller towns are based only on influenzal-pneumonia rates up to December 1, and returns for December and January (which have not been analyzed in this way) might show some change in the relative figures, due to slower spread of the disease in rural communities. As a matter of fact, however, a study of the figures for the early months of 1919 shows no such tendency to equalization of rural and urban rates, but rather the contrary. The rate for the entire state for January, 1919, was 19.8, and that for the towns under 5,000 only 17.5.

Dr. Raymond Pearl in his illuminating study "On Certain General Statistical Aspects of the 1918 Epidemic in American Cities,"[8] has

[8] Public Health Reports for Aug. 8, 1919.

TABLE 13

DEATH RATES IN FAIRFIELD COUNTY

Agricultural Towns	Population	Deaths
Darien	8,198	13
Easton	1,272	1
Monroe	1,364	4
New Fairfield	557	2
Sherman	525	1
Weston	734	2
Wilton	1,848	3
Totals	14,498 Death Rate, 7.2 (on annual basis)	26
Manufacturing and Agricultural Towns		
Bethel	3 046	4
Brookfield	986	1
New Canaan	4,852	10
Newtown	2,985	0
Redding	2,576	3
Ridgefield	3,576	16
Shelton	8,573	35
Trumbull	2,651	4
Westport	5,337	21
Totals	34,582 Death Rate, 11.6 (on annual basis)	94

TABLE 14

DEATH RATE FROM INFLUENZAL PNEUMONIA IN CONNECTICUT TOWNS UNTOUCHED BY STEAM RAILROAD

Towns	Population	Deaths
North Stonington	1,195	2
Voluntown	739	4
Salem	562	
Ashford	833	6
Union	345	
Eastford	534	2
Woodstock	1,955	4
Brooklyn	1,930	5
Hebron	1,048	
East Haddam	2,848	3
Lyme	878	
Killingworth	526	3
North Branford	1,150	1
Easton	1,272	1
Glastonbury	6,302	11
Marlborough	419	
Sharon	1,783	4
Goshen	599	1
Warren	476	
Bethlehem	625	
Hartland	539	2
Barkhampton	811	
Granby	1,425	5
Woodbury	1,854	3
Totals	30,649 Death Rate, 7.2 (on annual basis)	57

concluded that for 39 large cities in the United States there was no correlation between the explosiveness of the influenza outbreak and density of population. Dr. Pearl is, however, dealing with cities which were all sufficiently large to offer practically complete opportunities for contact infection, and it would appear probable from our study that in really rural communities, at least in Connecticut, conditions operated making for a distinctly less heavy incidence than occurred in cities.

An obvious explanation of this difference would be that under the conditions of rural life the opportunities for contact infection are diminished. It is quite possible, however, that the higher rates in the more urban communities may have been due to the age distribution and racial composition of the population, rather than to any factors directly connected with the transmission of the disease.

LOCAL VARIATIONS IN INDIVIDUAL TOWNS

Aside from the effect of exposure to the virulent original infection of the early weeks of the epidemic, and aside from the differences between rural and urban communities in general, there were enormous variations between the severity of the epidemic in individual communities. Returning to our general basis of the death rate from all causes for the last four months of 1918, the towns may be grouped in the following manner:

TABLE 15

DEATH RATE FROM ALL CAUSES

Group 1 Rate under 15	Group 2 Rates 15–19	Group 3 Rates 20–24	Group 4 Rates 25–29
Darien.......... 10	Glastonbury.... 15	Hamden........ 20	Enfield......... 25
Milford......... 13	Stafford........ 16	Wallingford.... 20	Bridgeport...... 26
	E. Hartford.... 17	Fairfield........ 21	Bristol.......... 26
	Manchester..... 17	Watertown..... 22	Stonington..... 26
	New Milford.... 17	Windsor........ 22	Danbury........ 27
	Stratford....... 17	Towns under 5,000........... 22	Plymouth....... 27
	Berlin........... 18	Branford....... 24	Southington.... 27
	Plainfield....... 18	Killingly........ 24	Stamford....... 27
		Torrington..... 24	New Haven..... 29
			Norwalk........ 29
			Orange.......... 29
			Shelton......... 29
Group 5 Rates 30–34	**Group 6 Rates 35–39**	**Group 7 Rates 40–44**	**Group 8 Rate over 45**
Ansonia......... 31	Waterbury...... 35	New London.... 40	Derby........... 56
Greenwich....... 31	Naugatuck...... 36	Seymour........ 40	
New Britain..... 31	Norwich......... 37	Middletown..... 42	
Groton.......... 32	Meriden......... 38	Windham....... 43	
Westport....... 32	Putnam......... 38		
Winchester...... 33			
Hartford....... 34			
Vernon.......... 34			
W. Hartford.... 34			

The variations are enormous, from towns like Darien and Milford which exhibited death rates that would be low in the absence of any epidemic, to New London, Seymour, Middletown, Windham and Derby with rates two or three times a normal figure.

Certain influences already discussed will help to some extent to explain these differences. Thus, the 15 very low rates are all in fairly small communities. All the rates below 24 are in towns of less than 12,000 population, with the exception of Manchester (19,590), Stratford (14,384) and Fairfield (12,187). On the other hand, of the ten towns with the highest rates (over 34) only 3 (Derby, Seymour and Putnam) had a population of under 12,000. Of these 10 communities which suffered most severely, 4—Waterbury, Naugatuck, Seymour and Derby—are closely grouped in the Naugatuck Valley, and apparently form a single focus of specially virulent infection.

One factor which appeared to affect the severity of the epidemic was proximity in time to the original New London outbreak. In table 16 we have classified the towns according to the week of maximum deaths; and it is apparent that while 10 out of 12 towns which reached their maximum during the first two weeks of October had a total death rate of over 24, not a single one of the 8 towns which showed their maximum in November attained this limit. Again, we have a strong indication that the virus of the epidemic was most virulent or most readily communicable when it first reached the state, and thereafter became gradually attenuated.

The differences between individual towns, like those between local and urban communities, is not reduced but accentuated by later figures. Thus, of the towns which escaped most lightly in the fall, Darien had a total death rate of 20 for January; Milford a rate of 18; Glastonbury a rate of 13; while the rate for New London was 37; for Seymour, 12; for Middletown, 26; for Windham, 18, and for Derby, 20.

Dr. Pearl's researches on the explosiveness of the influenza epidemic in 39 large cities of the United States indicated a distinct but not a high correlation between this factor and distance from the initial focus of the disease — the correlation being -0.348 ± 0.095. He is inclined, however, in his discussion to minimize somewhat the importance of this relation. Dr. Pearl assumed the primary focus to be Boston, and took as his factor for geographical position the linear distance in miles between Boston and the various other cities studied. It seems somewhat doubtful whether such linear distances constitute a fair measure of the rate of transmission of disease, which depends so much on the extent of travel between different points and other variable factors. For the group of communities that we have studied in Connecticut, we have compared the severity of the outbreak (not its explosiveness as measured by Pearl) with the week of maximum incidence, and the correlation obtained, based on the data given in table 16 (computations made through the courtesy of Dr. L. I. Dublin) is $r = -0.520 \pm 0.070$, a correlation which we consider distinctly significant.

TABLE 16

RELATION BETWEEN SEVERITY OF THE EPIDEMIC AND DATE OF MAXIMUM INCIDENCE

Death Rate	Period of Maximum Incidence, Week Ending					
	October 5	October 12	October 19	October 26	November 2	November 9
Under 25		Wallingford 20 Killingly.... 24	Manchester 17 Plainfield.. 18 Watertown 22	E. Hartford. 17 New Milford. 17 Stratford.... 17 Hamden..... 20 Torrington.. 24	Darien....... 10 Milford...... 13 Glastonbury 15 Stafford..... 16 Berlin....... 18 Windsor..... 22 Branford.... 24	Fairfield 21
25-34	Stonington.. 26 Groton...... 32	Shelton..... 27 Ansonia..... 31	Enfield-.... 25 Bristol..... 26 New Britain 31 Westport.. 32 Winchester 33 Vernon..... 34 Hartford.. 34 Plymouth.. 27	Bridgeport.. 26 Danbury..... 27 New Haven.. 29 Norwalk..... 29 Orange...... 29 Southington 29 Stamford.... 27 W. Hartford 34		
Over 34	New London 40	Norwich..... 37 Meriden..... 38 Windham... 43 Derby....... 56	Naugatuck 36 Putnam.... 38 Waterbury 35 Middletown 42	Seymour..... 40		

We have not found the study of the curves of the epidemic particularly significant. Figures 8 and 9 show typical curves for some of the smaller and larger communities, respectively, and are fairly illustrative of a large number we have plotted. Figure 8 is based on deaths from influenza and pneumonia alone; figure 9 on deaths from all causes. The outbreak in a given community generally occupied a period of from 6-8 weeks, and was steep and abrupt in communities which were badly hit; flatter and more gently sloping in those which escaped lightly.

Aside from the two facts mentioned above, that the outbreak was more severe in communities that received the infection early than in those later affected, and that it was on the average more severe in urban than in rural communities, we have found little clear evidence as to the factors associated with variations in local prevalence.

It is possibly significant that cities like New London, Derby, Waterbury and Seymour, which have been overcrowded by war workers, suffered severely, and it seems probable that unsanitary conditions may favor the spread of infection.

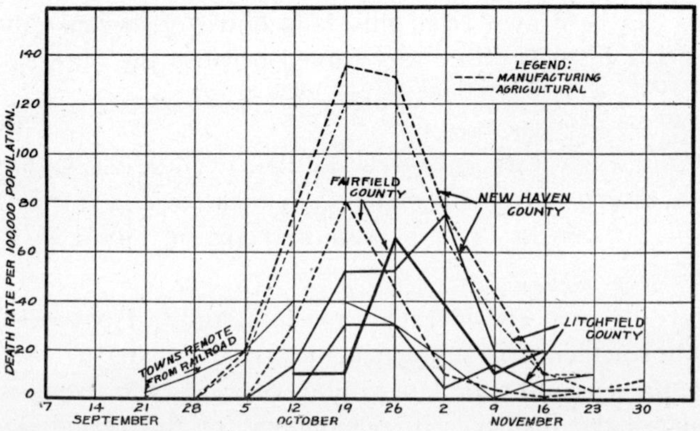

Fig. 8.—Weekly distribution of deaths from influenza and pneumonia in small manufacturing and agricultural communities and in towns remote from the railroad (actual weekly death rate, not on annual basis).

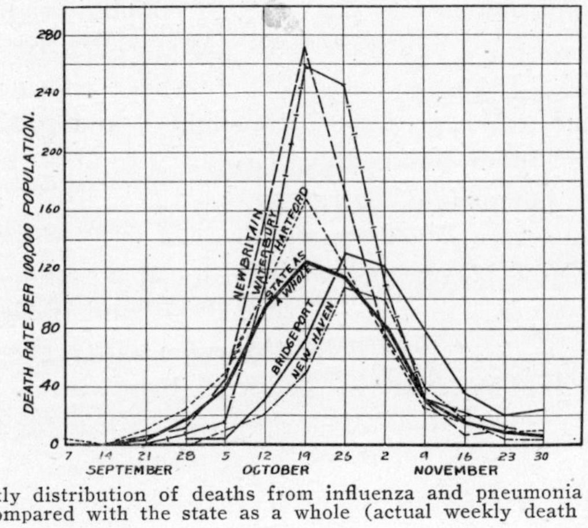

Fig. 9.—Weekly distribution of deaths from influenza and pneumonia in the larger cities of Connecticut compared with the state as a whole (actual weekly death rate, not on annual basis).

It seems quite certain that none of the orthodox methods of combating epidemics applied in Connecticut exerted any appreciable influence on the spread of influenza. The State Department of Health advocated the keeping open of schools under close medical supervision, and of theaters, provided persons who coughed and sneezed were excluded, and opportunities offered for educational addresses by local health officials. The three largest cities — Bridgeport, Hartford and New Haven—followed this policy, and suffered from death rates near the average for the state, lower than the rates which prevailed in cities like New London and Waterbury, which closed their schools. No deductions can be drawn from this fact, however, because the closing of the schools in most cases was forced because the outbreak was so severe.

RELATION BETWEEN THE SEVERITY OF THE INFLUENZA EPIDEMIC AND THE DEATH RATE FOR PREVIOUS YEARS IN CONNECTICUT AND IN CERTAIN LARGE CITIES OF THE UNITED STATES

We have devoted considerable time to a study of possible relations between the incidence of influenza in various towns in 1890-92 and during the present outbreak, but without very tangible conclusions. We also compared the incidence of pneumonia for the period, 1891-1916, with the incidence of the 1918 epidemic, but without striking results. Torrington has had a consistently low pneumonia record (102 was the average pneumonia death rate per 100,000 population for the period 1891-1916), and escaped lightly in 1918. Waterbury and Middletown (pneumonia rates 170 and 203, respectively) have had uniformly high rates (largely due to the presence of hospitals), and suffered severely in 1918. On the other hand, New Britain, Danbury and Norwalk, which had shown low pneumonia rates (134, 129 and 125, respectively) experienced a moderate incidence of influenza in 1918; while Bridgeport, Hartford, New Haven and Stamford (all hospital cities) which had shown consistently high rates (169, 203, 172 and 172, respectively), also suffered but moderately in 1918. Meriden with a good past record (129), and New London, Norwich and Windham with moderate pneumonia records (152, 144 and 137, respectively), had high death rates in 1918.

A study of the relation between the 1918 mortality and the general death rate from all causes in previous years proved more significant. We obtained from Mr. Balfe the annual death rates for the 49 large towns for 1915, 1916, and 1917, and averaged them to obtain the figures presented in table 17. Through the courtesy of Dr. L. I. Dublin, the correlation was calculated between these figures and the death rates from all causes for the period September-December, 1918, as given in the last column of table 11. The correlation worked out as follows: $r = +0.627 \pm 0.058$, which from the statistical standpoint is, of course, a highly significant figure. It might be suggested, since we dealt only with death rates from all causes, that such a correlation would naturally be expected between the death rates in a community during successive years. When, however, it is remembered that 60 per cent. of all the deaths in Connecticut during the last four months of 1918 were due to influenza and pneumonia (see table 4), it seems evident that in order to yield such a high coefficient of correlation the

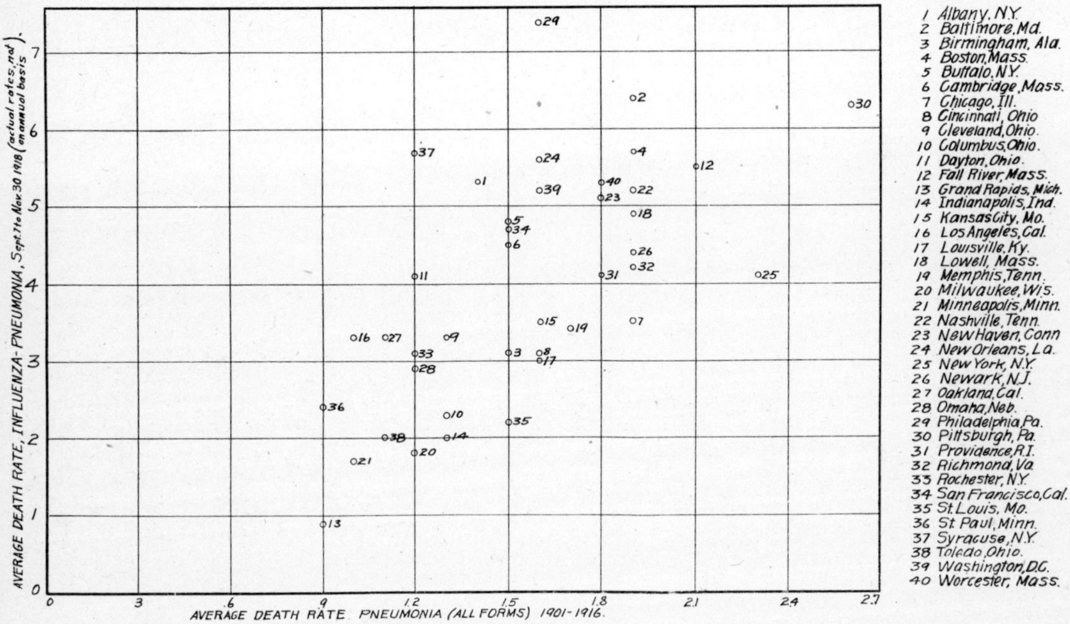

Fig. 10.—Relation of pneumonia death rate, 1901-1916, to influenza death rate, 1918, in certain large cities of the United States.

course of the influenza epidemic in 1918 must to a considerable extent have followed the variations in total death rate normal for the various communities affected.

Dr. Pearl, in the paper previously cited, has shown that for the larger cities of the country there were similar high correlations between his index of epidemicity of influenza and the 1916 death rates from all causes, from pulmonary tuberculosis, from organic heart disease and from acute nephritis and Bright's disease, while correlations with 1916 influenza and pneumonia were of lesser magnitude.

Before Dr. Pearl's report was published we had ourselves begun a tentative study of the relation between 1918 influenza-pneumonia and the death rate from pneumonia and other causes in the larger cities of the United States.

TABLE 17

AVERAGE DEATH RATE FROM ALL CAUSES, 1915-1917

Towns	Average Death Rate from All Causes, 1915-1917	Towns	Average Death Rate from All Causes, 1915-1917
Ansonia	13.9	New Milford	14.2
Berlin	9.0	Norwalk	14.6
Branford	12.2	Norwich	19.6
Bridgeport	15.7	Orange	12.4
Bristol	11.0	Plainfield	12.3
Danbury	15.6	Plymouth	9.0
Darien	14.2	Putnam	16.8
Derby	22.3	Seymour	13.2
East Hartford	10.6	Shelton	20.9
Enfield	13.7	Southington	12.8
Fairfield	12.9	Stafford	12.8
Glastonbury	9.7	Stamford	15.5
Greenwich	15.6	Stonington	13.6
Groton	14.8	Stratford	12.2
Hamden	11.9	Torrington	10.7
Hartford	15.8	Vernon	12.6
Killingly	15.0	Wallingford	12.0
Manchester	9.2	Waterbury	14.6
Meriden	17.2	Watertown	12.6
Middletown	23.1	West Hartford	20.8
Milford	15.8	Westport	18.2
Naugatuck	11.0	Winchester	17.2
New Britain	12.2	Windham	19.7
New Haven	16.3	Windsor	12.9
New London	18.2		

For 1918 data we used the number of deaths per 1,000 from influenza and pneumonia for the 12-week period from September 7 to November 30 as presented in a special summary of the Weekly Health Index of the U. S. Census Bureau. For early data we used the death rates from pneumonia (all forms) and from all causes. The fundamental data utilized in this study are presented in table 18, and the general relation between the pneumonia rates for the previous sixteen years and the influenzal-pneumonia rates for 1918 is brought out in figure 10. It is evident that there is a rather definite correlation indicated, the cities which have been characterized by a high pneumonia rate in the past being in general precisely the cities which suffered most severely in the 1918 outbreak. At this stage of the analysis we were inclined to suspect that the presence of particularly virulent types of pneumonia organisms in certain sections of the country might have played an important part in determining the fatality experienced in the influenza epidemic of 1918.

A comparison of the total death rates from all causes for the period 1901-16 with the influenzal-pneumonia death rate for the epidemic months of 1918, showed that such an assumption would be unwarranted. Figure 11 indicates that the correlation of the severity of the influenza epidemic with *total* death rates in the past was as close as with pneumonia death rates.

This correlation between 1918 influenza and previous mortality from other causes has been demonstrated by Dr. Pearl with a clearness

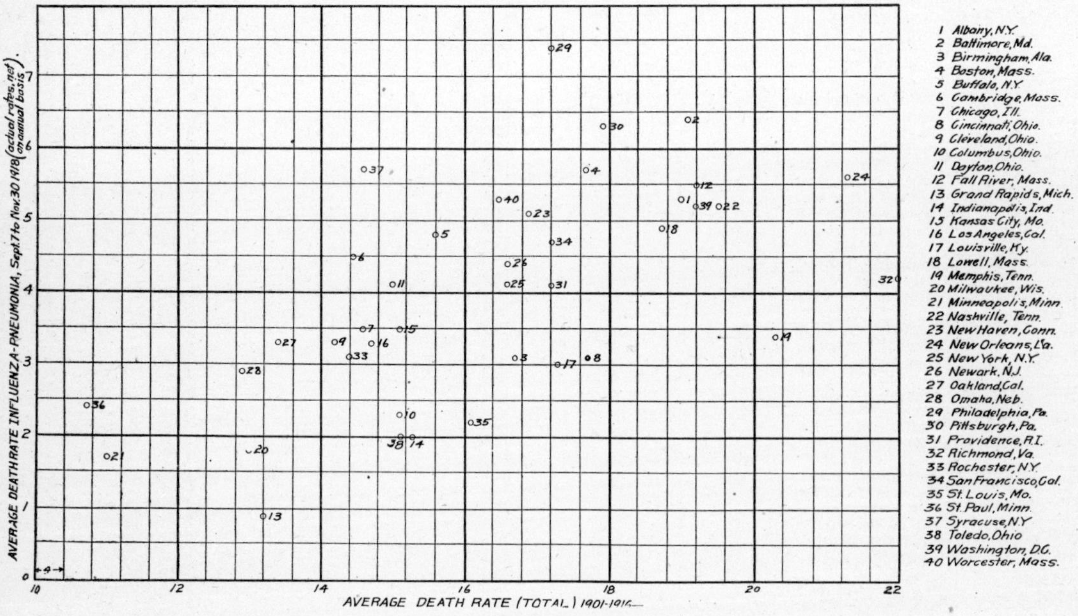

Fig. 11.—Relation of total death rate, 1901-1916, to influenza death rate, 1918, in certain large cities of the United States.

that made it seem unnecessary for us to carry out any detailed mathematical study of our own data. That the correlations found by him between the epidemicity of influenza in 1918 and the death rates from all causes, from pulmonary tuberculosis, organic heart disease and acute nephritis and Bright's disease, is a highly significant statistical correlation is quite certain. The interpretation of its significance is a much more complex matter and in this connection we have thought the graphic presentations contained in figures 10 and 11 worthy of brief consideration.

TABLE 18

AVERAGE TOTAL, PNEUMONIA, AND INFLUENZAL-PNEUMONIA DEATH RATES PER 1,000 FOR LARGE AMERICAN CITIES

Cities	Average Death Rate (Total) 1901-1916	Average Death Rate Pneumonia (All Forms) 1901-1916	Average Death Rate Influenzal-Pneumonia Sept. 7-Nov. 30, 1918 (Actual Rates, Not on Annual Basis)
Albany, N. Y.	19.0	1.4	5.3
Baltimore, Md.	19.1	1.9	6.4
Birmingham, Ala.*	16.7	1.5	3.1
Boston, Mass.	17.7	1.9	5.7
Buffalo, N. Y.	15.6	1.5	4.8
Cambridge, Mass.	14.5	1.5	4.5
Chicago, Ill.	14.6	1.9	3.5
Cincinnati, O.	17.7	1.6	3.1
Cleveland, O.	14.2	1.3	3.3
Columbus, O.	15.1	1.3	2.3
Dayton, O.	15.0	1.2	4.1
Fall River, Mass.	19.2	2.1	5.5
Grand Rapids, Mich.	13.2	0.9	0.9
Indianapolis, Ind.	15.3	1.3	2.0
Kansas City, Mo.	15.1	1.6	3.5
Los Angeles, Calif.	14.7	1.0	3.3
Louisville, Ky.	17.3	1.6	3.0
Lowell, Mass.	18.7	1.9	4.9
Memphis, Tenn.	20.3	1.7	3.4
Milwaukee, Wis.	13.0	1.2	1.8
Minneapoils, Minn.	11.0	1.0	1.7
Nashville, Tenn.	19.5	1.9	5.2
New Haven, Conn.	16.9	1.8	5.1
New Orleans, La.	21.3	1.6	5.6
New York, N. Y.	16.6	2.3	4.1
Newark, N. J.	16.6	1.9	4.4
Oakland, Calif.	13.4	1.1	3.3
Omaha, Neb.	12.9	1.2	2.9
Philadelphia, Pa.	17.2	1.6	7.4
Pittsburgh, Pa.	17.9	2.6	6.3
Providence, R. I.	17.2	1.8	4.1
Richmond, Va.	22.0	1.9	4.2
Rochester, N. Y.	14.4	1.2	3.1
San Francisco, Calif.	17.2	1.5	4.7
St. Louis, Mo.	16.1	1.5	2.2
St. Paul, Minn.	10.7	0.9	2.4
Syracuse, N. Y.	14.6	1.2	5.7
Toledo, O.	15.1	1.1	2.0
Washington, D. C.	19.2	1.6	5.2
Worcester, Mass.	16.5	1.8	5.3

* Death rates for Birmingham are the average for six years only, 1910-1916.

Granting that there was a distinct correlation, such as Pearl has demonstrated, between the epidemicity of influenza in various communities and the death rate from certain organic disorders in previous years, the phenomenon might in the first place be the result of a direct connection between the two correlated factors. In other words, the rapid explosive spread of the epidemic in Pearl's case, and the high mortality from influenza in the case of our Connecticut figures, may have been the result of weaknesses in the population due to high incidence of organic diseases and tuberculosis in earlier years. It is equally possible from a statistical standpoint, and inherently more probable, that the correlation is an indirect one, due to the relation between each of the factors studied and one or more underlying conditions affecting both. Thus the death rates from organic diseases and tuberculosis in previous years, and the incidence of influenza mortality in 1918, may both have been due to peculiarities in

a. Age distribution of the population.

b. Race distribution of the population.

c. Social and economic conditions in the various cities studied.

Or finally, it may be possible that the high rate from tuberculosis and organic disease in 1916 was due to the factors enumerated above and that the high incidence of influenza was due chiefly to proximity to the original focus of infection — the correlation being due merely to the accidental circumstance that the concentration of foreign race stocks living under poor economic conditions, and the original point of introduction of the influenza epidemic, both happened to be on the Atlantic seaboard.

Dr. Pearl has dealt with certain of these questions by calculating the correlation between his influenza epidemicity and the 1916 death rate from tuberculosis, organic heart disease and Bright's disease and nephritis—after correcting for age distribution and linear distance from Boston. He finds higher correlations after correction than before. The actual significance of such corrections, when made at the same time, as Pearl has made them, is, however, very difficult to interpret. The age distribution favorable to influenza is also favorable to tuberculosis, but unfavorable to organic heart disease and nephritis; while the factor of race, with its accidental relationship to geographical position, is almost impossible to evaluate in this way.

The broad fact, as indicated graphically in figures 10 and 11, would seem to be that eastern and southern cities with industrial populations, largely of Irish and Latin and Slavic stock, show high death rates from all causes, as well as from influenza and pneumonia, while western and middle western cities, with in general better living conditions and less Irish and Latin and Slavic stock, show lower death rates. In part, the greater severity of the influenza epidemic in the east may be attributed to the more unfavorable living condition in industrial communities and the higher proportion of Italian race stocks which we have shown favored high mortality in Connecticut. It is obvious, however, that the correlation indicated may in part be an accidental one. The low death rates characteristic of western cities in the past must no doubt be attributed to social and economic and racial factors; but the low influenza rates exhibited by the same cities in 1918 may in part be the result of the fact that they were exposed to the epidemic at a later period when, if the conclusions drawn in Connecticut are justified, it may probably have suffered from a natural decline in virulence or communicability.

SUMMARY AND CONCLUSIONS

The 1918 epidemic of influenza began in Connecticut with cases at the Naval Hospital in New London about September 1. From the naval base the disease spread rapidly to the civilian population. Other independent foci developed later at various points throughout the state, the source in several instances being the military population of Camp Devens, Mass.

The epidemic as a state-wide phenomenon lasted from September 14 to November 30, with recrudescences in December and January. Its height was reached between October 12 and October 26.

The epidemic cost the state about 7,700 lives, and was by far the most serious sanitary calamity from which Connecticut has ever suffered. The total death rate for the year was 19.4 per 1,000, a rate previously reached only in the earlier influenza epidemic year of 1892. The monthly rate for October was 63.9 (deaths per 1,000 population on an annual basis), double the rate for the worst single month in 1892.

It seems probable, from such imperfect data as are available, that the case rate in affected communities varied between 200 and 400 cases per 1,000 population, and the fatality rate between 2 and 4 deaths per 100 cases. Estimating on a basis of excess total deaths as compared with the corresponding months of 1917, the average excess mortality due to the epidemic for the state as a whole would be about 5.5 per 1,000.

The rapid spread of the disease throughout the state and the fact that quarantine completely protected isolated groups of individuals (so long as the quarantine was rigidly maintained) indicates clearly that it was transmitted by human contact, perhaps supplemented in certain cases by the use of infected food and utensils.

The mortality from the epidemic was proportionately higher among males than among females, and it was proportionately very much higher at ages under 5 years and at ages from 20-40 than at other periods of life. It seems somewhat doubtful whether the lower mortality in later adult life can be attributed to immunity acquired in the 1892 epidemic, since immunity due to this cause should have manifested itself in the age-period from 30-40 which, as a matter of fact, showed practically the same proportionate rate as the decade from 20-30.

The mortality was relatively low among persons of native Irish, English and German mother nativity. It was relatively high among persons of Canadian, Russian, Austrian and Polish mother nativity, and exceedingly high among persons of Italian mother nativity. The Italian race stock contributed nearly double its normal proportion to the state death roll during the epidemic period. The excessive incidence among the Latin and Slavic races mentioned (the Canadians being largely of French race stock) may in part be attributed to the age composition of these racial elements and perhaps to overcrowding and general poor economic conditions. This can hardly be sufficient, however, to account for such enormous differences as appear in the case of the Italians.

The mortality from the epidemic was lower in rural than in urban communities, lower in agricultural than in manufacturing communities, and very low in a group of small towns remote from any railroad.

The mortality was in general highest in those communities which were affected earliest. As the wave of infection passed westward and northward the mortality became less, strongly suggesting a progressive decrease in virulence or in communicability. The correlation between the mortality from all causes for September-December, 1918, and the week of maximum incidence of the epidemic was -0.520 ± 0.070.

The severity of the epidemic varied greatly in different communities. These variations are partly, but only partly, to be explained by the relations discussed under the foregoing conclusions. There is no evidence that variations in administrative procedure, such as the closing of schools, exerted any influence on the spread or the severity of the disease.

The severity of the epidemic in different communities in Connecticut showed no clear correlation with the severity of the 1892 epidemic or with the prevalence of ordinary pneumonias since that epidemic. The mortality from all causes for September-December, 1918 (of which influenza-pneumonia made up 60%), was however closely correlated with the average mortality for 1915-1917, the figure being

$+0.627 \pm 0.058$. A study of the census statistics for the larger cities of the United States as a whole showed a very definite relation between the severity of the 1918 influenza epidemic and both the pneumonia death rate and the total death rate for the sixteen years preceding. The relation is in general a geographical one, the eastern and south-eastern cities showing high death rates, the middle-western and western cities low death rates in each case. The higher pneumonia rates and total death rates in the eastern section may reasonably be attributed to unfavorable economic conditions associated with industrial life and presence of certain foreign race stocks always characterized by a high death rate. Whether the greater severity of the influenza epidemic in these same cities was due to the same causes or to a gradual loss of communicability or virulence as the infection passed westward from its point of introduction seems uncertain. In any case there are differences between individual cities (such as New York and Philadelphia) which cannot be explained on either assumption.

BACTERIUM ANATUM, N. S., THE ETIOLOGIC FACTOR IN A WIDESPREAD DISEASE OF YOUNG DUCKLINGS KNOWN IN SOME PLACES AS "KEEL"

LEO F. RETTGER AND MARGARET M. SCOVILLE

From the Sheffield Laboratory of Bacteriology, Yale University, and from the Storrs Agricultural Experiment Station

In the spring of 1918, the attention of the senior author was called to a disease affecting very young ducklings on a commercial duck farm in Connecticut. The mortality in a lot of 3,000 ducklings, all hatched at about the same time, was almost 100 per cent. The symptoms were noticeable soon after hatching, and were as a rule as follows: The affected individuals appeared weak and sluggish, and remained close to the heating pipes. They were not easily aroused, and did not go in search of food, as did the others. They ate at times, however, and their crops were distended. One of the marked symptoms was intense thirst. After drinking, some of the ducklings drew themselves to full height, staggered for a few seconds, keeled over and, after one or two gasps, died — hence the name "keel" for the disease. Few of the ducklings died after they were from three to four weeks of age, the greatest mortality occurring within the first week or ten days. Some of the symptoms may be lacking or obscured in the affected broods. Perhaps the large majority of the victims of the disease die without warning to the observer, and are found dead under the hover or occasionally out in the open. This is seen particularly when the ducklings die very soon after leaving the shell.

Examination of the dead ducklings revealed no lesions or any other pathologic condition except, perhaps, paleness of the tissues as a whole and light body weight. By the ordinary streak method on nutrient agar an organism was isolated without difficulty from the liver, heart and lungs, which resembled B. pullorum, and at once appeared to be a member of the coli-typhi-paratyphi group. This organism was obtained from the tissues and blood of the first two ducklings examined, from others which were sent in from time to time from the same farm, and from the ovary and from an abdominal cyst of two ducks from a large commercial plant in Massachusetts.

A rather extensive inquiry into the methods of duck farming and the conditions affecting the industry in the North Atlantic states revealed some interesting facts. The magnitude of this enterprise is indeed surprising to one who

Received for publication Nov. 1, 1919.

is not already familiar with the situation. A duck farm near Wrentham, Mass. (Weber Brothers), lays the claim to having reared 75,000 ducks to marketing age in a single season. Only a short distance away on the same road there is another farm, with a capacity of from 40,000 to 50,000. Numerous other places in New England, especially in Massachusetts and Connecticut, are with more or less success carrying on business on a somewhat similar scale, as for example the Conway Farm in Newington. Long Island has for some years been known as a very important duck-raising section of the state of New York. The annual production on Long Island farms, large and small, can be safely estimated at a million dollars at least.

Raising of Peking ducks on a large scale has been a most profitable enterprise, at least up to the years 1917 and 1918. Few diseases seem to affect this breed, and little trouble has been encountered until recently in the rearing of ducklings, when conducted by competent and skilled persons. Furthermore, the demand for ducks of marketable age has been such as to stimulate still greater production.

During 1917 and 1918, particularly in the season of 1918, however, serious reverses were reported from various duck farms. The hatchibility of the eggs was poor, and in many instances the ducklings that left the shell died while very young, apparently from the disease discussed in this paper. While the season was too far advanced, when the inquiries were made, to obtain specimens for examination from the various farms, descriptions of the symptoms and conditions by the owners and managers of the affected stock were such as to lead to but one conclusion.

The losses from this disease in 1918 were very great. Not over 10,000 ducks were raised on a farm which had a previous record and a capacity of at least 40,000. The largest farm visited fell short of its 1917 production by fully 50,000, and the owner appeared very much alarmed over the outlook for the future when he stated that, whereas two years before the fields were white with ducks, they were now green with grass. Similar reports came from other sources. The conditions were in all probability greatly aggravated by the severe winter of 1917-18.

Several points of similarity between the disease which affected so many ducklings and bacillary white diarrhea of chicks impressed themselves on the senior author, who alone was concerned with the investigation at this time. The greatest mortality occurred in ducklings less than three weeks old, and few deaths resulted after the fourth week. The disturbance appeared to be of an intestinal nature, although little or no diarrheal condition could as a rule be observed. The ducklings became very weak and clung to the hover, indicating subnormal temperature. No pathologic changes were apparent on dissection, except, perhaps, anemia and light weight. The deaths in a brood did not occur in large numbers at any one time, but extended over a period of several days or even a few weeks. Finally, an organism was obtained from the affected ducklings examined which in many ways bore a close resemblance to Bacterium pullorum, the causative agent in bacillary white diarrhea.

On account of these points of resemblance between the two diseases, it appeared probable that they were similar in their origin and methods of transmission. While sufficient data have not thus far been gathered to show that "keel" has the same cycle of infection as bacillary white diarrhea of chicks, that is, that the organism causing it is transmitted through infected eggs of breeding ducks whose ovaries are infected, certain observations strongly point to such a relationship between parent and offspring.

EXAMINATION OF BREEDING STOCK

Late in July, 1918, eight breeding ducks on an infected farm were killed and the ovaries in particular subjected to a thorough pathologic and bacteriologic examination. The following is a brief record:

DUCK 1.—The ovary was normal and well developed.

DUCK 2.—The ovary was well developed, with many large and small ovules. There were also three abnormal cysts which had once been ova; one of the size of a pea, and dark in color; another of about the same size, but firm, angular and discolored. Contents were composed of dried yolk-like material surrounded by an amber-colored clear fluid. The third cyst was smaller, discolored and slightly angular. The contents were semisolid. All three of these ovarian cysts yielded a pure, abundant growth of an organism apparently identical with that isolated from the original ducklings on the first farm.

DUCK 3.—The ovary was normal with the exception of one ovum of hazelnut size which was almost black and of a rubber-like consistency. The culture test was negative.

DUCK 4.—The ovary was well developed with three very small, slightly discolored ovules. One was negative; the other two were too small to culture.

DUCK 5.—The ovary was normal, but undeveloped.

DUCK 6.—The ovary was normal but undeveloped.

DUCK 7.—The ovary was normal with the exception of two very small opaque ovules. There was an abdominal cyst, dark and angular, resembling typical ovarian cyst of bacillary white diarrhea. The cyst was suspended by a light cord from the omentum, and contained cheesy matter mingled with clear amber-colored fluid. Culture tests were positive. The organism was identical with that obtained from the ovary of duck 2, present in contents in large numbers and unassociated with other bacteria.

DUCK 8.—The ovary was well developed. There was one dark, bloody ovule. The culture test was negative.

The other organs and tissues of the ducks examined were apparently normal, and hence require no comments.

One of the eight ducks (No. 2) examined had a distinctly pathologic ovary very closely resembling the typical white diarrhea ovary of hens, and contained an organism indistinguishable from the bacterium which was isolated at the outset of the investigation from the blood and organs of ducklings affected with the "keel," though on a different farm. A second duck (No. 7) showed little abnormality of the ovary, but harbored a characteristic cyst in the peritoneal cavity which contained the same organism as did the ovary of duck 2.

Unfortunately, it was too late in the season to obtain on this farm young ducklings that were affected or had died of the disease under observation. The greatest mortality occurred very early in the season, and the rate decreased until July, when there were apparently very few sick ducklings, and comparatively few eggs were being hatched. The same decrease in morbidity and mortality was reported from the other farms which were investigated. Attempts to fully demonstrate transmission of the disease from the ovary through the egg to the offspring were not as successful, therefore, as they would have been had they been begun early in the spring of the year. Further investigations along this line will be carried on as soon as conditions are again favorable.

CHARACTERIZATION OF THE ORGANISM CAUSING THE DISEASE—BACTERIUM ANATUM, NOV. SPEC.

In a preliminary report on the investigation (1919)[1] the name of the causative organism was given as Bacterium anatis, the word anatis being the genitive singular of the Latin *anas,* meaning duck. A survey of the literature showed that Cornil and Toupet[2] (1888) had applied this name to an organism which they isolated from diseased ducks, but which was indistinguishable from B. avisepticus, the organism of ordinary fowl cholera. The genitive plural has been substituted here for anatis, the name of the new micro-organism, therefore, being Bacterium anatum.

Five representative strains of the organism were used in all of the following characterization studies:

No. 1, isolated as 8C from one of a lot of ducklings received from C farm.
No. 2, isolated as cyst W from abdominal cyst of breeding duck on W farm.
No. 3, isolated as ovum W from ovarian cyst of breeding duck on W farm.
No. 4, isolated as IIC from second lot of ducklings received from C farm.
No. 5, isolated as VC from a third lot of ducklings received from C farm.

[1] Rettger, Leo F., and Scoville, Margaret M.: Bacterium anatis, Nov. Spec., an Organism of Economic Importance and a Member of the Paratyphoid Group of Bacteria. Paper presented before the Society of American Bacteriologists at the Annual Meeting, Baltimore, December, 1918.

[2] Cornil and Coupet: Sur une nouvelle maladie bactérienne du canard (cholera des canards), Compt. rend. de l'Acad. des Sciences de Paris, 1888, 106, p. 1737-50.

For purposes of convenience these different strains will be referred to as strains 1, 2, 3, 4 and 5.

It soon became apparent that the different strains revealed but very slight and insignificant differences among themselves, and that the organism, B. anatum, must be classed with the coli-typhi-dysenteriae group of bacteria, along the side of the well-known paratyphoid members. Hence, the investigation of the properties of B. anatum included a comparative study of this organism and B. typhi, B. paratyphosus A and B, B. enteritidis, B. pullorum (Rettger) and B. sanguinarium (Moore).[3]

MORPHOLOGY, STAINING PROPERTIES, ETC., OF BACTERIUM ANATUM

It is a short, rod-shaped, actively motile organism, in form resembling the shorter varieties of B. coli and B. enteritidis, rather than B. typhosus. It is actively motile, and possesses several peritrichiate flagella, although the exact number could not be definitely demonstrated. There are some variations in the length of the bacilli in the same culture medium. The average size may be stated approximately as 0.5 by 1 to 2 mikrons. It takes the ordinary stains readily, and is gram-negative.

The optimum temperature of B. anatum is 35-37 C., but it grows well at ordinary room temperature. It is a facultative anaerobe, having a very decided preference for atmospheric oxygen.

CULTURAL CHARACTERISTICS

Gelatin and Agar Plates.—The colonies have no characteristics that set them apart from the colonies of other members of the group. Growth is slightly heavier than that of B. typhosus, and less luxuriant than the colonies of B. coli.

Slant Agar.—Growth following inoculation with the needle by the single streak method is moderately abundant at the end of 24 hours at incubation temperature, and is indistinguishable from B. paratyphosus B and B. enteritidis. The growth becomes quite luxuriant and opaque after the first two days, and often shows more or less

[3] Smith, Theobald, and Ten Broeck, C.: Agglutination Affinities of a Pathogenic Bacillus from fowls (Bacterium sanguinarium, Moore) with the Typhoid Bacillus of Man, Jour. Med. Research, 1915, 31, p. 503-521.

Smith, Theobald, and Ten Broeck, C.: A Note on the Relation between B. pullorum (Rettger) and the Fowl Typhoid Bacillus (Moore). Idem, p. 547-555.

wrinkling eventually near the base. When the inoculation is made over the entire surface of the agar with a platinum loop, and with the blood from infected organs or with a light suspension of the organism in water or other liquid medium, discrete colonies are formed over the agar surface which in the early stages very closely resemble those of B. pullorum and which remain separate even after from 24 to 36 hours at incubation temperature. The older colonies are decidedly larger and more opaque than those of B. pullorum.

Gelatin Stab.—There is light growth along needle track, with little or no spreading on the surface. The gelatin is not liquefied.

Nutrient Broth.—Heavy clouding and surface pellicle occur in from 24 to 36 hours at 35-37 C. There is no appreciable odor.

Litmus Milk.—Faintly acid within 48 hours, but gradually changing to alkaline. Marked alkalinity at the end of 12 to 14 days. Reaction in litmus milk similar to that of strains of B. sanguinarium Moore and B. paratyphosus B employed in a series of comparative tests.

Potato.—The reaction on this medium differed more or less with the strains and with their viability. Strains 2 and 3 produced a scanty growth with no discoloration of the medium. Numbers 1, 4 and 5 developed a heavy, moist growth which in from 2 to 3 days became light brown, and brought about discoloration of the potato. After repeated transplantation on new medium, at intervals of 2 weeks, 5 was the only strain which discolored the potato.

No indol was produced in Dunham's peptone, nor in tryptophane broth, and all failed to give the Voges-Proskauer reaction.

Nitrates were reduced to nitrites by all five of the strains of B. anatum in 24 hours at 37 C.

All of the strains were able to utilize the nitrogen of ammonia, nitrate, urea, creatin and nucleic acid, but failed to attack uric acid.

ACTION ON CARBOHYDRATES AND OTHER FERMENTABLE SUBSTANCES

Gas production was determined in the double-barreled fermentation tube of Durham, the gas being measured by the Frost gasometer. Brom cresol purple was employed for the detection of acidity, only a P_H value of 5.6 or less being recorded. The cultures were incubated at 37 C.

The following fermentable substances were used; glucose, levulose, maltose, saccharose, lactose, galactose, inulin, dextrin, arabinose, rhamnose, raffinose, xylose, inosit, adonitol, dulcitol, mannitol, salicin and glycerol. Standard nutrient bouillon was the medium employed for the ordinary fermentation tests. The test agents were as a rule one per cent. strength. Some of the rarer substances (inosit, adonitol and dulcitol) were used in 0.25 per cent.

All of the five strains of B. anatum gave the same reaction, with the following exceptions: Number 2 failed repeatedly to produce acid or gas in xylose, and number 3 gas in the same medium, while the others acidified the medium and produced 10 per cent. of gas. The reactions may be summarized briefly as follows:

Substances acted on, with acid production — glucose, levulose, maltose, galactose, dextrin, arabinose, rhamnose, inosit, xylose (except strain number 2), dulcitol, mannitol and glycerol.

Substances acted on, with gas formation, and the percentage of gas produced — glucose 40, levulose 25, maltose 10, galactose 35, dextrin 5-10, arabinose 10-15, rhamnose 10-15, inosit 10, xylose 10 (excepting strains number 2 and 3), mannitol 20, and dulcitol 35-40. Neither acid nor gas is formed from lactose, saccharose, inulin, raffinose, adonitol and salicin.

A comparison of these reactions with those obtained with B. typhosus and the common members of the paratyphoid group revealed a very close resemblance between B. anatum and B. paratyphi A and B, and B. enteritidis (see tables 1 and 2).

TABLE 1

ACID PRODUCTION BY BACTERIUM ANATUM AND RELATED ORGANISMS

Fermentable Substances	B. anatum Strains					B. typhosus	B. paratyphosus A	B. paratyphosus B	B. enteritidis	B. sanguinarium	B. pullorum
	1	2	3	4	5						
Glucose	+	+	+	+	+	+	+	+	+	+	+
Levulose	+	+	+	+	+	+	+	+	+	+	+
Lactose	0	0	0	0	0	0	0	0	0	0	0
Galactose	+	+	+	+	+	+	+	+	+	+	+
Maltose	+	+	+	+	+	+	+	+	+	+	0
Saccharose	0	0	0	0	0	0	0	0	0	0	0
Arabinose	+	+	+	+	+	0	+	+	+	⊕	+
Rhamnose	+	+	+	+	+	0	+	+	+	0	+
Raffinose	0	0	0	0	0	0	0	0	0	0	0
Xylose	+	0	⊕	+	+	⊕	0	+	+	0	0
Dextrin	+	+	+	+	+	⊕	+	+	+	+	0
Inulin	0	0	0	0	0	0	0	0	0	0	0
Glycerol	⊕	⊕	⊕	⊕	⊕	⊕	⊕	⊕	+	0	0
Inosite	+	+	+	+	+	0	0	+	0	0	0
Dulcitol	+	+	+	+	+	0	+	+	+	+	0
Mannitol	+	+	+	+	+	+	+	+	+	+	+
Adonitol	0	0	0	0	0	0	0	0	0	0	0
Salicin	0	0	0	0	0	0	0	0	0	0	0

+ indicates acid production; 0 failure to produce gas; and ⊕ slight or doubtful reaction.

TABLE 2

GAS PRODUCTION BY BACTERIUM ANATUM AND RELATED ORGANISMS

Fermentable Substances	B. anatum Strains 1	2	3	4	5	B. typhosus	B. paratyphosus A	B. paratyphosus B	B. enteritidis	B. sanguinarium	B. pullorum
Glucose	40%	40%	40%	40%	40%	0	20%	35%	30%	0	25%
Levulose	25%	25%	25%	25%	25%	0	15%	30%	25%	0	15%
Lactose	0	0	0	0	0	0	0	0	0	0	0
Galactose	35%	35%	35%	35%	35%	0	20%	25-35%	25%	0	5-10%
Maltose	10%	10%	10%	10%	10%	0	30%	30%	30%	0	0
Saccharose	0	0	0	0	0	0	0	0	0	0	0
Arabinose	10-15 %	10-15 %	10-15 %	10-15 %	10-15 %	0	10%	20%	20%	0	—
Rhamnose	10%	15%	10%	10%	15%	0	10%	—	—	0	—
Raffinose	0	0	0	0	0	0	0	0	0	0	0
Xylose	10%	0	0	10%	10%	0	0	20%	40%	0	0
Dextrin	8%	8%	10%	10%	10%	0	5%	5%	5%	0	0
Inulin	0	0	0	0	0	0	0	0	0	0	0
Inosite	10%	10%	10%	10%	10%	0	0	10%	0	0	0
Glycerol	0	0	0	0	0	0	0	0	0	0	0
Dulcitol	38%	38%	40%	40%	40%	0	30%	35%	30%	0	0
Mannitol	20%	20%	20%	20%	20%	0	30%	30-35%	35%	0	5-10%
Adonitol	0	0	0	0	0	0	0	0	0	0	0
Salicin	0	0	0	0	0	0	0	0	0	0	0

HYDROGEN-ION CONCENTRATION OF BACTERIUM ANATUM AND RELATED ORGANISMS

The hydrogen-ion concentration was determined by the colorimetric method of Clark and Lubs. Both the peptone and the synthetic phthalate mediums of these authors were employed. The cultures were incubated at 37 C. for 5 days. Methyl red was used as the indicator, 5 drops of this reagent being added to 5 c c of the culture.

TABLE 3

RESULT OF TESTS

Organisms	Peptone Medium P_H =	Synthetic Medium P_H =
B. anatum 1	4.9	4.6
B. anatum 2	4.8	4.6
B. anatum 3	4.9	4.6
B. anatum 4	4.8, 4.9	4.6
B. anatum 5	4.9	4.6
B. typhi	5.2	5.4
B. paratyphi A	5.0, 4.9	4.9
B. paratyphi B	4.9	4.8
B. pullorum	4.9	5.1
B. sanguinarium	5.2	5.0

The uniformity of the P_H values of the different strains of B. anatum in both mediums, with a slightly higher hydrogen-ion concentration in the synthetic than in the peptone medium, is of some interest. In the peptone medium the figures for all of the organisms employed vary only within a few tenths, whereas the figures of the second column show somewhat greater irregularity among the different species.

AGGLUTINATION STUDIES

Agglutination experiments were conducted with the serum of rabbits which were immunized against one or another of the following organisms: B. anatum, 1, B. typhosus, B. paratyphosus A, B. paratyphosus B, B. pullorum, and B. sanguinarium.*

TABLE 4

AGGLUTINATION EXPERIMENTS WITH THE SERUM OF RABBIT IMMUNIZED AGAINST B. ANATUM, 1

Antigen	1:100	1:200	1:400	1:500	1:800	1:1,000	1:2,000	1:4,000
B. anatum 1	++++	++++	++++	+++	+++	+++	+++	+++
B. anatum 2	++++	++++	++++	++++	++++	++++	++++	++++
B. anatum 3	++++	++++	++++	++++	+++	+++	+++	+++
B. anatum 4	++++	++++	++++	+++	+++	++	++	+
B. anatum 5	++++	++++	++++	+++	+++	+++	+++	?
B. typhosus 3, Am. M.	++++	++	0	0	0	0	0	0
B. paratyphosus A, 228K	0	0	0	0	0	0	0	0
B. paratyphosus A, 258K	0	0	0	0	0	0	0	0
B. paratyphosus A, 287K	0	0	0	0	0	0	0	0
B. paratyphosus B. 225K	+++	+++	+++	+++	++	++	++	+
B. paratyphosus B, 234K	++++	+++	++	++	++	++	0	0
B. paratyphosus B, 232K	+++	++	++	+	+	+	0	0
B. sanguinarium, C.	0	0	0	0	0	0	0	0
B. pullorum, B'16	0	0	0	0	0	0	0	0

++++ indicates complete agglutination; +++, almost complete; ++, partial; +, slight; and 0, no agglutination.

TABLE 5

SERUM OF RABBIT IMMUNIZED AGAINST B. TYPHOSUS, 607, AM. M.

Antigen	1:100	1:200	1:400	1:500	1:800	1:1,000	1:2,000	1:4,000
B. anatum 1	0	0	0	0	0	0	0	0
B. anatum 2	0	0	0	0	0	0	0	0
B. anatum 3	0	0	0	0	0	0	0	0
B. anatum 4	0	0	0	0	0	0	0	0
B. anatum 5	0	0	0	0	0	0	0	0
B. typhosus 607, Am. M.	++++	++++	++++	++++	+++	+++	+	0
B. typhosus 3, Am. M.	++++	++++	+++	+++	++	++	+	0
B. paratyphosus A, 228K	0	0	0	0	0	0	0	0
B. paratyphosus A, 258K	0	0	0	0	0	0	0	0
B. paratyphosus A, 287K	0	0	0	0	0	0	0	0
B. paratyphosus B, 234K	0	0	0	0	0	0	0	0
B. paratyphosus B, 225K	0	0	0	0	0	0	0	0
B. paratyphosus B, 232K	0	0	0	0	0	0	0	0
B. sanguinarium, C.	0	0	0	0	0	0	0	0
B. pullorum, B'16	0	0	0	0	0	0	0	0

Slant agar cultures grown at 37 C. for 24 hours were employed. The growths were washed off with salt solution, and suspensions of definite density, in so far as these could be obtained by the nephelometer method, were administered subcutaneously. Four injections of heated vaccines, in doses of 0.5, 1.0,

* Since the rabbit which was inoculated with B. sanguinarium did not furnish a serum of marked agglutinating properties, this serum is not included in the following tables.

1.5 and 2.0 c c were followed by 0.5 c c of a living suspension, all at 4-5 day intervals. On account of the weak agglutination properties of the blood serums further subcutaneous injections of 0.25, 0.75, 1.25, and 2.0 c c of the suspensions were made. The final agglutination tests were conducted on blood samples drawn on the tenth day after the last inoculation.

In the agglutination tests the serum dilutions varied from 1 : 100 to 1 : 4,000. The antigens were prepared by washing off 24-hour agar cultures of the different organisms employed (B. anatum, B. typhosus, B. paratyphosus A, B. para-

TABLE 6

Serum of Rabbit Immunized against B. paratyphosus A, 228K

Antigen	1:100	1:200	1:400	1:500	1:800	1:1,000	1:2,000	1:4,000
B. anatum 1	0	0	0	0	0	0	0	0
B. typhosus, 607	0	0	0	0	0	0	0	0
B. paratyphosus A, 228K	++++	++++	++++	++++	++++	+++	+++	+++
B. paratyphosus B, 232K	0	0	0	0	0	0	0	0
B. sanguinarium	0	0	0	0	0	0	0	0
B. pullorum	0	0	0	0	0	0	0	0

TABLE 7

Serum of Rabbit Immunized against B. paratyphosus B, 232K

Antigen	1:100	1:200	1:400	1:500	1:800	1:1,000	1:2,000	1:4,000
B. anatum 1	+++	+++	++	++	+	+	+	+
B. anatum 2	0	0	0	0	0	0	0	0
B. anatum 3	++	++	0	0	0	0	0	0
B. anatum 4	++	++	++	+	+	+	0	0
B. anatum 5	+++	++	++	+	+	0	0	0
B. typhosus, 3	+?	0	0	0	0	0	0	0
B. typhosus, 607	++	0	0	0	0	0	0	0
B. paratyphosus A, 228	0	0	0	0	0	0	0	0
B. paratyphosus A, 258	0	0	0	0	0	0	0	0
B. paratyphosus A, 287	0	0	0	0	0	0	0	0
B. paratyphosus B, 225	++++	++++	++++	++++	+++	+++	+++	++
B. paratyphosus B, 232	++++	++++	++++	++++	+++	+++	++	+
B. paratyphosus B, 234	++++	++++	++++	++++	+++	+++	++	+
B. sanguinarium	0	0	0	0	0	0	0	0
B. pullorum	0	0	0	0	0	0	0	0

TABLE 8

Serum of Rarrit Immunized against B. pullorum

Antigen	1:100	1:200	1:400	1:500	1:800	1:1,000	1:2,000	1:4,000
B. anatum 1	0	0	0	0	0	0	0	0
B. anatum 2	0	0	0	0	0	0	0	0
B. anatum 3	0	0	0	0	0	0	0	0
B. anatum 4	0	0	0	0	0	0	0	0
B. anatum 5	0	0	0	0	0	0	0	0
B. typhosus, 3	++++	++++	+++	+++	++	0	0	0
B. typhosus, 607	++++	++++	+++	+	0	0	0	0
B. paratyphosus A, 228	0	0	0	0	0	0	0	0
B. paratyphosus A, 258	0	0	0	0	0	0	0	0
B. paratyphosus A, 287	0	0	0	0	0	0	0	0
B. paratyphosus B, 225	0	0	0	0	0	0	0	0
B. paratyphosus B, 232	0	0	0	0	0	0	0	0
B. paratyphosus B, 234	0	0	0	0	0	0	0	0
B. sanguinarium	++++	+++	++	+	+	+	0	0
B. pullorum	++++	++++	++	+	0	0	0	0

typhosus B, B. sanguinarium and B. pullorum) with carbolized salt solution. They were made to match in turbidity with 0.75 of the McFarland nephelometer scale.

The close relationship of B. anatum to B. paratyphosus B is again brought out vividly. Each of the three strains of B. paratyphosus B. employed was agglutinated in a dilution of at least 1:1,000 when tested with the serum of a rabbit which was immunized against B. anatum. Furthermore, four of the five strains of B. anatum reacted with the serum of the paratyphosus B rabbit, one in a dilution of 1:4,000. However, agglutination was in but one instance complete. B. anatum 2 failed to react. Excepting a reaction of B. anatum serum with B. typhosus in dilutions of 1:100 and 1:200, and a partial reaction in 1:100 of B. typhosus to the B. paratyphosus B serum, no other cross-agglutinations were observed.

All five of the B. anatum strains were agglutinated in high dilution by the serum of the rabbit immunized against B. anatum 1, strain 2 being completely clumped in a dilution of 1:4,000. The failure of B. pullorum and B. sanguinarium to react with the B. anatum serum is of particular interest, and further strengthens the view that B. anatum and B. pullorum are not only not identical, but that their relationship with each other is rather remote.

The cross agglutination of B typhosus and B. sanguinarium with the B. pullorum serum is in accord with the observations of Smith and Ten Broeck (1915) who demonstrated a very close relationship between these three organisms. The serum of the B. typhosus rabbit failed, however, to agglutinate B. sanguinarium and B. pullorum.

PATHOGENICITY OF B. ANATUM

Four chicks about three weeks old were inoculated with 0.25 c c of a suspension of B. anatum prepared by washing off a 24-hour slant agar culture with 20 c c of salt solution. The inoculations were made under the skin of the breast.

Within five hours after the injections, two of the chicks appeared decidedly lame. On the morning of the following day these chicks were found dead, and the other two unable to walk. Five hours later a third died. The remaining chick succumbed late in the afternoon two days later. All of the chicks died within 53 hours after inoculation. The quick response to the small doses administered must be regarded as an indication of a high degree of pathogenicity of the organism. Results obtained in later experiments were, however, not so striking; but this may at least in part be accounted for by the brief interval (2-3 weeks) which had elapsed after the isolation of the organism injected in the first series of experiments on young chicks and the time of later inoculations.

Aside from reddening of the area immediately surrounding the point of inoculation, no abnormal condition of the chicks as a whole or of the internal organs was apparent. On postmortem examination, B. anatum was recovered.

At the same time that the four chicks mentioned above were inoculated, a half-grown rabbit and an adult guinea-pig received a subcutaneous injection of 1.0 c c of the same bacterial suspension.

Five days after the injections, a large swelling was observed on the rabbit at the site of inoculation. This grew to about the size of a walnut, and was firm to the touch. It soon broke and yielded a fluid resembling ordinary pus. The abscess was treated daily with disinfectant, but persisted for several days. Healing was very slow. A similar reaction occurred on the guinea-pig, though the swelling was not as large and prominent as on the rabbit. Attempts to isolate B. anatum from the pus of the abscesses were unsuccessful.

Three chicks, 11 days old, and a fourth, 10 weeks old, were inoculated in the same manner as the preceding. The smaller chicks received from 0.25 to 0.5 c c of the bacterial suspension, and the older chick 1.0 c c.

Within from 24 to 36 hours the three small chicks showed indications of bodily disturbance. They were quiet and of subnormal temperature. They ate freely, and the crops were distended; they were thirsty also. The condition grew worse gradually. Four days after injection they were very weak and listless, their eyes closed, and they huddled together for warmth. One of the chicks died on the following day. Two days later a second died, and nine days after inoculation the third was found dead.

The tissues and organs of the three chicks showed no abnormal appearances except a slight swelling and the presence of a small amount of fibrous exudate at the site of inoculation in two of the chicks. B. anatum was recovered from the liver and heart blood in large numbers and unassociated with other organisms.

Fourteen ducklings, two days old, were divided into three groups of 4, 5 and 5. Four ducklings in each lot were given a subcutaneous injection of a salt solution suspension of B. anatum grown on slant agar for 24 hours. Lot 1 (4 in the group, and no control) received strain 3; 2, strain 1, and lot 3 strain 4. Lots 2 and 3 also contained an uninoculated control. The amount of bacterial suspension injected was 0.25 c c.

During the first 48 hours there was no visible change in any of the ducklings. On the third day a duckling was found dead in pen 2, and a little later on the same day one in pen 1. On the following day two others died in lot 1. On the fourth day but one remained alive in this pen. A second duckling was found dead in pen 2 on the fourth day after inoculation. On the same day the control bird of this lot was found dead in the feed dish which had become filled with water during a rain storm. The duckling had the appearances of being trampled on by the hen which was brooding them.

Lot 3 suffered its first loss on the fourth day. This duckling appeared abnormal, and the same staggering was observed as was seen on the farm where the first inquiry was made into the disease. The last survivor of lot 3 became lame on the third day after inoculation. A nodular swelling was observed at the site of inoculation which resembled those seen in the rabbit and guinea-pig. The swelling appeared to be painful, and the duckling moved about very little. It remained alive until 11 days after the injection. Postmortem examination revealed an abundance of fibrous exudate at the inoculation site, and for some distance over the right side of the breast and on the right thigh. The internal organs appeared normal. B. anatum was recovered from the liver and spleen in large numbers.

At the end of 11 days there were left of the original ducklings, 2 in pen 1, 3 in pen 2, and none in pen 3.

Culture tests on all of the dead ducklings yielded a pure growth of B. anatum from the blood of the internal organs in every instance except in the first victim and in the control. No pathologic changes could be observed except a swelling and accumulation of a fibrous exudate in the inoculation area on three or four of the ducklings.

SUMMARY

B. anatum, N. S., was isolated from the internal organs of young ducklings that died of a disease in some respects resembling bacillary white diarrhea of chicks and known in some sections as "keel." The disease is of apparently wide distribution, and the mortality may be very high.

The organism was obtained in pure culture also from ovarian cysts and from an abdominal cyst of breeding ducks on a large commercial duck farm which was very seriously affected by the duckling disease. It appears quite probable, therefore, that the disease is transmitted from the breeders through infected eggs in the same way as bacillary white diarrhea has been demonstrated to have its source in the ovaries of infected hens. Proof of such relationship in the duckling disease is, however, still lacking, owing to our inability to procure the necessary materials for a more extensive study of this point. It is planned to resume this phase of the investigation with the appearance of the next breeding season.

While B. anatum resembles B. pullorum in several particulars, it is more closely related, in so far as morphology, cultural, and fermentation properties are concerned, to B. paratyphosus A and B, and to B. enteritidis. Its agglutination reactions link it most closely with B. paratyphosus B; also its alkalinizing action in milk. Of the different organisms which have been used in the comparative study, namely, B. typhosus, B. paratyphosus A and B, B. enteritidis, B. pullorum and B. sanguinarium, B. anatum resembles B. typhosus least, and B. paratyphosus B most.

GROUPING OF BACILLUS INFLUENZAE BY SPECIFIC AGGLUTINATION

James C. Small and G. K. Dickson

From the Department of Pathology, Washington University, School of Medicine, St. Louis

Attention has recently been directed to the hemophilic bacteria in connection with the much discussed relation of Pfeiffer's bacillus to pandemic influenza. The present grouping of these organisms is unsatisfactory, being based largely on a consideration of the clinical conditions in which they are found. Slight differences in their cultural characters, in their pathogenicity for animals, and meager observations of their immunologic reactions play a secondary rôle in this classification. There has thus been designated: B. influenzae (Pfeiffer,[1] 1892); B. pertussis, the bacillus of acute contagious conjunctivitis, the bacillus of chronic conjunctivitis, a hemophilic bacillus isolated from urine (Davis,[2] 1910), as well as hemophilic organisms from various sources among lower animals. The pseudo-influenza bacillus of Pfeiffer has not been described with sufficient differential characters to warrant its separation from B. influenzae.

Davis,[3] in 1907, studied the immunologic reactions of a number of strains of hemophilic organisms, but was unable to establish by agglutination tests with immune rabbit serum a definite grouping among the strains studied. Park[4] and his co-workers have reported an extensive study of strains of B. influenzae isolated during the recent pandemic of influenza. No grouping of the strains studied was established by agglutination and by the absorption of agglutinins, using the serum of immunized rabbits. Specific agglutination with the homologous serum was obtained, but each strain appeared to be individual in its immunologic reactions. More recently Huntoon and Hannum[5] report work in which they obtained an "almost complete absorption of agglutinins for the immunizing strain and for heterogenous strains," and Roos[6] in collaboration with these workers concludes that "the various strains studied do not differ in kind."

Received for publication Nov. 6, 1919.

[1] Deutsch. med. Wchnschr., 1892, 2, p. 465; Ztschr. f. Hyg. u. Infektionskr., 1892, 13, p. 357.
[2] J. Infect. Dis., 1910, 7, p. 599.
[3] Jour. Am. Med. Assn., 1907, 48, p. 1563.
[4] Jour. Am. Med. Assn., 1919, 73,, p. 318.
[5] J. Immunol., 1919, 4, p. 167.
[6] J. Immunol., 1919, 4, p. 189.

We have had the opportunity to make a similar study of ten strains of hemophilic bacteria, all except one of which were typically B. influenzae from their cultural, morphologic, and staining properties. The tenth strain was an organism presenting the cultural and staining characters of B. influenzae, but it exhibited such fantastic pleomorphism that it would scarcely be classed with the B. influenzae group even by those fully appreciating the pleomorphic tendencies of this group. A rabbit was immunized with the organism with the idea of establishing its relationship to the typical strains studied. The results obtained differ from those previously reported in that a definite grouping of the strains studied was obtained.

ISOLATION AND ORIGIN OF STRAINS STUDIED

This study was begun in March, 1919, that is, after the passing of epidemic influenza. The strains were collected from various sources by culture on brown blood-agar plates. Several were from cultures of bronchial secretions made at necropsy at Barnes Hospital. The others were isolated by throat cultures from normal individuals, from influenza patients treated in the different wards of the St. Louis City Hospital, and from patients presenting themselves at the Medical Dispensary of Washington University Medical School.

The colonies of B. influenzae were picked from the mixed cultures after 24 hours' incubation and subcultured on brown blood agar. This medium was used throughout in isolating, in carrying along the strains and in growing the organisms for injection into rabbits and for antigen suspensions. It consisted of beef infusion agar neutral to phenolphthalein to which 5% defibrinated rabbit blood was added at 90 C. immediately before pouring the plates or slants.

IMMUNIZATION OF ANIMALS

Full grown rabbits were immunized by intravenous injection of living organisms from 48-hour growths of the different strains in pure culture. The agar slants or plates used for growing the organisms for the rabbit inoculations were seeded heavily with the different strains. After a 48-hour incubation period, the growth was washed off and emulsified in 5 c c of sterile normal salt solution. One or two cubic centimeters of the suspension was injected immediately into the ear vein of the rabbit. From time to time small amounts of blood were drawn from the ear vein and preliminary homologous agglutination tests were made.

The serums used in the titrations reported were obtained with blood drawn from the rabbit's heart by a syringe. All the animals survived this bleeding, and the yield of serum in every case was sufficient for complete agglutination, cross agglutination and absorption tests. From the protocols it will be noted that after a three or four day interval following the bleeding, the rabbits were reinoculated, using the same size dosage that each rabbit had last received. Within 12 hours following this injection, 4 of the rabbits died. At a previous time 10 c c of blood were drawn from rabbit 2, and immediately an inoculation was made. This rabbit also died following the inoculation. This experience is cited to emphasize the danger of inoculating large doses following the drawing of considerable blood from immune rabbits.

The blood as drawn was put in sterile centrifuge tubes, placed in the incubator at 37.5 C. for about 10 minutes when the clots were loosened from the sides of the tubes by means of a stiff wire. The tubes were allowed to stand in the icebox over night, then centrifugalized and the serum drawn off.

The following protocols give the details of the strains used and the progress of the animal immunizations.

STRAIN 1. — From necropsy, diagnosis, bronchopneumonia; isolated 4-28-19; antigen planted 5-10-19.

	Injections	Amount 24-Hour Culture	Date of Bleeding
Rabbit 1	3/30	1/5 agar slant	
	4/ 6	2/5 agar slant	
	4/12	1/5 agar plate	
	4/22	2/5 agar plate	
	5/ 3	2/5 agar plate	
	5/10	2/5 agar plate	
	5/24	1/5 agar slant	6/5 – 20 c c
	6/ 9	2/5 agar plate	

STRAIN 2.—From the normal throat of a medical student, exposed but no history of influenza; isolated 4-27-19; antigen planted 5-10-19.

	Injections	Amount 24-Hour Culture	Date of Bleeding
Rabbit 2	5/13	1/5 agar plate	
	5/16	1/5 agar plate	
	5/20	2/5 agar plate	5/24 bled 10 c c from ear vein
	5/24	2/5 agar plate	

STRAIN 3.—Isolated 4-10-19 from the throat of a girl aged 18 months; diagnosis, influenza; antigen planted 6-6-19.

	Injections	Amount 24-Hour Culture	Date of Bleeding
Rabbit 3	4/22	1/5 agar plate	
	4/28	1/5 agar plate	
	5/10	2/5 agar plate	
	5/20	2/5 agar plate	
	5/24	2/5 agar plate	6/6 – 20 c c from heart
	6/ 9	2/5 agar plate	

STRAIN 4.—From a medical student, ambulatory case of Vincent's angina; isolated 4-25-19; antigen planted 6-7-19.

	Injections	Amount 24-Hour Culture	Date of Bleeding
Rabbit 4	4/22	1/5 agar slant	
	4/26	1/5 agar plate	
	5/10	2/5 agar plate	
	5/20	2/5 agar plate	
	5/24	2/5 agar plate	6/5 – 20 c c from heart
	6/ 9	2/5 agar plate	

STRAIN 5.—Isolated from throat of girl, aged 8; diagnosis, influenza; 4-18-19; planting of antigen, 5-10-19.

	Injections	Amount 24-Hour Culture	Date of Bleeding
Rabbit 5	4/26	1/5 agar plate	
	5/ 5	2/5 agar plate	
	5/10	2/5 agar plate	
	5/20	2/5 agar plate	
	5/24	2/5 agar plate	6/5 – 20 c c from heart
	6/ 9	2/5 agar plate	

STRAIN 6.—From bronchial culture, necropsy, man; no history of influenza; diagnosis, terminal pneumonia following multiple fractures; isolated, 4-25-19; antigen preparation, 6-7-19.

	Injections	Amount 24-Hour Culture	Date of Bleeding
Rabbit 6	5/ 5	1/5 agar plate	
	5/10	2/5 agar plate	
	5/20	2/5 agar plate	
	5/24	2/5 agar plate	6/6 – 20 c c from heart
	6/ 9	2/5 agar plate	

STRAIN 7 (atypical morphologically).—From bronchial culture, necropsy, boy; acute osteomyelitis and staphylococcus septicemia; isolated, 4-19-19; antigen preparation, 6-7-19.

	Injections	Amount 24-Hour Culture	Date of Bleeding
Rabbit 7	5/10	1/5 agar plate	
	5/20	2/5 agar plate	
	5/24	2/5 agar plate	
	5/28	1/5 agar plate	6/6 - 20 c c from heart
	6/ 9	2/5 agar plate	

STRAIN 8.—From throat culture, woman, aged 46; influenza; isolated, 4-10-19; antigen preparation, 6-6-19.

	Injections	Amount 24-Hour Culture	Date of Bleeding
Rabbit 8	4/26	1/5 agar plate	
	5/ 5	2/5 agar plate	
	5/10	2/5 agar plate	
	5/20	2/5 agar plate	
	5/24	2/5 agar plate	6/5 - 20 c c from heart
	6/ 9	2/5 agar plate	

STRAIN 9.—From throat of a man, aged 42; influenza; isolated, 4-12-19; date of antigen preparation, 6-6-19.

	Injections	Amount 24-Hour Culture	Date of Bleeding
Rabbit 9	4/26	1/5 agar plate	
	5/ 5	2/5 agar plate	
	5/10	2/5 agar plate	
	5/20	2/5 agar plate	
	5/24	2/5 agar plate	6/5 - 20 c c form heart
	6/ 9	2/5 agar plate	

STRAIN 10.—From throat culture, woman, aged 29; influenza; isolated, 4-10-19; antigen preparation, 5-10-19.

	Injections	Amount 24-Hour Culture	Date of Bleeding
Rabbit 10	4/28	1/5 agar plate	
	5/ 5	2/5 agar plate	
	5/10	2/5 agar plate	
	5/19	2/5 agar plate	
	5/24	2/5 agar plate	6/5 - 20 c c from heart
	6/ 9	2/5 agar plate	

PREPARATION OF ANTIGENS

Twenty-four hour agar-slant cultures were emulsified in 2 or 3 c c of sterile infusion broth, and from this emulsion 15 or 20 petri dish agar surfaces were heavily seeded by means of a sterile cotton swab. After incubating 48 hours at 37.5 C., heavy growths were obtained. This growth was washed off with 0.9% sodium chlorid solution. Small amounts of the salt solution were used in this process, yielding a very heavy bacterial suspension. The operation was much facilitated by the use of a delicate glass scraper made from a capillary pipet by bending it in an "L" shape with the short arm of convenient length, which depended somewhat on the size of the plate surface used. This glass scraper when carefully made presents perfect contact with the agar surface, and can be used in removing the bacterial growth with little danger of removing particles of agar.

The concentrated bacterial suspension thus obtained was collected immediately in sterile centrifuge tubes, and the bacteria precipitated at moderate speed. High speed packs the bacteria too solidly and later renders emulsification more tedious. The supernatant liquid was then drawn off, and the bacteria were suspended in fresh salt solution. In this manner the greater part of the soluble elements from the surface of the agar was removed from the antigen suspension. Precautions to avoid contamination were observed throughout. To the concentrated antigen suspension, 0.5% of liquor formaldehydi was added and the containers thoroughly shaken to effect homogeneous suspension.

The antigen dilution used in the agglutination tests was more or less empirically determined for the first antigen. It was found that a turbidity amounting to little more than a perceptible opalescence in the small agglutination test tube gave very sharp and clear cut agglutination readings. Choosing this dilution as a standard, the other antigens were standardized to it by dilutions and direct comparison, as recommended in the turbidity standardization of antigen in the Dreyer method for agglutination within the typhoid group.

TECHNIC OF AGGLUTINATION TESTS

Agglutination tests were set up with final dilutions of serum of 1:20, 1:40, 1:100, and thence upward by increments of 100 as far as necessary to cover the agglutination zone of the serum tested. The serum dilutions and the antigen were used in 0.5 c c amounts each. The tests were read after 16 hours' incubation at 55 C. Complete agglutination with formation of large clumps is designated + +; complete agglutination with small clumps giving a granular appearance as +, and partial agglutination as ±. Naked eye readings were used, and partial agglutination dilutions disregarded in determining the serum titer.

Table 1 presents the agglutination and cross agglutination values obtained with the serums studied. The numbers given in the table represent the highest dilution which gave the 1 + reading as defined above.

TABLE 1

AGGLUTINATION AND CROSS-AGGLUTINATION TITERS

Immune Serum	Antigens										Normal Rabbit Serum Control	Normal Salt Solution Control
	1	2	3	4	5	6	7*	8	9	10		
1	900	20	40	0	0	40	0	800	700	40	—	—
2	40	1,000	1,900	0	1,400	700	0	0	0	2,000	—	—
3	20	0	20	0	0	0	0	0	0	20	—	—
4	0	0	0	700	0	20	0	0	0	0	—	—
5	40	1,100	1,900	0	1,700	400	0	20	20	1,800	—	—
6	0	100	200	0	200	1,300	0	0	0	400	—	—
7	20	40	40	0	40	600	0	0	0	200	—	—
8	800	0	0	0	0	20	0	600	700	20	—	—
9	400	0	20	0	0	20	0	400	500	20	—	—
10	0	1,300	2,200	0	1,400	100	0	0	0	2,400	±	—

* Antigen not agglutinable.

A definite pro-agglutinoid zone was observed in all the high titer serums. In several instances bacteriolysis was observed in the first dilution. It is suggested that this observation might have some bearing on the explanation of the so-called pro-agglutinoid phenomenon, that is, a sufficient concentration of bacteriolysins occurring along with the agglutinins may impede the action of the latter, or may cause disintegration of the bacterial clumps after they have formed.

DISCUSSION OF AGGLUTINATION TESTS

It will be noted in table 1 that serum 1 agglutinates strains 8 and 9 in about the same dilutions that it agglutinated the homologous strain. Serum 8 agglutinates strains 1 and 9, and serum 9 agglutinates 1 and 8. These three strains act nonspecifically with all other serums, while they appear to cross-agglutinate specifically and suggest their immunologic group identity.

Serum 2 agglutinates strains 3, 5, 6 and 10. In analyzing this group, it is noted first, that serum 3 contains practically no antibodies for its homologous antigen, and consequently must be ruled out as an immune serum.

Serums 5 and 10 contain a high titer of antibodies for strains 2, 3, 5, and 10, while there is a lower titer for strain 6 than appeared in serum 2.

Serum 6 agglutinates 2, 3, 5, and 10, but the antibody titer is low. The cross agglutination tests here place strains 2, 3, 5 and 10 in one group, and leave one in doubt about the placing of strain 6.

Serum 4 agglutinates only its own antigen, and strain 4 is unaffected by any of the other immune serums, suggesting the separate identity of strain 4 among these 10 strains.

Serum 7 shows considerable concentration of antibodies for strains 6 and 10, while the homologous antigen was not agglutinated. Antigen 7 was not affected by any of the immune serums. This result suggests at once that antigen 7 was a nonagglutinable bacterial suspension. This strain, it will be remembered, is the organism classified as "irregular" on account of its pleomorphism, and its great tendency to undergo autolysis. Suspensions of this organism were very difficult to make on account of the difficulty of breakng up the clumps of organisms as they were washed from the agar. That serum 7 contains antibodies is shown by its titer with antigens from other strains, for example 6 and 10.

The agglutination tests suggest:

Group 1.—Strains 1, 8 and 9.

Group 2.—Strains 2, 3, 5, 10, and perhaps 6.

Group 3.—Strain 4 only.

Strain 7 cannot be classified, but appears most nearly related to strains 6 and 10.

ABSORPTION TESTS

The absorption of agglutinins was conducted in the following manner: One cubic centimeter of a 1:10 dilution of the immune serum was mixed with 4 c c of the concentrated antigen in a sterile centrifuge tube. This amount of the antigen was found to be sufficient to absorb the homologous agglutinins after 4 hours' incubation at 37.5 C., the tubes being shaken at half hour intervals. After this period of incubation, the tubes were centrifugalized and the clear supernatant serum dilution (1:50) drawn off. Final dilutions of this were set up 1:100, 200, 400, 800 and 1,600, using all of the antigens which were agglutinated before absorption by the particular serum in dilutions above 1:100. The 16-hour incubation period at 55 C. was again used, and tests read as described under the agglutination tests.

The results of these tests are given in table 2. In the table + indicates an agglutination value, after exposure for absorption approximating serum titer before exposure, while — indicates no agglutination in the lowest dilution used (namely, 1:100). With the high titer serums used failure to show agglutination in 1:100 dilution after exposure for absorption definitely indicates specific absorption of agglutinins.

TABLE 2

AGGLUTINATION WITH TREATED SERUM

Serum	Absorbed with Antigen	Antigen									
		1	2	3	4	5	6	7*	8	9	10
1	10	+	..	..	..	..	..	..	+	+	..
	9	—	..	..	..	..	..	..	—	—	..
2	3	..	—	—	..	—	+	..	..	..	—
3†											
4	6	..	..	..	+	..	..	..	..	..	..
	7	..	..	..	+	..	..	..	..	..	..
5	3	..	—	—	..	—	+	..	..	..	—
	10	..	—	—	..	—	+	..	..	..	—
6	3	..	—	—	..	—	+	..	..	..	—
	4	..	+	+	..	+	+	..	..	..	+
	6	..	—	—	..	—	—	..	..	..	—
	7	..	+	+	..	+	+	..	..	..	+
7	6	..	..	..	..	..	—	..	..	..	—
	4	..	..	..	..	..	+	..	..	..	+
8	1	—	..	..	..	..	..	..	—	—	..
9	1	—	..	..	..	..	..	..	—	—	..
10	1	..	+	+	..	+	+	..	..	..	+
	2	..	—	—	..	—	+	..	..	..	—
	3	..	—	—	..	—	+	..	..	..	—
	5	..	—	—	..	—	+	..	..	..	—
	6	..	+	+	..	(?)	—	..	..	..	+

* Antigen not agglutinable.
† No agglutinins in serum.

The absorption tests definitely established two groups containing in the first instance strains 1, 8 and 9; and in the second, strains 2, 3, 5 and 10.

Strain 4 stood as an individual strain in the agglutination tests. Serum 4 had no agglutinins removed by absorption with strains 6 and 7. Conversely, serum 6 had no agglutinins removed by absorption with strain 4.

Strain 6, which by the agglutination tests showed a relation to the strains of group 2, by the absorption tests is shown to be outside of this group and represents another individual strain. Serum 7 agglutinated strain 6 in a dilution of 1:600. When this serum was absorbed with strain 6, this was removed. On account of the inability to prepare a satisfactory agglutinable antigen for strain 7, cross absorption tests could not be done to establsh the relation between strains 6 and 7.

The agglutination tests show some cross group agglutinins between groups 1 and 2, and also between strains 6 and 7, and the two groups. Strain 4 appears more strictly unrelated to the others, its antigen being agglutinated by none of the other serums, and its serum only agglutinating antigen 6 in a 1:20 dilution.

SUMMARY

From the results of these experiments it appears that four groups of B. influenzae have been identified, and that 70% of the strains studied fall into two groups:

Group 1.—Strains 1, 8 and 9.
Group 2.—Strains 2, 3, 5 and 10.
Group 3.—Strain 6.
Group 4.—Strain 4.

Strain 7 has not been proved to be distinct from strain 6, and is unclassified.

CONCLUSION

The hemophilic organisms (B. influenzae) can be grouped by immunologic methods, and four groups have been demonstrated.

THE CHEMOTHERAPEUTICS OF THE CHAULMOOGRIC ACID SERIES AND OTHER FATTY ACIDS IN LEPROSY AND TUBERCULOSIS

I. BACTERICIDAL ACTION; ACTIVE PRINCIPLE; SPECIFICITY

ERNEST LINWOOD WALKER
AND
MARION A. SWEENEY

From the George Williams Hooper Foundation for Medical Research, University of California Medical School, San Francisco

Chaulmoogra oil has an empiric reputation in the treatment of leprosy that extends back into antiquity. This reputation is supported by the experience of modern leperologists. The old and less effective method of oral administration of chaulmoogra oil has been replaced, first by subcutaneous and intramuscular injection of oil mixtures, and more recently by intravenous injection of salts of the chaulmoogric acids; and investigators almost unanimously agree that arrest of the disease, improvement, and frequently cure follows adequate treatment with chaulmoogra oil and its derivatives. The importance of the fatty acid therapy of diseases due to the acid-fast group of bacteria has been greatly increased by the report of Rogers[1] on the intravenous use of "sodium morrhuate," the sodium salts of the fatty acids of cod-liver oil, in the treatment of tuberculosis. Rogers maintains that there is nothing absolutely specific in the products of chaulmoogra oil for leprosy, but that the unsaturated fatty acids of both chaulmoogra and cod-liver oils, and by implication the unsaturated fatty acids of any oil, are equally efficacious in either leprosy or tuberculosis. He believes that the unsaturated fatty acids act in some way on the fatty coating of acid-fast bacilli, presumably by injuring the capsule of the bacillus and exposing it to the destructive action of the tissues.

These therapeutic claims for the chaulmoograte and morrhuates, if substantiated, would be of the greatest importance to medical science and human welfare. Further investigation is necessary, however, not only to confirm these claims, but also to discover the method of action of chaulmoogra and cod-liver oils, to identify and isolate the therapeutically active principle, if such exists, to determine its distribution in

Received for publication Nov. 9, 1919.

[1] Brit. Med. Jour., 1919, 1, p. 147; Indian Med. Gaz., 1919, 54, p. 165.

vegetable and animal oils, and to test the specificity of its action in leprosy, tuberculosis and other infectious diseases. Such an investigation conducted in the test tube, where the chemical and bactericidal aspects of the subject can be studied, and in animals in which the experiments can be adequately controlled, will, we believe, supply more precise information on at least some of the problems involved than would clinical observation alone. The scope of the experimental investigation which we have undertaken is indicated in the outline:

1. What is the method of therapeutic action, if any, of chaulmoogra oil in leprosy:
   - A. Direct or bactericidal
   - B. Indirect or physiologic
     - a. Stimulation of nonspecific lipolytic activity of the tissues which might attack the fatty capsule of acid-fast bacilli
     - b. Antigen for the production of more or less specific fat antibodies (Deycke,[2] Kleinschmidt,[3] Lucke,[4] Warden,[5] Young[6])
     - c. Disturbance of the ferment-antiferment balance of the body fluids (Jobling and Petersen[7])
     - d. Production of lymphocytosis, which might act as intermediaries in the defense of the host
     - e. Nutritional only
   - C. Inactive?
2. What is the active therapeutic principle of chaulmoogra oil:
   - a. Chaulmoogric acid
   - b. Hydnocarpic acid
   - c. Palmitic acid
   - d. Glycerol or other alcohols
   - e. Gynocardin
   - f. Unidentified substance?
3. Is the therapeutic action of chaulmoogra oil specific for:
   - a. Leprosy

   Or does its action extend to:
   - b. Tuberculosis and other infections with acid-fast bacilli
   - c. Infections with nonacid-fast bacteria
4. Is the therapeutically active principle peculiar to:
   - a. Chaulmoogra oil

   Or is it found in:
   - b. Cod-liver oil (Rogers[1])
   - c. Other oils
   - d. Nonfatty substances

DEVELOPMENT OF THE FATTY ACID THERAPY

Chaulmoogra oil was formerly administered as whole oil by mouth in the empirical treatment of leprosy, often accompanied by local applications of the oil to the skin lesions or combined with other treatment. The nauseating

[2] Deutsch. med. Wchnschr., 1907, 33, p. 89.
[3] Berl. klin. Wchnschr., 1910, 47, p. 57.
[4] Jour. Immunol., 1916, 1, p. 456.
[5] Jour. Infect. Dis., 1918, 23, p. 504.
[6] Jour. Path. & Bacteriol., 1919, 22, p. 224.
[7] Jour. Exper. Med., 1914, 19, p. 239.

property of this oil and the long course of treatment necessary to obtain therapeutic results seriously interfered with its efficient use. Nevertheless, improvement and even cure of leprosy attributed to chaulmoogra oil administered by this method have been reported (Dyer,[8] Hopkins,[9] Connel,[10] Hollmann and Dean[11]). The most comprehensive report published on the oral administration of chaulmoogra oil in leprosy is that of Hopkins, who gives the results of its use during fifteen years at the Leper's Home of Louisiana. Excluding cases on which a fair trial of the treatment had not been given, his figures are:

1. Incipient cases	82
Discharged cured	17%
Remaining at the Home, all lesions having disappeared	4%
Remaining at the Home in an improved condition	24%
Absconded in an improved condition	24%
Remaining at the Home, the disease apparently arrested	14%
Worse	8%
Died	4%
2. Advanced cases	88
Remaining at the Home in an improved condition	12%
Remaining at the Home, the disease apparently arrested	5%
Absconded in an improved condition	9%
Little change	28%
Disease became terminal	20%
Died in the terminal stage	23%

Since gastric disturbance and slowness of action are serious obstacles to treatment by oral administration, a number of mixtures of chaulmoogra oil with other substances have been proposed to render it more fluid, improve its absorption and reduce its irritating property, thus making it suitable for subcutaneous and intramuscular injection (Jeanselme,[12] Brocq and Pomaret,[13] Mercado and Heiser,[14] Hollmann and Currie[11]). Of these mixtures, that of Mercado and Heiser,[14] generally known as the Heiser mixture, has been used most extensively. This mixture consists of chaulmoogra oil, 60 c c; camphorated oil, 60 c c, and resorcin, 4 gm.

In 1913 Heiser[14] reported the apparent cure of two cases of leprosy by subcutaneous injections of this chaulmoogra oil mixture, combined with vaccine treatment, and in one case with the oral administration of chaulmoogra oil. Later[15] he reported the apparent cure of two other cases by subcutaneous injections of chaulmoogra oil mixture alone for a period of from 4 to 8 months. In a third communication[16] Heiser gave the results of this method of treatment in 12 additional cases. Some patients were apparently cured, others showed great improvement, and in all the disease had been arrested.

The subcutaneous or intramuscular injection of chaulmoogra oil mixtures has been used subsequently in the treatment of leprosy by Hopkins[9] in 9 cases,

[8] N. Y. Med. News, 1905, 87, p. 199.
[9] New Orleans Med. and Surg. Jour., 1916, 69, p. 223.
[10] Jour. Trop. Med. and Hyg., 1919, 22, p. 37.
[11] Jour. Cutan. Dis., 1919, 37, p. 367.
[12] Presse méd., 1911, 19, p. 989.
[13] Bull. Soc. franç. de dermat. et syph., 1913, 24, p. 70.
[14] U. S. Pub. Health Rept., 1913, 28, p. 1855.
[15] Ibid, 1914, 29, p. 21.
[16] Ibid., p. 2763; Am. Jour. Trop. Dis. and Prev. Med., 1914, 2, p. 300.

by McCoy and Hollmann[17] in 42 cases, by Armellini[18] in 1 case, by Bercovitz[19] in 14 cases, by Coghill[20] in 7 cases, by Hall[21] in 90 cases, by Cadbury[22] in 26 cases, by Connel,[10] Hollmann and Dean[11] and others, with encouraging results. The last named authors report 12 leper patients in Hawaii who became bacteriologically negative after treatment by intramuscular injections of chaulmoogra oil mixtures, of which only 2 subsequently had a recurrence, one within 7 months and the other within 2 years.

Recently Hollmann and Dean[11] have prepared and used by intramuscular injection the ethyl esters of fractions of the fatty acids of chaulmoogra oil in the treatment of leprosy in Hawaii. These acids, after isolation by the ordinary chemical methods, were separated into fractions by fractional crystallization and the fractions converted into their ethyl esters. The four fractions used in the experiments were:

A. Ethyl ester of chaulmoogric acid.
B. Ethyl ester of acids crystallizing from alcohol with chaulmoogric acid in the initial separation.
C. Ethyl ester of acids soluble in 92% alcohol in the first separation and which form soluble lead salts.
D. Ethyl esters of acids forming lead salts insoluble in ether.

These authors report 26 cases treated 4 months or longer by these several fractions. Patients receiving fractions C and D have shown the greatest improvement. Of these 26 cases, all have shown improvement—many, marked improvement. Eight have already become bacteriologically negative and have been paroled from segregation.

In this connection it is interesting to note that Brill and Williams[23] state that the ethyl esters of chaulmoogric and hydnocarpic acids, sometimes known as antileprol, were found to be ineffective on leprosy in the Philippine Islands.

The next advance in the chaulmoogra oil therapy of leprosy was the attempt to devise preparations suitable for intravenous injection. Vahram,[24] in order to avoid gastric disturbances resulting from the use of chaulmoogra oil by stomach and the pain and abscess formation incident to subcutaneous injection, prepared an emulsion of chaulmoogra oil for intravenous injection. The formula for this "pseudo-solution," as given by him is: gum acacia, 0.144 gm.; chaulmoogra oil, 0.00072 gm. The oil is added to the gum acacia. After desiccation cold, the mixture is submitted to long porphyrization, then put in suspension in the initial volume of liquid and sterilized at 110 C. The emulsion prepared in this manner is characterized by the minuteness of the suspended globules of oil, which are said to approach the dimensions of colloidal granules. Vahram thinks this property not only renders the emulsion suitable for intravenous injection but that it, in consequence of the great multiplication of surface, should produce an intensification of the therapeutic action. Stévenel,[25] in collaboration with Noc, prepared an emulsion for intravenous injection by shaking chaulmoogra oil with N/1 Na_2CO_3. Oil globules of emulsions prepared by this method are said to be as small or smaller than red blood corpuscles.

17 U. S. Pub. Health Bull., 1916, No. 75, p. 3.
18 Clin. Dermosifilopat. d. r. Univ. di Roma, 1917, 35, p. 103.
19 Jour. Am. Med. Assn., 1917, 68, p. 1960.
20 Ann. Trop. Med. and Parasit., 1917, 11, p. 205.
21 Trop. Dis. Bull., 1919, 13, p. 13.
22 China Med. Jour., 1918, 32, p. 226.
23 Philippine Jour. Sc., 1916, Sect. A, 11, p. 78; 1917, Sect. A, 12, p. 207.
24 Progrès med., 1916, 31, p. 19.
25 Bull. Soc. Path. Exot., 1917, 10, p. 684.

Vahram,[24] Hopkins[9] and Stévenel[25] each report improvement in two cases of leprosy undergoing intravenous treatment with these emulsions; but apparently these patients had not been under treatment long enough to determine the ultimate result.

Rogers[26] appears to be the first to use the soluble salts of the fatty acids of chaulmoogra oil intravenously in leprosy, although such salts and their administration by mouth are mentioned by Roux,[11] Trapezinkoff,[11] Dyer,[8] Desprex,[27] Amaral and Parambos,[28] and Hollmann and Currie.[11] Rogers separated the total fatty acids of chaulmoogra oil by the ordinary chemical methods. These crude fatty acids were then separated into fractions of different melting points by dissolving in hot alcohol and removing the acids that crystallized out at different temperatures as the solution cooled. The first fraction, which constituted about two thirds of the total, had a melting point of from 40.8 to 43 C. and is designated as fraction A; the second, with a melting point of from 37 to 40 C., is fraction B, and the remainder, which was liquid at room temperature (28 C.) in Calcutta, is fraction C. These fractions, which may be purified by dissolving in ether, were converted into water-soluble sodium salts by titrating with sodium hydroxid, using phenolphthalein as an indicator, and are called by Rogers "sodium gynocardates."

Rogers states that the sodium salt of fraction A is only slightly soluble in water, is unsuited for either subcutaneous or intravenous injection, and that it is doubtful whether it has any therapeutic value. He used the sodium salts of fractions B and C combined, first subcutaneously and later intravenously[29] in the treatment of leprosy. Still later Rogers[30] decided that the fraction of the fatty acids of chaulmoogra oil having a higher melting point of from 49 to 62 C. yield sodium salts sufficiently soluble and that they are more potent in the treatment of leprosy than the salts of fractions having lower melting points. After two years' experience with sodium gynocardate in leprosy he found that subcutaneous injections do not produce reactions in leprous tissues and are less effective therapeutically than intravenous injections. He employed the intravenous route very extensively, having given over 1,000 intravenous injections of the drug, without any ill effects beyond temporary giddiness and headache and occasional localized clotting in the veins, while the results have been most encouraging. All of the patients have shown improvement. The lesions have disappeared and become bacteriologically negative in 50% of the cases treated within 3 years of the onset of the disease, including cases treated for only from 3 to 12 months; while in cases of from 3 to 15 years' duration, 25% have cleared up under treatment.

Rogers' sodium gynocardate has been used subcutaneously and intravenously by Cadbury,[22] by Carthew[31] in 13 cases, by Muir[32] in 30 cases, by Peacock[33] in 6 cases, by Rogers in 36 cases, by Connel,[10] Muir,[34] in part combined with sodium morrhuate, in 23 cases of leprosy with equally encouraging results.

[26] Lancet, 1916, 1, p. 288.
[27] Lepra, 1900, 6, p. 218.
[28] Bull. gén. de therap., 1908, 155, 415; Lepra, 8, p. 249.
[29] Brit. Med. Jour., 1916, 2, p. 550.
[30] Ind. Jour. Med. Research, 1917, 5, p. 227.
[31] Ind. Med. Gaz., 1918, 53, p. 407.
[32] Ibid., p. 209.
[33] Ibid., p. 95.
[34] Ibid., 1919, 54, p. 130.

Spittle[35] alone reports unfavorably, stating that the reaction was always more or less severe even after small doses and in no case, even after several months, did benefit result.

Recently Rogers[36] reported the results of experiments with the sodium salts of the fatty acids of the oil from the seeds of Hydnocarpus wightiana, a plant closely related to Taraktogenos (Hydnocarpus) kurzii from which chaulmoogra oil is obtained. This oil is said to contain a larger proportion of hydnocarpic acid than chaulmoogra oil. The results of the treatment with these salts, which he now designates as "sodium hydnocarpate," Rogers considers very satisfactory. There was a great reduction and frequent total disappearance of the lepra bacilli, and the number of cases in which the lesions disappeared in less than a year is considered noteworthy. In only one of fourteen cases was the improvement slight.

The promising results obtained in the treatment of leprosy with chaulmoogra oil and its products would naturally suggest their trial in tuberculosis; yet there have been surprisingly few attempts to apply chaulmoogra oil therapy to this disease. Hernandez[39] gives an account of a few experiments, of which only a review has so far been available. He found that the addition of 2% of chaulmoogra oil to the culture medium inhibited the growth of B. tuberculosis, and that treatment of experimentally infected guinea-pigs seemed to confirm the destructive action of chaulmoogra oil on tubercle bacilli. Six patients suffering with tuberculosis were treated with small injections (subcutaneous?) of chaulmoogra oil, 1-2 c c at from 20 to 30 day intervals; all symptoms are said to have subsided in some of the patients.

Rogers[37] suggested the use of sodium gynocardate (chaulmoograte) in the treatment of tuberculosis in 1916; but, since in rare cases of leprosy prolonged febrile reaction and temporary exacerbation of the disease may follow intravenous administration of sodium gynocardate, he hesitated to use it in tuberculosis. For this reason he was led to try sodium morrhuate, the sodium salts of the fatty acids of cod-liver oil, in the treatment of tuberculosis. Without preliminary cultural or animal tests, Rogers has used this salt in the treatment of human tuberculosis, and has supplied it to several clinicians in India for trial, and sodium morrhuate has been put on the market as a specific treatment for tuberculosis.

Rogers[1] states that intravenous injections of sodium morrhuate produce a slight febrile and local congestive reaction, similar to that produced by sodium gynocardate in leprosy, which clearly points to a definite action on the tuberculous tissue. Improvement in phthisical cases is seen in the reduction and cessation of the fever, diminution of the expectoration and cough, and steady gain in weight. In addition, the tubercle bacilli in the sputum gradually decrease in number, and may in time disappear. Moreover, they commonly show deficient acid-fast staining and a granular or beaded appearance, indicating that they are actually being destroyed within the tissues. Furthermore, Rogers says that a year's experience has shown that sodium morrhuate is of great value in leprosy. He believes that the unsaturated fatty acids of both chaulmoogra and cod-liver oils act in some way on the coating of acid-fast bacilli, that of the tubercle bacillus having been shown to contain palmitic and other unsaturated fatty acids.

35 Ibid., 1918, 53, p. 33.
36 Brit. Med. Jour., 1919, 1, p. 147.
37 Jour. Am. Med. Assn., 1918, 71, p. 1177.

The Chemistry of Chaulmoogra Oil

Chaulmoogra oil is a fixed oil, expressed cold from the seeds of Taraktogenos (Hydnocarpus) kurzii King, a tree native of Burma. The most complete and trustworthy investigation of the chemistry of chaulmoogra oil is that by Power and collaborators (1904-1907).[38] Chaulmoogra oil has a melting point of from 22 to 23 C., a specific gravity of 0.951 at 25 C., an acid value of 23.9, a saponification value of 213.0 and an iodin value of 103.2. It is optically active, (a) $\frac{D}{150} = +52.0$ C. Like other fixed oils and fats, chaulmoogra oil consists essentially of glyceryl triesters of fatty acids. Of chief interest is the fact that Power and his collaborators have isolated from chaulmoogra oil and studied chemically a series of unsaturated fatty acids which have a structure and properties entirely different from all other known fatty acids. Although these fatty acids have the same empiric formula as the fatty acids of the linoleic series ($C_nH_{2n-4}O_2$) found in linseed and many other vegetable oils, they differ from these and all other fatty acids in their molecular structure. The fatty acids hitherto known are aliphatic or acyclic compounds, which are optically inactive and have their atoms or radicals arranged in an open chain, of which the following structural formula of oleic acid is an example:

$$CH - (CH_2)_7 - CH = CH - (CH_2)_7 - COOH$$

On the other hand, the fatty acids of the chaulmoogric series are optically active and have their atoms arranged in a closed carbon chain or ring; that is, they are cyclic compounds, as is illustrated by the structural formula proposed by Barrowcliff and Power for chaulmoogric acid:

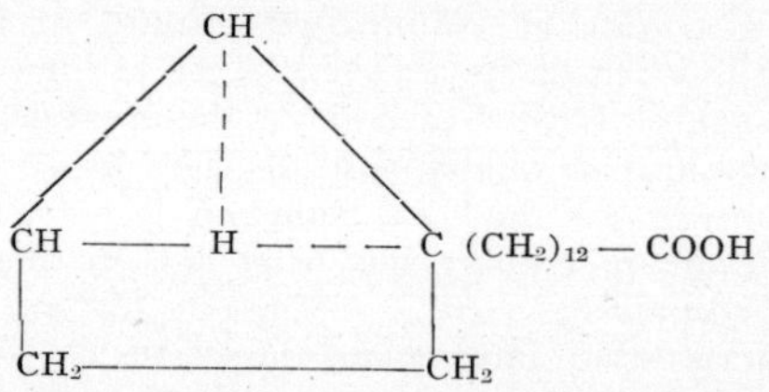

Power and his collaborators isolated two fatty acids of this cyclic series from chaulmoogra oil. One, constituting the larger proportion of the fatty acids, has a melting point of from 68 to 69 C., an empiric formula $C_{18}H_{32}O_2$, and is designated as chaulmoogric acid; a lower isomer, having a melting point of from 59 to 60 C. and an empiric formula of $C_{16}H_{28}O_2$, is designated as hydnocarpic acid. These authors also suggest that chaulmoogra oil may contain other lower isomers of this series of fatty acids. In addition to this series of cyclic fatty acids, chaulmoogra oil contains a small amount of a common, saturated, aliphatic fatty acid, palmitic acid, together with glycerol and phytosterol; and, since the oil is expressed cold from the seeds, it may possibly contain a small amount of the cyanogenic glucosid, gynocardin (Power and Lees) and other nitrogenous substances.

[38] Power and Gornall: Jour. Chem. Soc., 1904, 85, p. 851; Power and Lees: Ibid., 1905, 137, p. 349; Power and Barrowcliff: Ibid., 884; Barrowcliff and Power: Ibid., 1907, 91, p. 557; Power, F. B.: Am. Jour. Pharm., 1915, 87, p. 493.

Chattopadhyay[39] has taken exceptions to the conclusions of Power as to the cyclic structure of the chaulmoogric acid series; but Brill,[23] investigating the oil of Hydnocarpus venenata, a species closely related to Taraktogenos (Hydnocarpus) kurzii, has confirmed the presence of a fatty acid series in this group of plants having a closed carbon chain.

METHODS

The present report is concerned exclusively with a study of the antiseptic and bactericidal actions of chaulmoogra oil and its constituents, the identification and isolation of the bactericidally active substance of chaulmoogra oil, the determination of the specificity of its bactericidal action for acid-fast bacilli, and an investigation of the presence or absence of this bactericidal substance in cod-liver and other oils. The chemotherapeutic investigations on experimentally infected animals will be described separately in the near future.

The methods consist (1) in the separation of chaulmoogra and other oils into fractions and chemical constituents, (2) the preparation of water soluble salts of these fractions and constituents, and (3) tests of the antiseptic and bactericidal activities of these salts against acid-fast and other bacteria.

Since the fixed oils consist essentially of glyceryl triesters of fatty acids, the fundamental analytic procedure has consisted in the separation of the fatty acids from the glycerol and other nonsaponifiable constituents. The ordinary chemical methods of saponifying with alcohol-potash solution and recovering the fatty acids by decomposing the potassium soaps with dilute sulphuric acid were employed. In the case of chaulmoogra oil, the fatty acids, which are solid at room temperature, after being washed free from sulphuric acid, were sometimes purified by dissolving in ether and washing with water and then recovered by evaporating the ether. The fatty acids of cod-liver and linseed oils are fluid at room temperature and float on the surface of the solution as an oily layer; consequently, a slightly different procedure is necessary to recover the separated fatty acids. This was accomplished by dissolving the fatty acids in ether and washing in a separating funnel.

Rogers' fractions of the fatty acids of chaulmoogra oil, used by him in the treatment of leprosy, were prepared by a modification of the method described by this author. He dissolved the total fatty acids in hot 95% alcohol, and removed those that crystallized out at different temperatures as the solution cooled. The essential point is to obtain successive fractions of the total fatty acids crystallizing out of alcohol and having melting points of from 40.8 to 43 C., 37 to 40 C. and below 28 C., respectively. We have found it more practicable to obtain fractions having melting points within the required limits by fractional crystallization of the total fatty acids from cold solutions in three parts of 95% alcohol. Fraction A, with a melting point of 42 C., is a white crystalline solid; fraction B, with a melting point of 37 C., is a slightly yellowish, somewhat amorphous solid; and fraction C is a light brown fluid at 28 C. and a yellowish pasty mass at from 15 to 20 C.

The isolation and purification of the chemically distinct fatty acids of chaulmoogra oil was done by the methods described by Power and Gornall and Power and Barrowcliff.[38] Pure chaulmoogric acid was separated from the total fatty acids by repeated crystallization from 95% alcohol, followed by recrystallization from petroleum ether until a constant melting point of from 68 to 69 C. of the crystals was obtained. This acid, which constitutes the

[39] Am. Jour. Pharm., 1915, 87, p. 473.

greater part of the fatty acids of chaulmoogra oil, crystallizes in colorless glistening leaflets, insoluble in water, but sparingly soluble in and readily crystallized from ordinary organic solvents, with the exception of ether and chloroform in which it is readily soluble cold. Pure hydnocarpic acid was obtained from the noncrystalline residue from chaulmoogric acid by fractional precipitation with barium acetate, recovery of the fatty acids by decomposition of the barium salt fractions with dilute hydrochloric acid, and purification of the fractions last precipitated by crystallization from alcohol and finally from petroleum ether until a constant melting point of from 59 to 60 C. was obtained. This acid, like chaulmoogric acid, crystallizes as colorless, glistening leaflets. The palmitic acid fraction, remaining after the removal of the chaulmoogric and hydnocarpic acids, is a light brown oily fluid at room temperature. It undoubtedly contains small amounts of dissolved chaulmoogric and hydnocarpic acids or lower isomers, but it was not found necessary to purify this fatty acid for use in our experiments.

On account of the insolubility of the oils and their fatty acids in water, it was necessary to convert the fatty acids into water soluble sodium or potassium salts, in order to have solutions suitable for bactericidal tests. Rogers[29, 30] has shown that the therapeutic activity of chaulmoogra oil and its fatty acids is not decreased but rather increased by combining the fatty acids with sodium, due probably to the greater solubility and absorbability of the salts. These soluble salts were prepared by titrating the oil or its fatty acid fractions with half normal sodium or potassium hydroxid, using a suitable indicator. The standard chemical method requires that fatty acids be titrated in hot alcohol with phenolphthalein as an indicator because in aqueous solutions the salts of the fatty acids undergo hydrolytic dissociation. The fatty acid being insoluble is removed from the sphere of chemical action and the sodium ions combining with water interfere with the correct titration. The presence of ethyl alcohol in a concentration of 40% or higher prevents this hydrolytic dissociation and permits a correct titration. In our experience, however, the titration of fatty acids of chaulmoogra oil in 70% alcohol with phenolphthalein as an indicator gives a solution of the sodium or potassium salts which, when diluted with water, is strongly alkaline to litmus, is clear or only slightly clouded, but precipitates on standing and has a low bactericidal activity. On the other hand, when properly titrated in water the solution has a lower titer, is neutral or only feebly alkaline to litmus, is clouded but does not precipitate on standing, and possesses the maximum bactericidal activity. The practical difficulty in titrating in water is that phenolphthalein or any other of a series of indicators tested does not show a sharp end-point, and serves at best only as a rough control of the titration. Consequently, it was necessary to determine experimentally the titer of the chaulmoogrates giving the maximum bactericidal activity. The essential points in the titration are that all of the fatty acids are saponified, that the reaction to litmus is nearly neutral, and that the solution does not precipitate on standing. Since only the sodium and potassium salts of these fatty acids are soluble in water, our tests have necessarily been confined to them.

The correct titer of the oil or its fatty acids having been determined, a 1% solution for testing its antiseptic and bactericidal action was made up as follows: One gram of the oil or fatty acids was accurately weighed and placed in a 100 c c volumetric flask, and the required amount of normal sodium hydroxid and a little distilled water added; the flask and its contents were then heated over a water bath and repeatedly shaken until the fatty acids were completely saponified. The flask was then filled up to the graduation mark with distilled water and sterilized. This gave a 1% solution, not of the sodium chaulmoograte, but of the oil or fatty acids.

A 1% solution of the oil or fatty acids, instead of a 1% solution of the salts of the fatty acids, was made because we believe that in all comparative bactericidal and chemotherapeutic tests comparison should be made of the bactericidally and chemotherapeutically active atoms or radicals and not of the whole compound containing varying kinds and amounts of bactericidally and chemotherapeutically inert atoms and radicals. The latter serve to render the active atoms or radicals more soluble, absorbable and parasitotrophic, or less irritating and toxic to the host. The sodium in the sodium chaulmoogrates serves only to render the fatty acids soluble and plays no direct part in the bactericidal activity of the compound, as shown by the facts that potassium can replace sodium and that any excess of either base over that necessary to secure solution of the fatty acids, even within the limits of chemical combination with the fatty acids, depresses the bactericidal activity of the solution.

For testing the antiseptic and bactericidal activity of chaulmoogra and other oils and their constituents, cultures of the following acid-fast bacilli were employed: B. leprae muris (Hollmann); B. leprae hominis (Levy); B. smegmatis; B. lymphangitidis bovis (Traum); B. tuberculosis avis; B. tuberculosis bovis and B. tuberculosis hominis. Allied to the acid-fast bacilli are the streptothrices, filamentous branching fungi, often having a bacillary stage and a more or less acid-fast staining reaction, and causing streptothriciases in man and animals. A considerable series of these organisms have been used in our experiments, including one or more strains of the following species: Streptothrix asteroides, S. caprae, S. eppingeri, S. hominis, S. madurae and S. nocardi. For determining the specificity of the bactericidal action of the chaulmoogrates against acid-fast bacilli, cultures of the following nonacid-fast bacteria were used: B. coli, B. typhosus, B. dysenteriae Shiga, B. mucosus, B. pestis, Spirillum cholerae-asiaticae, Staph. aureus and Streptococcus (nonhemolytic). We are indebted to Dr. K. F. Meyer of this laboratory for many of these cultures, and to Dr J. Traum of the Veterinary Division of the Department of Agriculture, University of California, for a culture of Bacillus lymphangitidis bovis, a more or less acid-fast bacillus which he has found in and isolated from a type of chronic lymphangitis in cattle.

Our experiments with the cultures from human and rat leprosy are open to a certain criticism. A considerable series of more or less acid-fast organisms have been cultivated by different investigators from the lesions of human and rat leprosy, none of which have proved to be identical with B. leprae Hansen or the variety of it found in rat leprosy. The most that can be said of our cultures is that they are acid-fast bacilli cultivated by competent bacteriologists from the lesions or blood of human or rat leprosy, and, in the case of the culture from rat leprosy, that the organism was found to be pathogenic for rats, in which it produces a disease similar to rat leprosy. However, the criticism to which these cultures are open is largely, if not wholly, met by the fact that the bactericidal activity of the chaulmoogric acid series has been found to be specific for all members of the acid-fast group of bacteria.

The in vitro method of testing germicidal action of drugs as a guide to their use in chemotherapeutics has fallen into disfavor, because it has been found that germicidal action in the test tube does not always mean germicidal activity in the animal body in dosage within the limits of tolerance of the patient. However, sweeping criticism of this method is unjustified and is based on a misconception of its purpose and limitations. The in vitro method of testing germicidal action is an analytic method which enables us to exclude the organotrophic reactions of the host and consequently to obtain uncomplicated information on the action of the drug on the parasite. Moreover, and very important for our purpose, the use of this method has enabled us to exclude the possible indirect or physiologic actions of chaulmoogra oil in leprosy and obtain exact data on the bactericidal activity of this oil and its constituents against acid-fast bacteria.

The tests of the antiseptic action of chaulmoogric and other fatty acids were made by adding with a sterile pipet, graduated to hundredths c c, the required amounts of a sterile 1 or 0.1% solution of the salts to a series of tubes or flasks containing definite quantities of suitable fluid culture medium, so that dilutions of 1:1,000 up to the limits of antiseptic action were obtained. These culture tubes or flasks, together with controls of plain medium, were then inoculated with the organism to be tested, the openings sealed to prevent evaporation and incubated at 37.5 C. for at least twice the length of time necessary to obtain the maximum growth in the controls. These cultures were examined from time to time and the amount of growth or absence of growth recorded and, at the termination of the experiment, microscopic examination for purity was made of the cultures showing growth.

Another method was employed to determine the limits of bactericidal action, since in the antiseptic tests growth might be inhibited without the bacteria being killed. Culture tubes containing measured amounts of suitable culture medium were inoculated with the organism to be tested and incubated until a slight but distinct growth had developed; then the proper dilutions of the fatty acid salts were added to the growing cultures, excepting controls, the tubes replaced in the incubator, and at definite intervals transplants of one small loopful were made from each tube to tubes of fresh mediums, which were incubated and the growth results recorded. The amount of the bactericide transferred by this method to the transplant culture gave a dilution in every case far beyond the limits of antiseptic action. This method, instead of the standard method of testing bactericidal action, was used in our work because growth of the several varieties of tubercle bacilli after submergence and drying is uncertain. In the case of B. tuberculosis another method was used in an attempt to control the limits of bactericidal action. To a series of tubes containing 10 c c of a suspension of tubercle bacilli in salt solution definite dilutions of the chaulmoogrates were added, two tubes being reserved as controls. After incubation at 37.5 C. for 24 hours, 0.5 c c of the suspension of tubercle bacilli from each tube, well shaken up, was injected subcutaneously into guinea-pigs. The bactericidal action of the different dilutions of chaulmoogrates was determined by the absence or presence of infection at necropsy of the guinea-pigs several months after inoculation.

Experimental Data

1. ANTISEPTIC AND BACTERICIDAL ACTIONS OF THE TOTAL FATTY ACIDS OF CHAULMOOGRA OIL

Rogers,[31] Hollmann and Dean[11] and others claim superior therapeutic results in leprosy from the use of the salts or esters of the fatty acids of chaulmoogra oil; therefore it seemed probable that the active therapeutic principle of this oil must be contained in the fatty acid fraction. Consequently the antiseptic and bactericidal properties of the total fatty acids of chaulmoogra oil were first investigated. In our preliminary experiments the total fatty acids were titrated in water with N/1 Na_2CO_3, using phenolphthalein as indicator, and the tests were made on Hollmann's bacillus of rat leprosy cultivated in glycerol veal broth. The results of the first three experiments, in which successively higher dilutions were tested to determine the limits of antiseptic action, and in which transplants were made to determine whether or not the inhibited cultures were actually killed, are combined in table 1.

TABLE 1

PRELIMINARY TESTS OF THE ANTISEPTIC AND BACTERICIDAL ACTIONS OF THE SODIUM SALTS OF THE TOTAL FATTY ACIDS OF CHAULMOOGRA OIL ON B. LEPRAE MURIS

Proportion of Chaulmoogric Acids Added to Culture Medium	Growth in Treated Cultures		Growth in Transplant Cultures
	Macroscopic	Microscopic	
From 1:1,000 to 1:60,000	0	0	0
1:70,000	0	0	+
1:80,000	0	0	0
1:90,000	0	0	0
1:100,000	0	0	0
1:125,000	0	0	+
1:150,000	+	+	+
1:175,000	+	+	+
1:200,000	+	+	++
1:500,000	+	+	+++
1:600,000	++	++	+++
1:700,000	++	++	+++
1:800,000	++	++	+++
1:900,000	++	++	+++
1:1,000,000	++	++	+++
1:1,500,000	+++	+++	+++
1:2,000,000	++++	++++	++++
Controls	++++	++++	++++

From these results it appears that the sodium salts of the total fatty acids of chaulmoogra oil have markedly antiseptic and bactericidal actions on Hollmann's culture of rat leprosy bacillus. Growth of the cultures was totally inhibited up to the dilution of 1:125,000 and partial inhibition, as shown by feeble or delayed growth, extended up at least to the dilution of 1:1,000,000. Complete bactericidal action, as shown by absence of growth in transplants to fresh culture medium, extended up to the dilution of 1:100,000, with the exception of 1:70,000 which showed growth. The tendency of chaulmoogrates to skip antiseptic and bactericidal action is characteristic and will be discussed later.

In the next series of antiseptic tests of the sodium salts of the total fatty acids of chaulmoogra oil, the fatty acids were titrated in 70% alcohol with N/2 NaOH using phenolphthalein as indicator, according to the standard chemical method. The titer of 1 gm. of the fatty acids was 3.8 c c N/1 NaOH. The tests were made, as in the first series, against the bacillus of rat leprosy in glycerol veal broth. The antiseptic action of this solution proved by repeated tests to be only about one-half that of the first solution titrated in water. The cause of this depression of the antiseptic action of the fatty acids titrated in alcohol was obscure. It seemed possible that it might be due (1) to a higher initial acidity of the culture medium, perhaps increased by the growth of the cultures, sufficient to precipitate some of the fatty acids; or (2) to the high titer of the chaulmoograte solution titrated in alcohol. Titration of the culture medium before and after the growth of the cultures in it showed that the reaction was the same in both series of tests and that the growth of the rat leprosy bacillus decreased rather than increased the initial acidity of the medium. Comparative experiments were then undertaken to determine the influence of the reaction of the culture medium and of the titer of the chaulmoogrates on the antiseptic action of the sodium chaulmoogrates against B. leprae muris, the results of which are recorded in table 2.

TABLE 2

THE INFLUENCE OF VARIATIONS IN THE TITER OF THE FATTY ACIDS AND IN THE REACTION OF THE CULTURE MEDIUM ON THE ANTISEPTIC ACTION OF THE CHAULMOOGRIC ACIDS ON B. LEPRAE MURIS

Experiment	Titer of the Fatty Acids N/1 NaOH	Reaction of the Culture Medium	Dilution of the Chaulmoogric Acids Totally Inhibiting Growth*
5	1.1	+1.65	—1:20,000
6	1.8	+3.45	1:130,000
7	1.8	+1.7	+1:100,000
8	2.05	+1.65	1:90,000
9	2.05	+1.65	1:130,000
10	2.5	+2.0	1:40,000
11	3.0	+2.0	1:50,000
12	3.6	+1.65	+1:50,000
13	3.8	+1.7	—1:50,000
14	1.8	+1.7	1:100,000
	1.8	0	—1:70,000
15	3.8	+3.45	+1:50,000
	3.8	+1.65	—1:50,000
	3.8	0	+1:25,000
16	4.1	+1.7	1:30,000
	4.1	0	—1:30,000

* In this column the minus sign indicates lower and the plus sign higher than the figures.

From table 2 it is apparent, first, that there is some fluctuation in the antiseptic action with the same titer of the chaulmoogric acids and the same reaction of the culture medium. This fluctuation is due in part to the before-mentioned tendency of the chaulmoogrates to skip antiseptic action and is probably wholly explainable on the same grounds, which will be discussed later. But apart from these fluctuations there are more marked and constant variations in antiseptic action which plainly correspond to the difference in titer of the chaulmoogric acids and in the reaction of the culture medium. These variations would have shown up in greater contrast had it not been that some of the lower, higher and intermediate ranges of antiseptic action were not determined, owing to contaminations of the cultures or to the fact that lower or higher dilutions of the chaulmoogric acids were not included in the tests. It appears that a titer of 1.8-2.05 c c of N/1 NaOH per c c of the total fatty acids of chaulmoogra oil gives the maximum antiseptic activity against B. leprae muris, and other experiments have proved that this is true for other acid-fast bacilli. This is the titer obtained by titration in water. Any considerable increase or decrease in the titer from 2.0 markedly depresses the antiseptic and bactericidal activity of the chaulmoogric acids. These experiments also show that a reduction of the acidity of the culture medium to zero likewise depresses the antiseptic activity of the chaulmoogrates. This is brought out specially in Exper. 14, 15, and 16 (table 2), which are strictly comparative tests in the same lot of culture medium with the reaction modified.

This most active titer of 2.0 does not correspond to the titer required to convert all of the chaulmoogric acids into normal sodium salts, as indicated by their titration in alcohol with phenolphthalein as indicator, which requires a titer of 3.6-3.8. The hydrogen-ion concentration of 1% solutions of the chaulmoogrates at different titers, which were made by the colorimetric method of Clark and Lubs,[40] show the same divergence between the titer of 2.0 and the neutral point as does the titration method, but throws no light on the cause of the greater antiseptic and bactericidal activity of solutions of the lower titer.

TABLE 3

THE HYDROGEN-ION CONCENTRATION OF 1% SOLUTIONS OF SODIUM CHAULMOOGRATES AT DIFFERENT TITERS OF N/1 NAOH

Titer of Solution	Hydrogen-Ion Concentration with Indicators			
	Methyl Red (Range 4.4-6.0)	Brom Cresol Purple (Range 5.2-6.8)	Brom Thymol Blue (Range 6.6-7.6)	Phenol Red (Range 6.8-8.4)
2.0	5.6	5.4	...	...
3.0	...	6.4	6.4	...
3.8	...	...	7.6	7.7

From the tests in table 3 it appears that the solutions of a titer of 2.0 have a hydrogen-ion concentration well on the acid side, while the titer of 3.8 is slightly on the alkaline side.

A possible explanation of the greater antiseptic and bactericidal activity of the neutral solutions with a titer of 2.0 in water over the alkaline solutions with a titer of 3.8 in alcohol is supplied by Power and Gornall.[38] These authors found that in strongly alkaline alcoholic solutions of chaulmoogric acid the normal potassium salt ($C_{18}H_{31}O_2K$) was formed, while in neutral aqueous solutions the acid potassium salt ($C_{18}H_{31}O_2K - 2C_{18}H_{32}O_2$) was formed. Presumably the same reactions would hold true for the sodium salts, in which case the greater bactericidal activity of the neutral, water titrated solution would be due to the acid sodium salts of the chaulmoogric acids.

Having determined the titer of the total fatty acids of chaulmoogra oil that gave the highest antiseptic activity against B. leprae muris, we proceeded to test its antiseptic action on other acid-fast bacilli in cultures. In the case of the several varieties of B. tuberculosis certain technical difficulties were encountered. While our cultures of other acid-fast bacilli will grow in glycerol veal broth in intimate contact with the antiseptic solution, the human and bovine varieties of B. tuberculosis must be inoculated and grow only on the surface of the culture fluid as a waxy membrane. Owing to this growth requirement of tubercle bacilli and to the fatty nature of the bacilli, only the lower surface of the inoculated fragment of membrane comes in contact with and is made wet by the culture fluid and contained antiseptic. The chaulmoogrates are not freely soluble and gradually crystallize out of solution; it is remarkable that this tendency to crystallize out appears to be more marked in weaker solutions. Consequently, in such slow growing cultures as the tubercle bacillus, precipitation of the feebly soluble chaulmoogrates, and possibly also fixation by the contiguous layers of tubercle bacilli, will sufficiently reduce the concentration of the chaulmoogrates in the culture medium to enable the upper layers of tubercle bacilli in the inoculated fragment of membrane that have not been in contact with the antiseptic, to multiply. We have been able to overcome this difficulty in the case of the avian variety of tubercle bacilli which, unlike the human and bovine varieties, can be induced to grow at the bottom of the flask in intimate contact with the antiseptic solution.

[40] Jour. Bacteriol., 1917, 2, pp. 1-34.

In table 4 are collected the results of antiseptic tests of the sodium salts of the total fatty acids of chaulmoogra oil on different acid-fast bacilli, including comparative tests in surface and submerged cultures of the bacillus of avian tuberculosis. In order that the degree of antiseptic activity of the chaulmoogrates may be appreciated, we have included in another column of this table the antiseptic action of phenol tested under the same conditions on certain of these acid-fast bacilli. The figures are based in every case on the results of repeated tests.

TABLE 4

THE ANTISEPTIC ACTION OF SODIUM CHAULMOOGRATES AND OF PHENOL ON CERTAIN ACID-FAST BACILLI

Bacilli	Limits of Complete Antiseptic Action		
	Sodium Chaulmoogrates		Phenol
	In Cultures on the Surface of the Broth	In Cultures Submerged in the Broth	In Cultures Submerged in the Broth
B. leprae muris (Hollmann)	....	1:80,000 to 1:130,000	1:1,000
B. leprae hominis (Levy)	....	1:60,000 to 1:130,000	
B. smegmatis	....	1:80,000 to 1:110,000	1:1,000
B. lymphangitidis bovis	....	1:90,000 to 1:130,000	
B. tuberculosis avis	1:10,000	1:90,000 to +1:140,000	1:1,000
B. tuberculosis bovis	1:10,000 to 1:20,000	........*	
B. tuberculosis hominis	1:10,000 to 1:20,000	........*	

* Will not grow submerged in the broth.

These results show that the sodium salts of the total chaulmoogric acid have a high antiseptic action on all of the acid-fast bacilli tested, but that this antiseptic attains its full activity only when the organisms are growing in complete contact with it in submerged cultures. Comparison of the antiseptic action of the chaulmoogrates on the surface cultures of the human and bovine varieties with that on the surface cultures of the avian variety of B. tuberculosis, and of the surface cultures with the submerged cultures of the avian variety, apparently justifies the conclusion that the chaulmoogrates would have an equally high antiseptic action against the human and bovine varieties if they could be cultivated submerged in and in intimate contact with the antiseptic. Comparison of the chaulmoogrates with the standard antiseptic and bactericide, phenol, brings out in a striking manner the remarkably high antiseptic activity of the former against acid-fast bacilli.

Our experiments with the potassium salts of the total fatty acids of chaulmoogra oil have shown that their antiseptic activity is no greater than, and probably slightly inferior to, the sodium salts. The other ordinary salts of the chaulmoogric acids are insoluble in water and are consequently unsuited for experiments in vitro.

Having established the high antiseptic activity of the sodium chaulmoogrates against acid-fast bacilli, we attempted to determine whether this antiseptic action was merely an inhibition of growth or whether the bacilli were actually killed. We already had, it is true, some evidence that the chaulmoogrates are actually bactericidal and not merely inhibitory of growth. In our preliminary experiments in table 1 transplants from cultures containing chaulmoogrates up to a dilution of 1:100,000 (with the exception of 1:70,000) failed to grow. However, more accurate data on this subject can be obtained by adding the dilutions of chaulmoogrates to the tubes or flasks of culture medium after inoculation and incubation of the cultures until a definite growth has developed, and then transplanting from the treated cultures to fresh medium at definite intervals. The results on the bactericidal action of the sodium chaulmoogrates on B. leprae muris are given in table 5.

In this experiment the sodium chaulmoogrates killed the bacillus of rat leprosy in 24 hours up to a dilution of 1:75,000 but not at a dilution of 1:100,000 of the chaulmoogric acids. These results do not vary greatly from those obtained in connection with the antiseptic tests recorded in table 1, which gave a bactericidal action up to the dilution of 1:100,000. Probably the limits of complete bactericidal action in vitro of the chaulmoogric acids on this bacillus lie somewhere between 1:75,000 and 1:100,000. The experiment in table 5 also shows that action of the chaulmoogrates for a period of time longer than 24 hours does not increase its bactericidal range. No attempt was made to determine the bactericidal activity of the chaulmoogrates acting for a shorter time than 24 hours because there are reasons for believing that the bactericidal action of the chaulmoogric acids is biologic rather than directly chemical and is consequently slow in action.

An attempt was made to obtain data on the bactericidal action of the chaulmoogrates on B. tuberculosis hominis by the combined in vitro in vivo method. This consisted in subcutaneous inoculations into a series of guinea-pigs of 0.5 c c of saline suspensions of the tubercle bacilli which had been subjected to the action of definite dilutions of the chaulmoogrates for 24 hours at 37.5 C., together with controls inoculated with the same amount of untreated saline suspensions of the bacillus. The results of this experiment as determined by necropsies of the animals are given in table 6.

Some of the guinea-pigs in table 6 died from unknown cause too soon after inoculation to show tuberculous lesions, but these deaths occurred by chance at points in the series at which they do not interfere with the interpretation of the results. This experiment shows a complete bactericidal action of the sodium salts of the total fatty acids of chaulmoogra oil on B. tuberculosis hominis under the conditions of the experiments, only up to a dilution of 1:20,000. There is, however, a probable source of error in the conditions of the experiment that should be pointed out. There are reasons, which will be discussed more in detail later, for believing that the bactericidal action of the chaulmoogrates on acid-fast bacilli is not directly chemical by corrosive or fixative action on their protoplasm, as are salts of the heavy metals; but that its action is indirect or biologic, and is dependent on vital activities of the multiplying bacilli, which attach the chaulmoogric acids to themselves for the purpose of synthesizing their fatty envelopes, and that only when this assimilation has occurred can these peculiar fatty acids exercise the toxic action on the bacilli. Tubercle bacilli suspended in salt solution have their vital activities reduced to a minimum, and would consequently be capable of fixing but little of the chaulmoogrates; the bactericidal action would therefore be greatly reduced.

2. THE ACTIVE BACTERICIDAL PRINCIPLE OF CHAULMOOGRA OIL

Crude chaulmoogra oil has usually been recommended as more effective than the refined product in the treatment of leprosy. If this be true, and since the oil is expressed from the seeds, it might be that small amounts of nitrogenous or other nonfatty substances, such as the glucosid, gynocardin, would be expressed with the oil, and constitute the bactericidal and therapeutic active principle of chaulmoogra oil. Brill and Williams[23] found, on analysis of

TABLE 5

THE BACTERICIDAL ACTION OF THE SODIUM SALTS OF THE TOTAL FATTY ACIDS OF CHAULMOOGRA OIL ON B. LEPRAE MURIS

Dilution of Chaulmoogric Acids Added to 24-Hour Cultures	Growth in Cultures Transplanted at Intervals of		
	24 Hours	72 Hours	144 Hours
1:1,000 to 1:75,000	0	0	0
1:100,000	+	+	+
1:125,000	+	+	+
Control	+	+	+

TABLE 6

THE BACTERICIDAL ACTION OF THE SODIUM SALTS OF THE TOTAL FATTY ACIDS OF CHAULMOOGRA OIL ON B. TUBERCULOSIS-HOMINIS BY THE IN VITRO IN VIVO METHOD

Guinea-Pig	Inoculated with Tubercle Bacilli Incubated 24 Hours with Chaulmoogrates of a Dilution of	Fate of Animal	Tuberculous Lesions Found at Necropsy in				
			Point of Inoculation	Glands	Lungs	Liver	Spleen
12a	1:10,000	Killed 139th day	0	+*	0	0	0
12b	1:20,000	Killed 139th day	0	+*	0	0	0
12c	1:30,000	Killed 139th day	+	+	+	+	+
12d	1:40,000	Killed 139th day	+	++	++	+	+
12e	1:50,000	Died 10th day	—	—	—	—	—
12f	1:60,000	Died 132d day	0	++	+++	+	+
12g	1:70,000	Died 102d day	+	+	0	+	0
12h	1:80,000	Died 7th day	—	—	—	+ (?)	—
12i	1:90,000	Died 10th day	+ (?)	—	—	—	—
12j	1:100,000	Died 137th day	0	+	++	++	++
12k	Control	Died 14th day	+	+	+	0	0
12l	Control	Killed 139th day	+	++	++	++	+

* Inguinal gland proximal to inoculation slightly enlarged and caseous, due to the action of the dead tubercle bacilli.

TABLE 7

THE ANTISEPTIC ACTIVITY OF THE SODIUM SALTS OF CHAULMOOGRA OIL AND OF ITS FRACTIONS ON B. LEPRAE MURIS

Chaulmoogra Oil and Fractions	Growth of Bacilli lepræ muris in Dilution of														
	1:10,000	1:20,000	1:30,000	1:40,000	1:50,000	1:60,000	1:70,000	1:80,000	1:90,000	1:100,000	1:110,000	1:120,000	1:130,000	1:140,000	Control
Whole oil	0	+	+	+	+	+	+	+	+	+	+	+	+	+	+
Total fatty acids	0	0	0	0	0	0	0	0	0	0	0	0	0	+	+
Rogers' fraction A	0	+	0	+	0	+	+	+	+	+	+	+	+	+	+
Rogers' fraction B	0	0	0	+	0	+	+	+	+	+	+	+	+	+	+
Rogers' fraction C	0	0	0	0	0	0	0	+	+	+	+	+	+	+	+
Rogers' fraction B + C	0	0	0	0	0	0	±	0	+	+	+	+	+	+	+
Pure chaulmoogric acid	+	+	+	+	+	+	+	+	+	+	+	+	+	+	+
Pure hydnocarpic acid	0	+	+	+	+	+	+	+	+	+	+	+	+	+	+
Residue from the chaulmoogric and hydnocarpic acids	0	0	+	+	+	+	+	+	+	+	+	+	+	+	+

eight samples of chaulmoogra oil, a small amount of nitrogen present which would correspond to from 0.113 to 0.568% of gynocardin. However, our antiseptic and bactericidal tests and the therapeutic experience of Rogers and others indicate that the active principle resides in the fatty acid fraction of the oil; for the method of separation of the fatty acids and their purification by ether would exclude all but the smallest traces of other substances. In order to confirm this and to identify, if possible, the particular fatty acids that are active, the total fatty acids, the several fractions used by Rogers in the treatment of leprosy, and the individual fatty acids were separated by appropriate chemical methods; the whole oil was saponified, and the several fractions and pure fatty acids were converted into sodium salts and their antiseptic activity tested on acid-fast bacilli. The results of these comparative tests on B. leprae muris are given in table 7.

The data in table 7 do not give us the clean cut identification of the active substance of chaulmoogra oil expected from these comparative tests. From the uninterpreted results of these tests it would appear that the total fatty acids are more active than any of its fractions or constituent fatty acids. These apparently paradoxic results are due to certain physical properties of the fractions of higher melting points and of the pure fatty acids which modify the antiseptic and bactericidal activity of these fractions in solutions. Four factors must be considered for the proper interpretation of these data: (1) a bactericidally active fraction; (2) presumably one or more inactive fractions that dilute the active fraction; (3) the low solubility of the salts of fractions having high melting points (Rogers' fractions A and B) and of pure chaulmoogric and hydnocarpic acids, and their consequent tendency to precipitate out of solution; and (4) the well-known physical facts that in mixtures of fatty acids of different melting points, the melting points of the constituent fatty acids are lowered and the solubility of their salts increased.

With these complicating factors in mind the interpretation of the data in table 7 is less difficult. First, it is evident that the active bactericidal principle of chaulmoogra oil is contained in the fatty acid fraction because of the greatly superior activity of the total fatty acids over the whole oil. Second, the progressive increase in activity of Rogers' fractions A, B and C is due to a corresponding progressive decrease in the melting point and increase in solubility of their salts. The increase in the activity of fractions A to C is probably less than it would be if the activity of fractions B and C were not in part neutralized by the increasing proportion of the inactive fraction. Third, fractions B + C are slightly more active than either fraction B or C separately, because the mixture depresses the melting point and increases the solubility of the salts of fraction B which contains a larger proportion of the active fatty acids. Fourth, the last three fractions in table 7 contain together the total fatty acids of chaulmoogra oil which, as we have seen, must contain the active bactericidal substance; yet the activity of each of the three fractions by itself is greatly inferior to that of the total fatty acids. The residue consists chiefly of palmitic acid with some chaulmoogric and hydnocarpic acids or lower isomers that could not be crystallized out of solution. This palmitic acid or other unidentified constituent of the residue cannot be the active substance for the mixture is fluid and its salts freely soluble and, moreover, about 90% of the chaulmoogric and hydnocarpic acids, assumed for the purpose of our argument to be inactive, have been removed, therefore the remaining 10% of theoretical active substance, although not strictly pure, should have an antiseptic activity much greater than that of the total fatty acids. On the contrary, our tests show that its activity is feeble. The slight antiseptic activity the residue possesses is undoubtedly due to the small amounts of chaulmoogric and hydnocarpic acids contained in it. By this process of elimination we are forced to conclude that the bactericidal activity of chaulmoogra oil is a function of the chaulmoogric acid series, chaulmoogric acid and its isomer, hydnocarpic acid, which are of unique chemical structure among fatty acids, and which constitute about 90% of the total fatty acids of chaulmoogra oil. The feeble antiseptic and bactericidal activity displayed by salts of the pure acids is due to the relatively high melting points and low solubility of their salts, which tend to precipitate out of weak solutions before their bactericidal action becomes effective. When they, together with the small palmitic fraction, are mixed, the melting point of the mixture is depressed and their salts rendered sufficiently soluble to permit the chaulmoogric acid series to exert the high antiseptic and bactericidal activity characteristic of the total fatty acids of chaulmoogra oil.

3. SPECIFICITY OF THE BACTERICIDAL ACTION OF THE CHAULMOOGRIC ACIDS AGAINST ACID-FAST ORGANISMS

Our experiments have shown that the cyclic fatty acids of chaulmoogra oil have a high antiseptic and bactericidal activity against acid-fast bacilli. Is this action specific for acid-fast organisms, or is it general against all bacteria? In order to determine this important point experiments have been conducted with two groups of organisms, the streptothrices and nonacid-fast bacteria. The streptothrices are a group of branching, filamentous fungi, which may by fragmentation develop bacillary forms, and some of them are more or less acid fast. These organisms are regarded by recent investigators as phylogenetically related to the acid-fast bacilli which also, under certain conditions, develop branching forms. Because of this supposed relationship and the variable acid resistance of the different species, the antiseptic and bactericidal action of the chaulmoogrates on this group of organisms is of interest. Table 8 gives the antiseptic action of the sodium salts of the total fatty acids of chaulmoogra oil on different species of streptothrix, together with their morphologic characters and acid-resisting property.

It appears from the results in table 8 that the chaulmoogric acid series have some antiseptic action against streptothrices which is, however, less than against the acid-fast bacilli; that this antiseptic action varies for different species; and that in general the antiseptic action is greater against the bacillary and more or less acid-fast species than against the filamentous and nonacid-fast species.

More interesting and important are the tests of the antiseptic action of the chaulmoogric series on nonacid-fast bacteria (table 9).

These experiments show that the sodium chaulmoogrates are antiseptically and consequently bactericidally inert against nonacid-fast bacteria in dilutions as low as 1:1,000. At such a dilution the growth is usually as luxuriant as in the controls. Dilutions lower than 1:1,000 were not tested, since at this dilution the contrast between the inactivity against nonacid-fast bacteria and the activity against acid-fast bacteria is sufficiently well marked to prove the specificity of the bactericidal activity of the chaulmoogric acids for the latter group of bacteria.

Rogers[1, 36] has stated that therapeutic activity in leprosy and tuberculosis is not peculiar to the fatty acids of chaulmoogra oil, but is common to the unsaturated fatty acids of cod-liver, and presumably other oils. He suggests that the unsaturated fatty acids act on acid-fast bacilli, the coating of which

TABLE 8

THE ANTISEPTIC ACTION OF SODIUM CHAULMOOGRATES ON STREPTOTHRIX

Streptothrix	Morphology	Acid Resistance	Growth in Chaulmoogrates at Dilutions of										
			1:5,000	1:10,000	1:20,000	1:30,000	1:40,000	1:50,000	1:60,000	1:70,000	1:80,000	1:100,000	Control
S. eppingeri......	Rods and short filaments	Partial	0	0	0	0	0	0	0	0	+	+	+
S. caprae........	Rods and short filaments	Partial	0	0	0	0	+	+	+	+	+	+	+
S. norcardi......	Rods and short filaments	Partial	0	0	0	+	+	+	+	+	+	+	+
S. hominis.......	Long branching filaments	Vegetative	0	0	+	+	+	+	+	+	+	+	+
S. asteroides.....	Long branching filaments	Vegetative	0	0	+	+	+	+	+	+	+	+	+
S. albus..........	Long branching filaments	Vegetative	0	0	+	+	+	+	+	+	+	+	+
S. bovis..........	Long branching filaments	Vegetative	0	+	+	+	+	+	+	+	+	+	+
S. madurae......	Long branching filaments	Vegetative	0	+	+	+	+	+	+	+	+	+	+

TABLE 9

THE ANTISEPTIC ACTION OF SODIUM CHAULMOOGRATES ON NONACID-FAST BACTERIA

Bacterium	Growth in Sodium Chaulmoogrates: Dilutions from 1:1,000 to 1:100,000	Control
B. coli..	+	+
B. typhosus..	+	+
B. dysenteriae (Shiga)..............................	+	+
B. mucosus...	+	+
B. pestis..	+	+
S. cholerae...	+	+
Staphy. aureus..	+	+
Strep. sp. (non-haemolytic)........................	+	+

TABLE 10

COMPARISON OF THE ANTISEPTIC ACTIVITIES OF SODIUM CHAULMOOGRATES, SODIUM LINOLEATES AND SODIUM MORRHUATES ON ACID-FAST BACILLI

Bacilli	Dilutions Having Complete Antiseptic Action		
	Sodium Chaulmoogrates	Sodium Linoleates	Sodium Morrhuates
B. leprae muris................	1:80,000 to 1:130,000	—1:1,000 to 1:3,000	1:5,000 to 1:8,000
B. leprae hominis..............	1:60,000 to 1:130,000	1:1,000	1:7,000 to 1:9,000
B. smegmatis....................	1:80,000 to 1:110,000	1:1,000 to 1:4,000	1:8,000
B. lymphangitidis bovis.......	1:90,000 to 1:130,000	1:4,000	1:3,000
B. tuberculosis avis...........	1:90,000 to +1:140,000	—1:5,000 to 1:9,000	1:3,000 to 1:9,000

has been shown to contain unsaturated fatty acids. It is consequently of interest to compare the antiseptic and bactericidal activity of the fatty acids of cod-liver and other oils with those of chaulmoogra oil.

Linoleic acid, the principal fatty acid of linseed and certain other vegetable oils, has the same empiric formula ($C_{18}H_{32}O_2$) as has chaulmoogric acid, and differs from it only in the arrangement of the atoms in its molecule; the molecule of chaulmoogric acid has a carbon ring structure, while the molecule of linoleic acid has its atoms arranged in an open chain. Since the two fatty acids are the chief constituents of the respective oils, and since the salts of the total fatty acids of chaulmoogra oil have been proved to be more highly antiseptic and bactericidal in vitro against acid-fast bacilli than any of its fractions, it has been considered fair to use the sodium salts of the total fatty acids of both oils for comparative tests.

Rogers' sodium morrhuate consists of the sodium salts of the total fatty acids of cod-liver oil. Our knowledge of the chemistry of cod-liver oil is far from exact; but its composition, as is to be expected of an animal oil extracted from an organ having such metabolic activities as the liver, is very complex. A considerable number of fatty acids, including oleic, palmitic, steric, myristeric, palmitoleic, gadoleic, erucic and therapic acids, together with two alkaloids, asselin and morrhuin, traces of iodin and sometimes bromin, and butylamin, amylamin, herylamin and hydrodimethyl-pyridin, have been reported as occurring in cod-liver oil. However, all but traces of substances other than the fatty acids would be excluded by the method of preparation of Rogers' sodium morrhuate. So far as is known, cod-liver oil does not contain fatty acids of the chaulmoogric series nor any fatty acids having a cyclic structure.

In table 10 are collected the results of antiseptic tests of sodium linoleates and sodium morrhuates compared with sodium chaulmoogrates on various acid-fast bacilli. In this table, as in the preceding tables, where two figures are given they represent the lowest and highest range of antiseptic action obtained in repeated experiments.

These experiments show that the sodium linoleates and morrhuates have a slight antiseptic action on acid-fast bacilli. This is probably a nonspecific soap action—for the sodium salts of the fatty acids are soaps, of which dilutions up to 1:5,000 give decidedly soapy and up to 1:10,000 perceptibly soapy solutions—in which the fatty capsules of acid-fast bacilli are injured (emulsified) by the more concentrated solutions of the soaps. In consequence of this low antiseptic activity, and since bactericidal action is never greater, and is usually less, than antiseptic action, it has not been considered necessary to test the bactericidal actions of the linoleates and morrhuates on acid-fast bacilli. In strong contrast to this relatively feeble soap action of the linoleates and morrhuates stands the high antiseptic and bactericidal activities of the chaulmoogrates against acid-fast bacilli, activities which these comparative experiments indicate are specific to the cyclic fatty acids of the chaulmoogric series.

DISCUSSION

It is convenient in discussing the experimental data to follow the outline given in the introductory paragraphs, and to determine how much information we have obtained by these experiments in vitro bearing on the several problems involved in the fatty acid therapy of leprosy and tuberculosis.

The first problem was the method of therapeutic action of chaulmoogra oil in leprosy. This problem presented three chief possibilities: (1) that the reputed therapeutic effect is due to direct bactericidal action of chaulmoogra oil or some of its constituents on B. leprae; (2) that chaulmoogra oil acts indirectly by stimulating the tissues to react against the invading organisms, and (3) that chaulmoogra oil is inactive and improvement of patients following its use is spontaneous. The first of these possibilities, that of direct bactericidal action, was the simplest and most attractive one, and would place chaulmoogra oil or its active constituent among the true chemotherapeutic agents. For this reason the antiseptic and bactericidal activities of chaulmoogra oil and its constituents were first investigated. Our experiments have shown that the sodium salts of the total fatty acids of chaulmoogra oil have a very high antiseptic and bactericidal activity against acidfast bacilli. This bactericidal action extends to a dilution of about 1:100,000, and the antiseptic action is perceptible to a dilution of at least 1:1,000,000. In the light of these results and of the facts that these high antiseptic and bactericidal activities have proved to be peculiar to certain fatty acids of chaulmoogra oil and specific against acid-fast bacilli, as will be discussed, we have not considered it necessary or profitable to investigate hypothetical indirect action of chaulmoogra oil in leprosy; and we believe that it can be concluded with reasonable certainty that any therapeutic action which chaulmoogra oil may have in leprosy is due to its direct antiseptic and bactericidal action on B. leprae.

In this connection the question of the relation of bactericidal dilution in vitro to the therapeutic dosage in vivo of the chaulmoogrates naturally arises. If, as is true, the limits of complete bactericidal action in vitro is the dilution of about 1:100,000, but the therapeutic dosage intravenous in leprosy is in the proportion of from 1:2,000,000 to 1:500,000 of the body weight, how can we account for the therapeutic effect claimed in leprosy on the basis of even the high bactericidal action of the chaulmoogrates? Our experiments in vitro have, for the purpose of analysis, intentionally excluded the factors that may be supplied by the host in the action of the chaulmoogrates on acid-fast bacilli in vivo. There are three such factors which, individually or conjointly, might account for the apparent discrepancy between the bactericidally active dilution in vitro and the therapeutically active dosage in vivo. First, other chemotherapeutic agents are known, such as arsphenamin, which act therapeutically in the animal body at higher dilutions than they do germicidally in vitro. This intensified action in vivo is probably due to some chemical modification of the substance brought about by the tissues of the host. Second, fats and fatty acids are not, like some drugs, rapidly broken down and excreted by the animal body, but are stored in the tissues for metabolic use. Consequently, in the regular and long continued administration of the chaulmoogric acids in the treatment of leprosy there would be an accumulation of the chaulmoogric acids or their esters in the body that might well reach the concentration of bactericidal action. This might explain in part the slow action of the chaulmoogratés in leprosy. Third, the high antiseptic range of the chaulmoogrates, which is perceptible up to a dilution of at least 1:1,000,000, above the complete bactericidal activity may be an important factor in the therapeutic results. Such a high antiseptic action, although incomplete, might in conjunction with the tissue reactions be sufficient to restrain the multiplication of the bacilli; or the inhibitory action of the chaulmoogrates might so injure or reduce the vitality of the parasites that the natural resistance of the host would be able to overcome them. The experimental determination of the actual relation between bactericidal dilution in vitro and therapeutic dosage in animals will be considered in a later article.

The second problem was that of the active principle of chaulmoogra oil. Our experiments have shown conclusively that the bactericidally active principle is contained in the fatty acids of this oil. This is in accord with the experience of Rogers,[29, 30] Hollmann and Dean[11] and others that the fatty acid fraction of chaulmoogra oil is most active therapeutically in leprosy. But, whereas Rogers claims superior therapeutic results with first one fraction and then another of the chaulmoogric acids, we have obtained the highest bactericidal activity in vitro with the salts of the total fatty acids. Our results are due to the greater solubility of the salts of the mixed fatty acids, and do not indicate that all of the fatty acids of chaulmoogra oil are bactericidally active. The low solubility of the salts of the individual fatty acids and their consequent tendency to crystallize out of weak solutions have interfered with the direct identification of the specific fatty acids of chaulmoogra oil possessing this bactericidal property; but by indirect methods of exclusion we have been able to satisfy ourselves that the small palmitic acid fraction is inactive, and that the bactericidal activity is a function of the chaulmoogric acid series, chaulmoogric and hydnocarpic acids and possibly lower isomers of this series, which together constitute about 90% of the fatty acids of chaulmoogra oil. The chaulmoogric acid series, it will be recalled, have been shown by the researches of Power and Gornall,[38] and of Brill[23] to have a peculiar molecular structure containing a closed carbon chain, which is found in no other known fatty acids.

The third problem was the degree of specificity of the bactericidal activity of the chaulmoogric acid series. Bactericides may be either nonspecific, such as phenol and salts of the heavy metals, which act against all bacteria and show no marked variation in their action on different species, except in so far as it may be modified by the development of resistant spores by certain species; or they may be more or less specific and act more strongly against certain species or groups of bacteria, as is the case with ethylhydrocuprein against the pneumococcus group. Our experiments have shown that the chaulmoogric acids belong to the latter class of bactericides, and that they have a very sharply limited group specificity. They possess a high bactericidal activity against all members of the acid-fast group of bacilli and are inactive against all other bacteria tested. This group specificity is probably connected, not with acid-fastness as such nor with any protoplasmic relationship of the different acid-fast organisms, but with the fat metabolism of acid-fast bacilli and the mechanism of the bactericidal action of the chaulmoogric acids. It is known that growths of acid-fast bacilli contain large amounts of fats and waxes (20-37% in case of the tubercle bacilli), which are intimately connected with the bacterial cell in that they are a product of its metabolism, and constitute its protective capsule. Kendall, Walker and Day[41] have shown that acid-fast bacilli produce a soluble lipase in their growth, which is probably concerned in the metabolism of this fatty capsule. Rogers has suggested that the unsaturated fatty acids act on acid-fast bacilli by injuring the protective fatty capsules of acid-fast bacilli. This assumption, he believes, is supported by his observations that the bacilli excreted by patients undergoing treatment show irregular acid-fast staining. Such bacilli, deprived of their protective fatty capsules, would be exposed to the destructive action of the tissues and body fluids. Our experiments in vitro, however, have failed to show the slightest action of the sodium chaulmoogrates, in any concentration and acting for any length of time, on the staining characters or morphology of acid-fast bacilli.

[41] Jour. Infect. Dis., 1914, 15, p. 443.

An hypothesis which seems best to explain the mechanism of the bactericidal action of the chaulmoogric acids and their specificity for acid-fast bacilli is that these fat elaborating bacilli attempt to utilize the chaulmoogric acids to build up their fatty capsules, and that these cyclic fatty acids contain a group or an arrangement of atoms which is toxic for the bacterial cell. In the terminology of Ehrlich's side chain theory, we may express this reaction by saying that chaulmoogric acid possesses an haptophore group which becomes attached to the receptor or side chain of the acid-fast bacillus, and a toxophore group which, after attachment, exerts a toxic action on the bacillus. On the basis of this hypothesis, the chaulmoogric acids are not bactericidal against nonacid-fast bacteria because these organisms, not elaborating a fatty capsule, do not necessarily use fats in their metabolism, and consequently do not possess the proper receptors for the haptophore group of the chaulmoogric acids.

This hypothesis would also help to explain the irregularities encountered in our bactericidal experiments in vitro, such as skipping and variation in antiseptic and bactericidal action in different tests. It is well known that fat metabolism, as indicated by acid-fastness, is not a constant or even a vitally necessary function of acid-fast organisms, since there are usually a variable number of nonacid-fast individuals in young cultures of acid-fast bacilli, and it has been shown experimentally that acid-fastness can be modified and even wholly suppressed in some species by conditions of growth. In our experimental cultures such nonacid-fast individual bacilli, in which fat metabolism was temporarily dormant, would by our hypothesis be immune to the action of the chaulmoogrates. After the greater part of the chaulmoogrates in the culture had become fixed by the acid-fast organisms or precipitated in virtue of their slight solubility, these nonacid-fast individuals might be able to multiply and resume their fat metabolism and acid-fast property unrestrained.

The fourth and last major problem investigated was that of the presence of bactericidally active fatty acids in other oils. It will be recalled that Rogers has stated that the salts of the unsaturated fatty acids of both chaulmoogra and cod-liver oils, and by implication the unsaturated fatty acids of any oil, are equally efficacious therapeutically in either leprosy or tuberculosis. Our experiments do not support the claim of Rogers. They show that the high specific bactericidal activity against acid-fast bacilli is not a property common to unsaturated fatty acids, but that it is restricted to the cyclic fatty acids of the chaulmoogric series. The number of fatty acids that we have investigated is limited; but we believe that they have been particularly well chosen. Linoleic acid has an empiric formula ($C_{18}H_{32}O_2$) identical with that of chaulmoogric acid, and differs from the latter only in the arrangement of its atoms in an open chain instead of in a ring. Rogers' sodium morrhuate contains a considerable number of fatty acids, none of which are known to be of cyclic structure, and for which specific therapeutic action in leprosy and tuberculosis is claimed. We have demonstrated that neither of these have any marked bactericidal activity against acid-fast bacilli, but are relatively inert. Therefore we believe the conclusion to be warranted that the specific bactericidal activity of fatty acids against acid-fast bacilli is a function of the carbon ring structure of the molecules of the chaulmoogric acid series, a structure known to exist only in chaulmoogra oil and in oils of certain plants closely related to Taraktogenous kurzii from whence chaulmoogra oil is obtained.

These experiments in vitro supply certain definite information on the major problems of the purposed investigation of the fatty acid therapy of leprosy and tuberculosis, namely: (1) the method of therapeutic action of chaulmoogra oil in leprosy; (2) the active principle of chaulmoogra oil; (3) the specificity of its action on the acid-fast group of bacteria, and (4) the limitation of the active principle to the cyclic fatty acids of chaulmoogra oil. Much of this information could not have been obtained by other methods of experimentation; but the actual chemotherapeutic value of the chaulmoogric acid compounds in the treatment of infections due to the acid-fast group of bacilli, especially tuberculosis, remains to be proved by experiments on animals and by clinical experience. It is strongly recommended, however, that clinical trial of the chaulmoogrates in tuberculosis await the results of the animal experiments now in progress; for the indiscriminate use of this drug may arouse false hopes and be not without danger to the patients.

SUMMARY

Chaulmoogra oil contains bactericidal substances that are about one hundred times more active than phenol.

The bactericidally active substances of chaulmoogra oil are the fatty acids of the chaulmoogric series, chaulmoogric and hydnocarpic acids, and possibly lower isomers of this series.

The bactericidal activity of the chaulmoogric acid series is specific for the acid-fast group of bacteria, and inactive against all other bacteria tested.

This specific bactericidal activity against acid-fast bacteria is a function of the carbon ring structure of the molecule of the chaulmoogric acid series which, so far as known, is found only in chaulmoogra oil and in oils of certain plants closely related to Taraktogenous kurzii.

The fatty acids of cod-liver oil, the salts of which constitute Rogers' sodium morrhuate, used in the specific treatment of tuberculosis, do not possess the specific bactericidal activity of the chaulmoogric acid series.

These facts supply a scientific basis for the use of chaulmoogra oil and its products in leprosy.

Our experiments do not support the claims of Rogers for sodium morrhuate in the specific therapy of tuberculosis.

The bactericidal activity of the chaulmoogric acids against all members of the acid-fast group of bacilli, together with the clinical results obtained from their use in leprosy, furnish theoretical grounds for the application of the chaulmoogrates to the therapy of tuberculosis.

Experiments on animals are now in progress to determine whether or not the chaulmoogric acid series have any practical value in the chemotherapy of tuberculosis.

EXPERIMENTAL STREPTOCOCCUS EMPYEMA

ATTEMPTS AT PREVENTION AND THERAPY BY MEANS OF VACCINES AND SERUM *

F. P. Gay and R. L. Stone

An attempt was made in a recent survey of the literature to point out the great and growing importance of the streptococci in various human affections.[1] Emphasis was laid on the recently appreciated significance of hemolytic streptococci in bronchopneumonia and in the empyema which frequently follows it as it occurred in the early months of the late war in army camps. The importance of streptococcus empyema has not only not decreased, but has become intensified during the last year by its occurrence as a fatal sequel to influenza as well as in its previous relation to spontaneous bronchopneumonia and to bronchopneumonia after measles.

Our previous survey as to the actual accomplishment in the prevention and treatment of streptococcus infections by specific means, that is to say, by the use of vaccines and serum, gave us little encouragement. This study was undertaken not simply in an effort to proceed toward a possible practical method of treating streptococcus empyema, but in the desire to contribute some information to the larger question of streptococcus immunity as a whole.

THE GROUPS OF HEMOLYTIC STREPTOCOCCI

It was realized a few years ago that human pathogenic streptococci could be definitely divided by the blood plate method into hemolytic and nonhemolytic varieties. Of these two groups, the hemolytic organisms have been found associated with the more severe and generalized types of infection, such as septic sore throat, general septicemia, and the bronchopneumonia and empyema already mentioned. It was further known that the hemolytic streptococci may be divided

Received for publication Nov. 25, 1919.

* This study was begun while the senior author was in military service, and stationed at the laboratory of the Southern Department, Fort Sam Houston, Tex. It was continued at the Department of Research Medicine, University of Pennsylvania, and at the Yale Army Laboratory School, New Haven, Conn. The greater part of the experimental work was done in the Department of Pathology and Bacteriology, University of California. Thanks are due to a number of officers and enlisted men and assistants in civilian life, who under our direction have accomplished portions of the work described. In particular we wish to express our appreciation to Major J. S. Simmons and Lieut. W. C. Von Glahn, both of the Medical Corps, and to Lieut. J. J. Enright, and the late Paul D. Peltier, of the Sanitary Corps, to Sergt. F. Eberson, to Miss Dolores Bradley, and to Dr. Marjorie W. Cook.

[1] Gay, Frederick P.: Jour. of Lab. and Clin. Med., 1918, 3, p. 721.

on the basis of fermentation reactions in the sugars into some 8 or more groups (Holman). Of these latter it was estimated that only 2 or 3 varieties are numerically of great significance in human infections. There has seemed little evidence on which to associate any particular type of hemolytic streptococcus with any definite disease entity.

Until very recently the attempt to classify streptococci on an immunologic basis has simply indicated that the viridans, or the nonhemolytic group, in general is rather heterogeneous, whereas the hemolytic group seemed homogeneous. It is clear that the failure in preventive and therapeutic immunization against streptococci is due in large part to a failure to appreciate the diversity of the numerous types of organisms involved. Any progress is obviously dependent on the eventual recognition of the antigenic group varieties of the streptococci. In recent months, important contributions have been made toward the classification of the hemolytic streptococcus on immunologic lines by Hamilton and Havens,[2] Dochez, Avery and Lancefield,[3] and by Havens.[4] The work of Dochez, Avery and Lancefield in particular has brought out conclusively the fact that not only do such closely allied organisms as the hemolytic streptococcus pyogenes and the hemolytic Streptococcus infrequens (mannite fermenter) differ consistently and antigenically, but that Streptococcus hemolyticus itself contains three or more different immunologic types. Furthermore, these group varieties of Streptococcus pyogenes were isolated from the same group of empyema cases in the same locality (Fort Sam Houston). It is evident how markedly this subdivision of Streptococcus pyogenes in a given infection in the same locality will complicate any possibly successful vaccine or serum prevention, or treatment.
by Dr. Avery, to the culture numbered 136 in their series, and as yet

PERSONAL INVESTIGATIONS

Our own work, although undertaken in ignorance of the subsequently recognized antigenic varieties in a supposedly single organism, was fortunately carried out with a single pure strain isolated from successive single colonies of a culture from one of the Fort Sam Houston cases by the Rockefeller Commission. This organism ("H") was obtained from the lung in a fatal case of bronchopneumonia complicated by empyema and pericarditis and corresponds, we are informed by Dr. Avery, to the culture numbered 136 in their series, and as yet

[2] Jour. Am. Med. Assn., 1919, 72, p. 272.
[3] Jour. Exper. Med., 1919, 30, p. 179.
[4] Jour. Infect. Dis., 1919, 15, p. 315.

unclassified. It belongs to Streptococcus pyogenes group, that is to say, it is hemolytic, and ferments lactose and salicin, but not mannite.

There is some suggestive evidence from previous work in streptococcus immunity that success which may have been obtained was due to a strict observance of the relationship between the infecting strain and the immune serum employed. There is, further, some suggestion that the best results have been obtained in human infections by using a recently isolated or "humanized strain" of the organism in producing the immune serum.[1]

In order to test the possibility of the latter hypothesis we have employed in our experimental work on rabbits, strains of our streptococcus grown on the one hand in a medium containing rabbit serum, and on the other hand, in a glucose medium. Throughout our work we have utilized beef infusion broth for the growth of the organisms adjusted to a reaction of P_H 7.2-7.4, and containing either 1% glucose or 5% sterile, fresh rabbit serum. The streptococcus grows readily on both these mediums, and in 24 hours presents a general diffuse cloudiness. When, however, a culture is transferred from serum to glucose broth it fails to grow rapidly in the first few subcultures. In 2 or 3 days the growth in the glucose broth, owing to the more rapid production of acid, becomes granular and sediments to the bottom of the tube, whereas the growth on rabbit serum broth remains turbid for a longer period of time. The serum cultures remain alive at 37 degrees for at least 2-3 weeks; glucose cultures are dead at body temperature in from 3-5 days. They may be preserved for 10-14 days, however, by growth at 37 or 24 degrees and subsequent conservations in the icebox.

In our work both on infection and immunity it was necessary to have a fairly accurate enumeration of the number of bacteria contained in a cubic centimeter of either of these cultures. We had been somewhat skeptical of the strict accuracy of the Wright method of counting bacteria by comparison with red blood cells, but a careful check of the method in a number of instances by gravimetric tests has convinced us of its unusual accuracy. Counts made at intervals during the progress of the work by Wright's method have given very consistent results. The average of 26 counts of 24 hour H. R. S. cultures (by which is meant the "H" strain used for our work grown on rabbit serum broth) gave 1,207 million cocci to the cubic centimeter. Glucose cultures gave an average of 750 million per c c. The chains of organisms grown on the glucose medium are longer than those grown on the serum medium, and the individual cocci appear swollen and of greater diameter. As already stated, efforts have been made to check the accuracy of this simple method of enumeration of bacteria. The plating method, which is so successful in checking counts of this sort when carried out with organisms like the typhoid bacillus, appears to be quite valueless with the streptococcus. It has been found that succesful dilution beyond a certain point may continue to show as many or even more organisms than the next supposedly lower dilution in the series. It may be that this increasing count is due to the mechanical breaking up of the coccal chains. At all events, it was found necessary to abandon the plating method after numerous attempts; a gravimetric method was next tested, and found to show a striking correspondence of weight of dried streptococci as compared with the Wright method.

In table 1 are given several Wright counts as compared with the dried weight of the bacteria derived from 50 c c of the same culture from which the count had been made. The organisms were collected in the bottom of a tube by prolonged centrifugalization until the supernatant culture fluid was perfectly clear. After pouring off the supernatant fluid the sedimented culture was shaken in 10 c c of absolute alcohol, recentrifugalized, shaken and centrifuged again in 10 c c of absolute ether. A constant dried weight of baceria was obtained in 2 or 3 days by placing the tube in a partial vacuum over calcium chlorid.

TABLE 1

WRIGHT COUNTS AS COMPARED WITH DRIED WEIGHT OF BACTERIA

Culture	Wright's Count in Millions per c c	Milligrams of Bacteria in 50 c c	Millions of Bacteria per Milligram
H. R. S. 35*	459	6.8	3,381
H. R. S. 36	425	6.3	3.377
H. R. S. 41	619	8.1	3,821
H. R. S. 42	450	6.1	3,689
			Aver. 3,592
H. D. 27†	508	3.4	7,470
H. D. 32	833	5.3	7.871
H. D. 28	600	5.5	5,454
H. D. 36	760	5.6	6,800
			Aver. 6,898

* The serum broth employed of this serum was of slightly different composition which accounts for the lower counts as compared with the average found in later experiments.
† Cultures o f "H" on 1% glucose broth, with generation of culture.

An inspection of the table brings out not only the close correspondence between the direct counts of bacteria and their weight, but shows another interesting fact worthy of further consideration at some time, bearing on the metabolism of bacteria in culture media of different constitution. It will be noted that although in this particular series the counts of bacteria in the glucose cultures ran somewhat higher than those in the serum cultures, the weight of the organisms themselves was distinctly less when grown on glucose than when grown on serum. This observation should be still further correlated with the fact that the organisms in glucose cultures are distinctly larger than when grown in serum mediums. As a further check on the accuracy of the comparative estimates in these experiments, it should be stated that Wilson and Dickson[5] in their article on a "Gravimetric Method of Standardizing Vaccines" found that Streptococcus fecalis grown on agar contains 3,398 million streptococci to the milligram, which is in close correspondence with our averages.

EXPERIMENTAL EMPYEMA IN RABBITS

Our culture "H" of Streptococcus pyogenes agrees with the characteristics described by other investigators for organisms of this group. It is not markedly pathogenic for rabbits. Dochez, Avery and Lancefield found that 1 c c or more of a 24-hour broth culture administered intraperitoneally was necessary to kill rabbits. Davis[6] found that pathogenic human strains of the hemolytic streptococcus will rarely kill rabbits in a dose of less than 0.5 c c of a broth culture per kilogram of a rabbit, and the most pathogenic strains are apparently less fatal for these animals than the other strains. Our culture "H" soon after isolation would at times kill rabbits in from 2-4 days in a dose of approximately 0.5 to 1.0 c c per kilo administered intravenously. In successive subcultures on rabbit serum broth it became less pathogenic for rabbits, even when strains of the original "H" organisms that have been passed through the pleural cavity of rabbits for a number of generations are employed as the inoculum for broth cultures. When death does occur in these animals, the organism is found in the heart's blood, and in many instances produces a localized arthritis. An attempt to increase the general invasive properties of this culture, "H," for rabbits has been unsuccessful. It apparently cannot readily be induced to produce a general septicemia with uniformity.

[5] Jour. of. Hygiene, 1912, 12, p. 49.
[6] Jour. Am. Med. Assn., 1919, 72, p. 319.

We have, however, succeeded with great regularity in producing a streptococcus pleuritis or empyema in rabbits which we believe resembles in all respects its human analogue. In our early experiments we succeeded by the use of relatively large amounts of a culture of the "H" organism in producing pleuritis in a few rabbits, although somewhat inconstantly. When 1-3 c c of a 24-hour culture of "H" in its early generation on rabbit serum or blood broth was injected into the right pleural cavity or rabbits, 7 out of 10 animals showed at death, or when killed within a week, various stages of an extending pleurisy.

At this point it may be well to review our present conception of the pathogenesis of human empyema due to streptococci. It is clear from the observations of numerous investigators that the hemolytic streptococcus is present in the throat of from 20-50% of normal men in army camps. It has been found by Pilot and Davis[7] in 90% of the crypts in follicular tonsillitis, where it apparently serves as a potential focus for further invasion. It has further been evidenced by numerous observers since the work of Cole and MacCallum[8] that patients with measles who harbor these organisms in their throats are much more likely to suffer from the unfortunate sequels of bronchopneumonia and empyema than patients with "clean" measles. Streptococcus bronchopneumonia, whether or not complicated by empyema, has been found to occur in otherwise healthy individuals as well as a sequel to measles, scarlet fever and influenza. The bronchopneumonia frequently represents a transitory phase in the extension of the streptococcus from the nose and throat through the lungs to the pleura. There seems, further, little reason to question that this organism spreads by a process of direct extension rather than by metastasis. The extension may be extremely rapid as is evidenced by those instances of empyema which occur in individuals that were apparently well and working a day or two before. Bronchopneumonia is frequently not diagnosed if present until the occurrence of empyema. Blood cultures taken from human cases during the course of bronchopneumonia and empyema are almost always sterile except in the terminal phases of the disease (MacCallum[9]). Human streptococcus empyema in numerous cases continues its invasion by extension by involving first the pericardium and then the pleural cavity on the

[7] Jour. Infect. Dis., 1919, 24, p. 386.

[8] Jour. Am. Med. Assn., 1918, 70, p. 1146.

[9] The Pathology of the Pneumonia in the U. S. Army Camps During the Winter of 1917-18, Monograph No. 10, Rockefeller Institute for Medical Research, 1919.

opposite side. Metastatic complications are extremely rare; the process as a whole may be classified as infection by extension.

The experimental empyema in rabbits fulfills in every detail the human analogue as we have outlined it. We have not, however, succeeded in producing streptococcus bronchopneumonia in rabbits. It will be recalled in this connection that Lamar and Meltzer produced a typical lobar pneumonia in dogs by bronchial insufflation of cultures of pneumococcus. Winternitz and Hirschfelder[10] produced similar results with the same organism in rabbits. Wollstein and Meltzer[11] claim to have produced streptococcus bronchopneumonia in dogs, but so far as we are aware, no attempt has been made heretofore to produce it in rabbits. At all events, we have not succeeded in so doing, although we have insufflated large amounts (5-10 c c) of a culture into the bronchi through a rubber catheter inserted in the trachea, followed by a syringe full of air. The animals when killed in one or two days had normal lungs. In a few instances we tried to obtain results in rabbits that had been previously gassed with chlorpicrin. The three animals thus tested died under the anesthesia before the culture could be administered.

EXPERIMENTAL PROCEDURE

We have not, therefore, succeeded in producing the entire course of a human streptococcus empyema in rabbits. Empyema may be regularly produced, however, in rabbits by this streptococcus by direct injection of small amounts of culture into the pleura, particularly when the strain employed has been passed through the pleura of several rabbits. Small amounts of the culture, as will be discussed in detail, are injected in a volume of 1 c c through a buttonhole in the skin on the right side of the rabbit without anesthesia. The skin is painted with iodin and the fluid injected into the right pleural cavity, which is easily reached by pushing the needle gently through the muscles lying over the second and third interspace to a point about half an inch to the right of the sternum. Errors in technic which may occur in the first few animals are easily detected at necropsy by the occurrence of an abscess in the muscles on the one hand, or by an abscess in the lung when the needle has been pushed too far.

As already mentioned, even large doses (1-3 c c) of early "H" cultures grown on rabbit blood broth or rabbit serum broth did not uniformly produce a pleurisy in rabbits. Attempts were then made to produce pleurisy by injecting the pleural fluid from one animal, containing variable numbers of streptococci, into a second animal. These results were likewise inconstant. When subcultures were made from the pleural fluid of an animal that had suffered from fatal empyema, constant results were obtained, particularly if the fluid represented a strain that had been passed through the pleura of several (4 or more) animals. The pleural fluid from an infected rabbit can be preserved in a

[10] Jour. Exper. Med., 1913, 18, p. 657.
[11] Ibid., 1913, 16, p. 126.

sterile tube in the icebox for several weeks and used in numerous experiments. It has been found that the organisms in this pus remain alive for a long period of time. Twenty-four-hour cultures grown on 5% rabbit serum broth from a passage pleural fluid have therefore been used in numerous experiments. Such cultures in proper dosage produce a constant and characteristic extending empyema when injected into the pleural cavity of normal rabbits. The minimum infecting dose of a passage culture, as grown directly from pleural fluid for 24 hours in rabbit serum broth, is 0.1 or 0.2 c c. Thus, we find that of 16 normal rabbits that received intrapleural injections of 0.1 c c of passage pleural culture, 14, or 87%, showed a characteristic pleurisy. Of 14 animals given 0.2 c c of a 24-hour culture intrapleurally, all, or 100%, were positive.

The course of the pleuritis produced in rabbits by this means may properly be described as subacute, that is to say, it is sufficiently prolonged to resemble in some respects the human disease and to offer sufficient time for any therapeutic intervention that might avail. Death occurs in from 1-17 days in the numerous instances in which we have observed it. On an average it has occurred on the fifth day. There is no evidence that spontaneous recovery takes place, at least not in our later series in which a uniform passage culture in a constant dose was employed. The animals show progressive loss of weight, and if the disease is prolonged considerably, respiratory distress follows until death intervenes. Having determined that death is the invariable result of this infection, it has been found more expeditious in most experiments to kill all surviving animals in from a week to 10 days and to note their condition of recovery or advanced pleuritis, rather than to wait for death to intervene. This procedure has not only made a greater number of experiments possible, but has given information as to the destruction of the organisms during the course of the pleurisy.

As in human cases it was found that pleurisy usually spreads rapidly by extension, and involves the pericardium and the other chest cavity. Thus, of 103 animals examined, 47 (45%) were found to have both chest cavities and the pericardium involved, 23 (22%) were localized in one side alone, 17 (16%) involved both pleural cavities, and 15 involved one chest cavity and the pericardium. In a single instance the pericardium alone was involved, possibly through injection into this sac. Extension may be very rapid as was evidenced in a number of animals that died in 24 hours in which both pleural cavities and the pericardium were found involved. Mediastinal abscesses filled with thick yellowish pus are frequently found adjacent to the lower anterior margin of the lungs, as described by MacCallum[9] in the human cases.

The nature of the exudate likewise resembles in its appearance at successive periods the human empyema fluids as MacCallum has described them, except that it is never greenish in color. In earlier cases it is serous in nature, and in 2 or 3 days becomes seropurulent, then fibrinous or fibrinopurulent. As much as 15 or 20 c c of fluid may be found in one chest cavity. On examination the fluid contains large numbers of leukocytes and usually, but not always, numerous streptococci are seen in chains of varying length. The cultures from the pleural fluids irrespective of their appearance are always positive. The lung on the affected side is collapsed, atelectatic and covered with a thick matwork of fibrin, although it may be insufflated artificially as in the human cases described by MacCallum.

The leukocytic counts from the peripheral blood do not vary much from those in normal rabbits for several days, but when followed they show a sharp rise to from 20,000 to 30,000 two or three days before death. In one case, complicated by a broken leg, there was an immediate leukocytic increase and the formation of pus in the region involved. In animals that are killed in from 5-10 days while suffering from pleurisy, only 24% in a total of 41 have shown the presence of streptococci in the circulating blood, even when infecting doses as large as 1 c c are employed. In animals that are allowed to die spontaneously the blood cultures are more frequently positive, although even in these cases they were found in only 69% of 23 animals examined from this standpoint. There is evidence then that septicemia as in human beings is not characteristic, but that we are dealing rather with an infection by extension.

It should be clearly emphasized that there is no evidence in our own work to indicate an elective localizing affinity in the sense of Rosenow.[12] We tried, without success, in the early stages of our work, to obtain localization in the pleural cavities by intravenous injection, and in many attempts since subcultures from an empyema fluid given intravenously in amounts as large as 10 c c have failed in all cases to show localization in the pleura. Several cubic centimeters of the pleural fluid itself injected into the veins also failed to produce pleuritis.

ACTIVE IMMUNIZATION AGAINST EXPERIMENTAL EMPYEMA

We have seen in our previous review[1] that there is little evidence as to the effectiveness of active immunity in animals produced by

[12] Jour. Am. Med. Assn., 1915, 65, p. 1687.

injections of streptococcus vaccine. There was, until recently, no information as to the possibilities of systematic vaccine prophylaxis against this organism in human beings. In recent months several communications bearing directly or indirectly on this problem have appeared. Ely, Lloyd, Hitchcock, and Nickson[13] have attempted systematic immunization against streptococcus infections in the Puget Sound Navy Yard. They found hemolytic streptococci in the majority of their fatal cases of influenza, and after immunization of considerable numbers of men with these organisms they have apparently noted lessened incidence of influenza in the vaccinated as compared with the unvaccinated men, and a very striking decrease in the mortality in the former category. There were actually no deaths in over 4,000 vaccinated men, whereas deaths varied in from 4-12% of the cases of influenza that occurred among the unvaccinated. These authors do not speak of the instances of complications in either group, nor do they mention the existence of empyema. Rosenow, who believes a diplostreptococcus of the viridans type bears a causative relation to influenza, has advocated an immunization with a mixed vaccine containing those organisms present in the throats of influenza cases and including 30% of the viridans streptococci found there. His results indicate a lessened incidence of influenza in the vaccinated and a reduction in some of the complications, notably in the pneumonia which is only one third as frequent in the vaccinated as in the unvaccinated. No note is made as to the occurrence of empyema. Richey,[14] who was evidently dealing with a mixed vaccine similar to Rosenow's,[15] found that experimental tonsillitis was produced accidentally in a number of individuals who were given nasopharyngeal washings and bronchial secretions from cases of influenza in an attempt to produce the latter disease experimentally. This tonsillitis was found to be due to the hemolytic streptococcus present in such washings. He notes that "this tonsillitis occurred in three individuals who had received one month previously a vaccine containing, in addition to other organisms, three presumably adequate doses of haemolytic streptococci."

There is then no evidence to lead us to anticipate that either generalized or localized infections due to streptococci are prevented in human beings by the ordinary methods of vaccination which have been so successful in certain other bacterial infections.

[13] Jour. Am. Med. Assn., 1919, 72, p. 24.
[14] Jour. Infect. Dis., 1919, 25, p. 305.
[15] Jour. Am. Med. Assn., 1919, 72, p. 31 and p. 1604.

Rabbits may be treated with repeated injections of either killed or living "H" culture owing to the fact that it is not markedly pathogenic for these animals. An extensive series of animals has been treated in this manner not only in order to test their active protection against the pleurisy described, but also to test the properties of their serums in treating this infection. The animals were immunized, not only with serum broth cultures of streptococcus, but also in a few instances with glucose cultures in order to determine any possible influence of the immediate source of the organisms used in preparing the vaccine. Immunizations were usually carried out by gradually increasing the dose first of killed and then of living culture given at varying intervals and for periods extending for from one month to two and a half months. In some instances only living cultures were employed beginning with small doses. The animals lost weight during the course of immunization, but usually regained it if the series of inoculations was interrupted for a short time. A week or ten days after the last injection they were given intrapleural inoculations of the test dose of a subculture from the pleural fluid in the manner described. It will be recalled that 0.1 c c of a 24-hour serum broth culture almost invariably produces a progressive pleuritis and pericarditis (87% positive). In all instances tried 0.2 of a c c of a 24-hour culture has invariablly produced this syndrome. We are not only thus assured by the continued repetition of this experiment that it may be produced invariably in normal animals, but in each instance where two or more of the immunized animals to be tested were inoculated one or more control normal animals were run through at the same time. In every instance included in the following table the normal controls succumbed to the characteristic infection.

In table 2 are given the results obtained in producing an experimental empyema in rabbits previously immunized as outlined. They are arranged in order of the total amount of bacteria used in immunization. In the table is included, first the type of vaccine employed in immunization, whether obtained by growing the culture "H" on rabbit serum broth (vaccine "S") or on glucose broth (vaccine "D"). There is further mention here as to whether the animals received killed cultures alone or living cultures alone, or killed and living cultures. The number of injections and the total number of organisms used in the entire process of immunization, computed in billions, is then added. In the next column the infecting pleural dose is given and represents the amount of a 24-hour culture in serum broth from the pleural fluid of a rabbit previously dead of empyema. The time of death ("+") or killing ("X") is noted and the results found as regards the presence of pleurisy, and whether the latter is single or double (+ or + +), and also the occurrence of pericarditis.

TABLE 2

EXPERIMENTAL EMPYEMA IN IMMUNIZED RABBITS

No.	Vaccine	Injections	Total in Billions	Infecting Dose, c c	Killed or Dead	Pleurisy	Pericarditis
243	S killed	9	2¼	0.2	+ 7	++	+
244	S killed	9	2¼	0.2	+ 5	++	+
245	S killed	9	2¼	0.2	x 5	++	+
223	S killed and living	6	3	0.1	x 5	0	0
220	S killed	6	3	0.2	x 6	0	0
246	S killed	12	3¾	0.1	+ 4	++	+
251	S killed	14	4¾	0.1	x 6	0	0
229	S killed	9	6	0.1	+ 5	++	+
232	S killed	9	6	0.1	x 6	0	0
234	S killed	10	6	0.1	x 5	0	0
532	S living	9	6	0.2	x12	+	0
534	S living	9	6	0.2	x11	0	0
302	S killed and living	12	9	0.1	x 6	0	0
303	S killed and living	13	10¾	0.1	x 4	0	0
305	D killed and living	11	14	0.1	x 4	0	0
306	D killed and living	12	15	0.1	x 6	0	0
257	S living	15	26	0.2	x10	0	0

An inspection of this table shows clearly that a considerable number of injections of killed cultures can be used without producing protection against the experimental pleurisy and that killed cultures followed by living cultures must be given for a long period of time and in large aggregate amounts in order to assure complete active immunity against the localized infection. It is evident that if sufficient amounts of killed and subsequently of living cultures of streptococci are given over a considerable period of time, representing a large number of injections, protection against empyema is assured. The total number of bacteria employed in immunization rather than the number of injections given would seem to be the decisive factor. This would agree with the results attained in typhoid vaccination. There is apparently as good protection afforded by cultures of organisms grown on glucose as when they are grown on the serum of the animal in which protection is induced.

It seems evident that no optimistic conclusion can be drawn from these results in rabbits as to the possibility of protecting human beings against localized streptococcus infections, or specifically against empyema, owing to the large amount of vaccine and prolonged nature of the treatment required.

ATTEMPTS AT SPECIFIC THERAPEUTIC INTERVENTION IN EXPERIMENTAL EMPYEMA

Attempts to cure or prevent streptococcus infections by immune serum have been made almost entirely in generalized infections. This is true not only of the earliest work of Marmorek,[16] but also in the recent work of Dochez, Avery and Lancefield. We do not recall instances in which streptococcus immune serum has been utilized in treating local streptococcus infections either experimentally in animals or in human beings. Our results then are of interest not only as attempts to cure experimental streptococcus empyema, but as possible lines of attack on other localized infections due to this organism.

We have already recounted in some detail the methods employed in immunizing rabbits against our particular strain of streptococcus. Both glucose broth and serum broth cultures have been employed and the immunization was continued over a considerable period of time in varying doses, but, in all the completely protected animals, with large total amounts of living bacteria. As we have just described in the preceding section, we have succeeded by prolonged treatment in producing a very definite active immunity against intrapleural infections with this streptococcus. The animals that were tested for active immunity were killed by bleeding from 7-12 days after the trial intrapleural injection designed to test their protection and their serum employed in the curative experiments that follow. It is evident from the fact that they are obtained from actively immunized animals that they are, properly speaking, immune sera. In addition, we have tested the content of antibodies in these sera to determine the presence of antagonistic properties to the streptococcus used for immunization. Unfortunately, we have not hitherto been able to produce a constant septicemia in rabbits or mice with our strain "H" by which we could have tested the protective or curative properties of such serums in preventing generalized infections. The tests for antibodies employed have been principally for agglutinins, opsonins and precipitins, all of which have been positive in high degree.

Agglutinin Tests.—Much difficulty in the past has been found in demonstrating agglutinins in the serum of individuals suffering from streptococcus infections or in animals immunized against streptococci. The technical difficulties have been so great that many have been unable to satisfy themselves that agglutinins really are present under these conditions. In the light of our present knowledge, it would seem that failure to demonstrate agglutinins to streptococci is, however, a purely technical matter. The great difficulty has lain in obtaining cultures of streptococcus that are not spontaneously sedimented or flocculated, and various measures, such as mechanical attempts to

[16] Ann. de l'Inst. Pasteur, 1895, 9, p. 593.

break up the chains and the addition of alkali, have been tried to obviate this difficulty. Although we have succeeded in establishing a wholly satisfactory technic for agglutination tests of streptococci, it was done at first without appreciation of the mechanism involved, which has since become clear. It is desirable from every standpoint to have a standardized homogeneous suspension of organisms which can be used for considerable periods of time in making agglutination tests, and our efforts to obtain such suspensions were at first unavailing. We found finally, however, that a constant homogeneous suspension of streptococci may be obtained by adding phenol in a final dilution of 0.2 to 0.5% to a 24-hour serum broth culture. The cultures so treated are found sterile on the following day, after incubation at 37 degrees, and may then be concentrated by centrifugalization and resuspended in the same serum broth in which they have been grown in one-tenth the amount of the original fluid. This gives a thick suspension of the organisms which does not sediment except over a period of several days. The fact that complete and rapid sedimentation resulted when we first centrifuged the cultures and then suspended them in 0.5% phenolated salt solution led to the explanation of the success or the failure of these slight variations in technic. If phenol is added to carefully neutralized physiologic salt solution of a P_H of 7.2, the eventual 0.5% solution becomes approximately of a P_H of 6.9. If, however, the same amount of phenol is added to serum broth, it does not change more than to a P_H of 7.1. This slight difference in acidity then would seem to be the important factor in spontaneous sedimentation of these bacteria. We suspect, moreover, that it may have a more far reaching significance in those cultures described as "spontaneously" agglutinable. Physiologic salt and indeed distilled water, as prepared in the ordinary laboratory, is frequently not exactly at the neutral point, and very slight deviations in the acidity may give a flocculation of the type we have encountered in streptococci. Our work in preparing the antigen agrees completely with that of Dochez, Avery and Lancefield, and we further agree with them in obtaining far better agglutination results by incubating the agglutination tests at 55 C. instead of at 37. The results are more rapidly obtained, and the final reading is in higher dilution at the higher temperature. Controls with normal serum by this technic with the phenolated suspension of streptococci are uniformly negative even in low dilutions.

The immune serums we have produced gave positive agglutination reactions at 55 C. in dilutions of from 1:400 to 1:12,800. There is apparently no difference in the results of agglutination when the suspension of streptococci has been grown on glucose mediums, or when the serum of animals immunized by glucose cultures is employed with serum culture suspensions. Cultures of other streptococci of the pyogenes group obtained from the same group of empyema cases at Fort Sam Houston either gave slight agglutination or none at all with our antiserum to strain "H." This organism, it will be recalled, remains unclassified in the Dochez, Avery and Lancefield grouping, and our results, although largely negative for other strains, suggest findings similar to theirs.

Immune Opsonin Tests.—A 24-hour culture grown in serum broth was used. The culture was counted and diluted with broth, so that each cubic centimeter contained 500,000,000 organisms.

Leukocytes were obtained from the peritoneal fluid of a guinea-pig which had been injected intraperitoneally 24 hours previously with 10 c c of sterile broth. The peritoneal exudate was washed 3 times in 0.9% NaCl and the final sediment suspended in 0.9% NaCl.

The serum was inactivated for half an hour at 56 C., and used both undiluted and in dilutions of 1:50, 1:100, 1:200, 1:400, etc. In a control test with normal serum lower dilutions of 1:20, 1:40 and 1:80 were used.

An immune serum of known titer was included in each test to furnish a basis of comparison for the activity of each preparation of leukocytes.

In the case of the immune and normal sera, 0.1 c c each of serum dilution, culture, and leukocytes were mixed in small test tubes. As a control on the phagocytic activity of the leukocytes alone, the serum dilution was replaced by 0.9% NaCl, the tube containing only leukocytes, culture, and salt solution. All tubes were incubated for 2 hours at 37 C., the tubes being shaken frequently during the first hour.

At the end of the period of incubation, the supernatant fluid was poured off from each tube, leaving only a drop or two of fluid, in which the sedimented bacteria and leukocytes were thoroughly mixed. From this mixture smears were made with a loop on slides. The smears were fixed in picric acid and stained with alcoholic eosin and methylene blue.

Estimation of the opsonic properties of the immune serum was made as follows:

With each slide a count was made of the number of leukocytes which contained streptococci in a total of 100 cells. Counts of the leukocyte control tube gave the lowest percentage — about 12%. The dilution of serum which gave results comparable to the leukocyte control tube was considered the point of bacteriotropic extinction. In the case of normal serum this point was reached usually in a dilution of 1:40, rarely of 1:80. With the immune serums much higher dilutions, sometimes as high as 1:3,200, were required. The titer of the serum was considered to be the last dilution in which there was distinct evidence of phagocytosis above that shown in the leukocyte control. For a normal serum, as indicated above, this value was usually 1:20; for an immune serum anywhere from 1:200 to 1:1,600. By means of these figures, the activity of an immune serum was readily expressed as the multiple of the activity of a normal serum — an immune serum of 1:1,600 titer, for instance, being 80 times as active as a normal serum of 1:20 titer.

The serum of our animals in which active immunity had been proved by intrapleural inoculation was found to vary in tropin content from 5 to 80 times that of normal rabbit serum.

Precipitin Tests.—We have not obtained as good results in precipitin tests by the method described by Barnes[17] in this department who was working under somewhat different conditions with the larger group relations of streptococci. He employed the supernatant fluids of broth cultures of streptococci as antigen. We have, however, obtained constant precipitin results in our strictly specific relations as regards organisms and antiserum by employing extracts of dried "H" streptococci grown either in glucose or serum broth and ground in an agate mortar (operated by a mechanical ore grinder run by a small motor, for about one hour) until reduced to an impalpable powder. The immune serums employed by us for therapeutic purposes gave a marked precipitin reaction with these extracts of streptococci. The results were obtained by adding 0.5% carbolated salt containing an extract of from 1-10 mg. of dried ground culture to equal amounts of immune serum, both volumes used being 0.5 c c. No result was obtained with normal rabbit serum, even with the largest amounts of antigen employed. The results were usually positive at 37 C. by the ring test in from 15-30 minutes, but the ingredients were ordinarily mixed and allowed to stand over night in the incubator, and the final results read by sedimentation in the morning.

In general, the opsonin, agglutinin, and precipitin titers of our immune serum were found parallel, and in correspondence, so far as our figures go, with active protection, as illustrated by the following selected cases:

TABLE 3

RESULTS OF PRECIPITIN TESTS

Rabbit No.	Active Immunity	Agglutinins	Opsonin	Precipitins with Milligrams of Antigen
532	Negative	200	0	5
249	Not tested	200	25	5
304	Not tested	800	2.5	5
305	Positive	12,800	40	5
306	Positive	1,600	20	5
301	Not tested	6,400	80	1
251	Positive	12,800	20	—

Although we have made numerous attempts to demonstrate bactericidal properties in our immune sera after the manner described by Haven,[4] we have not succeeded in doing so. It should be remarked,

[17] Jour. Infect. Dis., 1919, 25, p. 47.

moreover, that our sera as measured by the agglutinin test were of greater potency than those employed by Havens.

Our antistreptococcus serum when mixed with a suspension of rabbit blood cells and living streptococcus culture has distinct antihemotoxic properties. The red blood cells of an immunized rabbit appear to be no more resistant to hemolysis than those of normal animals.

PREVENTION AND THERAPY OF EXPERIMENTAL EMPYEMA BY IMMUNE SERUM

A number of these immune sera produced in the manner described and containing strong antibodies have been tested for their preventive and curative action on experimental streptococcus empyema in rabbits. The injections of serum have been given before the intrapleural infecting dose, simultaneously with the dose, and at periods subsequent to it. One or two doses of 0.5 to 1 c c have been given, for the most part, into the infected pleural cavity, but in some instances intravenously. In each separate experiment results obtained by immune serum have been controlled by rabbits infected at the same time, but treated with normal rabbit serum.

Our results are distinctive, and indicate that experimental empyema may, in a definite though small percentage of cases, be prevented or even cured by the use of immune serum. They may best be summarized and then illustrated by an experimental protocol:

The immune serums from 10 different rabbits have been tested, most of them chosen as containing the highest content in antibodies. In 8 of the 10 rabbits furnishing this immune serum the active immunity against experimental empyema was tested and found to be complete. The other two were not tested. To repeat and add to the animals used as controls, it may be stated:

(1) That 14 normal rabbits inoculated with 0.2 c c of a 24-hour passage pleural culture of streptococcus "H" showed in every instance a positive empyema.

(2) 15 normal rabbits inoculated in the same manner and treated with normal rabbit serum in doses corresponding in amount and with the same routes of inoculation employed in the rabbits treated with immune serum, were also in every instance positive.

(3) In contrast to these 29 animals giving positive empyema in 100% of instances, we have succeeded in preventing or curing pleurisy by the use of rabbit immune serum in 5 of 20 animals when the

immune serum was given into the pleural cavity that contained the infecting dose, and in 1 of 3 animals in which the immune serum was given intravenously. Of the 5 animals in which the evolution of experimental pleurisy was prevented by the use of immune serum intrapleurally only two were, strictly speaking, cured, because in three instances 1 c c of serum was injected simultaneously with the culture and the treatment must be regarded as preventive. In the other two cured animals 1 c c of immune serum was in one instance given 24 hours after injection of the infecting dose, and in the other instance 0.5 c c of immune serum was given 6 and 24 hours after infection.

As an example of the experimental results obtained the full protocol of an experiment is herewith included:

Exper. 1.—A series of rabbits was given 0.2 c c of a 24-hour serum broth culture of passage pleural strain of streptococcus "H" intrapleurally. They were then treated with immune serum No. 305 or normal serum as follows:

TABLE 4

RESULTS OF IMMUNE SERUM TEST

No.	Serum Given	Death	Pleurisy	Pericarditis	Pleural Culture
584	1 c c Serum No. 305 simultaneously intrapleurally 1 c c 24 hours later intrapleurally	Killed 11 days	0	0	0
581	1 c c Serum No. 305 simultaneously intrapleurally 1 c c Serum No. 305 24 hours later intrapleurally	Killed 5 days	0	0	0
585	1 c c Serum No. 305 24 hours after culture intrapleurally	Killed 9 days	?*	0	+
586	1 c c Serum No. 305 24 hours after culture intrapleurally	Dead 2 days	++	+	+
583	1 c c Serum No. 305 simultaneously intravenously 1 c c Serum No. 305 24 hours later intravenously	Dead 4 days	++	+	+
587	1 c c normal serum simultaneously intrapleurally 1 c c normal serum 24 hours later intrapleurally	Dead 2 days	++	+	+

* The right pleural cavity showed firm fibrous adhesions between the partially collapsed lung and the parietal pleura. A very slight amount of bloody fluid was also present. The left pleural cavity and pericardium were normal. This finding is in sharp contrast to the double empyema usually found (++) and would indicate a healing process.

It is evident, then, that although distinct results in the prevention of experimental empyema and, in rare instances, the cure of experimental empyema, may be produced by the use of immune serum from rabbits, we have as yet no evidence of a sovereign or even encouraging serum therapy to offer. It would seem that the immune sera that we have employed, to judge from their antibody content, are not only as potent as those used by other investigators, but they would appear, moreover, to reach the limits of potency ordinarily to be obtained.

ATTEMPTS AT VACCINE THERAPY

In several animals an attempt has been made to influence the course of the experimental empyema we have described by giving injections to kill streptococcus culture intravenously, such injections beginning either on the day of the intrapleural inoculation or actually preceding it by 24 hours. In certain of these vaccinated animals the leukocyte counts reached very high figures—in one instance 64,000 to the cubic millimeter, and distinctly exceeded the counts made in control, unvaccinated, infected animals. In no instance, however, was the slightest effect produced on the evolution of the empyema. The vaccinated, infected animals died, not only as rapidly, but apparently even more rapidly than the unvaccinated controls.

A combination of vaccine and serum therapy seems worthy of trial, and our results in this respect may subsequently be given.

SUMMARY AND CONCLUSIONS

This experimental study was undertaken with the practical problem of human streptococcus empyema in mind. It may be regarded as bearing on the general question of streptococcus immunity, and particularly as indicating the possibilities of specific prevention or therapy of localized streptococcus infections of the empyema type.

Human streptococcus empyema may be regarded as an infection by extension in contradistinction to generalized streptococcus septicemia. From the beginning our work was carried out with a single pure strain of the streptococcus isolated from a case of human empyema, and thus we have inadvertently avoided the errors that have beset other workers in this field in view of the recently discovered fact that not only hemolytic streptococci in general but Streptococcus pyogenes in particular is divisible into several distinct immunologic types. This study has dealt with a strictly homologous infecting organism and corresponding immune principles. Still further possibilities of specific correspondence have been investigated by comparing the results from growing the organisms on the serum of the animal to be infected, in comparison with growth on media containing glucose. No differences in the antigenic property of the organisms grown on these two media, have been found.

Although the human strain of streptococcus employed in this study is not markedly pathogenic for rabbits, it has been found possible to produce a constant, characteristic, and fatal extending pleurisy or empyema in these animals by the use of a passage culture of the original strain carried through the pleural cavity of several animals. This empyema is produced by direct injection of a small amount of passage culture (0.1 to 0.2 c c) into the pleural cavity. Injections of large amounts of such a passage culture or of the original empyema fluid from which it is derived, are not fatal when given intravenously and the organisms do not show selective localization in the pleura. This experimental empyema resembles in appearance the human analogue, which it was aimed to simulate, except that the initial bronchopneumonia which may occur in the human cases has not been produced in rabbits. It is a streptococcus infection by extension and very rarely becomes generalized before death. It is invariably fatal, on an average in 5 days, thus allowing sufficient time for therapeutic intervention.

Experimental streptococcus empyema in rabbits may be prevented by previous immunization with killed, followed by living, cultures of the same strain of streptococcus, but only when repeated vaccinations have been practiced and in a total amount which would seem to preclude the practicability of such a preventive inoculation in human beings, provided the conditions are similar.

The serum of rabbits that have been successfully immunized against subsequent intrapleural infection with the streptococcus contains potent antibodies, particularly agglutinins, opsonins, and precipitins. As the technic of the determination of such antibodies in antistreptococcus serum has been questioned, it is herewith fully detailed.

The more potent of these antisera from rabbits when injected simultaneously with the culture into the pleural cavity may prevent the evolution of the otherwise invariable and fatal empyema. In a few instances subsequent injection of serum into the pleural cavity, or even intravenously, has cured the empyema.

No very optimistic conclusion on the practical use of an antistreptococcus serum in this type of localized infection can be drawn from our experiments as hitherto conducted.

Attempted vaccine therapy of the localized empyema has given consistently negative results.

STREPTOLYSIN

Paul H. de Kruif and Paul M. Ireland

From the Hygienic Laboratory of the University of Michigan, Ann Arbor, Mich.

The use of the blood-agar plate for the differentiation of alpha and beta hemolytic streptococci[1] has become general, and its value has been questioned by but few investigators. At the same time, a search of the literature on this subject reveals a distressing lack of uniformity of method and little attempt at standardization. Of 130 papers carefully summarized in the monograph of J. H. Brown,[2] no mention was made of the type of blood used in 29 instances. Human blood was employed in 35 cases, rabbit blood in 28, horse blood in 11, while the remainder of the trials were made with beef, sheep, guinea-pig, hog, dog, or goat blood. In many of the investigations where the species of blood used was named, no mention was made of the concentration of blood, or of the method of preparation of the plates.

It will be admitted that only by standardization of method can a profitable comparison of the results of various investigators be made. The most carefully standardized methods are those of Holman,[3] of Blake,[4] and especially that described in the recent monograph of Brown,[2] which came to hand just before the completion of the work about to be described.

This work has concerned itself almost entirely with the hemolysin of the beta type of streptococcus. It has been considered important to study carefully hemolysin production by this organism on blood accessible to general use, to find out whether variation in suitability exists among these bloods, and finally to determine their optimum concentration for maximum production of hemolysin.

It was apparent at once that such quantitative studies could best be carried out in fluid mediums. Hence the first part of this work is devoted to the investigation of hemolysin production by several strains of the beta streptococcus in a standard broth to which various con-

Received for publication Nov. 18, 1919.

[1] Jour. Med. Research, 1915, 31, p. 455.
[2] Monographs of the Rockefeller Institute, 1919, No. 9.
[3] Jour. Med. Research, 1916, 34, p. 377.
[4] Ibid., 1917, 36, p. 99.

centrations of the different serums studied were added. The second part concerns itself with the synthesis of a blood plate of maximal differentiating power, utilizing the quantitative data gleaned in the first part. It is considered superfluous to attempt a historical study of work previously done, since this is to be found in an admirably devised tabular form in Brown's monograph.[2]

Human, rabbit, sheep, and horse blood were used in this investigation. The first three are undoubtedly the most easily obtainable, and the first two have been the most widely used. Sheep blood has been employed by a few investigators but no claims have been made, to our knowledge, of a superiority of this blood over that of the human or rabbit. Horse blood was included because of the excellent results obtained with it by Smith and Brown,[1] and by Brown,[2] on blood-agar plates, and by M'Leod,[5] M'Leod and McNee,[6] von Hellens,[7] and others in the study of soluble hemolysin.

Part I

Streptolysin in Serum Broth Cultures

Streptolysin has been chiefly studied in two ways. The first and less frequently used consists in the filtration of ascites or serum broth cultures and the qualitative or quantitative investigation of such filtrates. This method was initiated by Besredka.[8] While streptolysin is undoubtedly filterable, the results from filtration have been uncertain and irregular. Certain makes of filter, such as the Maassen, are far more suitable than others, and even in the case of these, large amounts of hemolysin are lost during filtration.

This difficulty has caused the majority of investigators to employ another method—that of titration of whole cultures. The serum broth, with the organisms contained in it, is added directly to washed or unwashed red blood cells. Such use of whole cultures, while permissible for qualitative tests, is a method of dubious value for careful quantitative work. The reason for this opinion will become clear as the experimental results described below are studied. Two objections to the use of this method, which presented themselves before the experiments were begun, may be mentioned in this place. When dilutions of whole cultures are made, large numbers of organisms are carried over into the culture-red blood cell mixtures. When young cultures are being tested, these organisms will naturally continue to multiply and to secrete hemolysin. Hence, it would be very difficult to determine an end point in time of incubation. For example, a dilution might show a trace of hemolysis or none at the end of two hours at 37 C. Examined two hours later, the red blood cells in this tube might be found completely hemolyzed. Again, the tendency of streptococci to form clumps introduces a variable and unreliable factor into the study of closely graded dilutions of whole cultures.

In view of the objections to the two methods just described it was decided to use a third one. This method is not new. On the other hand it has been

[5] J. Pathol. & Bacteriol., 1912, 16, p. 321.
[6] Ibid., 1912-13, 17, p. 524.
[7] Centralbl. f. Bakt., I, O., 1913, 68, p. 602.
[8] Ann. de L'Inst. Pasteur., 1901, 15, p. 880.

very rarely used in the study of streptolysin. In our hands it has proved very satisfactory, and it certainly avoids the errors to which the first two are subject. It consists simply in the use of the supernatants of cultures centrifugated at high speed, i. e., 8,000 revolutions a minute. Such supernatants, while not sterile, contain minimal numbers of organisms. By their use quantitative results, suprisingly accurate and capable of exact reduplication, can be obtained.

The work outlined below had its inception in the observation that the hemolytic zones surrounding colonies of beta hemolytic streptococcus were much wider and clearer on 10% sheep blood-agar plates than on those prepared from similar concentrations of rabbit and human blood. The preliminary hypothesis as to the cause of this superiority of sheep blood involved the idea of a possibly greater susceptibility of the red corpuscles of the sheep to the streptolysin. To test this idea experimentally an attempt was at once made to obtain free hemolysin by the method of M'Leod, slightly modified by us.

The broth used in the work described was made in the same manner throughout. Beef infusion was employed in all cases. Parke, Davis & Co. bacteriologic peptone was added in a concentration of 2%. Normal $NaCO_3$ solution was added till a hydrogen-ion concentration of P_H 7.8 was obtained. The addition of 17-19 c c of alkali per liter was necessary to arrive at this H-ion concentration. The method used for the determination of P_H was that described by Clark and Lubs.[9]

Eighty c c of broth were placed in each of 4 small sterile Erlenmeyer flasks. Fifteen c c of fresh sterile horse serum (57 C. 60′) were added to each flask. These were now seeded with 0.1 c c each of a suspension in 2 c c of sterile NaCl solution, of 1 loop of a 24-hour blood-agar culture of streptococci, strains W-1, M, A-1, and V. The cultures used for seeding were 10% defibrinated rabbit blood-agar slants. The flasks, inoculated with the above strains in the order just mentioned, were labeled 1, 2, 3, and 4, placed in the water bath at 37 C. and incubated for 18 hours. Examination at the end of this time showed a heavy growth of streptococcus in each case. A portion of broth was removed by bulb pipet from each flask and centrifugated at 8,000 revolutions a minute. The clear supernatants were pipetted off and the following dilutions with 0.85% NaCl solution were made for each one.

TABLE 1

ILLUSTRATION OF DILUTION OF SUPERNATANTS FOR TEST OF HEMOLYSIN

Supernatant		NaCl Solution 0.85%	2.5% Suspension Red Blood Cells (3× washed)		
Undiluted	Diluted 1-10		Sheep	Rabbit	
1.0	—	—	0.5	0.5	Final vol. 1.5 c c
—	1.0	—	0.5	0.5	
—	0.8	0.2	0.5	0.5	
—	0.5	0.5	0.5	0.5	Water bath 37 C. 2 hours
—	0.3	0.7	0.5	0.5	
—	0.1	0.9	0.5	0.5	

No hemolysis was observed at the end of two hours in any of the eight series of dilutions made from the four strains. Repeated attempts to dis-

[9] Jour. of Bacteriol., 1917, 2, pp. 1, 109, 191.

cover traces of hemolysin in the supernatants of 18-hour cultures were made. Although we used all of the 6 strains of beta hemolytic streptococcus then at our disposal, these attempts invariably failed.

Besredka,[8] Braun,[10] M'Leod,[5] von Hellens,[7] and others, have laid stress on the instability of streptolysin. Making use of this fact, and of the observation firmly established by Chesney,[11] that broth cultures of various species of bacteria undergo the greater part of their multiplication at a period of from 4-10 or 12 hours' incubation, it occurred to us that the outpouring of hemolysin might be coincident with this logarithmic period of growth, and that when the rapid multiplication stopped, the free hemolysin might rapidly disappear.

A preliminary test of the validity of this hypothesis was made by cutting short the incubation of a serum broth culture of beta streptococcus, strain M, at 8 hours, centrifugating, and testing the supernatant at once against rabbits' and sheep's blood cells.

A small Erlenmeyer flask containing 50 c c of 15% horse serum broth (the serum previously heated to 57 C. for 45 minutes), was seeded with 0.1 c c of a suspension in 4 c c of broth, of 1 loop of 24-hour rabbit blood-agar culture of beta streptococcus M. The culture was incubated in the water bath for 8 hours at 37 C., centrifugated at 8,000 revolutions a minute for 3 minutes, the clear supernatant pipetted off, diluted in 0.85% NaCl solution and tested for the presence of streptolysin against 2.5% suspensions of 3 times washed rabbits' and sheep's red blood cells. The final volume in each tube was 1.5 c c. The tubes were thoroughly shaken, placed in a water bath at 37 C., incubated for 2 hours and readings made.

The degree of hemolysis in the various tubes will hereafter be designated by the following symbols:

C (complete)
C —
++
+
tr. (trace)
tr —
0

The minimal hemolytic dose of any supernatant will be abbreviated as MHD and will be understood as the smallest amount of supernatant giving complete hemolysis of 0.5 c c of a 2.5% suspension of 3 times washed sheep's red blood cells at the end of 2 hours at 37 C. The tubes, thoroughly shaken before incubation, are left undisturbed during the incubation. At the end of the 2 hours at 37 C. the racks are removed from the water bath, and each tube in turn carefully agitated. In tubes in which the reaction has fallen just short of complete hemolysis, a small deposit of red blood cells remains in the bottom. The agitation to which the tubes are subjected brings these cells into suspension. If this suspension is discernible, the tube is read "C —" (complete minus). Only tubes where there is no perceptible turbidity after thorough shaking are read as C (complete). The last tube, reading from low to high dilutions, giving this result, will naturally represent the MHD for the supernatant in question.

[10] Centralbl. f. Bakt., O., 1912, 62, p. 383.
[11] Jour. Exper. Med., 1917, 26, p. 503.

The result of this experiment is summarized in table 2.

TABLE 2

TEST OF SUPERNATANT OF EIGHT HOUR SERUM BROTH CULTURE FOR STREPTOLYSIN

Supernatant Undiluted	Supernatant 1–10	NaCl 0.85	Result (Hemolysis)	
			Sheep's Red Blood Cells 0.5 c c	Rabbit's Red Blood Cells 0.5 c c
1.0	—	—	C	C
—	1.0	—	C	C
—	0.8	0.2	C	C
—	0.5	0.5	C	C—
—	0.3	0.7	++	++
—	0.1	0.9	+	+

Contrasting with the inactivity of the supernatants of 18-hour cultures, this 8-hour supernatant is seen by the rough titration presented in table 2 to be actively hemolytic. The MHD against sheep red blood cells was 0.05 c c, that against the red cells of the rabbit 0.08 c c. It must be remarked here that the titration outlined in table 2 is only roughly quantitative. In experiments made hereafter dilutions between 0.01 and 0.1 c c are invariably graded by hundredths, e. g., 0.01, 0.02, 0.03, etc.

Similar tests were made with various strains of beta hemolytic streptococcus in both horse and sheep serum broth cultures of from 8 to 10 hours' incubation. Supernatants from such cultures were found invariably to be hemolytic. No great difference of resistance of like amounts of the washed red blood cells of the sheep and the rabbit could be discovered. It will be understood that in testing this point one and the same hemolysin was tested against the two kinds of cells, and that the tests were made at the same time. Occasionally a difference such as that noted in table 2 would appear. More often the MHD for the two species of cells would be identical. The same result was found when sheep's red blood cells were compared to those of the human. In this case the variability of result was still less marked, the MHD for the two, tested against the same hemolysin, being the same in every case.

CURVE OF STREPTOLYSIN PRODUCTION IN SERUM-BROTH CULTURES

Before proceeding further in the analysis of the cause of the superiority of sheep blood-agar plates over those made from human and rabbit blood it was considered important to study carefully the time at which a maximal production of hemolysin takes place. Taking the results outlined in the first two experiments into consideration, it should be possible to plot a curve of the appearance, crest, and disappearance of streptolysin from the serum-broth culture.

The broth used in these experiments was, as before, 2% peptone, beef infusion broth, P_H 7.8. The sheep serum employed had been drawn 24 hours previous to the experiment, and had been heated to 57 C. for 45 minutes.

A flask containing 170 c c of broth and 30 c c of heated sheep serum was seeded with 0.1 c c of an 18-hour serum broth culture of beta streptococcus M; 1 c c was removed at once after seeding and incubated for 2 hours at 37 C. with 0.5 c c of 3 times washed sheep red blood cells; 0.5 c c was removed and plated in 10% horse-serum agar for determination of the number of bacteria. The flask was then placed in a water bath at 37 C. and at 2-hour intervals 5 c c were removed under rigid aseptic precautions, centrifugated at

8,000 revolutions a minute for 5 minutes. The supernatants were then pipetted off, iced, diluted in iced 0.85% NaCl solution, and graded dilutions mixed with 0.5 c c of 3 times washed, 2.5% suspension of sheep's red blood cells. All tubes were brought to a final volume of 1.5 c c. The mixtures were incubated for 2 hours at 37 C., readings taken and MHD recorded. By MHD is meant the smallest amount of a supernatant which will completely lake 0.5 c c of a 2.5% suspension of 3 times washed sheep red blood cells. The end point of the reaction was determined in the manner described above.

At intervals identical with the test for hemolytic power of supernatant, small amounts of culture were removed, suitably diluted, and plated in 10% horse-serum agar for determination of the rate of multiplication of the streptococci. The result of the experiment just described is summarized in table 3.

The MHD found at succeeding 2-hour intervals are plotted in figure 1. The abscissae of this graph representing time in hours, and the ordinates the reciprocals of the MHD's. For example, an MHD of 0.04 would be recorded as 25, of 0.02 as 50, and so on.

TABLE 3

CURVE OF HEMOLYSIN PRODUCTION, BETA STREPTOCOCCUS M

Hours at 37 C.	Amount Super-natant	Result	MHD
0	1.0	0	—
2	1.0	0	—
	0.1	0	
	0.09	0	
	0.08	0	
4	1.0	0	—
	0.1	0	
	0.09	0	
	0.08	0	
	0.07	0	
	0.06	0	
	0.05	0	
	0.04	0	
	0.03	0	
	0.02	0	
	0.01	0	
6	1.0	C	
	0.1	C	
	0.09	C	
	0.08	C	
	0.07	C	
	0.06	C	
	0.05	C	
	0.04	C	0.04
	0.03	C—	
	0.02	++	
	0.01	tr.	
8	0.1	C	
	0.09	C	
	0.08	C	
	0.07	C	
	0.06	C	
	0.05	C	
	0.04	C	
	0.03	C	
	0.02	C	0.02
8 (cont.)	0.01	++	
	0.0075	++	
	0.005	tr.	
10	0.1	C	
	0.09	C	
	0.08	C	
	0.07	C	
	0.06	C	
	0.05	C	
	0.04	C	
	0.03	C	0.03
	0.02	C—	
	0.01	++	
	0.0075	tr.	
	0.005	0	
12	0.1	C	
	0.09	C	
	0.08	C	0.08
	0.07	C—	
	0.06	++	
	0.05	++	
	0.04	+	
	0.03	tr.	
	0.02	0	
	0.01	0	
	0.0075	0	
	0.005	0	
14	1.0	+	—
	0.1	0	
	0.09	0	
	0.08	0	
	0.07	0	
	0.06	0	
	0.05	0	
	0.04	0	
	0.03	0	
	0.02	0	
	0.01	0	

The results of this experiment indicate that the presence of streptolysin in the supernatants of serum-broth cultures is of short duration, and that the crest or maximum amount is attained at a very early period in the life cycle of the culture. The results of the bacterial counts, made coincident with the test for hemolytic power, are also instructive. The "lag" period described by Chesney,[11] was represented by a very slight increase in the number of organisms per c c for the first six hours. Very rapid multiplication then set in and continued through the 8, 10, and 12-hour tests, at which time the number of viable organisms per c c, as evidenced by the bacterial counts, reached its maximum. It would seem, then, from this experiment that the greatest outpouring of hemolysin occurs in the early stages of the logarithmic growth period. When multiplication comes to a standstill the free hemolysin deteriorates very rapidly.

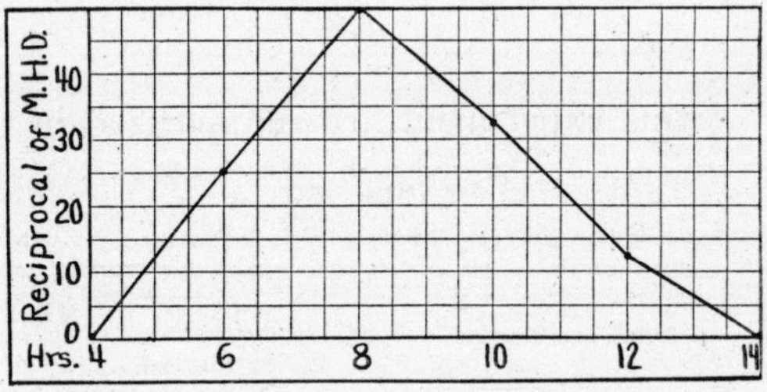

Fig. 1.—Curve of hemolysin production by streptococcus strain M.

Similar determinations of the curve of hemolysin production were made with other strains of beta hemolytic streptococcus. The conditions of these experiments were slightly modified. The sheep serum was used in concentration of 20, instead of 15%, the total volume of fluid in the culture flask was 100 instead of 200 c c, the test flasks were seeded with 9-hour blood-agar cultures instead of 18-hour serum-broth cultures.

Two small Erlenmeyer flasks were prepared, each containing 80 c c of the standard broth and 20 c c of 24-hour old sheep serum heated to 57 C. for 45 minutes. Flask 1 was seeded with 0.1 c c of a suspension in 4 c c of broth, of 1 loop of a 9-hour rabbit blood-agar culture of beta streptococcus A-1. Flask 2 was seeded with a like amount of a similarly made suspension of a 9-hour rabbit blood-agar culture of beta streptococcus V. Both of these flasks were placed in the water bath at 37 C., and at intervals of 2, 4, 5, 6, 7, 8, 9, 10, 12 and 13 hours, 5 c c portions were removed from each flask, centrifuged at 8,000 revolutions a minute for 3 minutes, the supernatant pipetted off, iced, and diluted with iced 0.85% NaCl solution. These were tested against 0.5 c c of a 2.5% suspension of 3 times washed sheep red blood cells. Incubation 2 hours at 37 C., water bath. The test series for amounts 0.1 to 0.01 c c were made from dilution 1 : 10. Those from 0.009 to 0.001 from dilution 1 : 100. All tubes were brought to volume of 1 c c with 0.85% NaCl solution, and 0.5 c c of the red blood cell suspension added at once. The test amounts were closely graded, being separated by hundredths from 0.1 to 0.01 c c, by thousandths from 0.009 to 0.001 c c. An illustration of the method of "set-up" is given in table 4.

TABLE 4

ILLUSTRATION OF ARRANGEMENT OF TEST DILUTIONS IN CURVE OF STREPTOLYSIN PRODUCTION FOR STRAINS A-1 AND V

Tube	Supernatant 1-10	Supernatant 1-100	NaCl 0.85	Actual Amount of Supernatant	
1	0.3	—	0.7	0.03	0.5 c c of 2.5% suspension of 3 times washed sheep's red blood cells added to each tube
2	0.2	—	0.8	0.02	
3	0.1	—	0.9	0.01	
4	—	0.9	0.1	0.009	
5	—	0.8	0.2	0.008	
6	—	0.7	0.3	0.007	
7	—	0.6	0.4	0.006	
8	—	0.5	0.5	0.005	
9	—	0.4	0.6	0.004	
10	—	0.3	0.7	0.003	
11	—	0.2	0.8	0.002	
12	—	0.1	0.9	0.001	

The results of this experiment are summarized in table 5.

TABLE 5

CURVE OF STREPTOLYSIN PRODUCTION, STRAINS A-1 AND V

Hours at 37 C.	Dilutions Tested	MHD	
		Strain A-1	Strain V
2	1.0 to 0.2	0	0
4	0.5 to 0.05	0	0
5	0.5 to 0.05	0	0
6	0.5 to 0.01	0	0
7	0.1 to 0.005	0.03	0.006
8	0.03 to 0.001	0.005	0.008
9	0.05 to 0.001	0.008	0.02
10	0.05 ot 0.005	0.02	0.04
12	1.0 to 0.007	0.1	0
13	1.0 to 0.5	0	0

The results represented in table 5 are plotted in curves in figure 2. The reciprocals of the MHD'S are plotted on the ordinates, the time of incubation in hours on the abscissae. The same phenomenon, rapid rise and early complete disappearance of streptolysin from the supernatants, is seen to occur in the case of strains A-1 and V, as that illustrated for strain M in table 3 and figure 1. The phenomenon for strains A-1 and V has been more closely studied than that for strain M, observations between 4 and 10 hours of incubation being made at one hour rather than 2 hour intervals.

The fulminating nature of the outpouring of hemolysin is especially noticeable in the case of strain V. At the end of six hours' incubation little or no free hemolysin had made its appearance; 0.5 c c of undiluted supernatant failed to cause even a trace of hemolysis, At seven hours it had risen from practically nil to an MHD of 0.006 c c. No larger amount than 0.5 c c was tested at the six-hour period. Assuming that 1.0 c c might have caused complete hemolysis of the usual amount of 0.5 c c of the red blood cell suspension, the hemolysin increased 165 times in strength in the course of an hour. Later curves will show increases still more remarkable than the one just described. It will be noted that the disappearance after a maximum has been reached is also very rapid, though it is not as sudden as the rise.

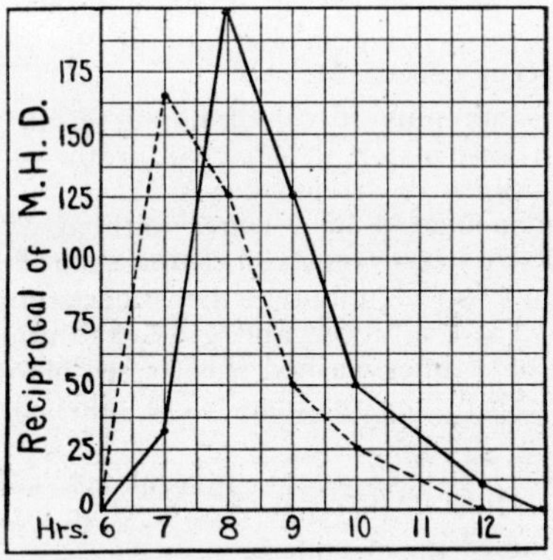

Fig. 2.—Curve of hemolysin production; continuous line, strain A-1; broken line, strain V.

In all three of the curves presented it will be observed that no free hemolysin is demonstrable in supernatants after 14 hours of incubation. On the other hand, M'Leod[5] found 16 to 18-hour serum-broth cultures to contain considerable amounts of the hemolytic principle. Closer examination of the experimental procedure resorted to by this author showed that he seeded his serum-broth flasks with small amounts of 24-hour plain agar cultures. In the experiment just described 9-hour blood-agar cultures were used as source of material for inoculation. This deviation in our technic, resulting from insufficiently close perusal of M'Leod's carefully outlined directions, was thought to be a possible cause of the discrepancy in result. It is to be expected that the older the culture used for seeding, the longer will be the period of lag preceding maximal rate of growth. This might have as a consequence a delay in the peak of hemolysin production and a corresponding retardation of disappearance.

This supposition was put to experimental test in the following way.

The conditions of experiment laid down by M'Leod were duplicated as nearly as possible. Broth rendered alkaline by the addition of 14 c c of normal Na_2CO_3 per liter was used, instead of the standard broth heretofore employed. Horse serum, heated to 57 C. for 45 minutes, was substituted for the heated sheep serum used in previous experiments. The organism employed in the test was beta streptococcus, strain M. This strain, with all others tested in this research, had been carried for months on 10% rabbit blood-agar slants. Ten days before the experiment about to be described, it was transferred to plain agar slants and underwent 6 transplants on this medium in the ensuing 9 days. The growth obtained on the plain agar was fair in amount, though not nearly as great as that on 12-hour rabbit blood-agar slants.

Two small Erlenmeyer flasks were prepared as follows:

FLASK 1.—40 c c of broth plus 10 c c of horse serum (56 C., 45 minutes), seeded with 0.1 c c of a suspension in 4 c c of broth, of 1 loop of a 24-hour plain agar culture of streptococcus M.

FLASK 2.—40 c c of broth plus 10 c c of horse serum (56 C., 45 minutes), seeded with 0.1 c c of a suspension in 4 c c of broth, of 1 loop of a 12-hour 10% rabbit blood-agar culture of streptococcus M.

Flasks 1 and 2 were incubated in a water bath at 37 C. for 8 hours. At the end of this time 3 c c were removed from each flask, centrifugated at 8,000 revolutions a minute for 3 minutes, the supernatants pipetted off, iced, diluted with iced 0.85% NaCl solution, and graded dilutions tested against 0.5 c c of a 2.5% suspension of 3 times washed sheep's red blood cells. The mixtures had a final volume of 1.5 c c; the readings were taken at the end of 2 hours' incubation at 37 C.

Similar procedure was resorted to at intervals of 2 hours until no more streptolysin was demonstrable in the supernatant from either flask. The result of this experiment is summed up in table 6.

TABLE 6

COMPARATIVE CURVE OF STREPTOLYSIN PRODUCTION IN SERUM BROTH SEEDED WITH 24 HOUR PLAIN AGAR AND 12 HOUR BLOOD-AGAR CULTURES

Hours of Incubation	Dilutions Tested*		MHD	
	Flask 1	Flask 2	Flask 1	Flask 2
8	0.1 to 0.005	0.05 to 0.003	0	0.004
10	0.1 to 0.005	0.05 to 0.001	0.01	0.008
12	0.05 to 0.001	0.2 to 0.01	0.005	0.03
14	0.05 to 0.01	0.2 to 0.01	0.01	0
16	0.1 to 0.005	—	0.03	—
18	0.2 to 0.01	—	0	—
20	0.5 to 0.01	—	0	—

* Dilutions graded by hundredths between 0.1 and 0.01, by thousandths between 0.009 and 0.001.

The results observed in table 6 are plotted in figure 3, the significance of the ordinates and abscissae being the same as in figures 1 and 2. The delay in production, peak and disappearance just predicted is shown by this experiment actually to occur. The 8-hour test of Flask 1 failed to demonstrate hemolysin in amounts up to 0.1 c c, while in Flask 2 the supernatant had already reached what was in all probability its maximum of streptolysin production — MHD of 0.004. In Flask 1 maximal production was reached at 12 hours — 4 hours after the probable peak in flask 2. In 14 hours no demonstrable lysin was present in 0.25 c c of supernatant of flask 2. On the other hand, flask 1, tested at the same time, showed an MHD of 0.01, and at 16 hours still contained lysin exhibiting a titer of 0.03.

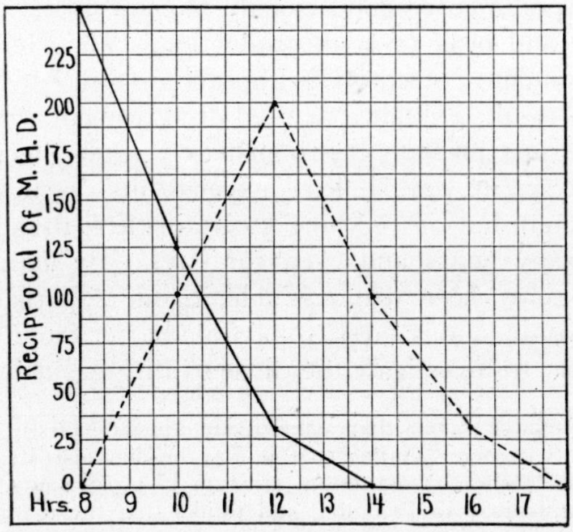

Fig. 3.—Comparative curves of streptolysin production in serum broth seeded with 24-hour plain agar and 12-hour blood-agar cultures of B. streptococcus M. Continuous line, 12-hour blood agar; broken line, 23-hour plain agar.

The persistence of streptolysin at 16 hours as described by M'Leod may be considered to be at least partially explained by the use of older, plain agar cultures for seeding. There still remains the necessity, however, of explaining why many investigators report a persistence of hemolysin not only at 16 to 18 hours, but even for several days.

At the time we first happened on the remarkably fulminating nature of hemolysin production and its correspondingly rapid disappearance from the supernatants of serum broth cultures, we were not aware of the researches made by von Hellens on this subject.[7] Examination of the work of that investigator showed that we were only confirming an observation already made by him. The technic of his experiments differed materially from that of ours, however. Von Hellens did not use the criterion of complete hemolysis in his quantitative measurements of streptolysin. Instead of this he made colorimetric measurements of amounts of hemoglobin released and reported these findings in terms of percentage of hemolysis. He used at one time 35%, at another 40%; at still others 45, 50, 55, etc. His results are therefore difficult to compare and to correlate. The strictly constant endpoint which is found in the experiments just described, as the smallest amount of supernatant completely hemolyzing a given quantity of red blood cells, is much to be preferred.

In spite of the wide variation of technic it is interesting to note that von Hellens' results correspond exactly to ours in the matter of time of appearance and peak of lysin production. Von Hellens finds that the maximal content of streptolysin appears at from 7 to 8 hours. After this period his results exhibit a marked disagreement with the observations we have just presented. Immediately after the peak has been reached, the lysin in von Hellens' experiments, as in ours, falls off rapidly in amount, but on reaching a certain titer, usually very low, it persists for many hours and even for days. By contrast, the lytic principle has never been demonstrable in our supernatants after 16 hours of incubation, and is rarely to be found after from 12 to 13 hours. It was necessary to investigate the cause of this marked difference.

Many authors have noted that streptolysin appears fairly early in serum-broth cultures. Sekiguchi[12] claims that it may be demonstrated in 3-hour cultures, and that it reaches its maximum in from 15 to 18 hours. M'Leod[5] notes its appearance at from 8 to 10 hours, and thinks that the maximum is reached at from 16 to 18 hours. Braun[10] thinks that the peak of production occurs at 10 hours. No matter what may be the opinion of these workers as to the maximum production time, they all agree that the lysin may persist, though in smaller amounts, for a considerable period of time.

The discrepancy in result is to be found in a difference in technic which has been discussed in the first part of this paper. The writers who have observed this persistence of streptolysin have tested whole cultures. We have been concerned only with supernatants of centrifugates of such cultures. It at once occurred to us that while the actually free hemolysin may have really disappeared from the serum-broth cultures within from 14 to 16 hours, the use of whole, uncentrifugated cultures might still reveal some of the lytic principle operating from the surfaces of the streptococci themselves. It is, indeed, reasonable to suppose that this labile principle might undergo much slower destruction when in contact with the organisms than when free in the

[12] Jour. Infect. Dis., 1917, 21, p. 475.

medium. And since there is every reason to think that streptolysin is a product of secretion of the organisms, it is logical to imagine that a large amount of it is adherent to the cell surfaces.

It was decided to compare experimentally the persistence of the hemolysin in whole cultures and in supernatants of 8,000 revolutions a minute centrifugation, the material for the parallel tests coming, of course, from one and the same flask.

A flask was prepared containing 40 c c of the standard broth described above (meat infusion, 2% peptone, P_H 7.8) and 10 c c of horse serum (56 C., 45 minutes). This was seeded with 0.1 c c of a suspension in 4 c c of broth, of 1 loop of an 8-hour rabbit blood-agar culture of streptococcus *M*. The flask was placed in a water bath at 37 C. and incubated at this temperature for 21 hours. At this point 14 c c were removed from the flask and examined microscopically—there was a growth of streptococcus but no apparent contamination. The portion of 14 c c which had been removed was divided into two equal parts, designated "A" and "B."

A was left at room temperature while B was centrifugated at 8,000 revolutions a minute for 3 minutes. Immediately after the removal of B from the centrifuge A and B were both iced and diluted in iced 0.85% NaCl solution. Graded quantities of each were tested against 0.5 c c of a 2.5% suspension of 3 times washed sheep's red blood cells. The final volume in all tubes was 1.5 c c. Incubation 2 hours at 37 C., water bath.

The results of this experiment are recorded in table 7.

TABLE 7

STREPTOLYSIN CONTENT OF WHOLE CULTURES AND SUPERNATANT AFTER 24 HOURS' INCUBATION AT 37 C.

A (Whole Culture)			B (Supernatant)		
Amount Culture	Result	MHD	Amount Supernatant	Result	MHD
1.0	C		1.0	0	—
0.75	C		0.75	0	
0.5	C		0.5	0	
0.3	C		0.3	0	
0.2	C		0.2	0	
0.1	C		0.1	0	
0.09	C		0.09	0	
0.08	C		0.08	0	
0.07	C		0.07	0	
0.06	C	0.06	0.06	0	
0.05	+		0.05	0	

This experiment and others with similar result seem completely to confirm the opinion expressed as to the cause of the persistence of lysin in comparatively old cultures. Lysin is still demonstrable in 21-hour whole cultures, the supernatants of which show no trace of hemolyzing power even in a dose of 1 c c. It seems to us that the only plausible explanation of this difference is to be found in the idea of residual streptolysin operating from the surfaces of the organisms.

Sachs[13] believes that the hemolysin of the streptococcus is almost completely, if not entirely, associated with the germ bodies. Lyall[14] also concludes from certain centrifugation experiments that the streptolysin is to be found in this location. This notion is without doubt erroneous. Free hemolysin does exist and in large quantities, but it must be sought for at a definite time in the life cycle of the culture. When bacterial multiplication is retarded, or stops altogether, the unstable hemolyzing principle rapidly disappears from the supernatant fluids; it may, however, persist for some time on the surfaces of the organisms.

Some observations concerning the hemolysis observed in part A, table 1, are worthy of mention here. The hemolysis in these tubes was very much slower than that ordinarily observed in dilutions of supernatant fluids. In the latter case the reaction invariably runs nearly to completion in from 30 to 45 minutes. Slight changes only occur after this time. In dilutions of from 0.01-0.001, graded by thousandths, an MHD might shift from 0.007 to 0.005 in the time elapsing between 45 minutes and 2 hours, but no greater change than this has been observed to take place after 45 minutes. On the other hand, in the case of the whole culture dilutions recorded in part A, table 7, complete hemolysis had appeared only down to 0.2 c c after 1 hour of incubation. Between 1 and 2 hours the higher dilutions (0.2-0.06) went to completion very gradually. The highest dilution, 0.05 c c, which showed only plus hemolysis at the end of 2 hours of incubation, was completely laked after standing over night on ice. Such marked shifts in readings have never been encountered in the case of supernatants.

Another serious difficulty was encountered in making the readings on the whole culture dilutions (part A). The turbidity due to the large numbers of streptococci in dilutions even as high as 0.05 c c rendered the macroscopic reading of "complete hemolysis" impossible. Microscopic examination of each tube had to be resorted to in order to be sure that this cloud was due to organisms and not to unhemolyzed red blood cells.

It will be understood that when one is dealing with a culture containing many millions of organisms per c c, dilution of 1:100 will leave an enormous number of organisms even in the fractions of a c c which represent amounts of 0.005, 0.004, etc. It was therefore thought

[13] Ztschr. f. Hyg. u. Infekt., 1909, 63, p. 463.
[14] Jour. Med. Research, 1914, 30, pp. 487, 515.

advisable to run parallel curves of lysin content in whole cultures and supernatants in order to determine whether the MHD of the former would far surpass that of the latter. It would appear that the lysin acting from the surface of the organisms in the whole culture dilutions would superpose itself on the free hemolytic principle and so produce a higher MHD. This point was put to experimental test.

A flask containing 200 c c of the standard 20% serum-broth mixture (horse serum, 56 C. 45 minutes), was seeded with 0.1 c c of a suspension in 4 c c of broth, of 1 loop of a 9-hour culture of beta streptococcus strain M. Parallel tests of the whole culture and of supernatants of 8,000 revolutions a minute centrifugates were made. These tests were run 4, 6, 8, 10, 12 and 14 hours after the beginning of incubation. The technic was in every respect the same as that of the test summarized in table 7. Definite amounts were removed from the flask and divided into 2 portions—A was subjected to 8,000 revolutions a minute centrifugation for 3 minutes while B was kept at room temperature during the centrifugation of A. Both A and B were then iced, diluted with iced 0.85% NaCl solution and tested in closely graded dilutions against 0.5 c c amounts of a 2.5% suspension of 3 times washed sheep's red blood cells. The final volume of all tubes was 1.5 c c; incubation 2 hours at 37 C. The results of this test are outlined in table 8.

TABLE 8

COMPARATIVE TITER OF HEMOLYSIN IN WHOLE CULTURE AND SUPERNATANTS

Hours at 37 C.	Amount Tested*		MHD	
	A (Supernatant)	B	A (Supernatant)	B
4	1.0 to 0.2	1.0 to 0.5	0	0
6	0.2 to 0.01	1.0 to 0.01	0.06	0.05
8	0.01 to 0.001	0.01 to 0.0005	0.004	0.004
10	0.05 to 0.0008	0.05 to 0.0008	0.008	0.003
12	0.05 to 0.005	0.05 to 0.003	0.01	0.005
14	0.1 to 0.01	0.05 to 0.005	0.04	0.01

* Dilutions between 1.0 and 0.2 graded by tenths.
Dilutions between 0.2 and 0.01 graded by hundredths.
Dilutions between 0.01 and 0.001 graded by thousandths.
Dilutions between 0.001 and 0.0005 graded by ten thousandths.

Table 8 shows a coincidence of MHD at the 8-hour period. This period of incubation has been found in the great majority of the numerous tests made to represent the peak of lysin production in 20% sheep or horse-serum broth for strain M. On the other hand, the whole culture (B) continues to increase in potency up to 10 hours, showing at this time an MHD of 0.003. At the 10-hour interval the supernatant had dropped to an MHD of 0.008, this decline taking place as it did in all other experiments of a similar nature.

Can it be concluded that the difference of 0.005 in MHD of A and B at the 10-hour interval represents a superposition of the "surface" lysin on that free in the broth? While it is possible that this is so, we do not think that such a conclusion can be safely made. Our doubt on this point is due to the fact that in testing a 10-hour whole culture one deals with organisms which are still in the logarithmic phase of growth. Those organisms, carried over into the dilutions for the lysin titration, will doubtless continue multiplication during incubation with the red blood cells. This factor, of course, is not present in the dilutions of supernatant (A). It is indeed this uncontrollable factor of continuance of multiplication in the whole culture-red blood cell mixtures which helps to make quantitative tests of whole cultures inaccurate.

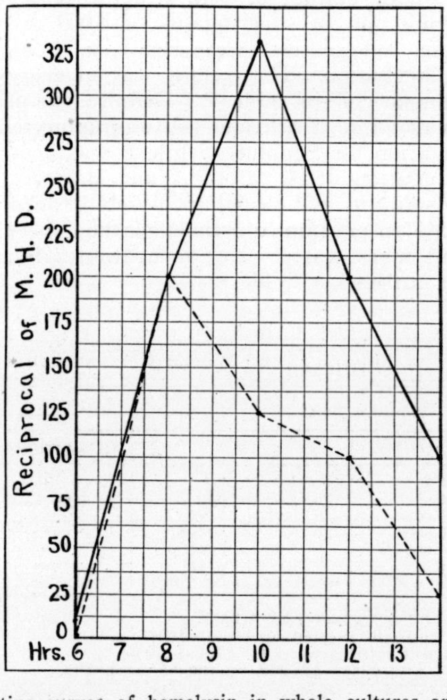

Fig. 4.—Comparative curves of hemolysin in whole cultures and supernatants; B. streptococcus M. Continuous line, whole culture; broken line, supernatant.

At no period in the test was the difference in titer between the whole culture and the supernatant of this culture great. It was greatest at the 10 and 12-hour incubations, being 0.005 at these times. The difference, while not striking, is greater than the experimental error encountered in these tests.

The period at which maximal streptolysin content is present in serum broth has been studied closely. This peak is found to take place in between 7 and 9 hours. The relation of the time of the crest of production and age of the culture used for seeding has been experimentally shown. The relatively short period of persistence of free streptolysin has been made clear, and in our opinion, a satisfactory explanation of the persistence of this principle in whole cultures has been given. We propose to take up now the amount of streptolysin produced in various concentrations of the serums of different species.

STREPTOLYSIN PRODUCTION IN VARIOUS CONCENTRATIONS OF THE SERUMS OF DIFFERENT SPECIES

The concentration of serum in broth used by the various investigators who have studied hemolysin has differed widely. Besredka[8] used undiluted rabbit serum; M'Leod[5] and M'Leod and McNee[6] employed 15 and 20% horse serum broth. Braun[10] obtained streptolysin from broth which contained 10% rabbit serum. Von Hellens states that 40% horse serum broth is most efficient. Other concentrations of numerous serums have been used by various workers, but it is true that at no time has a careful quantitative comparison of the different media been made. The work outlined below is the result of a careful comparison of sheep, rabbit, human, and horse serums in concentrations ranging from 2.5 to 40%. The majority of authors have employed serum heated to 56 C. in their tests. The comparative efficiency of heated and unheated serum has also been made the subject of study here.

The first experiment attempted concerned itself with a quantitative comparison of streptolysin in 20% sheep, horse, human and rabbit serum broth. The sheep, human and rabbit blood was obtained on the same day. The bloods were defibrinated by rod and the serum obtained by centrifugation. The horse serum used had been standing in the icebox for about one month. All of the serums were simultaneously inactivated by heat of 57 C. for 45 minutes. The following tubes were prepared:

TABLE 9

TUBES PREPARED FOR TEST

Standard Broth		Serum			
		Sheep	Horse	Human	Rabbit
1	8 c c	2 c c			
2	8 c c	.....	2 c c		
3	8 c c	.....	.....	2 c c	
4	8 c c	.....	.....	.....	2 c c

All tubes were seeded with 0.1 c c of a suspension in 4 c c of broth, of 1 loop of an 18-hour blood-agar culture of streptococcus M. They were placed in the water bath at 37 C. for 8 hours, centrifuged at 8,000 revolutions a minute for 3 minutes, the supernatants pipetted off, iced, diluted with iced 0.85% NaCl solution and the streptolysin determined quantitatively, against 0.5 c c amounts of 3 times washed sheep's red blood cells (2.5% suspension). The technic of making dilutions was in all respects the same as that previously employed. The final volume in all tubes was 1.5 c c incubation—water bath, 37 C. The results of the experiment are correlated in table 10.

Quantities of supernatant from 0.05 to 0.01 c c were made from dilution 1: 10 in 0.85% NaCl solution; from 0.01 to 0.001 c c from dilution 1: 100 in 0.85% NaCl solution.

The minimal hemolytic dose (MHD) is, as before, the smallest amount of supernatant causing complete hemolysis of 0.5 c c of a 2.5% suspension of washed sheep's red blood cells in 2 hours at 37 C.

TABLE 10

HEMOLYSIN PRODUCTION IN 20% HEATED SHEEP, HORSE, HUMAN AND RABBIT SERUM BROTH

Tube	Amount of Supernatant	Result	MHD	Tube	Amount of Supernatant	Result	MHD
1	0.05	C		3	0.05	C	
(Sheep)	0.04	C		(Human)	0.04	C	
Serum	0.03	C		Serum	0.03	C	
	0.02	C			0.02	C	
	0.01	C			0.01	C	0.01
	0.0075	C			0.0075	C—	
	0.005	C	0.005		0.005	++	
	0.0025	++			0.0025	0	
	0.001	+			0.001	0	
2	0.05	C		4	0.05	C	
(Horse)	0.04	C		(Rabbit)	0.04	C	
Serum	0.03	C		Serum	0.03	C	
	0.02	C			0.02	C	0.02
	0.01	C			0.01	C—	
	0.0075	C			0.0075	++	
	0.005	C	0.005		0.005	+	
	0.0025	++			0.0025	0	
	0.001	tr.			0.001	0	

The amount of streptolysin produced in 20% sheep and 20% horse serum was practically identical in this experiment. That in the human serum broth titrates about half the amount of the first two, while only one quarter as much could be demonstrated in 20% rabbit serum. Subsequent experiment has shown that the ratio of 4-2-1 for sheep, human, and rabbit serum in 20% concentration is a reasonably constant one. This is especially true of sheep and human. Rabbit serum tends to vary somewhat in its efficiency, the variation usually lying in the direction of a somewhat lower value as compared with the sheep and human serum. Horse serum 20% lies very close to sheep of a like concentration, not only in this, but in many other experiments. If any variation occurs it usually shows the horse serum to be slightly superior to the sheep, e. g., MHD 0.004 for horse as compared with 0.005 for sheep.

The experiment just recorded may be criticized because of the disparity in age between the horse and the other serum. This disparity was eliminated in subsequent tests in which 24-hour old horse serum was used in direct comparison with sheep serum of the same age. The difference between the two is quantitatively about that mentioned in the preceding paragraph. Fresh heated horse serum is slightly superior to that which has stood for some time. The difference does not appear to be sufficiently marked to make the older material unsuitable for use. The very best titer for streptolysin we have ever obtained was 0.03 (strain M.). This was secured with fresh heated horse serum. The same serum, used two days later, gave a titer of 0.004. Tested two weeks later the same MHD was obtained. Sheep serum in 20% concentration has never yielded a titer of streptolysin higher than 0.005. Consequently, horse serum broth may be said to have a slight but rather constant superiority to sheep serum broth. On the other hand, this titer for sheep serum (0.005), has been observed at least 8 times in 11 attempts. In all except one of these trials the test amounts were graded by thousandths, e. g., 0.007, 0.006, 0.005, 0.004, and so on. The titers attained in the three attempts which did not give MHD, 0.005 for strain M, were 0.0075, 0.01, and 0.02. It is very probable that these variations were due in at least two instances to the use of old broth, and in the other to the employment of a too old culture for seeding (24-hour blood-agar slant). In the latter case an MHD of 0.005 might very well have been obtained had incubation been continued to 10 or 12 hours, instead of being checked at 8 hours.

The next step taken was the systematic test of the four above named species of serums with a view to discovering their optimal concentration in broth for maximal streptolysin production, and to determine the amount of the lysin produced in low concentrations. The latter interested us particularly because the amount of serum in the broth (5%) approximated closely that used in 10% blood-agar plates. It was considered probable that the results of these tests would throw light on the disparity in size and quality of the hemolytic zones on blood-agar plates in which sheep, human and rabbit blood are used. The comparative efficiency of 5, 10, 15, 20, 25 and 30% heated sheep serum broth was first tested. Six tubes were prepared as follows:

TABLE 11

TUBES PREPARED FOR TEST

1.	9.5 c c standard broth + 0.5 c c 56 C. 45 minutes sheep serum, (5%)
2.	9.0 c c standard broth + 1.0 c c 56 C. 45 minutes sheep serum, (10%)
3.	8.5 c c standard broth + 1.5 c c 56 C. 45 minutes sheep serum, (15%)
4.	8.0 c c standard broth + 2.0 c c 56 C. 45 minutes sheep serum, (20%)
5.	7.5 c c standard broth + 2.5 c c 56 C. 45 minutes sheep serum, (25%)
6.	7.0 c c standard broth + 3.0 c c 56 C. 45 minutes sheep serum, (30%)

These were seeded with 0.1 c c of a suspension in 4 c c of broth, of 1 loop of a 16-hour culture of streptococcus V. All the tubes were placed in the water bath for 8 hours at 37 degrees, centrifugated at 8,000 revolutions a minute for 3 minutes, the supernatants pipetted off, iced, and diluted with 0.85% NaCl solution. The dilutions were tested against 0.5 c c of a 2.5% suspension of washed sheep red blood cells. The final volume of all tubes was 1.5 c c. The tubes were thoroughly shaken, incubated in the water bath for 2 hours at 37 C. and the MHD's read at the end of this time. The results of the experiment are summarized in table 12.

TABLE 12

STREPTOLYSIN PRODUCTION IN VARIOUS CONCENTRATIONS OF HEATED SHEEP SERUM BROTH

Tube	Serum Concentrations	Dilutions Tested*	MHD
1	5	0.06 to 0.005	0.04
2	10	0.06 to 0.005	0.03
3	15	0.06 to 0.005	0.01
4	20	0.06 to 0.005	0.005 or >
5	25	0.06 to 0.005	0.02
6	30	0.06 to 0.005	0.02

* Dilutions 0.06 to 0.01 graded by hundredths.
Dilutions 0.01 to 0.005 graded by thousandths.

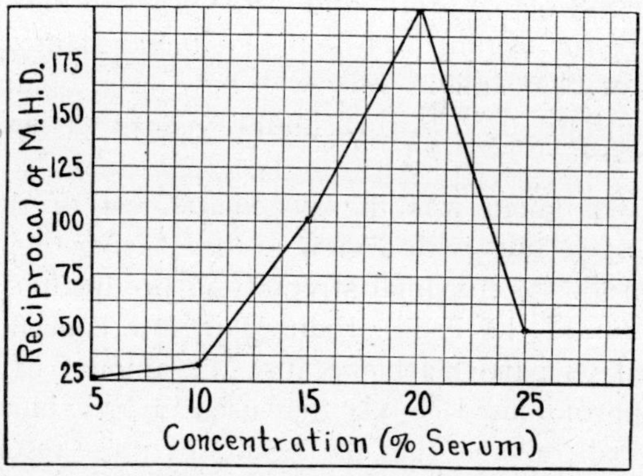

Fig. 5.—Streptolysin production in various concentrations of heated sheep serum broth, B. streptococcus, strain V.

The rise in efficiency as recorded in table 12 is strikingly presented in the curve of figure 5. The reciprocals of the MHD's are plotted on the ordinates, the concentrations of serum on the abscissae. A similar test made with beta streptococcus strain M gave values identical with those for V in concentrations of from 5 to 20%. The drop in potency occurring in 25 and 30% concentrations for V was not so clear in the case of strain M. With this strain 25% broth gave an MHD identical with that obtained at 20%, i. e., 0.005. The 30% concentration yielded a titer of 0.01.

The efficiency of heated human serum in various concentrations was next put to experiment. The concentrations studied in this experiment were those of 5, 10, 15 and 20%. The serum was inactivated at 57 C. for 45 minutes. Sheep serum, drawn on the same day as the human and heated to the same temperature was studied in parallel as control. The standard broth was used. All tubes, 8 in number, were seeded with 0.1 c c of a suspension in 4 c c of broth, of one loop of a 9-hour blood-agar culture of streptococcus M. Incubation, 8 hours in the water bath; dilutions were made and MHD determined as in all previous experiments against 0.5 c c of a 2.5% suspension of washed sheep's red blood cells. Table 13 summarizes the results of this experiment.

TABLE 13

STREPTOLYSIN IN VARIOUS CONCENTRATIONS OF HEATED SHEEP AND HUMAN SERUM BROTH

Tube	Serum Concentration		Dilutions Tested*	MHD
	Human	Sheep		
1	5	—	0.3 to 0.01	0.07
2	—	5	0.1 to 0.01	0.03
3	10	—	0.1 to 0.01	0.02
4	—	10	0.07 to 0.007	0.03
5	15	—	0.06 to 0.006	0.01
6	—	15	0.05 to 0.003	0.008
7	20	—	0.05 to 0.002	0.01
8	—	20	0.05 to 0.001	0.005

* Dilutions 0.1 to 0.01 graded by hundredths.
Dilutions 0.01 to 0.001 graded by thousandths.

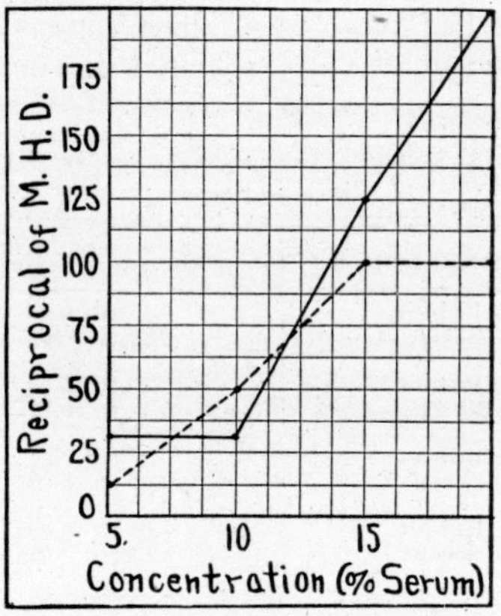

Fig. 6.—Streptolysin in various concentrations of heated sheep and human serum broth, B. streptococcus M; continuous line, sheep; broken line, human.

The results of this experiment are graphed in the curve presented in figure 6. It will be noted that for sheep serum there is very slight deviation from the curve of figure 5 which is plotted from a similar experiment with strain V. The 5% concentration shows a deviation of 0.01, the 10 and 20% concentrations give identical values while the

15% tubes show a difference of only 0.002. It will be noted further that the MHD for strain V in table 10 was 0.005 in the 20% concentration. Two other tests of 8-hour cultures in 20% sheep serum broth, using the same strain gave titers of 0.006 and 0.005, respectively. This result and the remarkable number of checks obtained in the case of strain M would indicate that under optimum conditions of test, hemolytic indices of great constancy for a given strain can be obtained. Since some investigators have made statements of an opposite nature we will return to the discussion of this question.

The experiment just recorded shows that the efficiency for hemolysin production increases directly with increase in concentration of both human and sheep serum up to at least 20%. The result of the use of higher concentrations of serum on streptolysin production will be discussed later, since we wish next to show the result of a comparative test of various concentrations of rabbit and sheep serum.

The rabbit and sheep blood used in this experiment were obtained on the same day, defibrinated, centrifugated, the serums pipetted off and heated to 57 C. for 45 minutes. Standard broth was used; 5, 10, 15 and 20% concentrations of each serum were employed. The tubes, 8 in number, were seeded with 0.1 c c of a suspension in 4 c c of broth, of 1 loop of a 9-hour blood-agar culture of streptococcus M. The cultures were, as usual, incubated 8 hours, at the end of this time centrifugated at 8,000 revolutions a minute, the supernatants pipetted off, iced, diluted, and graded amounts mixed with 0.5 c c of a 2.5% suspension of 3 times washed sheep's red blood cells. The final volume of all tubes was 1.5 c c. The result of the experiment is summarized in table 14.

TABLE 14

STREPTOLYSIN PRODUCTION IN VARIOUS CONCENTRATIONS OF HEATED SHEEP AND RABBIT SERUM BROTH

Tube	Serum Concentration	Dilutions Tested	MHD
1	5% Rabbit	0.2 to 0.05	>0.2
2	5% Sheep	0.2 to 0.03	0.04
3	10% Rabbit	0.2 to 0.03	0.2*
4	10% Sheep	0.1 to 0.01	0.03
5	15% Rabbit	0.2 to 0.01	0.05
6	15% Sheep	0.07 to 0.003	0.008
7	20% Rabbit	0.09 to 0.005	0.02
8	20% Sheep	0.07 to 0.001	0.005

* Complete hemolysis occurred in 0.2 c c, ++ hemolysis in 0.1 c c. No dilutions between these two figures were tested. Therefore it is possible that the real MHD may be somewhat lower than the figure recorded in the table.

The results tabulated in table 14 are plotted on the curve figure 7. The reciprocals of MHD's are plotted on the ordinates, the concentrations of serum on the abscissae. Marked differences will be seen to exist between this curve and that in figure 6. In 5% concentration of rabbit serum the largest amount of supernatant tested, 0.2 c c, failed to give complete hemolysis. The corresponding concentration of sheep serum gave an MHD of 0.04. This figure is identical with that for the 5% concentration in table 12, and only varies by 0.01 c c from that of table 13.

In 10% concentrations there is still a very marked discrepancy in the efficiency of the two serums, rabbit recording 0.2, as compared with 0.03 for sheep. It is interesting to note here that 5 separate tests of 10% sheep serum with strain M gave an MHD of 0.03 each time. This is a good example of the manner in which titers of supernatant fluids can be quantitatively reduplicated.

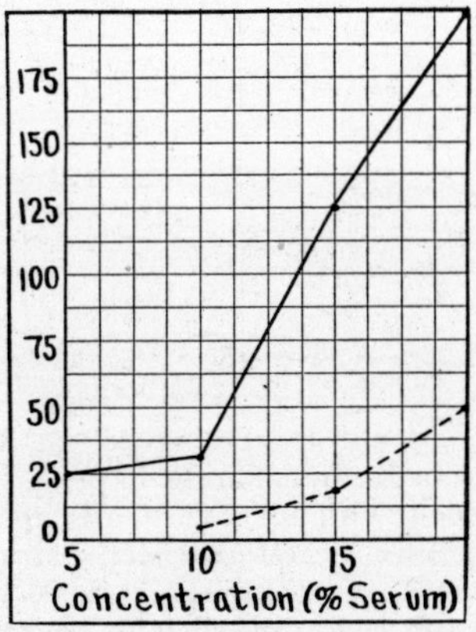

Fig. 7.—Streptolysin in various concentrations of heated sheep and rabbit serum broth, B. streptococcus M; continuous line, sheep; broken line, rabbit.

Rabbit serum, very poor in yield of streptolysin in 5% concentration and not much better in 10%, is shown by the table to be much more efficient in 15%, the MHD being in this case 0.05. The parallel tube for sheep serum exhibits an MHD of 0.008, a perfect check of the 15% concentration in table 13. Finally, 20% rabbit serum is better than 15, since an MHD of 0.02 is obtained for the former concentration. The sheep serum parallel checks that of table 13—0.005 c c.

It will be observed that the 20% concentrations of sheep, human and rabbit in tables 13 and 14 give titers of 0.005 in both cases for sheep and 0.01 and 0.02, respectively, for human and rabbit. In table 10 heated sheep, human and rabbit are compared in this concentration only. The same strain is used (M). The values are exactly the same, i. e., 0.005, 0.01, 0.02. This experiment was performed a month before that just recorded.

The experiment summarized in table 12 indicates that 20% serum concentration represents the optimum for streptolysin production in the case of strain V. The question arose whether this concentration was the optimum when rabbit and human serum were used, or whether the curves cross at higher concentrations.

Sheep, human, and rabbit was obtained on the same day, the serum pipetted off after centrifugation, and the serums, 24-hours old, were heated and added to the standard broth as follows:

TABLE 15

STREPTOLYSIN IN 20, 25, AND 30% HEATED HUMAN, RABBIT AND SHEEP SERUM BROTH

Tube	C C Standard Broth	Percentage	C C Serum 56 C. 45 Minutes		
			Human	Rabbit	Sheep
1	8.0	20	2.0	—	—
2	8.0	20	—	2.0	—
3	8.0	20	—	—	2.0
4	7.5	25	2.5	—	—
5	7.5	25	—	2.5	—
6	7.5	25	—	—	2.5
7	7.0	30	3.0	—	—
8	7.0	30	—	3.0	—
9	7.0	30	—	—	3.0

Tubes 1, 2, 3; 4, 5, 6; 7, 8 and 9 were seeded at 30-minute intervals. The three sets were removed from the incubating bath at similar intervals, 8 hours later. Each tube was seeded with 0.1 c c of a suspension in 4 c c of broth, of 1 loop of a 12-hour culture of streptococcus strain M. The tubes were incubated as usual for 8 hours, centrifugated at 8,000 revolutions a minute, the supernatants were pipetted off, iced, diluted with iced 0.85% NaCl solution and graded dilutions mixed with 0.5 c c of 2.5% suspension of washed sheep's red blood cells. The final volume in all tubes was 1.5 c c.

The entire series, which comprised 111 tubes, was incubated at 37 C. for 2 hours and readings taken. The results of the experiment are outlined in table 16.

TABLE 16

STREPTOLYSIN PRODUCTION IN 20, 25 AND 30% 56 C. HUMAN, RABBITT AND SHEEP SERUM BROTH

Tube	Heated Serum	Dilutions Tested*	MHD
1	20% Human	0.05 to 0.005	0.007
2	20% Rabbit	0.06 to 0.006	0.03
3	20% Sheep	0.05 to 0.003	0.005
4	25% Human	0.05 to 0.001	0.02
5	25% Rabbit	0.05 to 0.004	0.007
6	25% Sheep	0.05 to 0.003	0.005
7	30% Human	0.05 to 0.001	0.04
8	30% Rabbit	0.05 to 0.001	0.02
9	30% Sheep	0.05 to 0.001	0.01

* 0.05 to 0.01 graded by hundredths.
0.01 to 0.001 graded by thousandths.

Human serum broth shows a decided optimum at 20%, dropping from 0.007 at this concentration to 0.02 at 25% and 0.04 at 30%. Rabbit serum broth which gives an MHD of 0.03 at 20, jumps to 0.007 at 25, thus crossing the curve for human serum, but descends to 0.02 at 30%.

The MHD of 0.007 for 20% human serum, and for 25% rabbit serum represented the highest titer of streptolysin we have ever obtained from the serums of these two species.

The data summarized in table 16 are plotted in curves in figure 8.

It would be well at this point to summarize briefly the results gleaned from hemolysin production in various concentrations of heated sheep, human and rabbit serum broth. Sheep serum is distinctly superior to that of the human and rabbit in lower concentrations. It

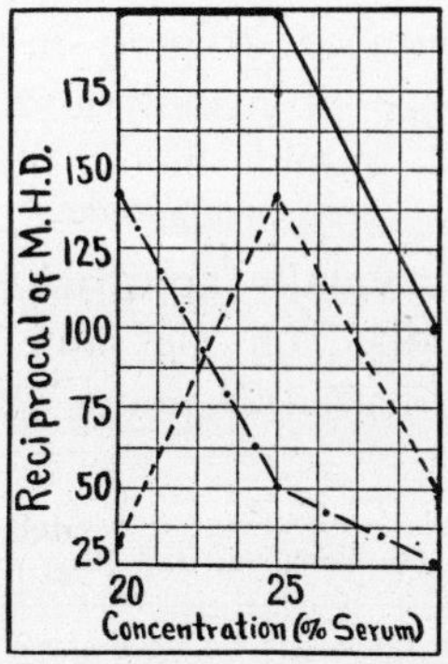

Fig. 8.—Streptolysin in 20, 25 and 30% heated human, rabbit and sheep serum broth, B. streptococcus M; continuous line, sheep; broken line, rabbit; dot and dash line, human.

reaches its optimum at from 20 to 25%, at which point it still retains its superiority over the other two species. Rabbit serum which is the poorest of the three in low concentrations rises rapidly through 15 and 20% to its optimum at 25% at which point it exhibits a titer nearly as high as that of sheep serum (0.007 as against 0.005 for sheep). Human serum, which is slightly inferior to that of sheep at 5% rises to its optimum at 20%. At higher concentrations its efficiency falls off to a point below that of rabbit and sheep.

It is important that any one of these three serums is suitable for securing streptolysin of high titer provided it is used in proper concentration. But in general, sheep serum is superior to the other two, and variation in lysin production according to concentration is not so great.

STREPTOLYSIN PRODUCTION IN FRESH UNHEATED SERUMS

It has been stated in a previous paragraph that this study of comparative quantitative hemolysin production in various concentrations of different serums had its inception in the observation of the marked superiority of sheep over rabbit and human blood agar in demonstration of hemolytic zones. The plates used in this test were prepared with fresh defibrinated blood. This fresh unheated blood was mixed in concentration of 10% with agar. In mixtures of this blood concentration, the serum present would amount to from 4 to 6% of the total volume, depending on the proportionate volume of red blood cells to serum. It was therefore considered that comparative hemolysin production with low concentrations of fresh unheated serum would be an important subject for study. The investigation of 5% fresh unheated sheep, human, and rabbit serum broth would approximate as closely as possible the conditions present in 10% blood plates. Possible differences in amount of streptolysin produced might explain the marked difference in size of hemolytic zones, on 10% sheep as compared with rabbit and human blood plates of a similar concentration.

The subject was experimentally approached thus: Sheep, human and rabbit blood were obtained on the same day, centrifugated, the serums pipetted off, iced and used 24 hours after bleeding. Six tubes were prepared as follows:

TABLE 17

Tubes Prepared for Test

1. 9.5 c c standard broth + 0.5 c c sheep serum (5%)
2. 9.0 c c standard broth + 1.0 c c sheep serum (10%)
3. 9.5 c c standard broth + 0.5 c c human serum (5%)
4. 9.0 c c standard broth + 1.0 c c human serum (10%)
5. 9.0 c c standard broth + 0.5 c c rabbit serum (5%)
6. 9.5 c c standard broth + 1.0 c c rabbit serum (10%)

All tubes were seeded with 0.1 c c of a suspension in 4 c c of broth of 1 loop of a 14-hour culture of beta streptococcus M., incubated 8 hours at 37 C., centrifugated at 8,000 revolutions a minute for 3 minutes. The supernatants were then pipetted off, iced, diluted with iced 0.85% NaCl solution and tested in graded quantities against 0.5 c c portions of a 2.5% suspension of three times washed sheep's red blood cells. Incubation of the test mixtures, 37 C., 2 hours. Results summarized in table 18.

TABLE 18

Streptolysin Production in Fresh Unheated 5 and 10% Sheep, Human and Rabbit Serum Broth

Tube	Unheated Serum	Dilutions Tested	MHD
1	5% Sheep	0.1 to 0.01	0.06
2	10% Sheep	0.1 to 0.01	0.03
3	5% Human	0.5 to 0.02	0.2
4	10% Human	0.5 to 0.02	0.08
5	5% Rabbit	1.0 to 0.04	—
6	10% Rabbit	1.0 to 0.04	—

The results just given in this table are most instructive. Five and 10% sheep serum broth yield fairly large amounts of streptolysin, the MHD's for these concentrations being, respectively, 0.06 and 0.3. These do not differ very greatly for those of heated sheep serum in like concentration. Human serum broth in the unheated condition yielded MHD's of 0.2 and 0.08 for 5 and 10% concentrations, respectively. Both figures are much lower than those for the respective concentrations of sheep serum and distinctly lower than for similar concentrations of heated human serum. Finally, unheated rabbit serum is seen to be extremely poor for streptolysin production in 5 and 10% concentrations. No complete hemolysis was obtained in any tube, despite the fact that as much as 1 c c of undiluted supernatant was tested against 0.5 c c of washed red blood cells. Subsequent results have shown that this almost total absence of hemolysin is not met with in all tests of a similar nature. We have observed MHD's of 0.5 and 0.6 for 5% concentrations of unheated fresh rabbit serum broth. This is still extremely low as compared with the titers from like concentrations of sheep or even of human serum. It was thought important to check carefully the comparative efficiency of heated and unheated human and sheep serums, the tests to be made simultaneously from the same batches of serum. Sheep and human serums obtained on the same day and iced for 24 hours were used in this experiment.

In all experiments with unheated rabbit and human serums, controls were made to rule out the possibility of normal antisheep red cell hemolysin.

The serums were divided into two parts, one portion of each serum being heated to 57 C. for 45 minutes, while the other was left on ice. The following tubes were then prepared:

TABLE 19

TUBES PREPARED FOR TEST

1.	9.5 c c standard broth + 0.5 c c unheated human serum (5%)
2.	9.5 c c standard broth + 0.5 c c 57 C. 45 minutes human serum (5%)
3.	9.5 c c standard broth + 0.5 c c unheated sheep serum (5%)
4.	9.5 c c standard broth + 0.5 c c 57 C. 45 minutes sheep serum (5%)
5.	9.0 c c standard broth + 1.0 c c unheated human serum (10%)
6.	9.0 c c standard broth + 1.0 c c 57 C. 45 minutes human serum (10%)
7.	9.0 c c standard broth + 1.0 c c unheated sheep serum (10%)
8.	9.0 c c standard broth + 1.0 c c 57 C. 45 minutes sheep serum (10%)

These tubes were then seeded with 0.1 c c of a suspension in 4 c c of broth of 1 loop of a 10-hour blood-agar culture of streptococcus strain M. The tubes were placed for 8 hours in the water bath at 37 C., centrifugated at 8,000 revolutions a minute for 3 minutes, the supernatants pipetted off and iced and dilutions made with iced 0.85% NaCl solution. These dilutions were tested in graded quantities against 0.5 c c of a 2.5% suspension of washed sheep's red blood cells, the final volume in all tubes being 1.5 c c. The results of the experiment are gathered together in table 20.

TABLE 20

STREPTOLYSIN PRODUCTION IN 5 AND 10% HEATED AND UNHEATED HUMAN AND SHEEP SERUM BROTH

Tube	Serum		Dilutions Tested	MHD
	Human	Sheep		
1	5% unheated	—	0.2 to 0.02	— (>0.2)
2	5% heated	—	0.2 to 0.02	0.1
3	—	5% unheated	0.1 to 0.02	0.08
4	—	5% heated	0.08 to 0.01	0.03
5	10% unheated*	—	0.1 to 0.01	0 04
6	10% heated	—	0.08 to 0.01	0.03
7	—	10% unheated	0.08 to 0.01	0.03
8	—	10% heated	0.08 t o 0.01	0.03

* Controlled for human antisheep red cell hemolysin.

The results presented in table 20 confirm those recorded in table 18. For 5% active human serum, no complete hemolysis occurred when as much as 0.2 c c of supernatant was added to the red blood cells. Therefore the MHD must have been greater than 0.2. The same concentration of sheep serum gave an MHD of 0.08 (tube 3, table 20). In the case of both human and sheep the heated 5% was more favorable for lysin production than the same concentration of unheated serum. For human this difference was expressed by MHD, 0.1 as against > 0.2, for the sheep by 0.03 as against 0.08. In the 10% concentrations, both of human and sheep, this marked difference was largely obliterated. Unheated 10% human had an MHD of 0.04 as against 0.03 for the 10% heated serum. Both unheated and heated 10% sheep serum broth yielded an MHD of 0.03.

It would be well to remark that a difference as striking as this between 5% unheated human and sheep serum cannot always be demonstrated. We have observed comparative tests of a nature similar to that just recorded in which 5% unheated sheep serum broth in an 8 hour culture, the same strain, M, being used, yielded an MHD of 0.07 as compared with 0.1 for a like concentration of unheated human serum.

On the other hand, this concentration of unheated sheep serum yields pretty constantly an MHD of 0.04 to 0.08, while similar concentrations of human serum may frequently give a titer of 0.2 or > 0.2. The foregoing indicates that considerable variations occur in streptolysin production in unheated sheep and human serums, when the serum is present in a small amount, but that the sheep is consistently more efficient than the human serum.

The same is true, only more strikingly so, of rabbit as compared with sheep serum. The differences in the case of rabbit serum are far greater than the ones just described for human and sheep. This is indicated clearly in the following experiment.

Twenty-four hour old rabbit and sheep serums were divided into two portions, one of each being iced and the other heated to 57 C. for 45 minutes. The following tubes were then prepared:

TABLE 21

TUBES PREPARED FOR TEST

Tube	Standard Broth	Serum Rabbit		Serum Sheep	
		Unheated	57 C. 45 Minutes	Unheated	57 C. 45 Minutes
1	9.5	0.5	—	—	—
2	9.5	—	0.5	—	—
3	9.5	—	—	0.5	—
4	9.5	—	—	—	0.5

These tubes were seeded with 0.1 c c of a suspension in 4 c c of broth of 1 loop of a 9-hour culture of beta streptococcus M, incubated for 8 hours at 37 C., centrifugated at 8,000 revolutions a minute for 3 minutes, the supernatants iced, diluted and tested against 0.5 c c of a 2.5% suspension of 3 times washed sheep's red blood cells.

The results of this experiment are presented in table 22.

TABLE 22

STREPTOLYSIN PRODUCTION IN 5% HEATED AND UNHEATED RABBITT AND SHEEP SERUM BROTH CULTURES

Tube 1 (5% Unheated Rabbit Serum)			Tube 3 (5% Unheated Sheep Serum)			Tube 2 (5% 57 C. 45 Minutes Rabbit Serum)			Tube 4 (5% 57 C. 45 Minutes Sheep Serum)		
Amount Super-natant	Result	MHD	Amount Super-natant	Result	MHD	Amount Super-natant	Result	MHD	Amount Super-natant	Result	MHD
1.0	C		1.0	C		1.0	C		0.1	C	
0.75	C		0.09	C	0.09	0.75	C		0.09	C	
0.5	C	0.5				0.5	C		0.08	C	0.08
			0.08	C—		0.3	C				
0.3	C—		0.07	++		0.2	C		0.07	C—	
0.2	++		0.06	+		0.18	C	0.18	0.06	++	
0.15	+		0.05	+					0.05	+	
0.1	tr.		0.04	tr.		0.16	C—		0.04	+	
			0.03	0		0.16	C—		0.03	tr.	
			0.02	0		0.12	C—		0.02	tr.	
			0.01	0		0.1	+		0.01	0	

The experiment just summarized confirms the quantitative relations indicated in tubes 1 and 2, 5 and 6, table 18. In the present experiment, however, the difference is not quite so marked, since the rabbit serum (unheated) shows a higher titer than in table 18, and the unheated sheep serum of this experiment is slightly lower in lysin content than that of the earlier test. The central fact is, nevertheless, clearly checked. Unheated sheep serum in low concentration is far superior to unheated rabbit serum for the production of streptolysin.

Higher concentrations of all three of the serums just studied have been investigated in regard to hemolysin production. Twenty per cent. heated and unheated sheep, rabbit and human serum broth was seeded with the usual amount of a 20-hour culture of beta streptococcus M. Test of the supernatants, after 8 hours of incubation at 37 C., gave the results summarized in table 23.

TABLE 23

STREPTOLYSIN PRODUCTION IN HEATED AND UNHEATED 20% SHEEP, HUMAN AND RABBIT SERUM BROTH

Tube	Serum, 20%			MHD
	Sheep	Human	Rabbit	
1	Unheated	—	—	0.01
2	56 C. 45 minutes	—	—	0.01
3	—	Unheated	—	0.02
4	—	56 C. 45 minutes	—	0.02
5	—	—	Unheated	>0.05*
6	—	—	56 C. 45 minutes	0.05

* Lower dilutions not made; ++ hemolysis in 0.05; MHD not obtained.

From this experiment one might be led to conclude that in 20% concentration no perceptible difference in efficiency exists between heated and unheated sheep, or heated and unheated human serum. For 20% rabbit serum heated is apparently somewhat superior to unheated serum, although the failure to use a dose higher than 0.05 c c made a strict quantitative comparison impossible in this experiment. It is quite probable that the low titer of lysin obtained in all cases is due to the use of a 20-hour culture for seeding. In cases of this kind the organisms transferred to the serum broth tubes would in all probability exhibit a longer period of lag. Consequently, the point of maximum production of streptolysin would have occurred at a time later than that at which incubation was cut off (8 hours). The experiment summarized in table 6 lays stress on the importance of the use of really young cultures for seeding when it is desired to secure an early peak of hemolysin content.

Similar experiments were made with fresh unheated horse serum, very kindly supplied to us by the research department of Parke, Davis & Co. The first experiment with this material concerned itself with the quantitative study of lysin produced in 5, 10, 15 and 20% concentrations of fresh unheated horse serum broth.

TABLE 24

TUBES PREPARED FOR TEST

1.	9.5 c c standard broth + 0.5 c c unheated horse serum (5%)
2.	9.0 c c standard broth + 1.0 c c unheated horse serum (10%)
3.	8.5 c c standard broth + 1.5 c c unheated horse serum (15%)
4.	8.0 c c standard broth + 2.0 c c unheated horse serum (20%)

All tubes were seeded with 0.1 c c of a suspension in 4 c c of broth of 1 loop of a 10-hour culture of beta streptococcus M. They were incubated for 8 hours at 37 C., centrifugated at 8,000 revolutions a minute for 3 minutes, the supernatants from this centrifugation iced, diluted with iced 0.85% NaCl; tested against 0.5 c c of a 2.5% suspension of washed sheep's red blood cells. Final volume in all tubes 1.5 c c. The results are given in table 24.

TABLE 25

STREPTOLYSIN PRODUCTION IN 5, 10, 15 AND 20% 24-HOUR, UNHEATED HORSE SERUM BROTH

Tube	Horse Serum, Percentage	Dilutions Tested*	MHD	Hemolytic Index
1	5	0.2 to 0.01	0.06	16.6
2	10	0.1 to 0.01	0.02	50.0
3	15	0.05 to 0.003	0.01	100.0
4	20	0.05 to 0.001	0.007	142.8

* From 0.2 to 0.1 dilutions graded by two-hundredths.
From 0.1 to 0.01 dilutions graded by hundredths.
From 0.01 to 0.001 dilutions graded by thousandths.

The results of table 25 indicate a very close correspondence in the amount of hemolysin produced between fresh unheated horse and fresh unheated sheep serum. This will be seen by comparing the results just summarized for horse serum with those for unheated sheep serum in tables 18 and 20.

It is unfortunate that no comparative test was made at this time of fresh unheated and heated horse serum broth, in 20% concentration. The same serum used in the experiment just described but aged for several days and heated to 56 C. for 45 minutes, gave an extremely potent lysin, the MHD reaching 0.003 in two instances. On the other hand, the 20% concentration of unheated serum (tube 4), table 25, gave an MHD of 0.007. This discrepancy was considered sufficiently wide to justify a parallel test of heated and unheated horse serum in the concentration of 20%. It was also attempted at this time to recheck the unheated 5% concentration.

The serum used in this test was 72 hours old, consequently the results cannot be strictly compared with those obtained from the experiment in which 24-hour serum was used. The findings observed are brought together in table 26.

TABLE 26

Streptolysin Production in 5 and 20% Unheated and 20% Heated Horse Serum Broth

Tube	Serum Percentage		Dilutions Tested*	MHD
	Unheated	56 C. 45 Minutes		
1	5	—	1.0 to 0.01	0.03
2	20	—	0.1 to 0.001	0.01
3	—	20	0.1 to 0.001	0.006

* Dilution 0.1 to 0.01 graded by hundredths.
Dilutions 0.01 to 0.001 graded by thousandths.

It will be observed (tube 1) that the MHD obtained for the 5% concentration was 0.03. This figure is 0.03 higher than that of the corresponding dilution in table 25. The serum used in the experiment just described was 72 hours old, as against 24 hours for that employed in table 25. Hence no strict comparison can be drawn. It is probable that the difference in age of serum is responsible for this difference in result. For it is quite likely that suitability of serum for hemolysin production might be increased by aging as well as by heat. This is true for other properties of serum. For example, heat of 56 C. and aging both have a deleterious effect on the alexic and the "serozyme" functions of serum.

Tubes 2 and 3, table 26, show a perceptible difference in titer. This would indicate a greater suitability for hemolysin production of heated horse serum in 20% concentrations. The result given in table 23 would indicate that this was not the case for similar concentrations of unheated sheep and human serum. It is true, on the other hand, that the comparative tests of heated and unheated human and sheep serum in this concentration were not exhaustive enough to allow one to draw sweeping conclusions. It may be remarked, too, that the difference in the case of horse serum, while perceptible, is not striking, since it shows 0.01 for the unheated, 0.006 for the heated serum.

It would be logical at this place to discuss the comparative value of horse and sheep serum broth for streptolysin production. Heated horse serum in 20% concentration has given in some instances MHD's higher than the best titer obtained with like amounts of heated sheep serum. Beta streptococcus, strain M, was used in all cases now under discussion. At the same time, it has been more difficult to obtain with horse serum the strikingly constant results observed in 20% heated sheep serum for strain M. The large number of times an MHD of 0.005 was obtained in this medium for strain M will be recalled. In similar concentrations of horse serum the MHD for this strain varied from 0.003 to 0.007.

Von Hellens[7] states that maximal hemolysin production occurs in concentrations of 30 and 40% horse serum broth. M'Leod[5] and M'Leod and McNee[6] assert that 15 to 20% is the optimum concentration. The following experiment strongly supports the latter opinion.

The usual amount of an 8-hour culture of streptococcus M was seeded into tubes, labeled 1, 2 and 3, containing respectively 20, 30 and 40% of heated horse serum broth. The broth was of the standard type used in all previous experiments. The usual 8-hour incubation, centrifugation at 8,000 revolutions a minute, and the dilution was carried out and tests were made of dilutions graded from 0.05 to 0.001 against 0.5 c c of a 2.5% suspension of sheep's red blood cell suspension. The final volume in all tubes was 1.5 c c; incubation, 2 hours at 37 C. The results are given in table 27.

TABLE 27

STREPTOLYSIN PRODUCTION IN 20, 30 AND 40% HORSE SERUM BROTH

Amount Super-natant	Horse Serum 56 C. 45 Minutes					
	20%		30%		40%	
	Result	MHD	Result	MHD	Result	MHD
0.05	C		C		C	
0.04	C		C		C	
0.03	C		C		C	
0.02	C		C		C	
0.01	C		C		C	
0.009	C		C		C	
0.008	C		C		C	
0.007	C		C		C	
0.006	C		C		C	
0.005	C		C		C	
0.004	C		C		C	
0.003	C	0.003	C	0.003	C	0.003
0.002	++		C—		C—	
0.001	+		++		++	

The striking reduplication of MHD occurring in all three concentrations does not argue for a marked superiority of the 30 and 40% over the 20% concentrations.

DISCUSSION OF RESULTS OBTAINED WITH VARIOUS CONCENTRATIONS OF UNHEATED AND HEATED SHEEP, HUMAN, RABBIT, AND HORSE SERUM

In all of the experiments described, eight-hour incubation was used. Beta streptococcus, strain M, was employed in all but a few instances. In these few the studies were conducted with strain V, which has a hemolytic index practically identical with that of M.

For all serums studied, heated serum, especially in the lower concentrations, yields better lysin than unheated fresh serum. This difference between heated and unheated serum is quantitatively most striking in a 5% concentration of rabbit serum. It is marked in 5% concentration of human serum; less so, but still perceptible in like amounts of sheep serum.

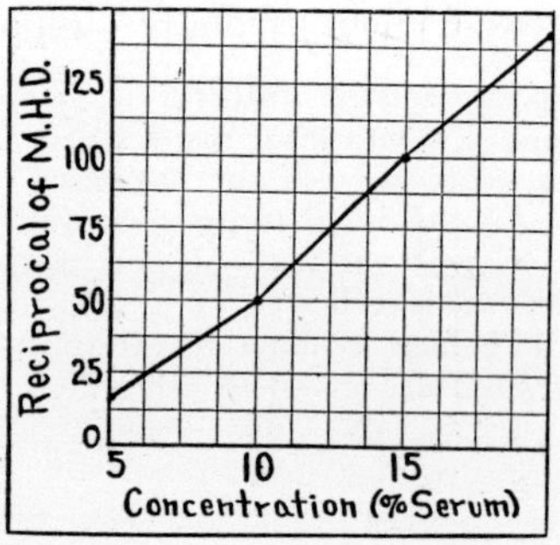

Fig. 9.—Streptolysin production in various concentrations of unheated horse serum broth, B. streptococcus M.

This difference in efficiency for streptolysin production becomes less as higher concentrations are reached. In 20% concentrations there is still a shade of superiority of heated over unheated horse and rabbit serum. Although the investigation of this point was not exhaustive, practically no divergence of titer is to be found in 20% concentration of sheep or human serum.

All serums, active or inactive, rise sharply from comparatively low titers in 5% concentration to high values which reach their maximum at 20% for horse, sheep and human, at 25% for rabbit. The curves for unheated horse and human serum, plotted in terms of MHD on the ordinates and concentrations of serum on the abscissae, have less steep slopes from low to high concentrations than those of human and rabbit (see figure 10). This means that the actual amount of hemolysin in unheated human and rabbit serum is far less in low concentrations than that produced in similar concentrations of sheep and horse. Study of the curves in figure 10 will make this clear. These curves indicate the actual amount of lysin present and not the proportionality expressed when reciprocals of the MHD are plotted. It will be seen that in the low concentrations, human and rabbit are far apart from sheep and horse. As the concentrations increase, the curves converge, which illustrates well the fact that all of the serums are fairly efficient for lysin production at a certain concentration. This explains, we believe, the marked difference in size of the hemolytic zones produced by beta streptococcus on horse and sheep as compared with human and rabbit 10% blood-agar plates, although in the case of human blood-agar plates another factor operates. This factor is discussed in the second part of this paper.

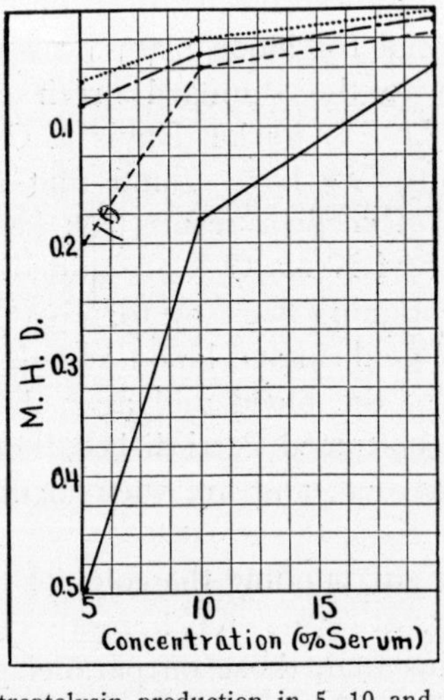

Fig. 10.—Comparative streptolysin production in 5, 10 and 20 concentrations of unheated horse, sheep, human and rabbit serum broth, B. streptococcus M; dotted line, horse; dot and dash line, sheep; broken line, human; continuous line, rabbit.

PART II

A NEW BLOOD-AGAR PLATE, DEVISED FROM THE DATA OBTAINED IN PART I

Holman[3] points out the necessity of a medium of maximal differentiating power for the fermentation reactions of streptococci. Brown[2] stresses a similar need in regard to blood plates as indicators of hemolysin and green production. He follows this demand by the description of a medium admirably suited to this purpose, i. e., horse blood agar. At the same time it would seem that the data obtained in Part 1 of this paper could be utilized in the synthesis of a plate which might present still further advantages, without introducing a too complicated technic.

Before describing the plate which has been devised on the basis of the experiments just mentioned, certain observations with the ordinary 10% horse, sheep, human and rabbit blood-agar plates will be recorded. These experiments, with very few exceptions, were carried out with poured plates. That is, dilute suspensions of beta streptococcus were transferred by platinum loop to liquid mixtures of blood and agar, the tubes thoroughly shaken to effect even mixture of the blood, agar and bacteria, and the plates immediately poured. The advantages of this procedure over the more facile streak method are fully explained by Blake[4] and by Brown,[2] and need not be dwelt on in this place.

The nutrient agar used for blood plates was made by adding agar in 1.5% concentration to the standard broth described in Part I. Reaction of broth P_H 7.6-7.8, Parke, Davis & Co., bacteriologic peptone, 2%. Very recently we have found that a lower alkalinity is perhaps more suitable. Excellent results can be obtained with broth to which 16 c c per liter of N Na_2CO_3 are added.

Large test tubes containing 8 c c of this agar are liquefied, cooled to 45 C., and 0.8 c c of defibrinated blood added. The tubes are then seeded with streptococci, the blood and agar thoroughly mixed, and poured at once into flat-bottomed Petri dishes, 9 cm. in diameter. The plates are allowed to harden, and are then incubated in an inverted position.

The hemolytic zones surrounding the colonies on sheep blood plates are considerably larger, are very much more clear, and have more cleanly scalloped margins than those on parallel plates of human and rabbit blood. The results of an experiment with beta hemolytic streptococcus M on parallel 10% sheep, human and rabbit blood-agar plates are summarized in table 28.

TABLE 28

DIAMETER OF HEMLYTIC ZONES ON 10% SHEEP, HUMAN AND RABBIT BLOOD AGAR

Plate	Kind of Blood	Percentage	Length of Incubation	Average Diameter of Hemolytic Zones in Millimeters
1	Sheep	10	14 hours	2.3
2	Human	10	14 hours	1.53
3	Rabbit	10	14 hours	1.5

Brown[2] notes that zones occurring on human blood-agar plates are cloudy, with indefinite borders. He does not think that this condition is due to unhemolyzed cells. In this opinion we differ with Brown. Microscopic examination of the zones surrounding colonies of beta streptococcus on human blood agar reveal residual, perfectly distinct clumps of unhemolyzed red blood cells. What is more, the vague, indefinite, fringed border of the zones is due to the same cause. This persistence of unhemolyzed clumps is undoubtedly the result of the strong hemagglutination occurring when human blood is mixed with agar in certain proportions. No matter how carefully and thoroughly these are mixed, microscopic examination of a poured plate reveals large numbers of small, closely packed clumps of red blood cells. It is probably the failure of the streptolysin to penetrate completely into these clumps that results in the incomplete laking of these masses, so giving the milky indefinite appearance to the hemolytic zones.

This observation led us to study quantitatively the hemagglutinative action of agar on the blood of different species. The method used was to mix decreasing quantities of 1.5% agar with constant amounts of the whole blood of various species. All tubes were brought to constant volume with 0.85% NaCl solution and the mixtures incubated at 45 C. While the quantitative amounts of agar able to cause agglutination of the different bloods did not vary widely, there was a marked difference in the speed and intensity of the reaction for different ones. Thus, while the smallest amount of agar able to produce agglutination might be approximately the same for all the kinds of blood tested, the reaction took place far more rapidly and completely in human blood than in the others.

What is more, the clumping of cells, once established, was much less easily reversible for human blood than for sheep or rabbit. When hemagglutination takes place in agar sheep blood mixtures, the cells can be brought to homogeneous resuspension by gentle tapping of the tube, and the subsequent reagglutination is slow. It is more difficult to break up the clumps of human cells, and reagglutination takes place much more rapidly. It will be understood that this fact makes it difficult to secure a human blood plate in which the cells are homogeneously distributed. The whole reaction takes place in a very few minutes, where blood plates are concerned, since the setting of the agar after pouring terminates the agglutination reaction.

Rabbit blood occupies a position midway between that of sheep and human in regard to agglutination by agar. Sheep blood agglutinates by far the most slowly of any of the three, with a resulting greater homogeneity of the blood-agar mixture.

Horse blood, as well as the others mentioned, is agglutinated by agar, although not with the intensity or rapidity of that of human. It must be remembered also, that the large amounts of streptolysin produced by streptococci, even in low concentrations of horse blood, as compared to the smaller amounts produced in human, are better able to penetrate and hemolyze the clumps that are formed.

The difference in size of the hemolytic zones on sheep, human, and rabbit blood-agar plate is explicable by consulting figure 10. The amount of hemolysin secreted in 5% concentrations of the different serums will be noted. Human serum occupies a position midway between the highly efficient sheep and horse serum and the unsuitable rabbit serum. In 10% blood plates, more lysin is doubtless manufactured from human blood than from that of the rabbit. Human blood is made less desirable, however, by the unevenness, due to hemagglutination, of the agar-blood mixtures.

To sum up, horse and sheep blood are distinctly superior to rabbit and human blood plates. The hemolytic zones produced by beta streptococcus on the former media are larger, clearer, and have more sharply defined borders. Human blood is inferior to sheep; first, because considerably less hemolysin is produced, in low concentrations used in plates; second, because of the energetic agglutination of human red blood cells when mixed with agar. The borders of the zones on human blood agar are so irregular that it is difficult to measure accurately the diameter of the hemolyzed area.

While hemagglutination is not a factor of importance in rabbit blood-agar plates, the small amount of lysin produced in low concentrations of rabbit blood causes hemolytic zones much inferior in size to those of sheep or horse blood. The zones on sheep and horse blood in plates with similar concentration of blood, using the same organism, are very nearly of the same size and quality. Slightly more lysin may be produced in these concentrations of horse blood. This is counterbalanced by the greater homogeneity of the sheep blood-agar mixtures. The suitability of sheep blood has been stressed only because it is more accessible to general use than horse blood.

A BLOOD PLATE GIVING MAXIMAL STREPTOLYSIN PRODUCTION

Analysis of the data obtained in Part 1 of this paper resulted in the synthesis of a blood-agar plate which should satisfy the demand for a medium of maximum differentiating power. Sheep blood was used in the majority of these experiments. It has the advantages of being easily obtainable, only slightly agglutinable by agar, and being highly potent as a pabulum for lysin production.

Taking advantage of the observation that maximal streptolysin production occurs in 20% concentrations of heated sheep serum (figures 5, 6, 7 and 8; Part 1), a plate was devised to contain serum in this amount. It will be obvious that if whole blood were used, a concentration of at least 40% would have to be employed to reach this amount of serum. If so much blood were used, the additional number of red blood cells added would offset the increased streptolysin produced in such serum concentration. Consequently, serum-blood cell mixtures were made. The red blood cells were combined with heated serum in such proportion that when mixed with the agar the final concentration of serum would be 20%; cells, 5%; agar, 75%.

This procedure is accomplished without great technical difficulty, and an example of the exact technic employed is given below.

Sheep blood is obtained, defibrinated carefully, centrifugated, the serum pipetted off aseptically and heated to 56 C. for 45 minutes. This serum is then recombined with the red blood cells in the proportion of four parts of serum to one part of cells. One part of this serum-cell mixture is then added to three parts of liquid agar, cooled to 45 C., the mixture seeded, the tube thoroughly shaken to secure even distribution of the agar, blood, and bacteria, and its contents immediately poured into plates.

It is desirable to ice the plates so made for some minutes previous to incubation, since the relatively large amount of the serum-cell mixture causes the agar to set rather slowly. Once set, these plates hold up perfectly, even in an inverted position.

To obtain good results it is necessary always to mix the cells and serum before addition of the agar. Red blood cells added alone are energetically agglutinated by agar. On the other hand, the preponderance of serum in the serum-cell mixture seems to protect the cells from agglutination, and perfect mixture can be secured.

The sheep serum-cell mixture plate just described is the most suitable of the plates we have studied, for the rapid diagnosis and differentiation of beta hemolytic streptococci. The organisms grow rapidly and abundantly on this medium, a maximal amount of hemolysin produced gives rise to large and clean-cut hemolytic zones, and the mixture of the blood and agar is homogeneous, provided proper precautions are taken. Table 28 gives some indication of the efficiency of this type of plate, compared to the ordinary 10% sheep, human and rabbit blood medium.

The technic used in this experiment was identical with that just described. Blood from all sources was obtained on the same day. Beta streptococcus, strain M, was used for seeding the plates.

TABLE 29

DIAMETER OF HEMOLYTIC ZONES ON 25% SHEEP SERUM-CELL MIXTURE PLATES AND ON 10% SHEEP, HUMAN AND RABBITT BLOOD-AGAR PLATES

Plate	Medium	Hours of Incubation	Diameter of Zones in Millimeters
1	25% sheep serum-cell	14	3.8
2	10% sheep blood	14	2.3
3	10% rabbit blood	14	1.3
4	10% human blood	14	1.5

Nine hours after seeding, the zones on Plate 1 had reached a diameter of 2.9 mm. Similar experiments with other strains of beta streptococcus show a like superiority of the special medium just described. If young cultures (8-12 hours) are used for the seeding of plates, diagnosis can be made at a very early period of incubation (5 to 7 hours).

The figures in table 29 represent the total diameter of the hemolytic zone, including the colony. It must not be inferred that this result represents the widest zone obtained. With heavy growing surface colonies, we have observed zones which attained diameters of 10 to 12 mm. in 24 hours. The deep colonies on such plates were, of course, much smaller, but the zones surrounding them measured in some cases 6 mm.

It is obvious that any of the four bloods studied can be treated similarly to that just described for sheep blood. In the case of horse and human blood the cell serum mixture which would be most desirable is identical with that just described (see figures 6, 8 and 9; Part I). For rabbit blood a still higher concentration of serum represents the optimum. In this instance 25% serum should be used.

While all of these bloods, combined in the manner described above, are far superior to 10% blood plates, sheep serum-blood cell mixture is especially recommended for a standard plate, for the reasons repeatedly mentioned in previous pages.

To sum up, an attempt has been made to devise a blood plate which will contain the optimum amount of serum necessary for maximum lysin production, and at the same time the number of red blood cells approximately equal to that of an ordinary 10% plate. To effect this purpose, artificial serum blood cell mixtures are made. This is done by centrifugating the blood, removing the supernatant serum, heating it to 56 C. for 45 minutes, and recombining this heated serum with the blood cells in the proportion of 4 parts of serum to 1 part of cells in sheep, horse and human blood. For rabbit blood the proportion of serum to cells would be 5 to 1.

Such serum cell mixtures are to be added to liquid agar in the proportion of 25 to 75 of agar for the first three kinds of blood, in proportion of 30 to 70 of agar for rabbit blood.

It may be remarked here that the factor of hemagglutination, so perceptible in the ordinary 10% human blood-agar plate, is much reduced in the human serum-cell mixture medium. The larger proportion of serum present in the latter would seem to exert some protective effect on the ability of agar to clump human red blood cells.

ALPHA-HEMOLYTIC STREPTOCOCCUS ON SHEEP SERUM-CELL MIXTURE PLATES

The formation of concentric rings of alternate methemoglobinized and hemolyzed corpuscles around colonies of alpha hemolytic streptococci is a phenomenon first observed by Konrad,[15] Sigwart[16] and Saito,[17] and afterward thoroughly studied by Brown.[2] The last named investigator came to the conclusion that this effect is due to the subjection of plates containing the alpha streptococcus to alternations of incubator and room or cold room temperatures. By resorting to successive incubation and icing, each interval lasting 48 hours, Brown was able to produce several concentric rings.

Immediately round the colony lies a zone of green unhemolyzed corpuscles, which is in turn surrounded by a hemolyzed area, appear-

[15] Beitr. Geburtsh. u. Gynäk., 1908, 9, 13, p. 364.
[16] Münch. Med. Wchnschr., 1909, 56, p. 1128.
[17] Arch. Hyg. u. Infektionskr., 1912, 75, p. 121.

ing when the plate is iced after the first incubation. Subsequent incubation results in a green zone outside of the hemolyzed one, which may be again surrounded by a hemolyzed area if one resorts to a second chilling of the plate.

We have studied this property of zone formation with a strain of alpha hemolytic streptococcus (viridans), on 10% rabbit, human and sheep blood plates, and compared the results with these mediums with those secured on the sheep serum-cell mixture described above. The concentric ring picture presented by this organism on the latter medium is a striking one and much superior to that on the ordinary 10% blood agar. Of the 10% blood-agar plates, human blood furnished the poorest medium for the demonstration of ring formation; rabbit blood presented a fair picture. Ten per cent. sheep blood agar was efficient, but far less so than the sheep serum cell mixture plate.

Twenty-four hours suffice for each period of successive incubation and icing when the special medium is used. The hemolytic zones are very clear, and the bands are sharply delineated, so that they can be easily distinguished by the unaided eye. The ring formation is much more marked in the deep than in the surface colonies. This alone forms a potent argument for pouring, rather than the surface streaking of plates.

There is no doubt that the investigations of Brown have changed materially the method of differentiation of green producing and hemolytic streptococci, since this worker has definitely shown that green production is not the sole thing to be looked for on blood plates seeded with viridans or pneumococcus. Given proper conditions hemolysis also makes its appearance.

The 25% sheep serum-blood cell mixture plate furnishes optimum conditions for hemolysin production by the beta hemolytic streptococcus. For the alpha hemolytic organisms, viridans and pneumococcus, the ring effect is striking and clean cut, it being possible to produce with ease quintuple zones by the use of this medium. Up to the present time this plate seems to us to satisfy better than any other the demand for a medium of maximal differentiating power for the different varieties of streptococcus.

Unfortunately, we have not had access to any strains of the alpha prime type described by Brown. It is this type and the beta types of very low hemolytic power that the serum-blood cell mixture plates will be of greatest use in picking up. It is well known that various strains of the beta type vary greatly in the amount of their hemolysin production. Those producing very small amounts, which might on 10% rabbit or human blood agar be confused with alpha prime or gamma would be exposed to optimum conditions for hemolysin production on the medium we propose.

It has not been possible for us to judge as to the relative merits of the blood plate and the blood broth medium in clinical investigations. The method of Lyall,[14] for the diagnosis of hemolytic streptococcus is at best qualitative and does not furnish adequate differentiation from the green producers. Throat cultures and study of the lungs and other organs at necropsy are best carried out in blood plates. For isolation from the blood stream it would seem best to utilize serum broth medium, following this by subplating at the moment cocci are demonstrated in the broth culture.

We have no opinion on the relation of hemolytic power of beta streptococcus to its virulence, and we do not think that this moot point has been satisfactorily settled. If this is to be done, liquid medium (serum broth) must be employed, since the evidence furnished by plates is qualitative only. In the employment of such serum broth for quantitative estimation of hemolytic power certain conditions should be secured. The data presented in Part I delineate quite clearly those conditions.

SUMMARY AND CONCLUSIONS

Hemolysin production in serum broth by beta hemolytic streptococcus has been studied. The amount of free hemolysin present at different intervals of incubation has been determined by the titration of the supernatants of high speed (8,000 revolutions a minute) centrifugation of serum broth cultures against constant quantities of washed red blood cells.

This method presents superiorities to those of titration of filtrates or of whole culture. These advantages are discussed in Part I.

Lysin production reaches its maximum for the strains studied at a very early period in the life of the serum broth culture. When the serum broth under test is seeded with young (8-12 hour) cultures, this peak is reached at from 7 to 8 hours. When older cultures are used for seeding, the crest may be deferred to 12 hours.

The outpouring of streptolysin occurs during the early part of the logarithmic growth period of the culture. When this growth period ceases, the free lysin begins to decrease rapidly, often disappearing completely in 14 hours.

When streptolysin has disappeared completely from the supernatants of high speed centrifugation (free lysin) whole cultures may still be hemolytically active in low titer. This activity is probably due to lysin operating from the surfaces of organisms, at which place it is destroyed less rapidly than in the free state.

These observations pave the way for accurate quantitative titration of the streptolysin produced by a given strain of beta streptococcus. One strain, tested frequently over a period covering several months, yielded remarkably constant titers of hemolysin.

The comparative efficiency of sheep, horse, human and rabbit serum broth for hemolysin production has been studied. Heated serums are in general superior to unheated. Sheep and horse serum are distinctly superior in all concentrations to human and far superior to rabbit serum broth. Curves of the relation of serum concentration to hemolysin production have been plotted and the optimum concentration for the various serums obtained.

The data gleaned in these quantitative studies have been used in the synthesis of a new blood-agar plate. This plate has been devised with the idea of using the optimum serum concentration for maximal lysin production of a blood which shall be efficient and at the same time accessible to general use.

Sheep blood is believed to fill this need. To obtain maximal lysin production rather high concentrations of serum are necessary (20%). The number of red blood cells is kept down by making artificial combinations of heated serum and cells.

The serum-cell mixture is made by combining 4 parts of heated serum with 1 part of cells. This mixture is then combined with liquid agar in proportion of 1 part of the mixture to 3 of agar. The final concentration therefore is: serum, 20%; cells, 5%, and agar 75%.

Rabbit and human serums can also be combined with their respective cells in a similar manner, the proportions being altered slightly in the case of rabbit serum. Plates made from these bloods, while superior to the ordinary 10% blood plates, are not as efficient as the sheep serum-cell mixture plate just described, for reasons given in Part II.

The proposed medium is not only a very suitable one for demonstration of the hemolytic zones of beta streptococcus, but is in addition very efficient in the demonstration of multiple concentric zones of green production and hemolysis for alpha streptococcus and pneumococcus.

THE INFLUENCE OF THORIUM X ON ANTIBODY-FORMATION

Ludvig Hektoen and H. J. Corper

From the John McCormick Institute for Infectious Diseases, Chicago

In 1902 Rutherford and Soddy[1] obtained a highly radioactive filtrate by precipitating thorium from solution with ammonia. Evaporated to dryness, the ammonia being driven off by ignition, this filtrate left a small residue, which weight for weight was several times more active than the original compound. The active constituent secured in this way they called thorium X.

In spite of the great activity of thorium X, its biologic effects were not studied to any extent until about 1912. At the present time we are interested especially in its action on the blood and its organs. Indeed, the most striking effect of thorium X when introduced into the body is leukopenia and disappearance of cells from the marrow. The changes have been studied mostly in the rabbit. Pappenheim and Plesch[2] concluded that it has a toxic effect on the leukocytes in the blood, the marrow cells, for both of which it seemed to have a direct selective affinity, the cells of the spleen, the lymph nodes, the liver and the kidney. Hirschfeld and Meidner[3] found that in large doses it affected all leukocytes practically alike and caused also a slight decrease in the red corpuscles and the hemoglobin. Arneth[4] and Rosenow[5] studied the changes in the leukocytes by thorium X, and Rosenow likened the effect to that of the roentgen ray, but Mello[6] maintains that thorium X has less effect on the lymphoid cells and more on the myelogenous than the roentgen ray. Pappenheim[7] has likened the action of thorium X on the blood to that of benzene. It is noteworthy that thorium X may cause an extreme leukopenia while the red corpuscles and hemoglobin appear to suffer but little, although it is possible that there may be

Received for publication Nov. 20, 1919.

[1] Rutherford: Radioactive Substances and Their Radiations, 1913.

[2] Folia Haematologica, 1912, 14, p. 172; Ztschr. f. exper. Path. u. Therap., 1912, 12, p. 185.

[3] Berl. klin. Wchnschr., 1912, 69, p. 1343.

[4] Deutsch. med. Wchnschr., 1913, 39, p. 733.

[5] Ztschr. f. ges. exp. Med., 1913, 3, p. 385.

[6] Ztschr. f. klin. Med., 1914, 81, p. 285; Arch. Brasil. de Med., 1919, 9, p. 123.

[7] Ztschr. f. exper. Path. u. Therap., 1914, 15, p. 39.

such effective stimulus of production as to conceal the destruction of red corpuscles going on at the same time (Mello[6]). With respect to the substances concerned in immunity reactions, Lippmann and Plesch[8] report that the complement remains apparently unchanged even when practically all the circulating leukocytes have been destroyed by thorium X. Fränkel and Gumpertz'[9] observations on the effect of thorium X on the production of typhoid agglutinin did not yield any striking results except that in animals receiving large doses the production seemed to be reduced. Corper[10] found that one-half the lethal amount of thorium X given seven days before or coincident with either the primary or secondary injection, had no effect on the anaphylactic reaction in guinea-pigs. Further, that repeated smaller doses, sufficient in many cases to maintain a leukopenia at about 2,000 during the incubation period, had no recognizable effect on anaphylaxis. Here may be mentioned too that Corper[11] could not influence the course of experimental tuberculosis in guinea-pigs by means of thorium X, and Hirschfeld and Meidner[12] did not succeed in modifying the growth of tumors with it. Corper, however, finds that thorium X in mice greatly increases the virulence of pneumococci and hemolytic streptococci (unpublished).

In connection with certain other experiments, we have made observations on the liberation of antibodies in rabbits under the influence, in varying degrees, of thorium X which is given easily in salt solution. The radiothorium from which the thorium X we have used was prepared was donated by Dr. H. W. McCoy, of the Carnotite Reduction Company, Chicago. The method of determination of dosage is described by Corper.[11] The antigen used was sheep blood, injected intraperitoneally in one dose of 25 c c, as we were familiar with its antigenic effects when so injected.

First, large doses of thorium X were given so that a marked reduction of leukocytes in the peripheral blood was maintained for a few days before the injection of the antigen as well as throughout the period ordinarily required by the antigen to produce its maximum effect as measured by newly formed lysin and precipitin in the blood. For this purpose one-fifth the lethal doses of thorium X was injected intravenously followed by further injections every two or three days

[8] Ztschr. f. Immunitätsforsch. u. exper. Therap., 1913, 17, p. 548.
[9] Berl. klin. Wchnschr., 1914, 51, p. 209.
[10] Jour. Infect. Dis., 1919, 25, p. 248.
[11] Am. Rev. Tuberc., 1918, 2, p. 587.
[12] Ztschr. f. klin. Med., 1913, 78, p. 407.

of from one-fifth to one-twentieth the lethal dose as required. The results, which were practically the same in the five rabbits studied, are illustrated in table 1, and they indicate that while lysin for sheep corpuscles was set free in large amounts, the production of precipitin for sheep protein was reduced very much.

TABLE 1

REPEATED LARGE DOSES OF THORIUM X BEGUN 8 DAYS BEFORE INJECTION OF SHEEP BLOOD

Days After First Injection of Thorium X	Days After Injection of Sheep Blood	Rabbit 2			Control	
		Precipitin	Lysin	Leukocytes	Precipitin	Lysin
0	..	...	......	15,000		
3	..	...	......	7,250		
5	..	...	......	3,500		
7	..	...	......	1,875		
8	0	0	192			
10	4	0	768	3,250	0	768
12	6	0	6,144	1,750	50	6,144
14	8	800	25,000	1,650	800	6,144
16	10	800	25,000	2,500	1,600	6,144
18	12	400	25,000	1,125	6,400	12,288
20	14	0	25,000	1,425	12,800	6,144
22	16	800	25,000	1,750	12,800	6,144
24	..	...	......	1,500		

TABLE 2

REPEATED SMALL DOSES OF THORIUM X BEGUN 3 DAYS BEFORE INJECTION OF SHEEP BLOOD

Days After First Dose of Thorium X	Days After Injection of Sheep Blood	Rabbit 1			Rabbit 5			Rabbit 6			Control	
		Precipitin	Lysin	Leukocytes	Precipitin	Lysin	Leukocytes	Precipitin	Lysin	Leukocytes	Precipitin	Lysin
1	..	....	......	7,750	......	......	13,250	....	......	9,750		
4	1	....	......	8,250	......	......	17,500	....	......	6,500		
6	3	....	......	15,000	......	......	......	....	......	7,000	200	
9	6	0	12,288	7.500	3,200	12.288	20,000	200	384	12,500	3,200	6,144
12	9	0	12,288+	6,250	3,200	6,144	8,000	800	192	10.000	6,400	12.288
15	12	400	12,288	6,500	3,200	3,072	12,500	400	96	8,750	9,600	6.144
18	15	800	6,144	7,500	6,400	3,072	18,500	800	192	15,000	4,800	6,144
21	18	800	12,288	10.000	12,000	1,536	11,250	800	1,536	10,000	4,800	6,144
24	21	200	12,288	8,250	6,400	6,144	13,250	200	384	12,500	4,800	6,144
27	24	200	12,288	8,750	3,200	6,144	11,250	200	384	7,500	3,200	3,072
30	27	200	6,144	8,000	3,200	12,288	6,750	200	768	8,500	1,600	3,072
33	30	200	1,536	10,000	3,200	6,144	10,000	200	384	8,000	1,600	3,072
39	35	200	768	12,500	800	6,144	9,500	200	384	14,000	800	3,072
	43	200	1,536	......	0	3,072	......	200	768	......	800	3,072
	50	0	384	......	400	3,072	......	0	384	......	400	1,536
	54	0	384	......	400	3,072	......	0	768	......	400	768

Rabbit 1 is an example of low precipitin and abundant lysin production.

Rabbit 5 shows a fairly abundant output of precipitin and lysin, the latter running a rather irregular course.

Rabbit 6 is an example of low production of both lysin and precipitin.

The figures in the tables give the highest active dilution of the rabbit serum in the lysin tests, and under precipitin the highest dilution

TABLE 3

LARGE SINGLE DOSE OF THORIUM X SIX DAYS AFTER INJECTION OF SHEEP BLOOD

Days after Injection of Sheep Blood	Rabbit 2			Rabbit 7			Rabbit 10			Rabbit 3			Rabbit 4			
	Precipitin	Lysin	Leukocytes	Precipitin	Lysin	Leukocytes	Precipitin	Lysin	Leukocytes	Precipitin	Lysin	Leukocytes	Precipitin	Lysin	Leukocytes	
0	0	192	10,400	0	96	10,000	0	192	11,600	0	96	10,800	0	96	12,800	
3	0	24	14,000	0	24	9,600	0	192	9,600	0	96	13,600	0	48	14,000	
5	0	3,072	9,800	0	1,536	8,800	0	3,072	10,800	0	3,072	8,200	0	3,072	8,600	
6	0	3,072	......	0	.....	......	200	6,144	......	0	3,072	.....	0	1,536	.....	Thorium X, one third of lethal dose
7	500	3,072	4,200	200	3,072	3,000	2,000	6,144	8,200	1,200	3,072	4,600	500	1,536	4,600	
8	800	6,144	3,600	1,600	3,072	2,800	2,000	6,144	5,400	1,600	3,072	3,600	500	3,072	2,600	
9	1,600	6,144	2,600	1,600	6,144	2,200	2,000	6,144	2,800	1,600	6,144	3,000	800	6,144	2,400	
10	3,200	6,144	1,700	3,200	6,144	1,500	2,000	6,144	1,800	1,600	6,144	1,400	1,600	6,144	1,300	
11	3,200	6,144	1,000	3,200	6,144	1,500	4,800	6,144	1,700	4,800	6,144	1,400	3,200	6,144	1,700	
13	6,400	3,072	2,000	1,600	6,144	1,200	3,200	6,144	2,000	3,200	3,072	2,100	6,400	3,072	1,800	
15	....	.....	1,400	6,400	3,072	1,100	3,200	6,144	2,700	1,600	3,072	2,200	12,800	3,072	1,000	
18	3,200	1,536	1,200	6,400	3,072	2,000	6,400	6,144	2,700	1,600	768	4,000	Died			
21	3,200	1,536	1,100	3,200	3,072	2,900	6,400	6,144	2,400	1,600	768	3,400				
24	3,200	768	1,700	800	1,536	3,000	3,200	3,072	4,200	800	768	4,100				
27	400	768	2,200	800	1,536	5,600	3,200	3,072	6,400	800	768	5,200				
30	200	768	2,700	800	1,536	5,300	3,200	3,072	5,200	800	768	6,000				
35	200	768	2,000	640	1,536	4,500	1,600	1,536	3,900	800	768	6,200				
40	160	384	......	640	1,536	......	800	768	......	400	768					
46	160	384	2,600	640	768	5,100	640	768	4,400	320	384	7,200				
49	160	192	3,000	640	384	5,200	640	768	4,400	320	384	9,200				
57	160	192	4,000	640	384	8,600	.....	.....	......	320	384					
63	160	192	4,800	320	192	8,000	320	768	4,600	320	384					

of sheep blood in which the rabbit serum caused precipitate by the contact method after two hours at room temperature. The lysin mixtures contained 0.2 c c of 5% suspension of washed corpuscles, 0.006 c c guinea-pig serum as complement, heated rabbit serum and salt solution, the total quantity of each mixture being 0.6 c c. The lysin mixtures were incubated for two hours and then put into the icebox until the next morning.

In the next experiment about one-half the lethal dose was given in a single intravenous injection at the same time as the sheep blood was injected into the abdomen. The leukocytes were reduced and the formation of precipitin restrained, but in neither case as much as in the first experiment; lysin was produced freely.

A series of 13 rabbits, all young and healthy, were injected intravenously, daily or every other day, with small doses of thorium X, mostly 1/500 of the lethal quantity, in some cases 1/200. These injections were started 48 hours before the sheep blood was injected in the usual way and continued until long past the high point of antibody production. The results are illustrated in table 2. In no case was there any marked change in the number of leukocytes; in 9 animals the production of lysin was abundant, in 4 the titer remained rather low; in all but 2 of the 13 rabbits the amount of precipitin in the blood was comparatively insignificant.

In still another series of 12 young and healthy rabbits, about one third of the lethal dose of thorium X was given on the sixth day after the intraperitoneal injection in each rabbit of 25 c c of sheep blood. The purpose of this experiment was to determine what effect if any thorium X would have when given after the production of antibodies was well under way. The results are illustrated in table 3. We note that while the leukocytes were greatly reduced by the thorium injection, there was no definite and clearly recognizable effect on either the amount of lysin and precipitin in the blood or on the length of time of their persistence.

SUMMARY AND DISCUSSION

In rabbits treated with thorium X in the early stages of antibody production, under the conditions described, the amount of precipitin in the blood may be reduced even when there is no definite reduction in the leukocytes in the peripheral blood. This result indicates that thorium X may act on the mechanism of production rather than on the precipitin itself, especially when taken in conjunction with the fact that thorium X seems to have no effect on the amount of precipitin in the blood if injected when the precipitin-production is well under way, that is, on the sixth day or so after the injection of the antigen. From our results it is uncertain whether the thorium X as given in these experiments exercised any definite effect on the formation of lysin. In this respect thorium X would appear to differ in effect from benzene [13] and the roentgen ray, which have been found to restrain the output of lysin as well as precipitin. It is noteworthy also that thorium X, like benzene and the roentgen ray, seems to be without effect on the antibody content of the blood when introduced near the height of the curve; but that unlike the other two agents, it causes leukopenia as promptly at this time as earlier. Further and more diversified experiments are required to determine whether these are constant and fundamental differences in the actions of agents which disturb in some way the production of antibodies at the same time they destroy leukocytes, marrow and lymphoid cells.

[13] Hektoen: Jour. Infect. Dis., 1916, 19, p. 69; 1915, 17, p. 415; 1918, 22, p. 28.

BACILLUS OF THE COLON-TYPHOID GROUP ISOLATED FROM A CASE OF FURUNCULOSIS

Wade W. Oliver and Alma F. Schwab

From the Department of Bacteriology, Hoagland Laboratory, Long Island College Hospital, Brooklyn, N. Y.

A colon-like organism has been isolated in pure culture from a case of furunculosis. The patient, who gave a history of annual or semi-annual crops of "boils," which had developed over a period of several years, presented, at the time of examination, three small acutely inflamed furuncles on the back of his neck. The largest lesion, which was red, indurated, and about the size of a dime, was punctured with a sterile needle, after preliminary cleansing of the skin with soap and water, mercuric chlorid (1: 1,000) and alcohol. A small amount of a moderately thick, gray-white pus was expressed. Aerobic and anaerobic cultures were made on human blood agar (+ 1) and Martin's ascitic agar (0.5), and incubated at 37 C. After 24 hours' incubation, single colonies from the aerobic blood agar were streaked across plates of human blood agar (+ 1) and incubated aerobically at 37 C. At the end of 24 hours single colonies were plated in plain agar (+ 1), and after 24 hours more at 37 C., single colonies were transplanted to slants of plain agar (+ 1).

Morphology.—The organism was a gram-negative, nonmotile, noncapsulated, nonsporogenous rod, averaging about 2-3 mikrons in length and of about the thickness of the colon bacillus. Like the latter, it exhibited rather marked variations in size when grown for from 24 to 36 hours in plain infusion broth (+ 1). The majority of the forms were short single rods, with rounded ends. However, thin rods and small coccoid bodies were not infrequently present. The latter were more numerous in cultures incubated for a number of days (7-10). Certain organisms, especially the medium sized rods, showed bipolar staining and others exhibited two or three irregularly placed granules within the body of the rod.

Biology.—Growth occurred readily on ordinary mediums. On plain infusion agar (+ 1), after 24 hours' aerobic incubation at 37 C. the colonies were medium sized, round, with regular edges, grayish-white in color and slightly viscous. A moderately marked growth occurred in gelatin, with no liquefaction, the gelatin showing a moderate diffuse clouding with a well defined thin line of growth along the line of inoculation, after seven days at room temperature. Plain infusion broth (+ 1) showed a diffuse uniform clouding, after 24 hours at 37 C. No pellicle formed even after two weeks' continuous incubation.

Received for publication Dec. 9, 1919.

After 2 days' incubation, a rather heavy gray-white collar of growth was visible on the sides of the test-tube immediately above the upper level of the broth, and in the bottom of the tube was present a moderate gray flocculent growth. No difference in the luxuriance of growth was noted in cultures incubated aerobically and at partial oxygen tension with the aid of B. subtilis. The organism was a facultative anaerobe, but even on human blood agar slants (+1), made anaerobic by the addition of pyrogallic acid and potassium hydroxid, the growth was delicate. The optimum growth temperature was 37 C.

Products of Growth.—When grown aerobically on 1% sugar litmus-agar slants (+1) acid, but no gas, was split off from lactose, galactose, maltose mannite and saccharose, but glucose and dextrin remained unchanged even after two weeks' incubation. This test was made on +1 beef extract agar, previously rendered sugar-free by incubation with B. coli. The sugars, etc., after being sterilized for 15 minutes at 20 pounds' pressure, were added aseptically to the medium just before it solidified. Inoculations were made on the surface of the slant, as well as by a stab into the depths of the medium. At partial oxygen tension,[1] glucose-agar slants showed a distinct acid reaction, but no gas, after 36 hours' incubation at 37 C., as did the lactose, galactose, maltose, mannite, and saccharose. Dextrin was not fermented. Aerobic transplants made from the respective sugars to a fresh series of sugar agars which were incubated aerobically, gave the same readings as on the first series. The same thing held true in the case of the partial tension series.

After being transplanted every week to glucose (+1) and plain (+1) agar slants for six months, the organism was planted on a plain (+1) agar slant. After 24 hours' incubation at partial tension at 37 C. the tube was placed in the icebox, with the tube of B. subtilis attached, and left continuously in the refrigerator for 17 months. At the end of this time, a transplant was made to plain (+1) broth and a heavy growth of the bacillus was obtained after 24 hours' incubation. After determining by plating that the culture was pure, the organism was planted into a series of peptone water tubes to which had been added the respective sugars to a concentration of 1%. The Andrade indicator was employed, and to detect gas small inverted tubes within the broth were employed. In this series, after 24 hours' incubation at 37 C., a marked acid reaction, which persisted after at least 10 days' continuous incubation, but no gas, was observed in glucose, levulose, galactose, salicin, raffinose, saccharose, maltose, lactose, mannite, and glycerin (5%). A faint trace of acid, but no gas, was observed in dextrin after 24 hours' incubation, but after 5 days' continuous incubation at 37 C., the faint reddish tinge had completely disappeared from this tube except for the broth within the small inverted tube. One per cent. potato starch remained unchanged until the fifth day of continuous incubation at 37 C., at which time a faint reddish layer, indicating acid, was observed at the bottom of the tube. No gas was formed from the starch. On 6 days' incubation the starch showed a moderate acid reaction throughout the tube. Inulin remained unchanged. Litmus milk exhibited acid coagulation after 48 hours' incubation at 37 C. No indol was produced. Gelatin was not liquefied.

A macroscopic agglutination test with known typhoid antiserum gave a positive agglutination in a 1:20 dilution, but no agglutination in dilutions of 1:40, 1:80, and 1:160.

[1] Wherry and Oliver: Jour. Infect. Dis., 1916, 19, p. 288.

Pathogenesis for the Guinea-Pig.—After continuous cultivation for 5 months 0.5 c c of a 24-hour plain infusion broth (+ 1) culture was injected intraperitoneally into about a 300 gm. guinea-pig. Death resulted within 15 hours, the animal giving evidence of a profound toxemia. From the peritoneal fluid, which was scant, straw-colored and viscous, as well as from the heart's blood, the organism was recovered in pure culture.

Vaccine Therapy.—A vaccine was prepared from plain infusion agar (+ 1) four days after the isolation of the organism. The cultures were incubated at partial oxygen tension for 24 hours at 37 C. The vaccine was killed by heating in the water bath at 55 C. for one hour. The bacterial count was approximately one-half billion per c c of vaccine.

The reaction obtained on administration of the vaccine was strikingly severe. The initial injection consisted of 1 minim injected subcutaneously into the forearm. Within 4 hours a marked, tender, reddened, swollen, area developed at the site of the inoculation. The local reaction increased in intensity, so that within 24 hours a painful, very red, indurated area of about the size of a half dollar had developed. With the local reaction occurred a rather marked constitutional reaction. By the end of 24 hours, the temperature had risen to 101.5 F. and the following day the patient was incapacitated from work, complaining of headache, malaise, and venturing the assertion "I feel exactly the way I do when I am getting a new crop of boils."

The second injection, given after three days, consisted of 1 minim, and evoked a slightly less marked local reaction. Then the dosage was increased 1 minim per injection at three day intervals, until 14 minims were being given at an injection. Injections of this maximum dosage were continued every three days until about 4 c c had been administered. After the first three injections the reaction was confined to a moderate local one.

The vaccine therapy seemed to abort the initial lesions, and no lesions have developed up to the present. It is now twenty months since the initial injection.

DISCUSSION

Pollitzer[2] says: "A boil is produced in one way and in one way only. It is the result of an infection of the skin with the staphylococcus aureus by way of the hair follicles." McDonald[3] reports twenty-eight cases of furunculosis, in all of which the staphylococcus aureas or albus was found. Similar findings were reported by Compton[4] and Harris.[5]

From its morphology and from certain of its cultural characters, the organism seems to belong within the colon group of bacteria. The finding of the bacillus in pure culture from the lesions of the disease and the marked reaction set up in the patient when treated with an

[2] The Post Graduate, 1914, 29, p. 825.
[3] Arch. Pediat., 1911, 28, p. 772.
[4] Lancet, 1918, 1, p. 99.
[5] N. Y. Med. Jour., 1911, 94, p. 984.

autogenous vaccine suggest an etiologic relation of the organism to the disease. The marked toxicity of the bacillus for a guinea-pig is also worthy of note.

The action of the organism on glucose merits notice. The fermentation of glucose at partial oxygen tension and its nonfermentation under aerobic conditions bears a resemblance to the fermentation reactions on this sugar of a bacillus isolated by one of us from the feces of a case of dysentery.[6] The production of acid in glucose broth is explainable possibly by the fact that in the depth of the broth the bacillus found conditions of diminished tension which favored splitting of the sugar.

SUMMARY

A member of the colon group of bacteria was isolated in pure culture from a case of furunculosis.

Intraperitoneal injection of 0.5 c c of a 24-hour broth culture, after the organism had been cultivated continuously for 5 months, resulted in the death of a guinea-pig of about 300 gm. in weight, in 15 hours.

Under aerobic conditions on solid media the organism failed to produce acid from glucose, even on prolonged incubation (14 days), but under conditions of partial oxygen tension, glucose was fermented with acid production, but no gas, within 36 hours. Under both aerobic and partial tension conditions, acid, but no gas, was formed from lactose, galactose, maltose, mannite, and saccharose.

The marked local and general reaction on the part of the patient following the initial injection of 1 minim of an autogenous vaccine (about one half billion bacilli per c c) followed by the patient's freedom from boils for almost two years since the vaccine was administered, suggest a relationship of the bacillus to the disease.

[6] Oliver and Perkins: Jour. Infect. Dis., 1918, 22, p. 507.

OBSERVATIONS ON PARATYPHOID BACILLI RECENTLY ISOLATED FROM ANIMALS

Robb Spalding Spray

From Purdue University, Agricultural Experiment Station, Lafayette, Ind.

In the recent study of an outbreak of highly infectious enteritis among swine a number of strains of the paratyphoid-enteritidis group were isolated, which offer excellent material for comparison with the reports of other investigators. Most of these strains conform to the standards at present accepted as diagnostic of the various groups, but there are numerous significant departures from these standards.

It is not the purpose to increase the now diminishing confusion in this intricate group, but to record certain striking deviations from type among recently isolated strains. That these variations are not to be regarded as resulting from conditions of artificial culture is evident by the fact that they appeared immediately on isolation and have been maintained through a number of generations. If the variations were limited to cultural characteristics they might be disregarded, but they are in all cases correlated with variations in agglutination.

In addition to the strains isolated from diseased swine, several others were isolated from hog cholera virus blood, in the course of routine serum production. These have been included for the purpose of comparison with the other strains.

Sources and Methods of Isolation

From Diarrheal Swine.—Routine inoculations were made from heart blood, lung, liver, spleen, kidney, and mesenteric glands. The identity of all paratyphoid strains isolated from the various organs of the same carcass may not be assumed, because in at least three instances two, or even three, distinct strains were isolated from the same body.

From Hog Cholera Virus.—(1) By Direct Plating: Samples of all lots of virus blood being tested for gas-producing bacteria by inoculation into glucose broth fermentation tubes. In case gas-formers were present a loop of the same blood was plated in litmus-lactose agar, and in most cases pure cultures of paratyphoids were obtained.

(2) From Rabbits: Whenever a loop of blood was plated a rabbit was inoculated subcutaneously with 0.25 c c of the same blood. When the plate showed paratyphoids the corresponding rabbit usually died within 14 days. Inoculations were made from heart, lung, liver, spleen, and kidney, and the resulting cultures compared, and all but one of a series of apparent duplicates discarded.

Received for publication Dec. 10, 1919.

The remaining culture was replated three times to insure purity. From the third plate two colonies were picked and grown on agar slants. At the end of 24 hours these two cultures were inoculated into glucose and lactose broth fermentation tubes, nutrient broth, milk, gelatin, and peptone water. All of the strains included in this paper displayed the accepted paratyphoid-enteritidis reactions in these mediums. If the two strains from the same source gave identical reactions one was discarded and the remaining one became the stock strain. From this culture the group determination was carried out by inoculation of a number of diagnostic mediums. Strains isolated from rabbits were compared with corresponding strains isolated by direct plating, When duplicates were evident the strain isolated by plating was retained and that from the rabbit discarded. Only when there was an evident difference were two strains kept from the same blood sample.

With few exceptions the strains were readily classified. Several, however, displayed such crossing of characters that it was impossible to determine their proper relative position, based on morphologic and cultural characteristics alone. These atypical strains were then used as a basis for classification on the evidence of agglutination and absorption tests.

Twenty-three of the strains discussed in this paper were isolated from the tissues of diseased swine; 8 by plating of hog cholera virus blood; 9 from rabbits that died following inoculation with virus blood known to contain gas-producing bacteria.

Included for comparison only, are two strains of B. paratyphosus A, two of B. paratyphosus B, and one of B. enteritidis, all of human origin.

Table 1 gives the essential diagnostic cultural reactions.

TABLE 1

ESSENTIAL DIAGNOSTIC CULTURAL CHARACTERISTICS

Cultures	Glucose Serum Water	Lead Acetate Agar	Milk Alkaline at	Translucent Opalescent at 90 days	Arabinose	Xylose	Dulcite	Inosite
B. suipestifer 49.....	+	—	4 days	+	— —	+ +	— —	— —
Intermediates....... Rabbit 91 Swine 163	—	+	6 days	+	— —	+ +	— —	— —
B. paratyphosus A Human A97 Swine 134 Virus 149	+	—	35 days	—	+ —	— —	+ +	— —
B. paratyphosus A Human A98	+	+	38 days	—	+ —	— —	+ +	— —
B. paratyphosus B Human B96 Rabbit 124, 135	—	+	3 days	+	+ +	+ +	+ +	+ +
B. enteritidis....... Human 117	—	+	2 days	+	+ +	+ +	+ +	— —

Glucose serum water: + = pink or red; — = decolorized.
Lead acetate agar: + = blackening; — = no black.
Various sugars in serum water: + + = acid, coagulation, and gas; — — = no change; + — = deferred reaction, gas not evident.

Strains from Diarrheal Swine.—Twenty-two of the 23 strains from diseased swine gave cultural reactions which clearly would classify them as B. suipestifer. All produced slight initial acidity in litmus milk in 24 hours, followed by alkalinity on the third to the twelfth day; they produced translucence and opalescence in milk at 35 to 50 days; and they did not blacken lead acetate agar.[1] They did not ferment arabinose, dulcite, nor inosite within 48 hours, but fermented xylose within from 6 to 18 hours, producing acid and gas. They fermented glucose serum water, producing acid and gas, without perceptible reduction of the Andrade indicator.[2]

Several strains showed latent and irregular fermentation of arabinose and dulcite, traces of acid appearing at from 5 to 8 days. In addition, the 22 strains formed a homogeneous agglutinating group.

The single remaining strain, 163, is of particular interest. While it is a B. suipestifer type, this strain showed striking variations immediately on isolation. Inoculation into lead acetate agar produced blackening second to none except that of B. enteritidis 117. Glucose serum water showed acid, gas and coagulation, with strong decolorization at 18 hours; mannite serum water showed decolorization to a degree; arabinose, dulcite and inosite were not fermented; xylose was fermented in 6 hours with the production of acid and gas.

Agglutination tests placed this strain with the other 22 strains. Absorption tests, however, showed it to be a distinct type, intermediate between the B. suipestifer type strain 49, and B. paratyphosus B human type strain B 96.

A strain, 91, discussed later, was isolated from a rabbit inoculated with hog cholera virus blood. This strain showed the same peculiarities as strain 163. Agglutination and absorption tests showed the two to be closely related, if not identical. As this paper is being prepared the same type has been isolated for the third time.

Six strains were tested for pathogenicity against rabbits. All killed in 72 hours when 0.2 c c of a 24-hour broth culture was injected intraperitoneally. The same amount injected subcutaneously on the abdomen caused death in 6 or 7 days. Three attempts to isolate the infecting organism resulted in the recovery of an organism culturally and agglutinatively identical with the strain used for inoculation.

[1] Jordan and Victorson: Jour. Infect. Dis., 1917, 21, p. 571.
[2] Krumwiede, Kohn and Valentine: Jour. Med. Research, 1919, 39, p. 453.

It is evident that the 23 strains isolated from diseased swine are, in spite of serious deviation from type in a single instance and frequent individual peculiarities, very closely related.

Strains Isolated by Plating of Hog Cholera Virus Blood.—Five of the 8 strains isolated by plating virus blood are typical B. suipestifers in all respects. Two strains, 125 and 146, are atypical only in the irregular fermentation of dulcite.

The single remaining strain, 149, is an "A" type, and is indistinguishable from the two human B. paratyphosus A strains, except as noted later for strain A 98.

Strains Isolated from Rabbits.—Four of the 9 strains isolated from rabbits are typical B. suipestifers in all respects. One strain, 126, is atypical only in the irregular fermentation of dulcite.

Two strains, 124 and 135, are "B" types, and are indistinguishable from the two human B. paratyphosus B strains B 95 and B 96. Conversely, they are sharply distinct from all the B. suipestifer strains, and absorption tests confirm the cultural and agglutination evidence beyond reasonable doubt.

One strain, 134, is an "A" type, and is indistinguishable from the two human B. paratyphosus A strains, except as noted later for A 98.

The single remaining strain, 91, was referred to as being apparently identical with strain 163. This strain, 91, was isolated early in the work, and was at first regarded as a typical B. suipestifer. Prompt blackening of lead acetate agar, and decolorization of glucose serum water, however, showed it to be atypical. Agglutination and absorption tests showed it to be sharply distinct from B. suipestifer 49, and from B. paratyphosus B 96. The same tests clearly indicate its close relationship, if not its identity, with strain 163.

From close observation it appears that these two strains should be regarded as atypical B. suipestifers, and the finding emphasizes the broad extent of possible variation toward the B. paratyphosus B type. It emphasizes further, the contention of Krumwiede[3] that B. suipestifer should be considered not as a "type," but as a "group," wherein wide latitude for variation should be allowed.

Human Strains Used for Comparison.—These five strains are old stock strains, and if variation may be induced by long continued cultivation on artificial mediums, every opportunity has undoubtedly been offered. However, only a single strain, A 98, showed such tendency.

[3] Personal communication.

Both "A" strains, A 97 and A 98, behaved according to the accepted standards, except that A 98 persistently caused immediate and extreme blackening in lead acetate agar.

Both "B" strains, B 95 and B 96, behaved in all respects according to the accepted standards.

The single B. enteritidis strain was culturally identical with the two "B" strains, except in its inability to ferment inosite, which confirms the observations of Krumwiede[4] and others[5] on the diagnostic value of inosite. Agglutinatively, this strain was distinct from all other strains encountered.

Agglutination and Absorption Methods

Rabbits were used for the production of antiserum. Intravenous injections of 0.5 to 1 c c of a moderately dense suspension of a 24-hour agar culture, heated and cresolized, at three day intervals produced a serum titer of 1:7,500 to 1:54,000.

Twenty-four hour broth cultures, diluted to uniform density with formaldehyd-salt solution, were used as antigen.

The absorption tests were performed by a slight modification of the method of Krumwiede, Kohn, and Valentine.[6] The absorbing cultures were grown on agar in pint whisky flasks. Four flasks were inoculated and incubated for 24 hours.

A stock dilution of the antiserum in salt solution, 1:15, was prepared, and 5 c c used to wash off the growth of the first flask. This washing was transferred to the second flask, and the process repeated for the other two. The four flasks were rinsed with a second 5 c c portion of dilute serum, and the rinsing added to the first washing. About 8 c c of a very dense suspension was recovered.

This suspension was incubated from 2 to 3 hours, then centrifugalized at high speed till clear. It was found that the proportion of sedimented bacteria to serum was between 1:3 and 1:4, and that the agglutinins for the absorbing strain were exhausted or reduced to barely a trace where the serum was of very high titer.

This absorbed antiserum was then preserved with a drop of chloroform, and stored in the refrigerator, where its agglutinating powers were retained for as long as four months.

Agglutinations were carried out by the macroscopic method, and when peculiarities were observed the tests were repeated.

The results of the agglutination tests are summarized in table 2. It was found that all strains culturally B. suipestifer agglutinated identically with the type strain 49, and the record of this strain may be accepted as the summary for the group.

[4] Jour. Med. Research, 1918, 38, p. 112.

[5] Tenbroeck: Jour. Exper. Med., 1918, 28, p. 764.

[6] Jour. Med. Research, 1918, 38, p. 105.

TABLE 2

HIGHEST SERUM DILUTION SHOWING PERCEPTIBLE AGGLUTINATION

Cultures	Serums				
	B. suipestifer 49	Intermediate 91	B. paratyphosus B B96	B. paratyphosus A A98	B. enteritidis E117
B. suipestifer 49	1:30,000	1:15,000	1:3,000	....	....
Intermediates Rabbit 91 Swine 163	1:15,000	1:30,000	1:7,500	....	....
B. paratyphosus A Human A98 Swine 134 Virus 149	....	....	....	1:15,000	....
B. paratyphosus B Human B96 Rabbit 124, 135	1:3,000	1:3,000	1:15,000	....	....
B. enteritidis Human E117	....	....	....	....	1:7,500

Rabbit strain 91 and swine strain 163 are not only agglutinatively identical, but have affinities for both B. suipestifer and B. paratyphosus B, and should be regarded as intermediates.

The agglutination tests of rabbit strains 124 and 135 confirm the cultural evidence of their identity with human B. paratyphosus B 96. Rabbit strain 134 and virus strain 149 are likewise identical with B. paratyphosus A strain 98.

Absorption tests were set up whenever necessary to clear up the confusion of group agglutination. These results are summarized in table 3. Only the essential ones are recorded.

TABLE 3

ABSORPTION TESTS SHOWING RELATIONSHIP BETWEEN INTERMEDIATES AND B. SUIPESTIFER

Cultures	Serums					
	B. suipestifer 49		Intermediate 91		B. paratyphosus B B96	
	Absorbed by Intermediate 91	Absorbed by B. paratyphosus B B96	Absorbed by B. suipestifer 49	Absorbed by B. paratyphosus B B96	Absorbed by B. suipestifer 49	Absorbed by Intermediate 91
B. suipestifer 49	1:30,000	1:30,000	1:750	1:15,000	....	....
Intermediates Rabbit 91 Swine 163	....	1:15,000	1:7,500	1:30,000	....	....
B. paratyphosus B Human B96 Rabbit 124, 135	....	....	....	....	1:15,000	1:15,000

The record of type strain B. suipestifer 49 may again be accepted as representative of the strains culturally B. suipestifer.

Intermediate strains 91 and 163 are evidently identical and distinct alike from B. suipestifer and B. paratyphosus B. At the same time the absorption of antiserum 91 by B. suipestifer 49 antigen indicates close relationship.

Rabbit strains 124 and 135 are identical with B. paratyphosus B 96.

SUMMARY

An intimate study of the tissues of carcasses of several hundred swine dying of enteric diseases has shown the predominating bacterial flora to be members of the paratyphoid-enteritidis group.

Thirty-four out of 40 strains studied in detail were typical B. suipestifers; two were identical with human B. paratyphosus A; two were identical with human B. paratyphosus B; two were intermediate between B. suipestifer and B. paratyphosus B. B. enteritidis was not encountered at any time.

No true representative of the paratyphoid-enteritidis group has been isolated from feces nor from the lumen of the intestine in a large number of attempts. This fact is very striking in view of the predominance of this group in the tissues.

It has been possible in this work to confirm in all respects the reports of other workers on the value of arabinose, xylose, dulcite, inosite, lead acetate agar, and glucose serum water as diagnostic mediums for the differentiation of the members of the paratyphoid-enteritidis group.

AN INTRACELLULAR PROTOZOAN PARASITE OF THE DUCTS OF THE SALIVARY GLANDS OF THE GUINEA-PIG

WITH ONE PLATE

LEILA JACKSON

From the John McCormick Institute for Infectious Diseases, Chicago

In the course of an examination of the various salivary glands of the guinea-pig for an entirely different purpose, a peculiar protozoan infection of the ducts was observed, which seemed of sufficient interest to warrant further study. Accordingly, a microscopic examination was made of the salivary glands of 48 guinea-pigs. Through the kindness of Dr. H. J. Corper, I was able to secure salivary glands from 18 tuberculous guinea-pigs that came originally from Pennsylvania and had been brought here but a few days before they were killed. The kidneys of most of these animals were also examined as they are sometimes the seat of a coccidial infection. The intestines, unfortunately, were examined in only a few cases. The disease apparently causes the animal very little, if any, inconvenience and no gross pathologic changes were distinguished in the glands. On microscopic examination it was found that glands from 26 of the 48 guinea-pigs were infected. The infection occurred in about the same proportion of cases in the guinea-pigs obtained from Dr. Corper and in those from our own laboratory. The ducts of the serous portions of the glands are the favorite location of the parasite, but they are occasionally found in the ducts of the mucous glands, especially if the infection is severe. Many of the guinea-pigs had very mild infections, and the chief change aside from the presence of parasites in the cells of the ducts was a small amount of mononuclear infiltration about affected ducts, and in presumably early cases even this was lacking. In the cases in which the process was advanced, considerable portions of the gland were involved and more or less destruction of ducts and glandular tissue was evident.

The protozoan, as it most often appears in the cells of the ducts of the salivary gland, is an encysted organism of irregular, round or oval contour. In its most conspicuous and fully developed form it

Received for publication Dec. 16, 1919.

practically replaces the host cell which still retains its relations to the duct wall. The center is occupied by a round or oval body of irregular outline which stains deeply and unevenly. Around this central or restiform body is a rather wide, lightly stained zone, and outside of this a peripheral zone or capsule which may vary considerably in width, the widest part being that directed toward the lumen of the duct.

From a study of the parasite it appears that the chromatin condenses at various points on the surface of the central body, and smaller bodies bud off and proceed through the intermediate zone to the periphery where they possibly undergo further division. These smaller, deeply stained bodies of irregular outline and unequal size, are seen in various stages of separation from the central body and in various positions in the intermediate zone, and in some instances the chromatin material forms bands of considerable width extending from the central body to the border of the peripheral zone (Fig. 5). The appearance of radiating lines from the central body to the periphery at a certain stage of development is evidently the result of this budding off process.

Considering the large number of round, lightly stained bodies, which appear in the peripheral zone of the parasite at a certain stage of its development, and the comparatively few more deeply stained, irregularly shaped bodies seen in the process of separation from the central body and in the various stages of progress toward the peripheral zone, it seems not unlikely that further division of the latter bodies takes place when they reach the outer part of the intermediate zone; this, however, cannot be stated with certainty. The peripheral zone, as previously stated, varies considerably in width and stains more deeply than the intermediate zone, and in the later stages of development it contains large numbers of round bodies which collect for the most part in the portion of the capsule nearest the lumen of the duct. I have not been able to satisfy myself as to the exact number of these bodies, if indeed there is a definite number given off by each parasite. As counted in the stained preparations, they vary in number in the apparently fully developed forms from 30-40 or more. A form of the parasite which differs somewhat from that just described is seen only occasionally (Fig. 4). It is about the size of the large forms just described. In the intermediate zone is a band apparently made up of small, elongated bodies which seem to radiate from the central body. This band nearly or entirely encircles the restiform body, and is separated from it and from the peripheral zone by a clear space. No rounded bodies are seen in the peripheral zone. Just what is the significance of this form is not evident.

The earliest form of the parasite observed is a small, round, deeply stained body embedded in the cytoplasm of the epithelial cell of the duct (Fig. 3). As the parasite grows it develops an enveloping membrane or capsule, and later a definite intermediate zone appears between the deeply stained restiform body and the capsule. A form frequently seen is one in which the central body is elongated with the chromatin massed at the two poles.

In infections of long standing one may often find the cast off restiform body in the lumen of the duct and occasionally in the tissue just outside the duct. It appears as a pink stained vacuolated body of irregularly round or oval shape. That the parasite penetrates to the tissues about the ducts in the severed infections seems probable. I have observed what I believe to be young forms in the infiltrated regions about the ducts in which the epithelium has largely been destroyed and occasionally young forms appear in the glandular cells in these cases, but no fully developed types have been observed in these locations. In the severe infections one may find four or five of the organisms in a cross section of a duct, or if the section is lengthwise of the duct, the parasites are arranged side by side, and projecting into the lumen present a sawtooth-like appearance.

It seems evident from the foregoing that we are concerned with the vegetative cycle of an intracellular protozoan, the sexual cycle of which does not occur in this location. Since during this stage of development apparently no organs of locomotion are produced and the parasite becomes encysted, it probably belongs to the class protozoa and from its intracellular position most likely among coccidia. This being the case, we may consider the small round bodies in the peripheral zone of the parasite as merozoits.

Whether the parasite gains entrance to the salivary gland by way of the ducts from the oral cavity or by way of the blood stream is not obvious. If infection takes place by way of the ducts, the progress of the parasite up the duct is against the flow of saliva as the epithelial cells of the distal portions of the ducts are never invaded. Whatever the mode of entrance, it is evident that the larger ducts do not offer favorable conditions for the growth of the parasite.

The parasite stains fairly well by the ordinary staining methods, hematoxylin and eosin, methylene blue and eosin, polychrome methylene blue and eosin and Giemsa.

A routine microscopic examination of the other organs of guinea-pigs was not carried out, except in a few cases in which the results were negative, with the exception of the kidneys. The kidneys of 44 of the 48 guinea-pigs were examined for protozoa, and 12 were found positive. The organisms present were usually few in number and apparently correspond with the forms of Klossiella muris described by Smith and Johnson[1] and Louise Pearce,[2] but appear to have no relation to the parasites in the salivary gland.

[1] Jour. Exper. Med., 1901-5, 6, p. 303.
[2] Ibid., 1916, 23, p. 431.

Explanation of Plate

Fig. 1.—Area of infiltration in which are infected ducts, × 130.

Fig. 2.—A duct containing four large parasites, in three of which merozoits are easily distinguished, × 650.

Fig. 3.—A duct containing two large forms and an early form of the parasite, × 680.

Fig. 4.—A duct containing four parasites, the lower one of which is a form seen only occasionally, × 680.

Fig. 5.—A large form of the parasite showing budding of small bodies from the restiform body, × 680.

Plate

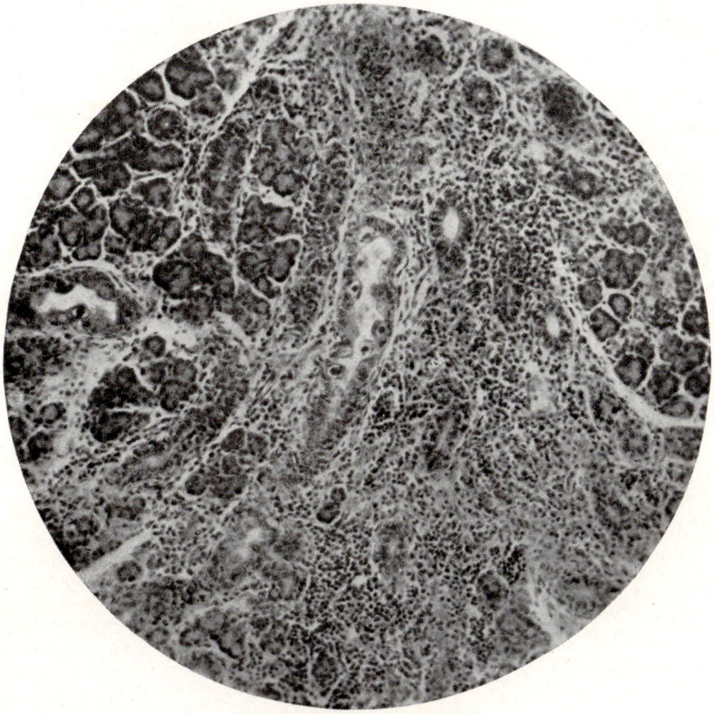

1

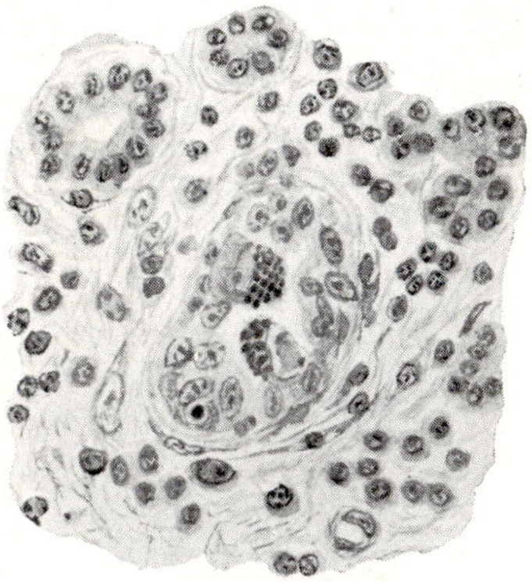

3

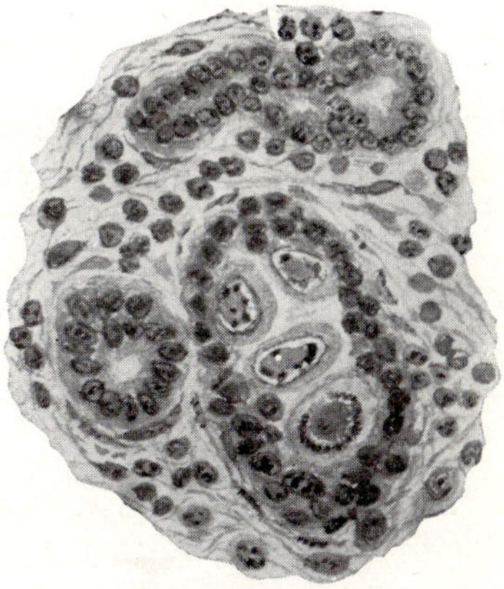

4

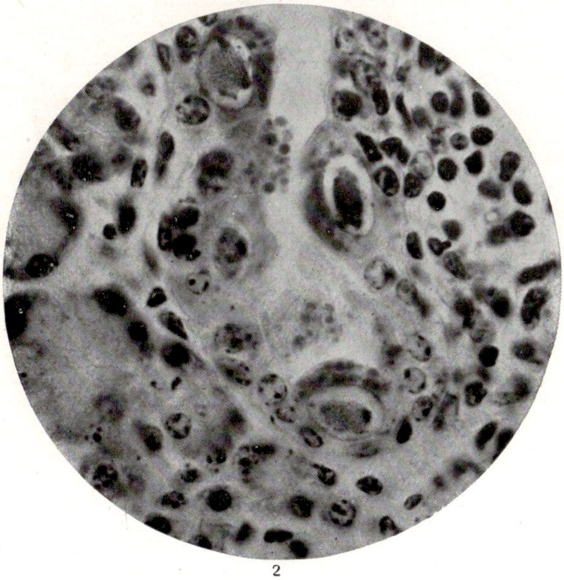

2

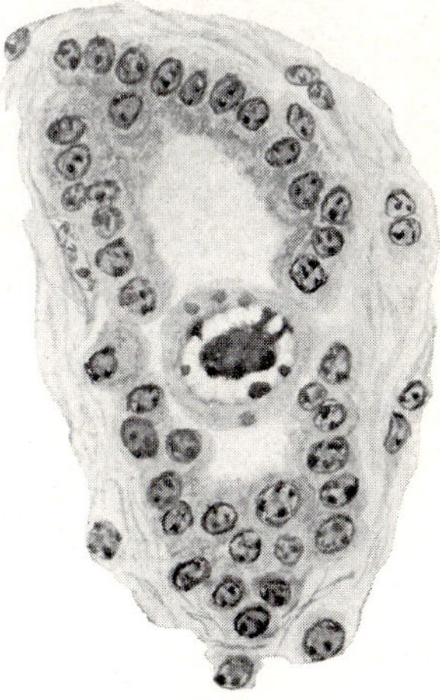

5

Jackson: Intracellular Protozoon Parasite of Ducts of Salivary Glands of Guinea-Pigs

AN INQUIRY INTO THE CAUSES FOR VARIATION IN DETERMINATIONS OF DISINFECTING VALUE *

Bernard Fantus and Florence Rumry

From the John McCormick Memorial Institute for Infectious Disease, Chicago

Having noted discrepancies in results of experiments for the determination of the disinfecting value of chemicals, especially in tests made on different days, we attempted to determine the reason for these variations. Difference in number of organisms in the culture on different days was the first thing that suggested itself as a cause. We therefore purposely varied, to a considerable degree, the number of organisms added to the water prior to disinfection.

Technic.—A 24-hour typhoid culture grown in standard broth of a reaction of + 1.5 acid to phenolphthalein was filtered through paper and, in different experiments, quantities varying from 0.1 ml. to 3 ml. were discharged into 75 ml. of water contained in wide-mouthed sterile glass-stoppered bottles. Samples from each of these were taken for counting the number of bacteria by the usual technic. The infected bottles were brought to a temperature of 20 C. and kept at this temperature by means of a water bath. To each bottle was then added 25 ml. of N/1 citric acid solution so that the resulting dilution represented N/4 strength; the contents of the bottles were then shaken, and subcultures taken at intervals. The results were read after 48 hours' incubation by noting the turbidity of the tubes in which growth had taken place.

The results are given in table 1, from which it will be seen that the length of time required for disinfection is not in proportion to the number of bacteria present, in variations between 10 to 1,000 millions per ml.

We next tested the theory that clumps were responsible for the variation in results, having noted that, at times, pellicles were present on the surface of the 24-hour cultures. The filtered culture that was used for inoculating the water to be disinfected being quite turbid, we modified the technic in the next experiment by centrifuging the culture at moderate speed for from one half to one hour, or until it was clear. We employed 1 and 3 ml. of centrifuged culture for the various tests. Our aim was to present single bacterial bodies to the action of the dis-

Received for publication Dec. 16, 1919.

* Aided by a grant from the Fenger Memorial Fund.

TABLE 1

RESULT OF EXPERIMENTS. NUMBER OF BACTERIA SEEMS TO HAVE NO DETERMINING EFFECT ON TIME REQUIRED FOR DISINFECTION

Millions per ml.	10.0	12.5	15.0	20.0	25.0	30.0	40.0	50.0	63.0	80.0	100.0 Min.
1000.0											
800.0							x				
630.0							x x				
500.0						x x					
400.0							x				
300.0							x	x			
250.0											
200.0						x					
150.0											
125.0					x			x			
100.0											
80.0											
63.0							x				
50.0						x			x		
40.0						x					
30.0											
25.0											
20.0											
15.0										x	
12.5											
10.0											

TABLE 2

DISINFECTION OF WATER INOCULATED WITH CENTRIFUGED CULTURE. AVERAGE DISINFECTING TIME 15 MINUTES

		x				
		x				
	x	x				
	x	x				
	x	x	x			
x	x	x	x			
x	x	x	x			
x	x	x	x			
x	x	x	x			
x	x	x	x	x		
5	10	15	25	40	60	Minutes

infectant. The results shown in table 2, in which each x represents the end point in one experiment, show that centrifugalization lessens the disinfection time, but does not contribute to much greater constancy of results. That the lessening of the disinfection time was not due to numbers, was shown by the following facts: 1. No consistent differences were found between those experiments in which we used 1 ml. and those in which we used 3 ml. for inoculating the water. 2. A few counts showed the bacteria present in the water to be well above the lower count of our previous experiment.

TABLE 3

DISINFECTION OF WATER INOCULATED WITH CULTURE CENTRIFUGED WITH COTTON. AVERAGE DISINFECTING TIME 25 MINUTES

			x			
			x			
			x			
			x			
			x			
			x			
	x	x	x			
	x	x	x			
	x	x	x			
	x	x	x			
	x	x	x	x	x	
	x	x	x	x	x	
5	10	15	25	40	60	Minutes

As it was found difficult to be absolutely certain that the clumps were entirely excluded in the experiments shown in table 2, owing to the fact that some of the sediment at the bottom of the centrifuge tube would tend to float upward into the liquid during the subsequent manipulations, we placed, in our next series of experiments, sterilized absorbent cotton in the bottom of the centrifuge tube, so as to entangle the sediment. This was quite successful as far as eliminating visible clumps was concerned. That this modification had no effect on constancy of results is shown in table 3. For the fact that, in this set of experiments, the disinfection time was actually somewhat lengthened—to an average of 25 minutes as compared with an average of 15 minutes in experiment 2—we have no explanation to offer.

CONCLUSIONS

Within the limits of the observations made, neither variations in the numbers of bacteria nor the presence of clumps are the determining factors for variations in results in observations on disinfecting time.

The reason for these variations has not been determined.

To command confidence in results in experiments of this kind, a much larger number of observations is required than are usually made; the average might then be noted, and only large differences in disinfection time considered conclusive evidence of difference between different agents.

CHEMOTHERAPEUTIC STUDIES WITH ETHYLHYDRO-CUPREIN AND MERCUROPHEN IN EXPERIMENTAL PNEUMOCOCCUS MENINGITIS IN RABBITS

John A. Kolmer and Goro Idzumi

From the McManes Laboratory of Experimental Pathology of the University of Pennsylvania, Philadelphia

Pneumococcus meningitis, whether originating as a local infection of the cerebral meninges by extension from the ear and accessory nasal sinuses, during pneumonia, or developing as a spontaneous infection without a discoverable primary lesion, is a highly fatal disease; in the experience of one of us with fourteen cases of this infection, death resulted in all. Fortunately the disease is not common and does not occur in epidemics; reliable statistics are not available, but an analysis of the available literature shows that the mortality is over 90%.

Serum treatment of this infection either with polyvalent serums or the monovalent serum for type 1 infections, has failed materially to influence the disease; the studies of Lamar[1] with experimental pneumococcus meningitis in monkeys, have shown that the serum alone has but slight curative value, although encouraging and frequently brilliant results were observed with mixtures of serum, sodium oleate and boric acid, the sodium oleate rendering the organisms more vulnerable to the serum. These results were observed only when specific serum was employed, that is, the serum corresponding to the type of pneumococcus producing the disease; the antiserum for type 1 was ineffective for type 2 infections even in the presence of sodium oleate.

Systematic studies in the chemotherapy of pneumococcus meningitis do not appear to have been made; owing to the comparative ease with which the disease may be produced experimentally, providing highly virulent cultures are available, it would appear a particularly interesting field for experimental study under conditions closely resembling a disease occurring among persons. The fact that the subarachnoid space is practically a closed one with circulation of the cerebrospinal

Received for publication Jan. 3, 1920.

[1] Jour. Exper. Med., 1912, 16, p. 581.

fluid resulting in a diffusion of substances introduced in the lumbar regions until such time as inflammatory changes interfere, renders experiments in meningitis particularly serviceable in chemotherapeutic studies in bacterial infections.

PURPOSES OF INVESTIGATION

In the chemotherapy of pneumococcus infections various compounds of quinin, and particularly the optochin of Morgenroth and Levy,[2] have given the most encouraging results. As a result of the work of these investigators in addition to that of Moore[3] and Cohen, Kolmer and Heist[4] in this country, showing the high pneumococcidal activity of ethylhydrocuprein hydrochlorid in test tube experiments and some protective and curative activity in experimental pneumococcus infections in mice,[5] we decided to study the probable influence of this substance alone and in combination with antipneumococcus serum and sodium oleate on pneumococcus meningitis experimentally produced in rabbits. Additional experiments were conducted with some of the ordinary soluble salts of quinin, notably the hydrobromid, and also with sodium oxymercury ortho-nitro-phenolate prepared by Schamberg, Kolmer and Raiziss,[6] a mercurial designated "mercurophen" and possessing certain superior properties as high germicidal activity for pathogenic cocci notably staphylococci and pneumococci, lesser toxicity as compared with other mercurials on the basis of content of mercury, and remarkable freedom from precipitating influence on serum proteins.

Our experiments were conducted by first determining the toxicity of these various substances by subthecal injection in rabbits followed by a study of their influence in varying dosage on the course of infections produced by the subthecal injection of virulent pneumococci; the object of this paper is to record briefly the results of these experiments with ethylhydrocuprein hydrochlorid and mercurophen inasmuch as the former particularly yielded encouraging results and may prove of some aid in the treatment of pneumococcus meningitis during the early stages of this highly mortal disease.

[2] Berl. klin. Wchnschr., 1911, 48, pp. 1561, 1650, 1779, 1983.
[3] Jour. Exper. Med., 1915, 22, p. 269.
[4] Jour. Infect. Dis., 1917, 20, p. 272.
[5] Moore, H. F.: Jour. Exper. Med., 1915, 22, p. 551 Cohen, S. S.: Kolmer, J. A., and Heist, G. D.: Jour. Infect. Dis., 1917, 20, p. 313.
[6] Jour. Infect. Dis., 1919, 24, p. 547.

EXPERIMENTAL PNEUMOCOCCUS MENINGITIS

The lesions were produced in rabbits by the subthecal injection in the lumbar region of virulent pneumococci suspended in physiologic salt solutions; as to be described,[7] a definite train of lesions and symptoms follow in the nature of an acute suppurative leptomeningitis involving the spinal cord and base of the brain accompanied by cloudy spinal fluid, fever, leukocytosis, hyperesthesia, opisthotonus and convulsions.

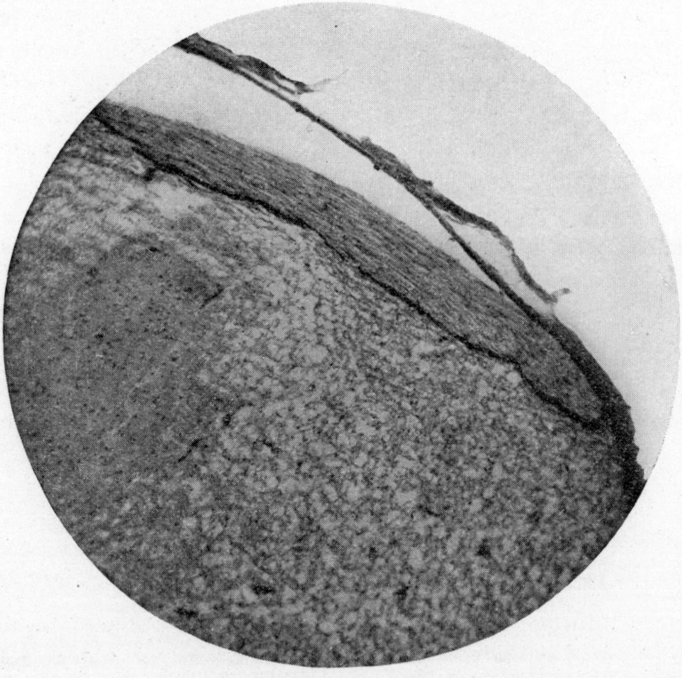

Fig. 1.—Section of spinal cord in dorsal region of a rabbit succumbing 36 hours after the subthecal injection in the lumbar region of 0.5 c c of 1: 100 ethylhydrocuprein per kilogram of weight; shows slight hyperemia and leukocytic infiltration of the meninges with involvement of the adjacent cord substance; × 70.

Types 1 and 2 strains of pneumococci were used; the latter were freshly cultivated from the spinal fluid of a fatal case of meningitis. The type 1 strain proved fatal for white mice of about 20 gm. in weight in 48 hours in a dose of 0.001 c c of 18 to 24 hour broth culture; the type 2 strain was more virulent inasmuch as it regularly killed mice in 48 hours in a dose of 0.00001 c c of 24-hour broth cultures. According to body weight, rabbits required about ten times larger doses injected subthecally to produce a fatal leptomeningitis accompanied by pneumococcus bacteremia; for example, rabbits weighing about 2,000 gm. required 0.01 c c of type 2 to produce a fatal meningitis in about 48 hours, which calculated on the base of body weight, is ten times greater

[7] Idzumi, G.: Experimental Pneumococcus Meningitis in Rabbits and Dogs. This journal.

than the minimum lethal dose for mice by intraperitoneal injection (table 1). Smaller doses of these cultures produced milder forms of meningitis and prolonged life for one or more days.

TABLE 1

VIRULENCE OF TYPE 2 PNEUMOCOCCUS FOR RABBITS BY INTRASPINAL INJECTION

Weight in Grams	Dose in c c	Results	Necropsy	Cultures at Necropsy	
				Heart	Spinal Fluid
2,300	1.0	Died in 12 hours	Acute meningitis	+*	+
1,800	0.5	Died in 12 hours	Acute meningitis	+	+
2,000	0.1	Died in 26 hours	Acute meningitis	+	+
2,100	0.01	Died in 38 hours	....	+	+
1,800	0.001	Died in 72 hours	Acute meningitis	+	+
1,700	0.0001	Lived			

Virulent for mice by intraperitoneal injection 0.00001 c c in 48 hours.
* + = pneumococci in cultures; — = sterile.

TOXICITY OF ETHYLHYDROCUPREIN HYDROCHLORID FOR RABBITS BY SUBTHECAL INJECTIONS

According to Moore,[5] solutions of ethylhydrocuprein hydrochlorid slowly injected intravenously into rabbits proved immediately fatal in doses of about 0.06 gm. per kilo of body weight, the tolerated dose being 0.02 to 0.05 gm. per kilo; Cohen, Kolmer and Heist[5] found the immediate lethal dose about 0.06 gm. per kilo and the highest tolerated dose about 0.02 to 0.04 gm. per kilo of body weight in a period of 10 days. As is well known, the drug may produce a toxic amblyopia in persons, and its therapeutic usefulness has been thereby reduced.

TABLE 2

TOXICITY OF ETHYLHYDROCUPREIN HYDROCHLORID BY INTRASPINAL INJECTION

Weight in Grams	Dose per kilo	Equivalent in Grams	Results	Necropsy
1,700	0.5 c c of 1:50	0.01	Died in 12 hours	Acute congestion; meningitis
2,300	0.5 c c of 1:100	0.005	Died in 36 hours	Acute meningitis
2,400	0.5 c c of 1:500	0.001	Lived indefinitely	
1,800	0.5 c c of 1:500	0.001	Killed in 48 hours	Mild meningitis
2,000	1.0 c c of 1:500	0.002	Killed in 96 hours	Mild meningitis
2,000	0.5 c c of 1:1,000	0.0005	Lived indefinitely	
1,800	0.5 c c of 1:1,000	0.0005	Killed in 48 hours	No meningitis
2,000	1.0 c c of 1:1,000	0.001	Killed in 96 hours	No meningitis
2,500	0.5 c c of 1:2,000	0.00025	Lived indefinitely	
1,700	0.5 c c of 1:5,000	0.0001	Lived indefinitely	

Solutions of the drug in salt solution injected subthecally in rabbits have proved fatal in doses of 0.03 to 0.05 gm. per kilo of body weight in 48 hours as shown in table 2. These amounts dissolved in 0.5 c c salt solutions per kilo of weight produce paralysis of the hind legs in the majority of animals and an acute meningitis characterized by marked hyperemia and slight leukocytic infiltration of the meninges, especially in the lumbar region near the site of injection, but also extending to the base of the brain. Smaller doses as 0.001 gm. in 0.5 c c of salt solution per kilo of body weight usually do not produce symptoms, but may produce slight congestion of the meninges at the site of the injection; 0.0005 gm., equivalent to 0.5 c c of a 1:1,000 dilution per kilo, did not produce any symptoms or discernible changes in the meninges and has been generally employed by us in the therapeutic experiments. This dose corresponds to 30 c c of a 1:1,000 dilution per 60 kilo of weight and represents a safe dose of ethylhydrocuprein hydrochlorid for adult persons by subthecal administration.

Toxicity of Mercurophen for Rabbits by Subthecal Injection

Schamberg, Kolmer, Raiziss and Trist have found the tolerated dose of mercurophen for white rats by intravenous injection to be 0.006 to 0.008 gm. per kilo of weight over a period of 10 days; by subthecal injection in rabbits we have found the lethal dose of mercurophen about 0.002 to 0.004 gm. per kilo of body weight in about 48 hours (table 3); these doses produce paralysis of the hind legs and a severe meningitis characterized by intense hyperemia and hemorrhagic extravasation in the meninges, particularly in the neighborhood of the site of injection in the lumbar regions. In dose of 0.0005 gm. per kilo of weight, equivalent to 1 c c of a 1:2,000 dilution, mercurophen does not produce paralysis or prove fatal for normal rabbits but may produce slight hyperemia of the meninges in the immediate site of injection; when injected subthecally in rabbits with pneumococcus meningitis the toxic effects are more marked and may hasten the death of the animal as compared with untreated control animals.

TABLE 3

Toxicity of Mercurophen for Rabbits by Intraspinal Injection

Weight in Grams	Dose per Kilo	Equivalent in Grams	Results	Necropsy
1,700	1 c c of 1:500	0.002	Paralysis; died in 58 hours	Acute hemorrhagic meningitis
1,900	1 c c of 1:1,000	0.001	Slight paralysis; lived*	Mild meningitis at site of injection
2,200	1 c c of 1:2,000	0.0005	No paralysis; lived*	No meningitis
2,100	1 c c of 1:5,000	0.0002	No paralysis; lived*	No irritation of meninges

* Killed after 96 hours.

Therefore, both ethylhydrocuprein and mercurophen are equally or probably slightly more toxic when injected subthecally than when introduced directly into the venous blood; probably this is due in part to the local injury consequent to lumbar puncture and more especially to the direct effect of these substances on the delicate nervous structures with which they are brought into immediate contact.

The Pneumococcidal Activity of Ethylhydrocuprein Hydrochlorid and Mercurophen in the Spinal Fluid of Acute Meningitis

While both ethylhydrocuprein hydrochlorid and mercurophen possess extremely high germicidal values for pneumococci in a broth or salt solution, this activity is materially reduced in the presence of large amounts of serum proteins and it was necessary to determine their pneumococcidal activity in the spinal fluids of acute meningitis before undertaking experiments on their influence in experimental pneumococcus meningitis.

For this purpose turbid spinal fluids containing many thousands of pus cells per cubic millimeter and yielding strongly positive Pandy and Noguchi reactions for proteins were used. In one of these fluids within a few hours after removal from a person with meningitis, type 2 pneumococci identified by serologic methods were present in large numbers and were mostly extracellular; in other experiments spinal fluid containing type 1 pneumococci (extracellular) was employed.

In the tests varying amounts of spinal fluid were mixed with a solution of the drugs in sterile salt solution and the mixtures kept on a water bath at 38 C.; at varying intervals from 2 to 4 loopfuls of each mixture were subcultured in tubes of glucose blood broth and observed over a period of 72 hours to determine germicidal activity. The results of several experiments shown in tables 4, 5 and 6 give the amounts of spinal fluid and drug employed and the final dilutions.

TABLE 4

GERMICIDAL ACTIVITY OF ETHYLHYDROCUPREIN AND QUININ HYDROBROMID FOR TYPE 2 PNEUMOCOCCI IN SPINAL FLUID

Drug 1 c c	Spinal Fluid	Final Dilution	Results of Subcultures after Exposure for Minutes at 28 C.					
			5	15	30	45	60	90
Ethylhydrocuprein 1:1,000	1 c c	1:2,000	+*	+	—	—	—	—
Ethylhydrocuprein 1:2,000	1 c c	1:4,000	+	+	+	+	—	—
Ethylhydrocuprein 1:5,000	1 c c	1:10,000	+	+	+	+	+	—
Ethylhydrocuprein 1:25,000	1 c c	1:50,000	+	+	+	+	+	+
Quinin hydro. 1:100	1 c c	1:200	+	+	+	+	—	—
Quinin hydro. 1:200	1 c c	1:400	+	+	+	+	+	+
Salt solution	1 c c	....	+	+	+	+	+	+

* + = pneumococci; — = sterile.

TABLE 5

GERMICIDAL ACTIVITY OF MERCUROPHEN FOR TYPE 2 PNEUMOCOCCI IN SPINAL FLUID OF MENINGITIS

Spinal Fluid, c c	Mercurophen, 0.1 c c	Final Dilution	Results of Subcultures after Exposure for Minutes at 38 C.					
			5	15	30	45	60	120
0.3	1:250	1:1,000	—*	—	—	—	—	—
0.3	1:500	1:2,000	—	—	—	—	—	—
0.2	1:1,000	1:3,000	+	—	—	—	—	—
0.3	1:1,000	1:4,000	+	+	+	+	—	—
0.5	1:1,000	1:6,000	+	+	+	+	+	+
0.7	1:1,000	1:8,000	+	+	+	+	+	+
1.0	None	....	+	+	+	+	+	+

* — = sterile; + = pneumococci.

TABLE 6

GERMICIDAL ACTIVITY OF MERCUROPHEN FOR TYPE 1 PNEUMOCOCCI IN SPINAL FLUID OF MENINGITIS

Spinal Fluid, c c	Mercurophen, 0.1 c c	Final Dilution	Results of Subcultures after Exposure for Minutes at 38 C.					
			5	15	30	45	60	120
0.3	1:250	1:1,000	—*	—	—	—	—	—
0.3	1:500	1:2,000	—	—	—	—	—	—
0.2	1:1,000	1:3,000	—	—	—	—	—	—
0.3	1:1,000	1:4,000	+	+	—	—	—	—
0.5	1:1,000	1:6,000	+	+	+	+	+	+

* — = sterile; + = pneumococci.

As shown in table 4 ethylhydrocuprein hydrochlorid proved germicidal for type 2 pneumococci in dilutions of 1 : 2,000 in 30 minutes; in 1 : 4,000 in one hour and 1 : 10,000 in 1½ hours; quinin hydrobromid was much less active proving germicidal in but 1 : 200 in an hour. Inasmuch as ethylhydrocuprein could be used in rabbits in a dose of 0.5 c c of 1 : 1,000 dilution per kilo of weight, and assuming that there are about from 2 to 3 c c of spinal fluid per kilo of weight equivalent to from 120 to 180 c c per adult of about 125 pounds, the final dilution of the drug in the spinal fluid of normal rabbits was about 1 : 6,000 providing diffusion occurred. Experiments with dye stuffs have shown that 0.5 c c of 1% solutions injected subthecally in the lumbar region of rabbits diffuse along the entire cord and base of the brain within from 3 to 6 hours, but may not be found in the ventricles; accordingly the final dilution

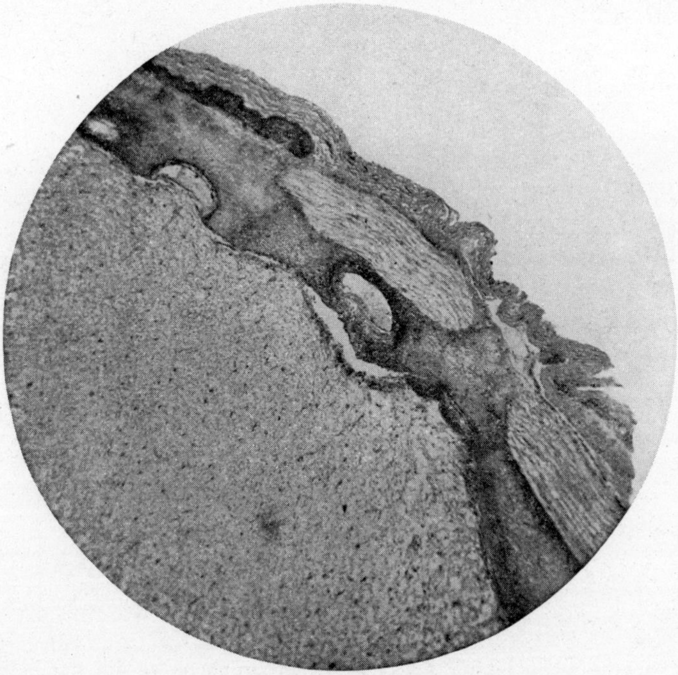

Fig. 2.—Section of spinal cord of rabbit in dorsal region succumbing 48 hours after the subthecal injection in the lumbar region of 0.5 c c of 1 : 500 mercurophen per kilogram of weight; shows marked hemorrhagic meningitis; × 70.

of drug in the subarachnoid space may not be as high as stated, and in view of the results observed with germicidal tests in vitro with purulent spinal fluids it was reasonable to expect that sufficient amounts of ethylhydrocuprein hydrochlorid could be injected subthecally to influence the course of a pneumococcus meningitis even though the amount of spinal fluid was increased by the inflammatory processes. In view of the much lower pneumococcidal activity of the ordinary soluble salts of quinin in purulent spinal fluids and since their toxicity is close to that of ethylhydrocuprein,[5] we did not regard it possible to influence the course of experimental meningitis and experiments subsequently showed the truth of this assumption.

Similar experiments with mercurophen have shown a well defined pneumococcidal activity; as shown in table 5, this substance proved completely germicidal in 5 minutes in a final dilution of 1:2,000 and in 60 minutes in a final dilution of 1:4,000 employing the same purulent spinal fluid used in the tests with ethylhydrocuprein hydrochlorid. Similar results were observed with type 1 pneumococci (table 6) and indicate that while mercurophen acts somewhat more quickly and is more germicidal than ethylhydrocuprein hydrochlorid in short exposures, the latter excels somewhat in the larger exposures. Owing,

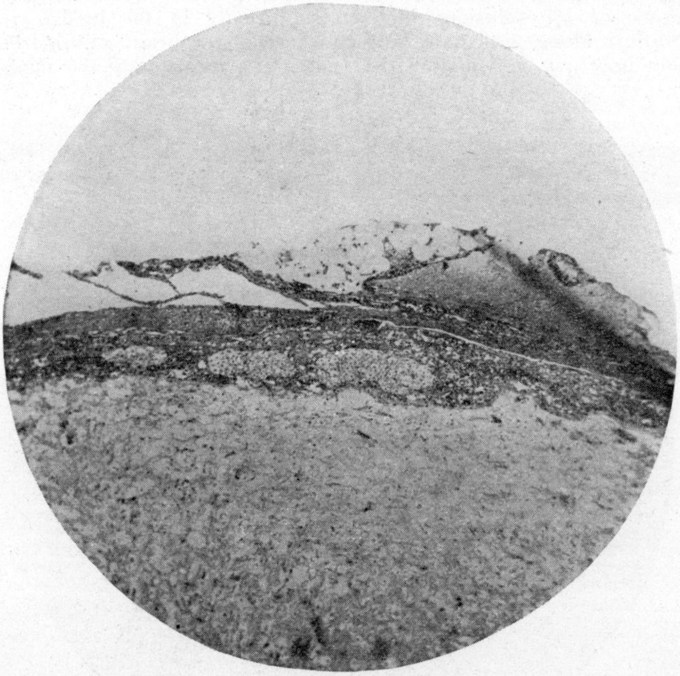

Fig. 3.—Section of spinal cord of rabbit in dorsal region succumbing four days after the subthecal injection of type 1 pneumococci in the lumbar region; shows purulent leptomeningitis; × 70.

however, to the much higher toxicity of mercurophen, we did not believe that a sufficient amount could be injected subthecally in one dose to impart to the spinal fluid well defined germicidal activity. Subsequent experiments have shown this to be true.

THE INFLUENCE OF ETHYLHYDROCUPREIN HYDROCHLORID ON EXPERIMENTAL PNEUMOCOCCUS MENINGITIS

With these preliminary experiments finished, the study was continued by producing severe leptomeningitis in rabbits by the subthecal injection in the lumbar region of type 1 or type 2 pneumococci suspended in warm salt solution. At varying intervals the drug was injected subthecally about two interspaces higher in the lumbar region and the animals carefully observed over a period of several days. Temperature observations and leukocyte counts were made at regular intervals and the influence of ethylhydrocuprein determined by these observations in addition to the clinical condition of each animal and the duration of its life as compared with numerous controls. Owing to the small size of the animals, it was not always possible to secure spinal fluid for examination; a drop or two was the largest amount that could be secured suitable for films and permitting observations on the nature of the exudate in the spinal fluid and the degree of phagocytosis. The clinical symptoms, duration of life and results of complete postmortem examinations, including a histologic examination of the cord and brain of each animal, were the chief criteria for judging the results which are presented in the form of tables and omitting detailed descriptions of individual animals for the purpose of brevity.

Table 7 shows the results of one experiment employing type 1 pneumococci; the control died on the fourth day with well defined leptomeningitis. A large dose of ethylhydrocuprein as 0.5 c c of a 1:100 dilution per kilo of body weight produced paralysis in a control and hastened the death of an infected animal; smaller doses of the drug, however, prolonged the lives of several animals over an indefinite period when injected within 4 hours of the pneumococci. When the infection had been given a 24 or 48-hour start, the influence of the drug in prolonging life was not evident.

TABLE 7

INFLUENCE OF ETHYLHYDROCUPREIN HYDROCHLORID ON TYPE 1 MENINGITIS OF RABBITS

Weight in Grams	Dose of Drug per Kilo	Time of Injection of Drug in Relation to Infection	Result in Days							Lesions
			1	2	3	4	5	6	7	
1,600	0.5 c c of 1:100	At once	T	D	...	...	...	...	...	Acute congestion
1,500	0.5 c c of 1:500	4 hours	T	T	T	R	R	R	R	Paralysis
1,900	0.5 c c of 1:1,000	4 hours	T	T	R	R	R	R	R	
2,000	0.5 c c of 1:5,000	4 hours	T	T	T	T	T	R	R	
2,000	0.5 c c of 1:500	24 hours	T	T	T	T	D	...	...	Meningitis
2,100	0.5 c c of 1:500	48 hours	T	T	T	D	...	...	...	Meningitis
1,700	0.5 c c of 1:100	Control	T	T	R	R	R	R	R	Paralysis; recovered
1,800	1.0 c c salt sol.	Control	R	R	R	R	R	R	R	No paralysis
2,000	Control (culture)	....	T	T	T	D	...	...	...	Meningitis

Culture used in dose of 0.5 c c.
T = toxic; R = recovered; D = died.

These results are illustrative of those obtained in similar experiments employing this culture which possessed a moderate degree of virulence; even as small doses of drug as 0.5 c c of 1:5,000 dilution per kilo of body weight exerted a well defined protective value, providing the administration was within a few hours of the injection of cocci. These results were probably due to the actual destruction of the pneumococci while the organisms were confined to the subarachnoid space of the spinal cord; when well defined and widespread inflammatory changes became apparent with an increased volume of spinal fluid containing numerous pus cells, flakes of fibrin and great numbers of pneumococci, the curative influence of a single dose of ethylhydrocuprein was greatly reduced.

With the more virulent type 2 strain the curative value of a single dose of ethylhydrocuprein hydrochlorid was feeble, as shown in table 8; this culture in the dose employed, produced a particularly severe form of leptomeningitis and rendered the experiments unfavorable for the discovery of minor degrees of curative activity of the drugs studied. The controls usually died in about 48 hours with suppurative leptomeningitis; a single dose of ethylhydrocuprein would prolong the life for 1 or 2 days providing the drug was administered within 4 to 6 hours after the cocci.

TABLE 8

INFLUENCE OF ETHYLHYDROCUPREIN HYDROCHLORID ON TYPE 2 MENINGITIS OF RABBITS

Weight in Grams	Dose of Drug per Kilo	Time of Injection of Drug	Results in Days			Necropsy
			1	2	3	
1,700	1 c c of 1:1,000	2 hours after cocci	T†	T	D	Acute meningitis
1,500	1 c c of 1:1,000	6 hours after cocci	T	T	D	Acute meningitis
2,000	1 c c of 1:1,000	24 hours after cocci	T	D	..	Acute meningitis
2,000	0.5 c c of 1:1,000‡	2 hours after cocci	T	D	..	Acute meningitis
1,500	Control	....	T	D	..	Acute meningitis

* Culture used in dose of 0.005 c c of 24-hour culture intraspinally.
† T = toxic; D = died.
‡ Administered intravenously.

In other experiments consisting in the repeated injection of smaller doses of pneumococci followed 6 hours later by a subthecal injection of ethylhydrocuprein, in order to avoid an overwhelming infection and to similate more closely the method of procedure in the treatment of human infections, ethylhydrocuprein hydrochlorid showed a well defined curative or protective activity inasmuch as the treated animals generally survived for longer periods than the controls. As shown in tables 9 and 10, the repeated injection of the drug in dose of 0.5 c c of 1:1,000 solution per kilo of weight had no discernible injurious effect; several injections of cocci alone generally produced a fatal meningitis whereas in animals receiving the same doses of culture followed after an interval by a subthecal injection of the drug life was prolonged, in one instance for 12 days beyond the life of the control.

TABLE 9

INFLUENCE OF ETHYLHYDROCUPREIN HYDROCHLORID ON TYPE 2 MENINGITIS OF RABBITS

Weight in Grams	Culture c c*	Drug, Dose per Kilo†	Results
1,800	0.0001	None (control)	Died on 6th day
2,000	0.0001	0.5 c c of 1:1,000	Died on 12th day
2,000	0.0001	0.5 c c of 1:1,000	Died on 18th day
2,000	None	0.5 c c of 1:1,000	Lived indefinitely

* Culture 0.0001 c c given intraspinally on 1st, 3rd, 5th, 7th, 9th and 11th days.
† Administered intraspinally 6 hours after each injection of cocci.

TABLE 10

THE INFLUENCE OF DAILY INJECTIONS OF ETHYLHYDROCUPREIN HYDROCHLORID ON TYPE 2 MENINGITIS OF RABBITS

Weight in Grams	Culture c c	Drug, Dose per Kilo*	Results
2,000	0.0001	0.5 c c of 1:1,000	Died on 6th day
2,000	0.0001	None	Died on 3rd day

* Daily subthecal injections.

Experiments consisting in the intravenous injection of ethylhydrocuprein had no appreciable effect on the course of experimental meningitis.

Since the investigations of Kolmer, Cohen and Steinfield[8] have shown that the presence of ethylhydrocuprein hydrochlorid in leukocytic mixtures increases the phagocytosis of pneumococci, certain experiments were specially planned employing large rabbits for the purpose of conducting repeated examinations of the spinal fluids during the course of meningitis produced by the type 2 strain with and without treatment with ethylhydrocuprein. As previously stated, only sufficient fluid could be obtained during life for films; total cell counts were generally inaccurate owing to the presence of traces of blood.

Within a few hours after the injection of pneumococci many polymorphonuclear leukocytes were to be found in the spinal fluid; at the end of 24 hours these numbers had increased so rapidly along with an enormous proliferation of the organisms as to render the fluid distinctly turbid. Within 48 hours the fluid was rich in fibrin and particles of plastic exudate were to be found attached to the meninges, cord and base of the brain. The pneumococci were invariably extracellular; only occasionally would a pair or two be found within a polymorphonuclear leukocyte.

Films of fluid removed at varying intervals after the injection of ethylhydrocuprein frequently showed numerous phagocytes and at times swollen diplococci retaining the Gram stain poorly or not at all; evidence of the influence of ethylhydrocuprein on the organisms and the phenomenon of phagocytosis were especially marked when spinal fluid was secured within 4 to 6 hours after the injection of the drug.

Influence of Antipneumococcus Serum Alone and in Combination with Ethylhydrocuprein Hydrochlorid on Experimental Meningitis

Moore[9] has shown that mixtures of antipneumococcus serum type 2 and optochin (base) injected subcutaneously are more protective for mice infected by intraperitoneal injections of virulent pneumococci than either substance alone and beyond what could be expected as the summation of the protective value of each; Kolmer and Steinfield[10] have likewise found that ethylhydrocuprein injected subcutaneously usually increased the protective value of antipneumococcus serum for type 1 infections of mice.

Accordingly, we thought it of interest and value to study the influence of mixtures of antipneumococcus serum and ethylhydrocuprein on type 1 meningitis inasmuch as type 1 infections are occasionally encountered among persons suffering with pneumococcus meningitis.

The serum employed was not as good as it should have been but was the best obtainable at the time these experiments were conducted; this serum agglutinated the type 1 strain in final dilution of 1:32 and in dose of 0.2 c c protected mice against about 10 minimal lethal doses of culture, both tests being conducted after the Rockefeller Institute methods.

Experiments consisting in the treatment of meningitis with the serum alone administered subthecally in single dose of 1 c c per kilo of weight corresponding to 60 c c for a person weighing about 125 pounds and at intervals varying from 2 to 72 hours after the injection of the pneumococci, have generally

[8] Jour. Infect. Dis., 1917, 20, p. 334.
[9] Jour. Exper. Med., 1915, 22, p. 389.
[10] Jour. Infect. Dis., 1918, 22, p. 492.

yielded negative results as shown in one experiment in table 11; in other experiments some slight influence of the serum was apparent on the basis of prolongation of the lives of the experimental animals for 1 to 3 days beyond the duration of the lives of the controls, as shown in an experiment in table 12.

TABLE 11

THE INFLUENCE OF ANTIPNEUMOCOCCUS SERUM ON TYPE 1 MENINGITIS OF RABBITS

Weight in Grams	Serum, Dose per Kilo	Results
1,800	1 c c 2 hours after cocci	Lived 4 days; acute meningitis
2,000	1 c c 24 hours after cocci	Lived 5 days; acute meningitis
2,000	1 c c 48 hours after cocci	Lived 4 days; acute meningitis
1,800	1 c c 72 hours after cocci	Lived 4 days; acute meningitis
2,000†	2 c c 24 and 48 hours after cocci	Lived 9 days; acute meningitis
2,000	None (control)	Lived 5 days; acute meningitis

* Minimum lethal dose for mice 0.001 c c in 60 hours; rabbits injected with 0.5 c c.
† Serum administered intravenously.

TABLE 12

INFLUENCE OF ETHYLHYDROCUPREIN AND ANTIPNEUMOCOCCUS SERUM ALONE, AND IN MIXTURE ON TYPE 1 MENINGITIS OF RABBITS

Weight in Grams	Injection	Time of Injection of Serum or Drug or Mixture after Infection	Days							Necropsy
			1	2	3	4	5	6	7	
1,900	Culture alone* (control)	....	T†	T	D	...	...	...	...	Meningitis
2,500	Serum alone‡	24 hours	T	T	T	D	...	...	...	Meningitis
1,900	Serum alone	48 hours	T	T	T	D	...	...	...	Meningitis
1,900	Serum alone	24 and 48 hours	T	T	T	T	D	...	...	Meningitis
2,000	Ethylhydrocuprein alone§	24 hours	T	T	T	T	D	...	...	Meningitis
2,000	Ethylhydrocuprein alone	48 hours	T	T	T	D	...	...	...	Meningitis
2,300	Ethylhydrocuprein alone	24 and 48 hours	T	T	T	T	D	...	...	Meningitis
2,100	Mixture¶	24 hours	T	T	T	T	D	...	...	Meningitis
1,900	Mixture	48 hours	T	T	T	T	T	T	D	Meningitis
2,100	Mixture	24 and 48 hours	T	T	T	D	...	...	...	Meningitis

* Minimum lethal dose for mice 0.001 c c in 60 hours; rabbits infected with 0.5 c c subthecal injection.
† T = toxic; D = died.
‡ Serum alone injected subthecally in dose of 1 c c per kilogram of weight.
§ Ethylhydrocuprein hydrochlorid alone injected subthecally in dose of 0.5 c c of 1:1,000 dilution per kilo of weight.
¶ Serum 0.5 c c and ethylhydrocuprein 0.5 c c of 1:1,000 dilution per kilo of weight.

On the other hand, the repeated intravenous injection of the serum occasionally resulted in prolonging the lives of our rabbits, in one instance for 4 days as shown in table 11; we have not followed out this plan of treatment with a sufficiently large series of animals to determine more definitely the influence of intravenous injection of serum, but it is probable that these effects are due to the influence of the serum on the pneumococcus bacteremia, which invariably accompanies experimental pneumococcus meningitis in rabbits.

Mixtures of serum and ethylhydrocuprein hydrochlorid in preparation of 0.5 c c serum and 0.5 c c of 1: 1,000 solution of drug per kilo of body weight, yielded irregular results in the treatment of experimental meningitis difficult to evaluate, but as a general rule these results were not superior to those observed with the drug alone, as shown in an experiment in table 12.

THE INFLUENCE OF ETHYLHYDROCUPREIN HYDROCHLORID, SODIUM OLEATE AND BORIC ACID ON EXPERIMENTAL PNEUMOCOCCUS MENINGITIS

Lamar having shown that sodium oleate in 0.5 to 1% solution is destructive for pneumococci and that weaker solutions as 0.1 to 0.001% lessen the virulence of these organisms and increase their susceptibility to the destructive action of antipneumococcus serum, boric acid overcoming the inhibitory influence of the protein constituents, we have included a study of these substances alone and in combination with ethylhydrocuprein, on the pneumococcus in

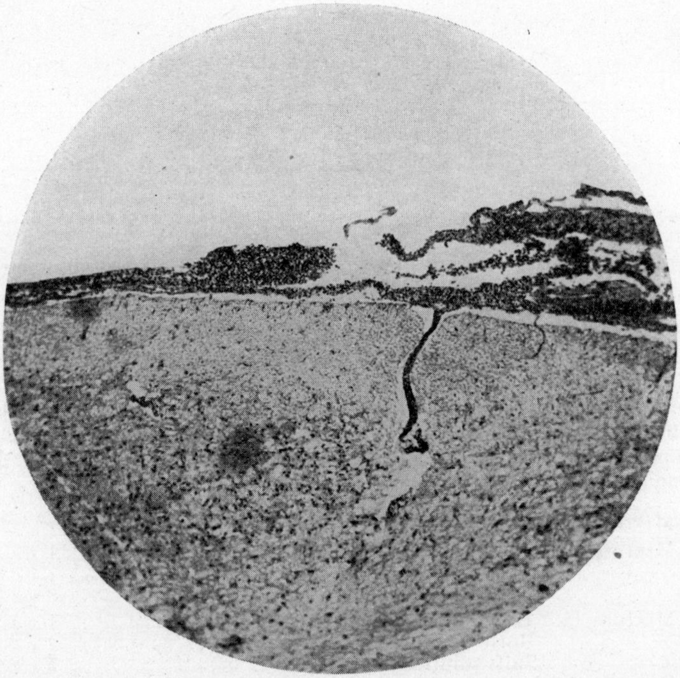

Fig. 4.—Section of spinal cord of rabbit in dorsal region removed seven days after the injection of the same culture in similar dosage employed in the infection of the meninges shown in figure 3, but followed four hours later by an injection of 0.5 c c of 1: 1,000 ethylhydrocuprein per kilogram of weight; shows slight leukocytic infiltration of the meninges. This animal was rapidly recovering when killed for microscopic study; × 70.

infected mice and in rabbits with pneumococcus meningitis, to determine whether sodium oleate increases the susceptibility of virulent pneumococci to the destructive activity of ethylhydrocuprein.

Exposure of virulent pneumococci to solutions of sodium oleate appeared to increase their susceptibility to the pneumococcidal activity of ethylhydrocuprein; the experiment shown in table 13 was conducted by cultivating the type 2 strain in glucose blood broth for 24 hours and dividing it into two parts of 4 c c each; to one part was added 0.5 c c of a 1: 1,000 solution of Merck's sodium oleate and to the second part 0.5 c c of salt solution as a control. Both mixtures were placed in an incubator for an hour followed by thorough centrifuging and resuspension of the cocci in 2.5 c c of warm physiologic salt solution. Both emulsions were then injected intraperitoneally in mice in equal doses followed in an hour by the intraperitoneal injection of varying doses of ethylhydrocuprein. The controls receiving the soaped and plain or untreated diplococci died in about 12 hours; mice receiving ethylhydrocuprein lived for varying periods up to 6 days and longer, and while the results were not regular, a larger percentage of mice infected with soaped pneumococci survived than of those infected with untreated cultures, indicating the protective value of ethylhydrocuprein especially against pneumococci exposed to sodium oleate.

TABLE 13

THE INFLUENCE OF ETHYLHYDROCUPREIN HYDROCHLORID ON SOAPED AND PLAIN PNEUMOCOCCI (TYPE 2)

Mouse Weight	Culture 0.5 c c	Ethylhydrocuprein	Results
18	Soaped	0.5 c c of 1:500	Lived over six days
22	Soaped	0.5 c c of 1:1,000	Lived over six days
20	Plain	0.5 c c of 1:500	Lived three days
21	Plain	0.5 c c of 1:1,000	Lived over six days
20	Soaped	None	Died in 12 hours (culture control)
20	Plain	None	Died in 12 hours (culture control)

In pneumococcus meningitis in rabbits the results were even more irregular than with mice, as the lesions were more involved; subthecal injection of mixtures of ethylhydrocuprein and sodium oleate appeared to prolong the lives of some infected animals and not of others as compared with animals receiving ethylhydrocuprein alone. These results are expressed quite well in the experiment shown in table 14 in rabbits with type 2 meningitis treated by the subthecal injection of various mixtures prepared as follows:

Mixture A:	Ethylhydrocuprein 1:1,000	
Mixture B:	Ethylhydrocuprein 1:100	1 c c
	Sodium oleate (Merck), 0.5%	1 c c
	Sodium solution	8 c c
Mixture C:	Ethylhydrocuprein 1:100	1 c c
	Boric acid (5%)	2 c c
	Salt solution	7 c c
Mixture D:	Ethylhydrocuprein 1:100	1 c c
	Sodium oleate (0.5%)	1 c c
	Boric acid (5%)	1 c c
	Salt solution	7 c c
Mixture E:	Sodium oleate (0.5%)	5 c c
	Boric acid (5%)	5 c c

Mixtures of ethylhydrocuprein and sodium oleate in salt solution were turbid; mixtures of ethylhydrocuprein and boric acid were quite clear.

Rabbits were infected by the subthecal injection of 0.01 c c of 24-hour broth cultures of virulent type 2 pneumococci, followed 2 hours later by the subthecal injection of 1 c c of each of the above mixtures.

As shown in this particular experiment, the control died in 48 hours with suppurative leptomeningitis and the animal receiving ethylhydrocuprein alone (A) survived longer than the animal receiving a mixture of ethylhydrocuprein and sodium oleate. Curiously, the animal receiving a mixture of ethylhydrocuprein and boric acid (C) survived indefinitely as did the animal receiving a mixture of sodium oleate and boric acid (E).

TABLE 14

INFLUENCE OF SODIUM OLEATE, BORIC ACID AND ETHYLHYDROCUPREIN HYDROCHLORID ON TYPE 2 MENINGITIS OF RABBITS

Weight in Grams	Drug†	Results
1,700	1 c c mixture A	Lived 9 days
2,000	1 c c mixture B	Lived 3 days
2,000	1 c c mixture C	Lived indefinitely
1,500	1 c c mixture D	Lived 5 days
2,000	1 c c mixture E	Lived indefinitely (control)
1,800	Cultured control	Died in 48 hours

* Rabbits infected by intraspinal injection of 0.01 c c of a 24-hour broth culture of type 2 (fatal for mice of 20 gm. in a dose of 0.0001 c c in 48 hours).

† Injected subthecally 2 hours after injection.

While sodium oleate undoubtedly reduces the vitality of pneumococci or at least increases their susceptibility to the destructive influences of ethylhydrocuprein when the organisms are exposed to the oleate in vitro, our results in the treatment of experimental pneumococcus meningitis in rabbits with mixtures of ethylhydrocuprein and sodium oleate have not yielded the encouraging results observed by Lamar in the treatment of experimental meningitis in monkeys with mixtures of specific antipneumococcus serum, boric acid and sodium oleate.

THE INFLUENCE OF MERCUROPHEN ON EXPERIMENTAL PNEUMOCOCCUS MENINGITIS IN RABBITS

As previously stated, the irritant properties of sodium oxymercury ortho-nitro-phenolate (Mercurophen) on the meninges following subthecal injection in rabbits, has not permitted the injection of a single dose sufficiently large to raise the germicidal activity of the spinal fluid to such a degree as will influence the course of a pneumococcus meningitis. Assuming that a 2,000 gm. rabbit has at least 2 c c of cerebrospinal fluid, the subthecal injection of 0.5 c c of a 1:2,000 solution of mercurophen which is the largest dose producing no irritation of the meninges, results in a final dilution of about 1:8,000 mercurophen which is too high for marked pneumococcidal activity on the basis of the results of germicidal tests in vitro with purulent spinal fluid, showing that mercurophen in dilutions higher than 1:4,000 exerts slight or no germicidal effect on pneumococci (table 5) under these conditions.

Experiments consisting in the infection of rabbits by subthecal injection of the type 2 pneumococcus followed 1, 4 and 24 hours later by the subthecal injection of solutions of mercurophen as high as 1:1,000 have had no appreciable effect on the course of the meningitis, the treated animals dying with leptomeningitis and showing pneumococci in the spinal fluid and blood of the heart. These results agree with those reported by Kolmer and Steinfield[10] showing that the intravenous and intramuscular injections of single doses of various mercurials including mercurophen, alone and in combination with pneumococcus serum, had no appreciable effect on prolonging the lives of mice infected by the intraperitoneal injections of type 1 pneumococci lethal in 72 hours; with the repeated subthecal injection of smaller doses of mercurophen in the treatment of a milder form of experimental meningitis as that produced by our type 1 strain of pneumococcus, some effect on the course of the meningitis was usually apparent, as best shown by the prolongation of the lives of the treated animals (table 15).

TABLE 15

THE INFLUENCE OF MERCUROPHEN ON TYPE 1 PNEUMOCOCCUS MENINGITIS

Weight in Grams	Culture*	Mercurophen		Results
		Dose	Injected	
1,200	0.01 c c	0.5 c c of 1:5,000	1st and 3rd days	Lived 8 days; acute meningitis
1,200	0.01 c c	None	....	Lived 4 days; acute meningitis
1,000	None	0.5 c c of 1:5,000	1st and 3rd days	Developed paralysis after second injection; recovered

* Minimum lethal dose for mice 0.001 c c in 48 hours; rabbits injected intraspinally on first, second and fourth days.

DISCUSSION

Our experiments have been severe tests for the protective and curative properties of the drugs included in this study, because it was necessary to infect the subarachnoid space with relatively large doses of virulent pneumococci in order to produce a definite train of lesions and symptoms, and owing to the marked susceptibility of the rabbits to invasion by the pneumococcus, the experimental infection was usually severe and rapidly fatal. The effects following the administration of the medicaments were judged mainly on the basis of duration of life of the treated animals as compared with the untreated controls; owing to the difficulty of securing spinal fluid from rabbits during life repeated chemical, cytologic and bacteriologic examinations of the fluid could not be made which would have yielded more evidence of a valuable character on the progress of the infection and effect of treatment. Histologic examinations of the brain, cord and meninges were made of every animal, but we have found these changes too irregular at different levels and areas to permit comparative studies and deductions.

Owing to the highly fatal nature of pneumococcus meningitis, the subject is particularly worthy of investigation, and we believe that ethylhydrocuprein has given some encouragement, providing the drug is injected subthecally early in the disease. According to the results of toxicity tests, it would appear safe to inject persons subthecally with 0.5 c c of a 1: 1,000 dilution per kilo of weight once or twice in 24 hours for a period of several days following the withdrawal of spinal fluid; this treatment in conjunction with appropriate surgical measures to effect local drainage in those cases of meningitis following a primary infection of the mastoid cells, frontal sinus or other accessible areas, is likely to modify the severity of the infection and may result in lowering the mortality of the disease.

The dose of ethylhydrocuprein advised would amount to 30 c c of a 1:1,000 solution for a young adult weighing 60 kilo or about 125 pounds; this is equivalent to 0.0005 gm. of the drug per kilo of weight, and being at least 60 times less than the toxic dose, may be accepted as safe even when given once or twice a day for 4 or 5 days. With the withdrawal of spinal fluid and the injection of this amount of drug, a distinct pneumococcidal activity is imparted to the spinal fluid, the duration depending on absorption and requiring further study.

SUMMARY

Both ethylhydrocuprein and mercurophen are slightly more toxic by subthecal injections in the lumbar regions of normal rabbits than by intravenous injection.

Ethylhydrocuprein hydrochlorid in a dose of 0.03 to 0.05 gm. dissolved in 0.5 c c saline solution per kilo of body weight of rabbits produces leptomeningitis especially well defined at the site of injection, and is lethal in about 48 hours; in a dose of 0.5 c c of a 1:1,000 solution per kilo of body weight the drug produces no irritation of the meninges, and is well borne by normal rabbits.

Mercurophen in a dose of 0.002 to 0.004 gm. in 0.5 c c salt solution per kilo of body weight, produces severe hemorrhagic leptomeningitis in rabbits and is lethal in about 58 hours; 1 c c of a 1:2,000 dilution per kilo of weight injected subthecally produces slight or no irritation of the meninges, and is well borne for an indefinite period of time.

Germicidal tests in vitro with purulent spinal fluids containing virulent type 2 and type 1 pneumococci, have shown ethylhydrocuprein and mercurophen pneumococcidal in final dilution of 1:4,000 in an exposure of one hour at 37 C.; the latter acts somewhat more rapidly than the former.

The subthecal injection of single doses of ethylhydrocuprein in amounts of 0.5 c c, of 1:500 and 1:1,000 solutions per kilo of body weight, had a distinct beneficial effect on the course of experimental meningitis in rabbits produced by a type 1 pneumococcus of moderate virulence, when administered not later than 4 to 6 hours after the injection of organisms; when given 24 hours after the pneumococci this effect was not apparent. With a meningitis produced by a more virulent culture of type 2 pneumococci, single doses of this drug had but slight or no effect on the duration of the lives of the experimental animals.

In experiments consisting in the repeated subthecal injection of smaller doses of pneumococci followed in a few hours by ethylhydrocuprein, the protective and curative effects of the drug were more apparent.

Mixtures of specific antipneumococcus serum and ethylhydrocuprein did not yield results in the treatment of experimental meningitis produced by type 1 pneumococci, superior to those observed with the drug alone; the serum alone was without appreciable effect on the course of the experimental lesions.

Exposure of virulent pneumococci to solutions of sodium oleate in vitro increased their susceptibility to the germicidal activity of ethylhydrocuprein, but the subthecal injection of mixtures of sodium oleate and ethylhydrocuprein did not yield results in the treatment of experimental pneumococcus meningitis superior to those observed with ethylhydrocuprein.

The subthecal injection of single doses of mercurophen in amounts as large as 0.5 c c of 1 : 1,000 solution per kilo of body weight was without appreciable effect on the course of experimental meningitis.

The repeated injection of smaller doses of type 1 pneumococci of moderate virulence followed in a few hours by the subthecal injection of smaller doses of mercurophen, resulted in prolonging the lives of some of the experimental animals.

In the treatment of pneumococcus meningitis of persons it is recommended that spinal puncture be made once or twice every day during the acme of the infection with the withdrawal of spinal fluid followed by the injection of a sterile and warm solution of ethylhydrocuprein hydrochlorid in physiologic salt solution in a dose of 0.5 c c of 1 : 1,000 per kilo of body weight; in cases of meningitis following infection of the mastoid cells and accessory nasal sinuses, local drainage should be instituted by surgical measures.

EXPERIMENTAL PNEUMOCOCCUS MENINGITIS IN RABBITS AND DOGS

Goro Idzumi

From the McManes Laboratory of Experimental Pathology of the University of Pennsylvania, Philadelphia

Three forms of pneumococcus meningitis may occur in human beings: First, that due to direct infection of the meninges from a primary focus in the ear, mastoid cells, nose and accessory sinuses; second, that arising during the course of pneumococcus pneumonia, and third, that developing spontaneously and without a discoverable primary focus of pneumococcus infection elsewhere in the body. The first form of the disease is usually a localized infection of the cerebral meninges, while the other two types are likely to prove to be generalized infections of the cerebral and spinal meninges; all forms are accompanied by a high mortality, as the majority of patients succumb to the infection. During the course of labor pneumonia delirium may develop, and spinal puncture reveals an increased volume of sterile cerebrospinal fluid; this condition is due to an acute meningeal congestion erroneously designated as "serous meningitis," and is not to be confused with pneumococcus meningitis. Recently mixed meningococcus and pneumococcus meningitis has been described by Netter and others and the mortality apparently is not as high as in pneumococcus meningitis.

How the meninges become infected with pneumococci in those forms of the disease with no discoverable primary focus of infection or with a primary focus situated remotely from the meninges, as in the lungs, pleura and pericardium, is unknown; it is possible that the pneumococci gain access to the blood and localize in the meninges as a metastatic lesion or, having gained access to the upper respiratory passages and particularly to the nasal mucous membrane, find their way to the meninges at the base of the brain in a manner analogous to infection with meningococcus by this route, as described by Flexner.[1] Bull[2] has reported the development of meningitis in dogs receiving

Received for publication Jan. 3, 1920.

[1] Jour. Exper. Med., 1907, 9, p. 142.
[2] Jour. Exper. Med., 1916, 24, p. 7.

large doses of virulent pneumococci by intravenous injection whereas in experimental meningococcus meningitis, it would appear, according to the experiments of Austrian,[3] that the intravenous injection of virulent meningococci in normal rabbits is not followed by meningitis unless local injury is produced and conditions disturbed by the withdrawal of spinal fluid with or without the subthecal injection of some bland irritant as normal serum.

According to Amoss and Eberson,[4] meningococcus meningitis in monkeys and rabbits cannot be produced by the intravenous injection of meningococci alone; in their experiments such attempts were fruitless unless spinal puncture was conducted during the bacteremia with the subthecal injection of some irritant, as normal serum, which produced physical injury of the meninges and reduced the local mechanism of defense. In the experiments of Weed, Wegefarth, Ayer and Felton[5] meningitis in cats was produced by injecting cultures of B. mucosus intravenously followed by spinal puncture and the removal of spinal fluid during the bacteremia.

PURPOSE OF INVESTIGATION

Similar experiments in the production of pneumococcus meningitis have not been made. For the production of experimental pneumococcus meningitis Lamar has used monkeys injected subthecally in the lumbar region with virulent cultures. Owing, however, to the relatively high cost of these animals and the difficulty of obtaining them in sufficient numbers for extensive chemotherapeutic studies, Dr. Kolmer requested me to make a series of experiments for the twofold purpose of throwing additional light on the mechanism of infection of the meninges with pneumococci and of determining whether a definite form of pneumococcus meningitis could be produced in dogs and large rabbits by

(1) The intravenous injection of virulent pneumococci.

(2) The intravenous injection of virulent pneumococci combined with spinal puncture and the subthecal injection of sterile, bland irritants.

(3) The subthecal injection of virulent pneumococci in the region of the spinal cord.

[3] Bull. Johns Hopkins Hosp., 1918, 29, p. 183.
[4] Jour. Exper. Med., 1919, 29, p. 605.
[5] Jour. Amer. Med. Assn., 1919, 72, p. 190.

The rabbit is known to be highly susceptible to the pneumococcus and doubt was entertained regarding the successful production of meningitis before death was produced by a bacteremia, but according to Lamar's experiments, pneumococcus bacteremia frequently followed the subthecal injection of pneumococci in monkeys, and it was hoped that the dosage for rabbits could be so regulated as to permit the development of meningitis before the rabbits succumbed. This has been found possible in these experiments.

The dog, on the other hand, is known to be highly immune to virulent pneumococci injected intravenously, and our main interest was centered on the possibility of producing a localized infection of the subarachnoid space without generalized infections; as will be shown, considerable difficulty was encountered in the production of pneumococcus meningitis in dogs, the resistance of this animal being unusually high to the effects of virulent pneumococci injected not only intravenously but subthecally as well.

TECHNIC

The experiments were made with three strains of pneumococci; type 1 strain was obtained from Dr. Avery of the Rockefeller Institute, type 2 from Dr. Berta Meine and type 3 from Dr. Kolmer.

The type 2 strain came from the spinal fluid of a child of 14 years suffering with pneumococcus meningitis of spontaneous development and ending fatally; the type 3 strain came from the spinal fluid of an adult of 56 years suffering with meningitis secondary to a pneumococcus infection of the mastoid cells and ending fatally. Naturally most interest centered on the results of experiments with type 2 and type 3 strains and especially type 2, inasmuch as both produced meningitis in human beings.

The virulence of these strains was maintained by animal passage and usually killed mice of 17 to 22 gm. in weight in the following doses of 24-hour blood-broth cultures:

Strain	Minimal Lethal Dose			
	In 18 Hours	In 24-30 Hours	In 48 Hours	In 72 Hours
	cc	cc	cc	cc
Type 1..........	....	0.001	0.0001	0.00001
Type 2..........	0.01	0.001	0.0001	0.00001
Type 3..........	0.1	0.1	0.001	0.0001

Twenty-four hour blood-broth cultures were used, and in order to reduce the volume of fluid to be injected subthecally and to avoid the irritant properties of the broth alone for the meninges, the cultures were pipetted into sterile tubes and centrifugated at high speed, the cocci being resuspended in warm, sterile salt solution just prior to injection. The disadvantage of this procedure consisted in the varying dosage from day to day depending on the thoroughness with which the cocci were removed from the broth cultures.

Successful spinal puncture is not a difficult procedure in rabbits and dogs, providing large animals are employed and the back well arched. An ordinary Babcock spinal puncture needle cut off to a length of 4 cm. was used; this needle is of small caliber and when properly pointed serves well for the puncture of animals. In the first experiments each animal was etherized, but after experience had been gained it was proved possible to conduct the operation quickly and with a minimum of discomfort, rendering anesthesia unnecessary. In the operation each animal was placed on its right side and firmly held by an assistant with the back arched; the needle was entered slowly and cautiously in the lower lumbar region in the median line. Entrance into the subarachnoid space is felt by the hand of the operator in much the same way as experienced in conducting lumbar puncture on persons. On the withdrawal of the stylet, spinal fluid may not appear from rabbits and small dogs for a minute or more, owing to the slight pressure of the fluid under normal conditions and the length of needle to be traversed.

As preliminary experiments had shown that the subthecal injection of solutions of dyes in an amount of 0.5 c c in the lumbar region of rabbits is followed within 3 hours by diffusion along the entire length of the cord and base of the brain with slight diffusion over the cerebrum, all injections were made in the lower lumbar region instead of in the region of the occipito-atlantoid ligament. This is probably a somewhat easier route for puncture, but the animal is more likely to be injured. Experiments have shown that the amount of fluid injected subthecally in rabbits weighing from 1,500 to 3,000 gm. should not be more than 0.5-1.0 c c; even when these amounts are used a temporary paralysis of one or both hind legs may follow the operation. In dogs weighing 6 kilo or more, about 1 c c of fluid may be injected without harm, but it appeared advisable in our experiments never to inject more than 1.5 c c.

In all experiments careful records were kept of the temperature and clinical condition of each animal and changes in the total number of leukocytes in the blood; owing to the small size of the majority of rabbits, it was difficult to secure during life more than a drop or two of spinal fluid for cytologic and bacteriologic examinations, although as much as 0.5-1 c c may be obtained from large dogs.

EFFECT OF INTRAVENOUS INJECTION OF VIRULENT PNEUMOCOCCI IN NORMAL RABBITS

The intravenous injection of virulent pneumococci into a series of normal rabbits was never followed by the development of meningitis. The doses were so regulated according to body weight as to prolong the lives of many of the animals for at least three days. Necropsy examination was made immediately after death, but without exception it failed to disclose any macroscopic or bacteriologic evidence of invasion of the meninges or cerebrospinal fluid. Most interest centered in

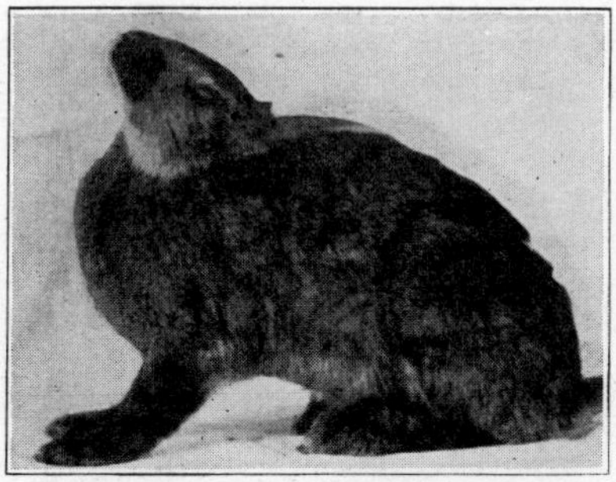

Fig. 1.—Opisthotonos in a rabbit 48 hours after the subthecal injection of 0.01 c c of type 2 pneumococci in salt solution.

the type 2 strain because it produced a fatal spontaneous meningitis in a child. It was employed in some of these experiments in the first broth culture from fresh spinal fluid, but the results were negative and showed that an induced bacteremia was not followed by an invasion of the normal meninges and spinal fluid of rabbits as shown in the following protocol:

A rabbit, weighing 2,000 gm., with a temperature of 38 C., with a leukocyte count of 10,200, received intravenously 0.5 c c of a suspension of type 2 pneumococcus secured by centrifuging 5 c c of an 18-hour broth culture and resuspending the cocci in 5 c c of salt solution. Twenty-four hours later the temperature was 40 C. and the leukocyte count was 20,600. The animal was very ill but presented no evidence of hypersensitiveness or increased reflexes. It died three days after the injection showing no evidence of involvement of the brain and cord. A culture of the heart's blood showed pneumococci; smears and cultures of the spinal fluid were sterile.

EFFECTS OF INTRAVENOUS INJECTION OF VIRULENT PNEUMOCOCCI IN NORMAL DOGS

Similar results were observed in normal dogs; the intravenous injection of large doses of pneumococci did not produce meningitis in any of our animals. A dog weighing 6,000 gm., with a rectal temperature of 36.5 C., and with a leukocyte count of 10,200, received an intravenous injection of 30 c c of a 24-hour broth culture of type 2 strain which killed mice weighing 17 to 20 gm. in 48 hours when given a dose of 0.0001 c c. Twelve hours later the temperature was 41 C. and the leukocytes numbered 21,900; the animal appeared sick and refused food. Twenty-four hours later the temperature was 39.5 C., the leukocytes numbered 20,200, and the animal was quite active and had a good appetite. Seventy-two hours later the temperature was 38 C. and the leukocytes numbered 15,000; the animal was active, had a good appetite and appeared normal. Necropsy revealed a clear, sterile spinal fluid of normal amount in the ventricles and subarachnoid space with no macroscopic changes in the spinal and cerebral meninges; smears and cultures of the heart's blood were sterile.

A dog weighing 7,000 gm., with a temperature of 37 C. and a leukocyte count of 10,000, received intravenously 30 c c of a 24-hour broth culture of type 3 strain of pneumococcus in the first culture from the cerebrospinal fluid of a fatal case of meningitis in an adult person; 0.001 c c killed mice weighing about 20 gm. in 24 hours. Twelve hours later the temperature was 39 C. and the leukocytes numbered 17,600; the animal refused food and appeared ill. Twenty-four hours later the temperature was 39.5 C. and the leukocytes numbered 18,000; the animal still appeared ill, was quiet and refused food. Forty-eight hours after injection the temperature was 38.5 C. and the leukocyte count was 16,400. The animal had a good appetite, moved about freely and actively and appeared to have fully recovered. Necropsy revealed no macroscopic changes in the abdominal and thoracic organs; the brain, cord and meninges appeared normal. The cerebrospinal fluid was clear, sterile and of normal volume; the heart's blood proved sterile.

These two protocols are typical of the results observed; it is possible that more virulent cultures injected intravenously would have produced meningitis as reported by Bull, but the three cultures of pneumococci employed in these experiments and in rather large doses (about 5 c c per kilo of weight of 24-hour blood-broth cultures) showed no evidence of localization of the diplococci in the tissue of the central nervous system.

EFFECT OF THE INTRAVENOUS INJECTION OF VIRULENT PNEUMOCOCCI FOLLOWED BY THE SUBTHECAL INJECTION OF STERILE SERUM OR BROTH

In experiments with rabbits and dogs, consisting in the intravenous injection of pneumococci followed immediately by the subthecal injection of sterile serum or broth, well developed meningeal irritation was produced in rabbits, but not in dogs, providing virulent cultures were employed. As shown by Flexner and Amoss,[6] the subthecal injection

[6] Jour. Exper. Med., 1917, 25, p. 525.

of sterile normal serum lowers the resistance of monkeys to the virus of acute anterior poliomyelitis, and Kolmer and Sekiguchi [7] have found that the subthecal injection of sterile normal serum into dogs facilitates the passage of antibodies from the blood into the cerebrospinal fluid.

A rabbit weighing 2,000 gm., with a temperature of 38 C. and a leukocyte count of 12,000, received intravenously 0.5 c c of a 24-hour broth culture of the type 2 strain; one hour later 1 c c of sterile rabbit serum was injected subthecally in the lumbar region. Twenty-four hours later the temperature was 39 C. and the leukocytes numbered 16,000; the animal appeared ill, but showed evidence of meningitis. Forty-eight hours after the injections the tempera-

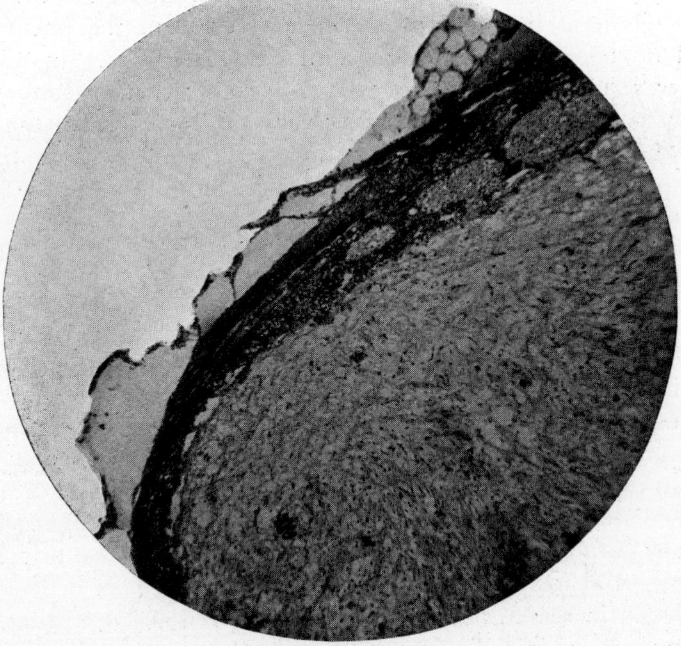

Fig. 2.—Section of the spinal cord in the dorsal region of a rabbit 48 hours after the subthecal injection in the lower lumbar region of type 1 pneumococci in salt solution; acute hyperemia and leukocytic infiltration of the meninges; × 70.

ture was 40 C. and the leukocyte count was 20,000; the animal was very sick, refusing food and presenting opisthotonos with greatly increased reflexes. On the third day death occurred. Necropsy revealed no gross lesions in the abdominal or thoracic organs except enlargement of the spleen. The cerebrospinal fluid was increased in amount and slightly cloudy; the spinal and cerebral meninges were hyperemic, especially the cervical portion of the cord. Hyperemia was more marked at the base than in the convex portions of the brain. Smears showed the presence of polymorphonuclear leukocytes and

[7] Jour. of Immunology, 1918, 3, p. 101.

extracellular diplococci; cultures of the heart's blood and spinal fluid showed the presence of pneumococci. A control rabbit receiving a similar injection of pneumococci intravenously but without the subthecal injection of serum, presented absolutely no evidence of involvement of the meninges. A second control receiving 1.5 c c of the same serum subthecally in the lumbar region of the cord developed a temporary paralysis of both hind legs, but three days later was in normal condition and presented no discernible evidence of meningeal involvement.

The above protocol is illustrative of the results obtained in rabbits with pneumococci of such virulence that 0.0001 c c or less killed mice within 40 hours. Similar experiments with pneumococci of less virulence, requiring from 0.01 to 0.001 c c as the lethal dose for mice, invariably yielded negative results; that is, when injected intravenously with a subthecal injection of sterile rabbit serum the pneumococci showed no tendency for localization in the meninges. In dogs the results were generally negative, even with highly virulent cultures; the intravenous injection of doses of pneumococci as high as 0.5 c c per kilo of weight of 24-hour broth cultures followed one hour later by the subthecal injection of from 1 to 3 c c of sterile broth in the lumbar region of the cord, was not followed by any evidence of pneumococcus meningitis.

Effect of the Subthecal Injection of Virulent Pneumococci in the Lumbar Region of the Spinal Cord of Rabbits

Well developed suppurative leptomeningitis was produced with regularity in rabbits following the subthecal injection of relatively large doses of virulent type 1 and type 2 pneumococci suspended in warm normal salt solution; the best results were observed with the type 2 strain, probably because of its greater virulence.

Immediately following the injections many of the animals showed temporary paralysis of one or both hind legs probably due to pressure. Within from 12 to 18 hours the temperature and number of leukocytes of the blood increased and the animals appeared sick, refusing to eat or to move about in their cages. Within 24 hours hypersensitiveness was generally apparent; many of the animals sat with their heads retracted in the position of opisthotonos and tapped the forehead or produced muscular tremors or convulsions along the vertebrae. Usually the animals remained in this condition, and it was accompanied with high fever, leukocytosis, loss in weight and increasing apathy until death occurred on from the second to the fifth day following the lumbar puncture. Spinal puncture on the second day usually showed an increased volume of cloudy spinal fluid, as several drops could be obtained, whereas in normal rabbits not more than a drop or two appeared at the end of the needle after an interval of a minute or more. Smears of the fluid showed large numbers of polymorphonuclear leukocytes with a few mononuclears and large numbers of diplococci, which were almost invariably extracellular.

At necropsy the abdominal and thoracic organs appeared normal except for acute hyperemia of the spleen, which was frequently noted; culture of the heart's blood invariably showed the presence of pneu-

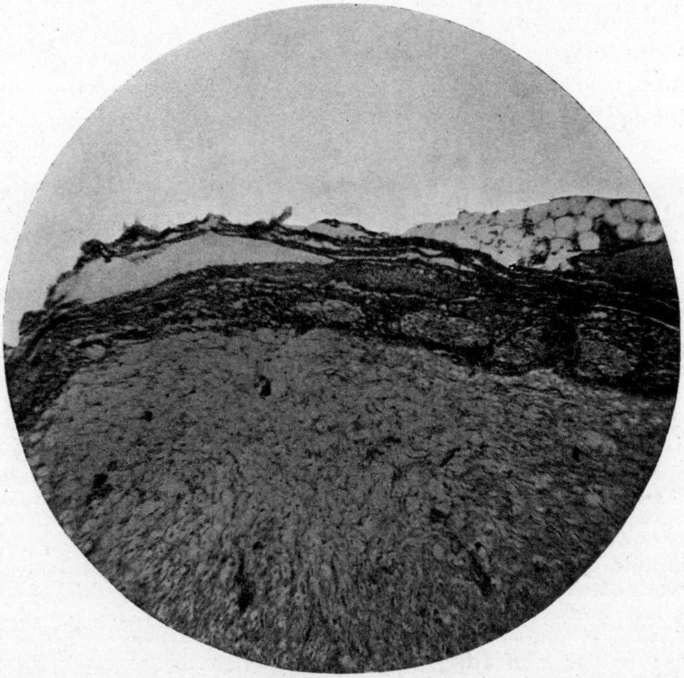

Fig. 3.—Section of the spinal cord in the dorsal region of a rabbit 48 hours after the subthecal injection in the lower lumbar region of type 2 pneumococci in salt solution; acute hyperemia and marked leukocytic infiltration of the meninges with extension in the cord; × 70.

mococci. The meninges of the cord and usually of the brain, particularly at the base, showed well defined hyperemia with an increase of spinal fluid filling the sulci of the brain. The pia mater was usually dull and flakes of exudate composed of fibrin, polymorphonuclear leukocytes and extracellular pneumococci were found plastered to the pia of the cord and occasionally at the base of the brain; in a few instances portions of exudate were found over the convex portions of the cerebrum. The spinal fluid was cloudy and contained large numbers of polymorphonuclear leukocytes and extracellular diplococci. Hyperemia and exudation were invariably most marked over the first 4 to 6 cm. of the cord and near the site of the lumbar puncture; in a few instances injury of the spinal cord was found, due to piercing with the spinal puncture needle. Not infrequently marked hyperemia and exudation were apparent in the cerebral portion of the cord, which was some distance from the site of injection of the pneumococci.

Histologic examination of the spinal cord and meninges at different levels showed well marked hyperemia and intense leukocytic infiltration of the meninges with slight edema of the substance of the cord adjacent to the pia mater and extension of the leukocytic infiltration along the perivascular spaces for some distance into the cord.

These changes were most marked in sections of the cord and meninges removed within 4 cm. or less of the site of injection; smaller, but well defined and similar, changes were frequently present in sections removed from the cervical portion of the cord and base of the brain. The following protocols of two experiments are illustrative of the results observed:

A rabbit weighing 2,000 gm. with a temperature of 38.5 C. and a leukocyte count of 11,200, received a subthecal injection in the lumbar region of 1 c c of a suspension of type 1 pneumococci in salt solution secured by centrifuging 5 c c of a 24-hour broth culture and resuspending the cocci in 5 c c of salt solution. Immediately after the injection the animal showed slight paralysis of the left hind leg. Twenty-four hours later the temperature was 41.5 C. and the leukocytes numbered 18,200. The animal presented increased reflexes and opisthotonos. On handling, generalized convulsion occurred. Necropsy showed no changes in the abdominal or thoracic organs; the cerebrospinal fluid was increased in amount, slightly cloudy and showed numerous polymorphonuclear leukocytes and extracellular diplococci. The meninges of the cord were hyperemic, particularly in the lumbar region near the site of injection. Small amounts of exudate were found along the cord and base of the brain; the meninges over the convex portion of the cerebrum showed hyperemia but no exudate. Cultures of the spinal fluid and heart's blood showed the presence of pneumococci in pure culture. Histologic examination of the cord and brain revealed marked hyperemia with infiltration of the meninges. There were moderate numbers of polymorphonuclear and mononuclear leukocytes. No changes in the substance of the brain and cord could be discovered.

A rabbit weighing 2,700 gm., with a temperature of 37.5 C. and a leukocyte count of 10,200, received a subthecal injection in the lumbar region of 0.5 c c of a suspension of type 2 pneumococci in physiologic salt solution recovered by centrifuging 3 c c of a broth culture. Six hours later the temperature was 40.5 C. and the leukocytes numbered 14,000. Twenty-four hours later the animal was hypersensitive and presented muscular weakness and beginning paralysis of both hind legs. The temperature rose to 41.5 C. and the leukocytes numbered 22,000. Forty-eight hours after the injection the animal was very ill with retention of urine, complete paralysis of the hind legs and marked opisthotonos. The temperature rose to 41 C. and the leukocytes numbered 12,000. It died about 60 hours after receiving the injection. At necropsy the abdominal and thoracic organs showed no gross changes except acute hyperemia of the spleen. There was an increase of cloudy spinal fluid in both lateral ventricles and the subarachnoid space with a patch over the convex portion. A smear of the spinal fluid showed pus cells and numerous pneumococci, mostly extracellular. Cultures of spinal fluid and heart's blood showed pneumococci in pure culture. Histologic examination of sections of the brain and spinal cord revealed an acute suppurative leptomeningitis with extension into the substance of the cord and brain.

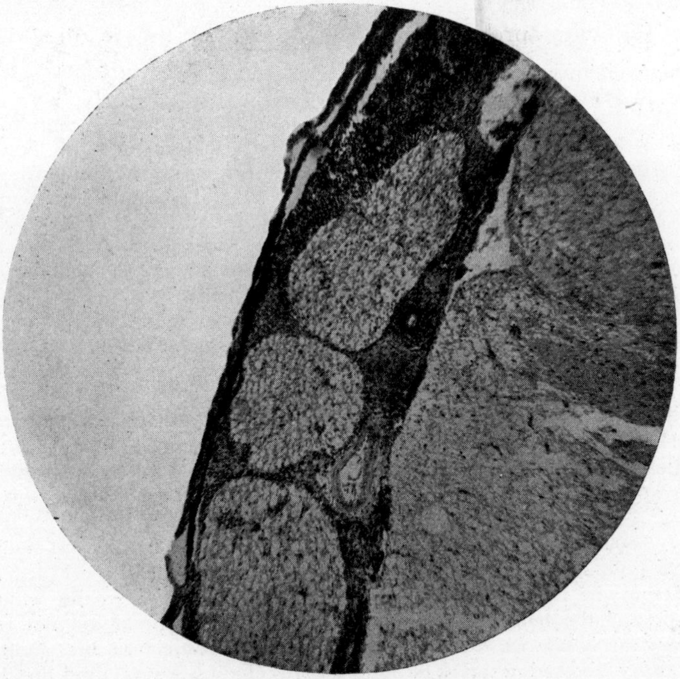

Fig. 4.—Section of the spinal cord in the dorsal region of a rabbit 48 hours after the subthecal injection in the lower lumbar region of type 2 pneumococci in salt solution; acute hyperemia and marked leukocytic infiltration of the meninges with extension in the cord; × 70.

EFFECT OF THE SUBTHECAL INJECTION OF VIRULENT PNEUMOCOCCI IN THE LUMBAR REGION OF THE SPINAL CORD OF DOGS

In similar experiments with dogs meningeal irritation and actual suppurative leptomeningitis were produced, but much less regularly and only with large doses of pneumococci. Acute hyperemia of the meninges of the cord, especially near the site of injection in the lumbar region extending to the base of the brain, with an increased volume of slightly cloudy spinal fluid in the ventricles and subarachanoid space, were the usual changes encountered. Flakes and patches of inflammatory exudate were rarely found, although histologic examination of the cord and meninges at different levels usually revealed some leukocytic infiltration confined to the meninges. Smears of the spinal fluid usually revealed a few polymorphonuclear and mononuclear leukocytes with scattered extracellular diplococci. Cultures of the spinal fluid were generally positive whereas cultures of the heart's blood were generally sterile.

The following protocols are illustrative of the results observed.

A dog weighing 6,500 gm., with a temperature of 38 C. and a leukocyte count of 14,200, was injected subthecally in the lumbar region with 2 c c of suspension of type 1 pneumococci in salt solution secured by centrifuging 10 c c of a 24-hour broth culture. This culture killed mice in 48 hours in a dose of 0.001 c c of 24-hour broth culture injected intraperitoneally. Forty-eight hours later the temperature rose to 39 C. and the leukocyte count was 19,200. The animal was very sick with ruffled hair, loss of appetite, some hypersensitiveness on handling, and he was too weak to stand. Spinal puncture removed about 0.5 c c of cloudy spinal fluid which revealed large numbers of pus cells and extracellular pneumococci; blood culture proved sterile. The animal died during the night. Necropsy disclosed a small patch of consolidation in the right lung with no other gross changes in the abdominal and thoracic viscera. On removal of the brain and cord there was found marked hyperemia of the meninges, particularly of the spinal portions, with marked increase of spinal fluid in the ventricles of the brain and subarachnoid space. Histologic examination revealed marked hyperemia of the meninges with leukocytic infiltration. Smears and cultures of spinal fluid showed polynuclear pus cells and extracellular diplococci; a culture of the heart's blood was sterile.

A dog weighing 10 kilo, with a temperature of 37.5 C. and a leukocyte count of 9,800, received a subthecal injection of 8 c.c. of a 24-hour broth culture of type 2 pneumococci of such virulence that 0.00001 c c killed mice of about 20 gm. in from 50 to 60 hours. Twelve hours later the temperature was 39 C. and the leukocytes numbered 16,800. The animal did not have the appearance of being ill. Twenty hours after the injection the animal died and necropsy showed a marked increase of cloudy spinal fluid in the ventricles and subarachnoid space with marked hyperemia of the meninges, especially in the lumbar region of the spinal cord near the site of injection of the pneumococci and in the cervical portion where petechial hemorrhages also were found in the pia mater. Smears of the spinal fluid showed large numbers of polymorphonuclear leukocytes and extracellular diplococci free of clumping; cultures of the spinal fluid and of the heart's blood were positive.

The following experiment yielded peculiar and interesting results as the animal appeared to recover from the immediate effects of a subthecal injection of pneumococci with the development of a well marked meningitis fourteen days later:

A dog weighing 7,000 gm., with a temperature of 38 C. and a leukocyte count of 10,200, was injected subthecally in the lumbar region with 2 c c of a suspension of type 1 pneumococci in physiological salt solution recovered by centrifuging 10 c c of a 24-hour broth culture. Twenty-four hours later the temperature was 38.5 C. and the leukocyte count was 22,400. During the following four days the dog appeared well but the number of leukocytes continued to be slightly increased—from 15,000 to 16,000. Fourteen days after the injection the animal became ill, showing these symptoms: ruffled hair, loss of appetite and beginning paralysis of the hind legs. The next day the animal was unable to stand, the hind legs were completely paralyzed. The bladder was also paralyzed leading to complete retention of urine; catheterizattion was necessary. The temperature was 39.5 C., and the leukocyte count was 15,400. The animal was killed with ether. Necropsy disclosed no gross changes in the abdominal and thoracic organs except an enlarged spleen. The meninges of the brain showed no changes except possibly an acute hyperemia, especially in the lumbar region. There was no visible exudate although the spinal fluid was slightly turbid and showed numerous pus cells and extracellular diplococci; culture of the spinal fluid and of the heart's blood showed the presence of pneumococci in pure cultures. Sections of the brain showed no histologic changes except slight hyperemia of the vessels of the pia mater; sections of the cord taken about 2 inches above the level of injection showed well marked hyperemia of the meninges and scattered areas of well marked infiltration with polynuclear and mononuclear leukocytes.

SUMMARY

These experiments show that pneumococcus cerebrospinal meningitis may be produced in rabbits by injecting virulent cultures directly into the subarachnoid space of the spinal cord. The reaction is much less marked in dogs, and usually takes the form of hyperemia without well defined suppurative changes, owing to the high resistance of this animal to the pneumococcus.

It would appear that large rabbits may be utilized in chemotherapeutic studies in pneumococcus meningitis because spinal puncture of this animal is not difficult; a definite series of pathologic changes in the spinal fluid and meninges with well defined symptoms of meningitis follows the subthecal injection of adequate doses of virulent pneumococci; and the supply of animals is unlimited. Furthermore, their carriage is generally semierect, as the majority sit up in their cages following spinal puncture. The disadvantages of using this animal are: its relatively small size; the difficulty in securing, during life, sufficient spinal fluid for examination, and the development of bacteremia, which probably is largely responsible for the early death of a majority of the animals. Monkeys are preferable because of their large size and erect carriage. Not infrequently, however, as in the rabbit, it is difficult to secure, during life, sufficient spinal fluid for examination. They also develop bacteremia, which probably is an important factor in shortening the duration of life and the period of observation. Furthermore, these animals may not be available in sufficient numbers for extensive chemotherapeutic experiments, or they may be too costly. Dogs are less satisfactory than monkeys and rabbits, owing to their high general resistance.

Intravenous injection of pneumococci alone into rabbits and dogs in our experiments has not resulted in the production of meningitis. Intravenous injection of pneumococci, followed by spinal puncture and the injection of sterile serum and broth, has usually elicited changes in the spinal meninges, chiefly in the nature of an acute hyperemia with slight or no leukocytic infiltration of the meninges and spinal fluid.

Subthecal injection of virulent pneumococci, however, produces a well marked suppurative leptomeningitis involving the entire spinal meninges, particularly in the immediate vicinity of the injection; the cerebral meninges, especially the basilar portions, are likewise involved, providing the animal survives at least 48 hours. What mechanism is involved in the production of acute hyperemia of the meninges or meningitis by the intravenous injection of pneumococci followed by the subthecal injection of the sterile broth or serum, is a matter of conjecture. That the subthecal injection of serum alone may produce hyperemia is a matter of direct observation as is also the fact that there is danger of direct injury to the meninges and cord which would permit the access of infected blood to the tissues and subarachnoid space. With small animals it is almost impossible to avoid producing considerable injury, and in some instance in our experiments the injections were made into the substance of the cord despite a considerable degree of care in conducting the spinal puncture.

CONCLUSIONS

The intravenous injection of virulent pneumococci, including two strains producing fatal meningitis in persons, into normal rabbits and dogs was not followed by the development of meningitis.

The intravenous injection of these virulent pneumococci into rabbits, followed by spinal puncture and the subthecal injection of sterile broth and serum, was usually followed by the production of acute meningeal congestion and occasionally by suppurative leptomeningitis. In dogs there was invariably acute congestion with no evidence of suppurative changes.

The subthecal injection of virulent pneumococci into the lumbar region of the spinal cord of rabbits is usually followed by the development of a fatal suppurative leptomeningitis accompanied by definite changes in the tissues and spinal fluid, fever, leukocytosis and clinical symptoms of meningitis, such as hyperesthesia, opisthotonos and convulsions. These changes appear to be sufficiently definite to permit the use of large rabbits for chemotherapeutic experiments in pneumococcus meningitis when they are infected by the direct subthecal injection of virulent pneumococci.

Spinal meningitis may be produced in dogs by the subthecal injection of large amounts of highly virulent pneumococci, but the results are more irregular than those observed in rabbits, and generalized suppurative changes occur only occasionally.

BIOLOGIC STUDIES OF THE DIPHTHERIA BACILLUS

Leon C. Havens

From the Division of Preventive Medicine and Hygiene, State University of Iowa, Iowa City, Ia.

1. THE SPECIFICITY OF THE MORPHOLOGIC TYPES

There has been considerable uncertainty evidenced concerning the variability of the morphologic characteristics of B. diphtheriae with reference to Wesbrook's types. The general opinion appears to be that these types are to a great extent, at least, immutable. If a particular form is found it is assumed that the strain remains constantly of that type of morphology. It has, furthermore, been assumed that the solid staining forms, D_2 and E_2, are relatively avirulent strains, and are usually reported avirulent or even negative in diagnostic laboratory reports.

The literature on the subject is not by any means in accord with these views. Almqvist and Koraen [1] report observations of one strain of diphtheria bacillus over several years, and they found no marked change in its morphology at any examination. However, Denny [2] found that strains of types C_2 and D_2 tend, on prolonged cultivation, to become clubbed and to stain irregularly; in other words, to approach the barred and granular forms in their staining properties. He concludes that the solid types are young forms. Wherry[3] arrives at the same conclusion from a study of the retarded growth of the organism under conditions of lowered oxygen tension. When growth takes place under such conditions it is retarded, and only the solid staining forms are found, principally D_2 and E_2. However, if such a culture is allowed to grow at normal oxygen tension barred and granular types soon develop.

In connection with other problems, the question of the specificity of the morphology arose and studies were consequently made to determine whether variations in morphology and staining properties were common and if so, under what conditions these changes take place. Accordingly, a detailed study has been made of a series of strains with reference to their morphologic characteristics, to determine the specific or nonspecific nature of their morphology and the

Received for publication Jan. 5, 1920.

[1] Ztschr. f. Hyg. u. Infektionskr., 1918, 85, p. 347.
[2] Jour. Med. Research, 1913, 9, p. 117.
[3] Jour. Infect. Dis., 1917, 9, p. 27.

relation of morphologic characteristics to certain biologic properties, such as virulence, toxin production and agglutinability. These strains were obtained through the courtesy of R. L. Laybourn, bacteriologist of the Iowa State Board of Health.

The bipolar or granular types, C and possibly D of Wesbrook's classification, have been regarded as the typical form of the diphtheria bacillus and are the forms, together with type A, most frequently encountered. Type A, composed of organisms with clubbed or swollen ends, are not so often found, and have been regarded as involution forms. The barred forms are more rare, but are usually considered typical virulent forms, with the exception of those which fall into types E_1 and F, which are usually found to be of questionable virulence.

In a study of 154 strains of the diphtheria bacillus the relative numbers of the different morphologic types have been noted, their tendency to remain constant has been studied and the relation of the culture to its morphology has been considered.

It is impossible to make a definite statement of the relative proportions of the several types as they occur under natural conditions as it has been found that in a considerable number of cases the age of the culture determines the morphology of the organisms. This is illustrated in the following series of cultures studied.

The cultures obtained were streaked on blood serum plates and individual colonies isolated and subcultured at the end of 4 to 8 hours. These were examined for morphology and then transferred to slants of the same medium for further study.

TABLE 1

RELATIONSHIP OF MORPHOLOGY TO AGE OF CULTURES

Culture	4 Hours	8 Hours	24 Hours	Subculture, 4 Hours
21	D_2	D_2	C	D_2
124	D_2	D_2	C	D_2
168	D_2	C and D_2	C	D_2
215	E_2	E_2 and C	C	E_2 and D_2
216	D_2	C	C	D_2
218	D_2	D_2	C	D_2
219	E_2	E_2 and C	C	E_2
220	D_2	D_2	C	D_2
224	E_2	E_2	C	E_2

From the table it is evident that 9 strains of the series, or about 6%, were of the solid types at the end of short periods of incubation, but at the end of 24 hours they had assumed the typical granular appearance. The morphology and staining characteristics of the so-called atypical bacilli had changed to that of the typical virulent organism. In most cases a period of from 12 to 24 hours was required to produce the change from the solid type to the granular and, as appears in the table, all of these 9 strains on subculture reverted to the solid form.

That the morphologic characteristics of the solid forms are not always reversible is shown in Table 2. The strains in this series, having once become granular, remained so in subsequent subcultures at all examinations.

TABLE 2

GRANULAR AND BIPOLAR FORMS INITIALLY OF SOLID TYPES

Culture	4 Hours	12 Hours	24 Hours	Subculture, 4 Hours
181	D_2	D_2	C	C
209	D_2	D_2	D	D
211	E_2	E_2	C	C
214	D_2	D_2	C	C
217	E_2	E_2	C	C
222	D_2	D_2	D	D

Further subculture showed that these strains remain of the bipolar or granular types indefinitely.

This apparent change in types has usually been from solid to granular. However, 3 strains were encountered in this series which were type C forms initially but which on further subculture were found to be solid staining forms, D_2 or E_2. The most striking tendency noted in this study has been a change from the types which are assumed to be of low virulence to the typically virulent types of the organism. Of 19 originally solid forms, it will be seen from tables 1 and 2 that 15 were found to become granular or bipolar on prolonged cultivation. Four strains remained solid at all examinations.

That changes due to the growth of the organisms are a factor in determining morphology and staining properties seems possible. A study of these conditions is being made at the present time in this laboratory and will be made the subject of a future report.

From an epidemiologic standpoint it is improbable that the morphologic types of the diphtheria bacillus are biologically specific. Unlike the types of the pneumococcus and meningococcus which rarely occur but singly in the nasopharynx, the cultures of the nasopharynx in active cases and carriers of diphtheria regularly show a mixture of morphologic forms. The predominating type in the active case has no bearing on the type found in a contact.

The observations here recorded corroborate the findings reported by other investigators that the solid staining types are young forms that later develop the granules and polar bodies characteristic of the other types. If this is the case, caution should be used in reporting a diagnostic culture negative when only solid forms are found. Such cultures should be incubated a longer period of time and subcultures studied before a negative report is made. If necessary, tests for virulence would seem to be advisable. To report such a culture negative, a priori, merely because the morphology fails to conform to that of the accepted virulent types, is, in view of the observations reported here and elsewhere, hazardous.

2. THE RELATION OF MORPHOLOGY TO VIRULENCE

It is common practice in diagnostic laboratories to regard the solid staining bacilli of the diphtheria group and certain of the barred and granular types as being avirulent and to render a negative report on cultures which show only these forms. In view of numerous instances in which strains have been reported to change their morphology from time to time under certain conditions, a study of these strains seemed advisable.

Bunker [4] reports an observation of a single strain which showed all the morphologic types at different intervals. Meader,[5] in a study of 25 strains, found variations in morphology and virulence in subcultures, and concluded that the virulence of a strain is not closely correlated with the morphology. In the series of strains just described by me, variations were found to occur among certain groups. Wayson [6] found that solid staining bacilli were sometimes virulent, and states that morphology alone is an insufficient index of virulence.

This study was undertaken to determine the virulence of certain solid staining strains, both those that remained solid at all observations and those that on longer incubation and prolonged growth became granular or bipolar in their morphology. Since the change from uniformly staining organisms to those with granules depends, in some cases at least, on the age and the products of growth of the culture, it was interesting to determine whether those cultures which eventually become typically granular were virulent.

It was shown in the preceding section that since there is a tendency for solid staining forms to develop on further cultivation into the characteristic type C organisms, care should be taken in studying such cultures and the virulence of the individual cultures should, if necessary, be determined before they are reported as negative.

Table 3 shows the results of virulence tests with guinea-pigs with strains which were initially of types D_2 and E_2. With the first six strains of the table the tests were made by the subcutaneous method using 1 c c of culture. With the last five strains the intracutaneous method was used.

It is evident that many of the uniformly staining strains are virulent for guinea-pigs. It is interesting to note that strains 222 and 223, which were originally solid but which on longer cultivation developed granular characteristics, remained avirulent.

[4] Abstracts of Bacteriology, 1, p. 31, 1916.
[5] Jour. Infect. Dis., 1919, 24, p. 145.
[6] Public Health Reports, 1916, 31, p. 3113.

TABLE 3

VIRULENCE TESTS WITH STRAINS INITIALLY OF TYPES D_2 AND E_2

Culture	Morphology		Result		
	Diagnostic Culture	Pure Culture	24 Hours	48 Hours	72 Hours
181	D_2	D_2	......	......	Death
219	D_2	D_2	Local edema	......	Death
221	D_2	C	Negative	Local edema	Death
222	D_2	C	......	Negative	
223	D_2	C	......	Negative	
224	D_2	C	......	......	Marked edema of abdominal wall
226	D_2	D_2	+	++++	++++
227	D_2	C	++	++++	++++
228	D_2	C	++	++++	++++
229	D_2	D_2	Negative	++	++
230	D_2	D_2	Negative	Negative	Negative

From the evidence presented here and elsewhere, it seems that morphology bears little relation to toxin production. It is undoubtedly true that the greater proportion of virulent strains show granular or bipolar staining characteristics and are the typical forms of diphtheria bacilli in that they occur in by far the greater number of instances. However, to regard so-called solid staining forms as avirulent on the basis of morphology and staining characteristics as the sole criteria, is open to serious question.

Weaver[7] found, from a study of a series of strains isolated from patients and from contacts, that the majority of these strains are virulent. No observations are recorded concerning the morphology of these strains, but his conclusion is that such strains are usually virulent. A much better criterion of virulence, from the standpoint of prevention, is the history of the carrier state. If a history of contact with an active case is obtained, the strain should be regarded as virulent until proved otherwise. If there are cases in which no history of such contact can be obtained—usually a small minority of cases—a test for virulence should be made regardless of morphology before such individuals are allowed to become a potential menace to the community. It would seem that morphology as a criterion of virulence has no more foundation in connection with the diphtheria bacillus than does the morphology of the pneumococcus, for example, in ascertaining its virulence.

To determine the virulence of the strain harbored by a carrier requires the detention of the individual for from 48-72 hours longer, but this inconvenience is more than compensated by the benefit to the

[7] Jour. Infect. Dis., 1917, 20, p. 145.

community from a definite knowledge of the virulence or lack of virulence of the organisms which he carries. In the case of a carrier with a definite history of contact with a patient the organisms should be considered virulent until proved otherwise. It is far better to cause one individual a slight inconvenience than to run the risk of inflicting unnecessary cases on the community. In reporting on release cultures after convalescence from diphtheria, the morphology should bear still less weight. A negative report based on the fact that the culture shows only solid forms at the time of examination should not be made until the virulence has been determined. The fact that the source is a recently active case should carry more influence than the staining properties.

3. BIOLOGIC GROUPS AS EVIDENCED BY AGGLUTINATION TESTS

Attention has been primarily devoted, in immunologic studies of B. diphtheriae, to the toxin and the production of antitoxin. The unity of all strains in their immunologic properties has been assumed rather than definitely determined and, in consequence, a single strain, if it forms a potent toxin, is considered sufficient for the production of antitoxin for therapeutic purposes.

The few studies of the agglutinability of the diphtheria bacillus which have been made in the past have shown certain variations in this respect between different strains of the organism. Langer,[8] using a monovalent serum, found that certain strains were not agglutinated. These nonagglutinating strains were otherwise typical diphtheria bacilli and he states that they represent, clinically, cases of mild infection and healthy carriage. Mason[9] used the agglutination test as a means of diagnosis and found in a study of 65 strains that, with a serum of relatively low titer (1:320), differences in degree of agglutinability exist among the individual strains.

It appears, then, that differences in immunologic properties exist among the various strains of the diphtheria bacillus. In order to determine the degree and specificity of these differences, a series of 206 different strains has been studied with regard to their agglutinability. These represent diagnostic cultures from acute cases of diphtheria, release cultures and cultures from healthy carriers. The morphologic types represented in the series were quite universal, most of the types given in Wesbrook's classification being included. As

[8] Centralbl. f. Bakteriol., II, 78, p. 117, 1916.

[9] Military Surgeon, 1919, 45, p. 560.

pointed out in the preceding part on the specificity of the morphologic groups as evidenced by their tinctorial properties, it was found that the morphology tends to vary, the tendency, in brief, being toward the granular types, especially in old cultures. Consequently, in the study of the agglutinability of the strains in this series detailed attention was not paid to the morphologic characteristics. It was found, however, that morphology bears no observed relation to agglutinating properties.

A monovalent serum was produced in rabbits, using for its production, a granular form corresponding to type C. This strain had shown no variations in morphology, being typically granular at all observations. The growth of a blood serum slant, incubated for 24 hours and suspended in 10 c c of salt solution, was used for injecting the rabbit, the injections being made intravenously in increasing amounts. An agglutinating serum was obtained in this way with a titer of 4,860 for the homologous strain. Using this serum, the members of the series were tested for their agglutinating properties.

Of the series of 206 strains, 169 were found to agglutinate with this monovalent serum; 37 failed to agglutinate. The agglutinating members of the series showed no variations in degree of agglutinability. All were agglutinated in a dilution of serum of 1:4,860 as did the strain used in the production of the serum. The 37 strains which failed to agglutinate in any dilution of serum showed no differences morphologically or culturally from the agglutinating strains.

A member of this group of nonagglutinating strains was used to produce a second agglutinating serum in a rabbit. This serum also had a titer of 4,860 or higher for the homologous strain. Using this serum, agglutination tests were made on the members of the series which failed to agglutinate with the first serum. All of these strains were found to agglutinate with this serum in high dilution (1:4,860).

Judging by the evidence furnished by the agglutination test there are two biologic groups of the diphtheria bacillus, one including 82% of the series of 206 strains studied, the other containing the remaining 18%. No evidence of cross-agglutination was found among the members of this series. The specific agglutinating serum for the second group showed no agglutinating power for any of the members of the first group. Members of the second group were likewise not agglutinated in any dilution by the first group serum. In this respect the two groups are distinct.

The members of the second group show no peculiarities of morphology, staining properties or toxin production, which differentiate them from strains of the first group. Typical granular organisms of high virulence for guinea-pigs are found in both groups and the proportions of the morphologic types are about the same. No marked preponderance of any one form is found in either group.

As pointed out already, solid forms occur which possess a high degree of virulence for guinea-pigs. Such strains have been found to exist in both of these groups. These strains in the majority of instances eventually show granules and swollen forms characteristic of the diphtheria bacillus. Some, however, retain their solid staining characteristics indefinitely. There seems to be no more reason for using tinctorial characteristics as a criterion for virulence than for using them as a guide to the serologic grouping.

There seems, furthermore, to be no reason for believing that the members of the second group should show any marked differences in virulence as compared with the first. As a matter of fact, of 24 strains of the second group which were tested, 18 were found to be highly virulent for guinea-pigs. It is necessary to show, in order to prove that a case of an infectious disease is the result of contact with a particular carrier, that the two strains are identical serologically. Consequently, it is highly improbable that a serologic group should exist composed entirely of avirulent organisms. Serologic properties are independent of virulence, rather than dependent on that property.

In this series of 206 strains no individuals were encountered which were inagglutinable. All the members of the series fell into one of the two groups with no differences observed in degree of agglutinability. As judged by the results of agglutination, two groups exist which include all strains of the diphtheria bacillus.

4. THE PROTECTIVE PROPERTIES OF DIPHTHERIA ANTITOXIN WITH REFERENCE TO BIOLOGIC GROUPS

It seems from the preceding evidence that two definite groups of the diphtheria bacillus exist, in so far as agglutinins are concerned. The experiments described in this section deal with the relationships of other properties of the two groups, notably their toxins and the corresponding antitoxins. It does not necessarily follow that other antigenic properties would be analogous to those responsible for agglutinin formation. The protective properties of standard diphtheria antitoxin are well known, and it was consequently deemed advisable to test the protective properties of this antitoxin against strains of the two groups which were ascertained by the agglutination test.

Besides the standard antitoxin obtained from the Hygienic Laboratory of the U. S. Public Health Service, through the courtesy of the director, Dr. G. W. McCoy, specimens of antitoxin were obtained from six different commercial houses. All of these were tested against a culture of the strain of diphtheria bacillus known as "Park No. 8," which is the strain used extensively in the production of antitoxin and which was found by agglutination to fall into the first or larger group. The protective properties of these different brands of antitoxin against this strain were found to be effective and the number of units per c c essentially as stated on the label.

Experiments were then made to determine the comparative value of the protective properties of these various antitoxins against strains of the second group as well. In the following protocols, unless otherwise stated, the amount of culture injected is that amount of a 24-hour blood serum slant suspended in 5 c.c. of salt solution.

G. pig 1. Control. 1.0 c c subcutaneously of culture 210 (group 1). Dead in 48 hours. Lesions characteristic of diphtheria.

G. pig 2. 1.0 c c subcutaneously of culture 210 (group 1). 100 units antitoxin 18 hours previously. Remained normal.

G. pig 3. Control. 1.0 c c subcutaneously of culture 221 (group 2). Dead in 36 hours. Lesions characteristic of diphtheria.

G. pig 4. 1.0 c c of culture 221 (group 2). 100 units of antitoxin 18 hours previously. Dead in 36 hours. Lesions characteristic of diphtheria.

G. pig 5. 1.0 c c of culture 141 (group 2). Dead in 48 hours. Lesions characteristic of diphtheria,

G. pig 6. 1.0 c c of culture 141 (group 2). 100 units of antitoxin 18 hours previously. Dead in 48 hours. Lesions characteristic of diphtheria.

From this experiment, using two strains of group 2 organisms, there seems to be no evidence that any degree of protection was furnished against strains of group 2 by the standard antitoxin which protected satisfactorily against a virulent strain of group 1. It is at least probable from this experiment that two of the group 2 cultures differ from the group 1 organisms in their toxin production as evidenced by protective tests.

It seemed desirable to test the protective property of the standard antitoxin against a representative number of the members of group 2 and for this experiment, in order to conserve guinea-pigs, the intracutaneous method [10] was used. Previous experience has shown this method to be satisfactory for virulence tests, and it has the advantage that several tests can be made simultaneously on the same animal. The following table shows the results with 18 strains of group 2 and 6 of group 1 to serve as controls.

[10] Zingher, A., and Soletsky, D.: Jour. Infect. Dis., 1915, 17, p. 455.

TABLE 4

RESULTS OF TEST

No. of Culture	Group by Agglutination	Result in 72 Hours—Degree of Local Edema and Necrosis	
		Antitoxin	No Antitoxin
173	1	0	++
59	1	0	++++
223	1	0	++++
34	1	0	++++
119	1	0	++
24	1	0	++++
185	2	++++	++++
207	2	++++	++++
118	2	++++	++++
170	2	++++	++++
83	2	++++	++++
74	2	++++	++++
69	2	++	++++
60	2	++++	++++
57	2	++	++
53	2	++++	++++
43	2	++	++++
40	2	++++	++++
208	2	+	++
181	2	+	+
219	2	++++	++++
168	2	++++	++++
141	2	++++	++++
95	2	++++	++++

The results obtained by subcutaneous injection are thus corroborated by intracutaneous tests with a larger series of strains. It is seen from the table, however, in the case of two strains, 69 and 208, that while a certain amount of necrosis was produced at the site of inoculation, it was not so marked as in the control animal. However, in these experiments a large amount, 100 units, of antitoxin was used, a much larger amount than is necessary to protect a guinea-pig against the amount of culture injected. Consequently in order to determine more accurately the relative differences between the two groups and to graduate the dosage more nicely, in the following experiments the pure toxin was used instead of the culture of the bacilli. Two strains were selected from each group, strains which were found to produce a potent toxin, the MLD for the toxin produced by these cultures being found to be from 0.005-0.01 c c. With these toxins the following experiment was made.

G. pig 1. Injected subcutaneously with the following mixture: 2 MLD toxin 34 (group 1) and 10 units standard antitoxin, incubated 2 hours at 37 C. Remained normal.

G. pig 2. Control. Injected subcutaneously with the following mixture: 2 MLD toxin 34 (group 1) and 1.0 c c salt solution incubated 2 hours. Guinea pig dead in 48 hours.

G. pig 3. Injected subcutaneously with the following mixture: 2 MLD toxin 74 (group 2) and 10 units standard antitoxin, incubated 2 hours. Dead in 48 hours.

G. pig 4. Control. Injected subcutaneously with the following mixture: 2 MLD toxin 74 (group 2) and 1.0 c c salt solution. Dead in 48 hours.

G. pig 5. Injected subcutaneously with the following mixture: 2 MLD toxin 53 (group 2) and 10 units standard antitoxin. Dead in 72 hours.

G. pig 6. Control. Injected subcutaneously with the following mixture: 2 MLD toxin 53 (group 2) and 1.0 c c salt solution. Dead in 72 hours.

It appears from these results that guinea-pigs injected with the toxin of strains of group 2 are not protected by five times the corresponding amount of standard antitoxin. It was thought possible that larger amounts of antitoxin might show a protective action, especially if group antitoxins were found to be present in highly potent antitoxins. In order to determine whether this were so a series of guinea-pigs were injected with increasing amounts of antitoxin, the amount of toxin remaining constant — two minimal lethal doses being the amount injected. The following protocol illustrates the results obtained.

G. pig 1. Control. 2 MLD toxin 34 (group 1) and 5 units standard antitoxin. Survived.

G. pig 2. 2 MLD toxin 74 (group 2) and 5 units standard antitoxin. Dead in 48 hours.

G. pig 4. 2 MLD toxin 74 and 20 units antitoxin. Marked local edema and toxemic symptoms. Survived.

G. pig 5. 2 MLD toxin 74 and 25 units antitoxin. Local edema. Survived.

G. pig 6. 2 MLD toxin 74 and 50 units antitoxin. Survived. No local reaction.

There seems, therefore, to be present in the standard antitoxin a certain amount of group antitoxin which protects against both groups of the diphtheria bacillus. This is not present apparently in sufficient amounts to exert its action until many times the number of units of antitoxin as of toxin are present. Furthermore, different brands of antitoxin vary in their content or their titer in respect to this characteristic. Two antitoxins, designated "A" and "D," failed to show this protective action until 100 units were injected for every MLD. One antitoxin, (C), failed to protect up to 1,000 units, which was as far as the experiment was carried.

Evidence having been obtained that the standard diphtheria antitoxin showed group antitoxins in small amounts the question arose whether an antitoxin produced with a group 2 strain of the diphtheria bacillus would likewise show this characteristic, possibly more markedly. In other words, group antitoxins might be present in higher titer. A rabbit was injected with gradually increasing amounts of group 2 toxin and also virulent cultures of group 2 bacilli. However, a highly potent antitoxin was not obtained. The serum from this animal had a titer of about 50 units per c c. While this was a relatively low titer no evidence was obtained that group agglutinins were developed in any greater concentration than in the standard antitoxin. The following experiment illustrates the relative protective properties of the two group antitoxins:

G. pig 1. 1 MLD toxin 34 (group 1) and 5 units standard antitoxin. Survived. No local reaction.

G. pig 2. 1 MLD toxin 53 (group 2) and 5 units standard antitoxin. Dead in 96 hours.

G. pig 3. 1 MLD toxin 34 (group 1) and 5 units group 2 antitoxin. Dead in 96 hours.

G. pig 4. 1 MLD toxin 53 (group 2) and 5 units group 2 antitoxin. Survived. Slight local edema.

G. pig 5. Control. 1 MLD toxin 34 (group 1). Dead in 96 hours.

G. pig 6. Control. 1 MLD toxin 53 (group 2). Dead in 96 hours.

It seems from the experimental evidence that the toxins produced by the two groups of diphtheria bacillus, in so far as can be judged by the corresponding antitoxins, are not so sharply defined as are the agglutinins. No evidence was obtained of agglutinins common for both groups. Strains which were agglutinated by one agglutinating serum were not agglutinated by the serum of the other group even in low dilution (1:20). The standard antitoxic serums, however, show some evidence of containing antitoxins common for both groups. These are not, it is true, present in any large quantities, but undoubtedly they occur to some extent. The minimum amount of the standard antitoxin which was found to protect against one minimal lethal dose of the group 2 toxin was 20 units and 5-10 units regularly failed to protect.

The results of these experiments may throw some light on those cases of diphtheria which are not benefited except by large amounts of antitoxin. It is entirely possible that such cases are due to infection with a strain belonging to the second or smaller group of the diphtheria bacillus and consequently a large amount of the standard antitoxin is necessary to obtain the benefit of the small amount of antitoxin common to both groups.

Furthermore, the death rate from diphtheria, in spite of the increasing use of antitoxin and in spite of its use early in the disease, is still about 10%.[11] How many of such fatal cases are due to infection with organisms of group 2 it is, of course, at the present time, impossible to say. A study of these stubborn cases which fail to yield to liberal doses of antitoxin would seem advisable and might throw light on the use of antitoxin.

In view of the experimental evidence here set forth it would seem that the inclusion of a representative of group 2 in the production of therapeutic antitoxin would greatly increase its efficiency and should be an influence in lowering the mortality of diphtheria in proportion to the frequency of the occurrence of strains of group 2. The occurrence of such strains is, judging from the series of 206 strains studied, about 18%.

It is possible that the use in the Schick test of a mixture of the two toxins including both groups will make this test of more universal value. An individual may be immune to infection with the larger group and yet be susceptible to members of group 2. It is probable, however, that the antitoxin which such an individual possesses contains certain group protection properties similar to the artificially produced antitoxin in the horse. On the other hand, if the antitoxin is not present in considerable amounts the experimental evidence suggests that the protection against the second smaller group will be inadequate. That immunity to infection with group 1 protects against all infection with diphtheria for practical purposes is probable, due to the fact that the second group occurs more rarely.

Likewise, active immunization with toxin-antitoxin mixtures would probably be made more complete by the use of mixtures of the two group toxins and antitoxins or a polyvalent antitoxin. That some protection is furnished against group 2 by the production of a high degree of immunity against group 1 is probably true. The degree of protection, however, against the second group is problematic and at best, is incomplete.

The presence of group antitoxins in certain small amounts in the standard antitoxin saves it from being valueless in group 2 infections, but in all cases, its value for such infections could be enhanced by the inclusion in its production of group 2 toxin.

[11] Carey, B. W.: Bost. Med. and Surg. Jour., 1919, 181, p. 92; Public Health Reports, 1919, 34, p. 1063.

SUMMARY

The morphologic characteristics of the diphtheria bacillus show a tendency to variations from time to time. The morphologic types are, therefore, apparently nonspecific. The solid forms corresponding to types D_2 and E_2 are probably young forms of the more common granular types.

Solid staining types of the diphtheria bacillus are sometimes virulent. They should not be regarded as avirulent on the basis of morphology alone. Virulence tests should be made to determine the status of carriers.

Instead of placing undue emphasis on morphology, more attention should be paid to the history of the carrier state, whether a convalescent or a contact with an active case. Such cultures should be considered virulent, regardless of morphologic characteristics, until proved otherwise.

By the use of the agglutination test two groups of the diphtheria bacillus have been determined. These groups are distinct, showing no evidence of cross-agglutination.

The members of the two groups show no differences in morphology or in relative virulence.

The results of agglutination tests in determining two groups of the diphtheria bacillus are corroborated by protective tests with antitoxin against the two group toxins.

Evidence is presented showing that the antitoxins of these groups are not so sharply differentiated as are the agglutinins. Group antitoxins seem to exist in small amounts common to both groups.

The effectiveness of therapeutic diphtheria antitoxin could probably be enhanced by the inclusion in its production of a member of the second or smaller group.

BACILLUS ENTERITIDIS INFECTION IN LABORATORY RATS

Paul R. Cannon

From the Department of Hygiene and Bacteriology, University of Chicago

Spontaneous infections among laboratory rodents, associated with organisms of the paratyphoid-enteritidis group, are not uncommon. Such epidemics have been described by many observers.[1] Unfortunately, there is much confusion in regard to the identification of the organisms concerned in many of the epidemics, as exact cultural and serologic tests were not always used. Consequently, it is not certain whether the bacilli isolated from these epidemics were strains of B. enteritidis, suipestifer or true paratyphoid bacilli.

An epidemic associated with organisms of this group recently developed in this laboratory in a stock of white rats, 6 days after the animals had been received. During a period of 4 weeks, 45 rats of 52 died. Previous to the outbreak there had been no deaths among the 24 rats then in stock. The rats were obtained from various places in the city and were apparently in healthy condition when received.

The rats, when infected, became listless and showed no inclination for food. Shortly before death, they were unable to sustain their own weight and were found in a sprawling position. In practically every case, there were evidences of diarrhea, and in some cases the rectum was bloody. The eyes also were affected, bloody crusts usually forming around them just before death.

The spleen was usually enlarged, in some cases being almost twice its normal size. The surface of the liver was, in many instances, dotted with small, milky areas, evidently small foci of necrosis. Frequently the small intestines were filled with bloody material and Peyer's patches were prominent.

ORGANISMS ISOLATED

A paratyphoid-like organism was isolated from the heart blood of 31 rats of 35 examined. B. proteus was obtained in 2 cases, and B. coli in 2. The predominant organism was a gram-negative, motile bacillus

Received for publication Jan. 17, 1920.

[1] Loeffler: Centralbl. f. Bakteriol., 1892, 11, p. 129; Danysz: Ann. de l'Inst. Pasteur, 1900, 14, p. 193; Issatschenko: Centralbl. f. Bakteriol., 1898, 23, p. 873; Trautmann: Ztschr. f. Hyg. u. Infectionskr., 1906, 54, p. 104; Savage: J. Hygiene, 1912, 12, p. 1; Bainbridge: J. Path. & Bacteriol., 1909, 13, p. 443; Petrie and O'Brien: J. Hygiene, 1910, 10, p. 287; Pappenheimer and Von Wedel: J. Infect. Dis., 1914, 14, p. 180.

which fermented the following carbohydrates, with the formation of gas: glucose, maltose, levulose, mannite, galactose and dulcite, but had no effect on lactose, saccharose, dextrin, inulin and salicin. In lead acetate agar, there was a browning of the medium at the end of 24 hours. In litmus milk the reaction, at the end of 24 hours, was slightly acid, but after 3 or 4 days it became markedly alkaline. Gelatin was not liquefied in 30 days. No indol was produced in trypsinized casein medium by any of these organisms.

AGGLUTINATIONS

As shown by the table, the organism (R. 1) is B. enteritidis serologically, since it is agglutinated by B. enteritidis serum to the full titer of the serum, absorbs B. enteritidis agglutinin, is not agglu tinated by B. paratyphosus B or suipestifer serum, and does not absorb B. paratyphosus B or suipestifer agglutinins from their respective serums. Furthermore, the immune serum from this organism agglutinates B. enteritidis to the full titer of the serum, but does not agglutinate B. suipestifer or B. paratyphosus A or B.

TABLE 1

AGGLUTINATION TESTS

Organisms	B. Enteritidis 52 Serum	B. Enteritidis 52 Serum after Absorption with R. 1	B. Paratyphosus B 12 Serum	B. Suipestifer 118 Serum	B. Paratyphosus B 12 Serum after Absorption with R. 1	B. Suipestifer 118 Serum after Absorption with R. 1	R. 1 Serum
R. 1	12,800	400	0	0	0	0	6,400
B. suipestifer 118	0	0	6,400	1,600	3,200	800	0
B. paratyphosus B	0	0	6,400	200	3,200	0	0
B. enteritidis 228	12,800		0		0		6,400
B. enteritidis 52		400	0	0		0	6,400
B. paratyphosus A4		0	0	0			
B. paratyphosus A212							0

The figures give the highest dilution of the serum causing definite agglutination.

The tests were made with 24-hour growths of organisms from agar slants, suspended in salt solution. Saturations were made by adding scrapings of 5 agar slants to a 1:100 dilution of serum, incubating for two hours at 37 C., centrifuging, repeating with 5 more slants and then using the clear supernatant serum for agglutination. The known strains of B. enteritidis, B. suipestifer and B. paratyphosus A are from Jordan's collection.[2] The B. paratyphosus B (Asam) strain was isolated by the writer from a case of paratyphoid fever and has proved by absorption tests to be a typical strain of B. paratyphosus B.

A survivor of the epidemic, rat 40, could not be infected by feeding the organisms, and was killed. The blood of this rat did not coagulate in 15 minutes and the Peyer's patches in the ileum were very thin as though the mucosa had sloughed off, in marked contrast to those in a normal young rat.

[2] Jordan: Jour. Infect. Dis., 1917, 20, p. 457.

The serum agglutinated both R. 1 and B. enteritidis but not B. suipestifer, B. paratyphosus A or B. This rat had, undoubtedly, had the disease and recovered. As focal necrosis of the liver is a usual condition in B. enteritidis infection in rats, the decreased coagulability of the blood may have been due to a decrease in fibrinogen.

Pathogenicity

A male rat, weighing 127 gm. injected intraperitoneally with 0.5 c c of a 24-hour broth culture, died at the end of 72 hours. A 94 gm. rat, injected in a similar manner with 1 c c died within 16 hours. A rat injected subcutaneously with 1 c c of a 24-hour broth culture died at the end of 5 days. A rat fed with 24-hour broth cultures died at the end of 7 days. In all cases, B. enteritidis was recovered from the heart blood and spleen.

Mode of Spreading

Flies doubtless played a part in spreading the infection, as they were very numerous. After screening the cages, the epidemic came to an end. Most of the rats were infested with fleas, and in two instances in which fleas were put into broth, B. enteritidis was recovered. However, fleas from infected rats, when placed on other rats, did not cause infection. Food, which was constantly being contaminated by the rats themselves, may also have furthered the spreading of the disease.

Summary

In an epidemic among white laboratory rats, extending over a period of four weeks, 45 of 52 died. An organism which is culturally and serologically identical with B. enteritidis was isolated from the heart blood of 31 of 35 rats examined. This organism, when injected intraperitoneally or subcutaneously into other rats, or when fed, caused the death of the rats, and the organism was recovered from the heart blood and spleen.

OBSERVATIONS ON GREEN PRODUCING COCCI OF INFLUENZA

Ruth Tunnicliff

From the John McCormick Institute for Infectious Diseases, Chicago

During the recent (1918-1919) influenza epidemic the majority of observers isolated diplococci from the sputum and from material obtained at necropsy. The organisms were classed generally as pneumococci of type 4 on account of their being soluble in bile and not agglutinated by pneumococcus serums of types 1, 2 and 3. Pneumococci of types 2, 3, and more rarely of type 1, were also isolated. Other workers, notably Mathers,[1] MacDonald,[2] Rosenow,[3] Howell and Anderson,[4] Jordan,[5] isolated bile-insoluble diplococci or streptococci from the nasopharynx, sputum, blood and necropsy material, which in 24 hours produced large, flat, moist, green colonies on blood-agar plates. MacDonald describes his colonies as slightly hemolytic. Rosenow [6] says his strains acquired hemolytic power. Howell and Anderson describe their cocci as nonhemolytic during the 10 days in which they were observed. Bernhardt and Meyer [7] isolated a bile-insoluble, gram-positive diplococcus, "Diplococcus epidemicus," which on human agar produced very minute, slightly hemolytic colonies with a black-greenish tinge. In 1917 Stephan [8] described as the agent of a clinically typical endemic of influenza in Leipzig a "diplococcus mucosus," which he isolated from the sputum and the blood, and which was agglutinated specifically by an immune serum as well as by patient and convalescent serum. It produced a capsule in the body and mucus in some mediums, was variable in its retention of Gram's stain, nonpathogenic to animals, insoluble in bile, but not identical with Str. mucosus of Schottmüller or pneumococcus mucosus. As the original article cannot be obtained now it is impossible to say whether this diplococcus and the coccus

Received for publication Jan. 26, 1920.

1 See Tunnicliff: Jour. Am. Med. Assn., 1918, 71, p. 1723.
2 Brit. Med. Jour., 1918, 2, p. 481.
3 Jour. Am. Med. Assn., 1919, 72, p. 31.
4 Jour. Infect. Dis., 1919, 25, p. 1.
5 Ibid., p. 28.
6 Jour. Am. Med. Assn., 1919, 72, p. 1604.
7 Med. Klin., 1918, 14, p. 683; abst., Jour. Am. Med. Assn., 1918, 71, p. 1573.
8 München. med. Wchnschr., 1918, 65, p. 257; abst., Jour. Am. Med. Assn., 1918, 71, p. 1573.

described by Mathers are identical. Howard [9] isolated green streptococci from the majority of his cases of influenza, but found the colonies smaller and less moist than typical pneumococcus colonies, and not different from colonies isolated from control cases. Cocci described as Str. viridans and nonhemolytic streptococci were isolated by Keegan,[10] Nuzum,[11] Blanton and Irons,[12] Deven,[13] Meyer,[14] Dick and Murray [15] and others, but the colonies are not described in such a way that they may be compared with those of other observers.

In the observations under consideration solubility in bile is the main criterion whether a coccus belongs to the pneumococcus or streptococcus groups, but unfortunately, as a rule, no description is given of the methods used in determining bile solubility. The ability of bile to dissolve influenzal cocci is recorded differently by different workers. Keegan [10] found it difficult to differentiate pneumococci of type 4 from Str. viridans, the bile test of broth cultures not being found reliable. Nuzum [11] found that pneumococci of type 4 and allied green producing organisms varied greatly as regards bile solubility. Dunn [16] also mentions that the bile solubility of his cultures of diplococci varied, 40% being soluble. Some of Howard's [9] strains were partially bile soluble.

On account of the difficulty in differentiating these organisms by the bile test, I have made immunity experiments to determine particularly whether various green-producing cocci, isolated from influenza and its complications, soluble and insoluble in bile, are in any way related.

I have shown [1] that specific opsonin for the peculiar green-producing streptococci from influenza developed during the course of the disease. A specific opsonic decrease was observed in the pneumonia following influenza, which persisted unless the patient recovered, when the opsonins rose to normal or above. No agglutinins could be demonstrated in the case of 3 strains tested, with the serum of 5 influenza and 2 pneumonia patients examined during the attack and convalescence. On the other hand, Rosenow found that the serum of patients convalescent from influenza agglutinated specifically some of the more sensitive of his green-producing streptococcus strains, but that some

[9] Bull. Johns Hopkins Hosp., 1919, 33, p. 13.
[10] Jour. Am. Med. Assn., 1918, 71, p. 1051.
[11] Ibid., p. 1562.
[12] Ibid., p. 1988.
[13] Ibid., 1919, 72, p. 265.
[14] Cal. State Jour. Med., 1919, 17, p. 216.
[15] Jour. Infect. Dis., 1919, 25, p. 6.
[16] Jour. Am. Med. Assn., 1918, 71, p. 2128.

strains were not agglutinated at all. A monovalent horse serum prepared by him with one of these strains specifically agglutinated 65, that is 66%, of 98 strains studied, most of the negative results being obtained with cultures made during convalescence. Other streptococci from a wide range of sources were rarely agglutinated by this serum. As stated, many of his strains acquired hemolytic power on cultivation. The close relationship of the green-producing strains to hemolytic streptococci was indicated, moreover, he says, by the fact that hemolytic streptococcus serum commonly manifested decided agglutinating power for the green producers. He concludes that his experiments show that green-producing strains of streptococci or diplostreptococci from influenza are immunologically identical or closely related. The results of his absorption tests were in harmony with this conclusion.

Howell and Anderson [4] obtained a large number of fixation reactions with influenza serums and strains of green-producing streptococci from influenza at Camp Meade and in Chicago. The serum of the convalescent influenza patients came from a wide range of localities.

Here it may be noted that various observers have tried to differentiate green-producing streptococci into groups by various immunity reactions, the opsonic probably being the most successful. Kinsella and Swift [17] believed they could classify nonhemolytic streptococci by complement fixation tests, but Howell [18] concluded that the organisms could not be classified by that method. Agglutination tests were found useful by Rosenow and Gray [19] for differentiating the poliomyelitis streptococcus from streptococci and pneumococci from other sources. Mathers and Howell [20] obtained better results in differentiating the poliomyelitis coccus with immunized rabbit serum when opsonins were studied rather than agglutinins, on account of spontaneous agglutination. Nuzum and Willy [21] found that by means of opsonic determinations of immune horse serum, they were able to separate strains of poliomyelitis cocci from other strains of cocci presenting more or less confusing cultural and morphologic similarities. Later Davis [22] found well-marked specific increase in opsonins for the poliomyelitis streptococcus in the serum of monkeys with experimental poliomyelitis. Opsonic determination of specific immune rabbit serum

[17] Jour. Exper. Med., 1917, 25, p. 877.
[18] Jour. Infect. Dis., 1918, 22, p. 230.
[19] Ibid., 1918, 22, p. 345.
[20] Ibid., 1917, 21, p. 292.
[21] Ibid., 1918, 22, p. 258.
[22] Ibid., 1919, 24, p. 176.

was found by Tunnicliff and Brown [23] to be an easy and reliable method to differentiate the diplococci found in measles and rubella from each other and from other nonhemolytic diplococci and streptococci. These cocci when first isolated were not suitable for agglutination tests because of spontaneous clumping.

The thirty-four strains of green producing cocci from influenza used in these experiments were isolated by the late Captain George Mathers at Camp Meade, by Major E. F. Hirsch at Camp Grant, by Dr. Nuzum in Chicago, and by myself at Camp Meade and in Chicago. All of these strains were isolated during the early months of the epidemic (September, October and November, 1918).

Bile solubility was determined by adding one-fifth the volume of sterile ox-bile to a broth culture; the mixtures were incubated for two hours as some strains were found to dissolve slowly in bile, and compared macroscopically with a broth culture without bile. Suspensions of the cocci in salt solution gave results similar to those in broth cultures. Of the 34 strains, 23 were insoluble in bile and consequently would be classed as streptococci, but seven of them were agglutinated by pneumococcus serum of types 2 and 3 (Rockefeller). The 11 bile-soluble strains belonged to pneumococcus groups of types 2, 3 and 4, according to their agglutination reactions.

All of the 34 strains produced green colonies on goat blood agar, and after 48 hours' incubation and 24 hours' refrigeration showed partial hemolysis of the corpuscles immediately surrounding the colony. The majority of the strains produced large, moist colonies, similar to the colonies described by Mathers.[1] The Camp Grant cultures, as a rule, gave rise to smaller and drier colonies than the others. Some of the strains which on isolation produced large, moist colonies, after six months cultivation grew in much smaller and less moist colonies, but without change in their hemolyzing power.

The eight strains which were agglutinated by pneumococcus serum of type 3 were moister than the other strains, but not mucoid. These cocci were larger and rounder and possessed a wider capsule than the others.

The strains isolated by me in Chicago were obtained from the edematous brain in ten cases of influenzal bronchopneumonia in adults. The brains were removed by Dr. E. R. LeCount immediately after death, the surface seared, the brain substance broken up and removed with a large sterile pipet and the material added to broth, cultures being made from this mixture. At first both aerobic and anaerobic cultures were made on human blood agar, but as the same organisms were found in both, the anaerobic cultures were discontinued. The blood-agar plates were made by adding 5% blood to 12 c c beef extract agar (Fairchild Culture Peptone), which was 0.8% acid to phenolphthalein. After the original culture was made goat blood was used instead of human. The cultures from one brain were sterile. Gram-positive diplococci in medium long chains were grown from the other

[23] Ibid., 1918, 23, p. 572; 1919, 24, p. 181.

9, in pure culture except for staphylococci in 2 broth cultures which also contained a rapidly growing bacillus. In no instance was the Pfeiffer bacillus cultivated. Twice the cocci grew in the original broth culture, but not on the aerobic blood-agar plate. Two strains would not grow in subculture, possibly due to their not being transferred at the end of 24 hours' incubation. From 5 to 10 colonies grew on the original plates. The 2 strains of diplococci isolated in broth and then grown on blood agar, produced green colonies, which were drier and smaller than those isolated from the spinal fluid of the same patient in one case and from the brains and fluids of the other 5, grown originally on blood agar. After 24 hours' incubation these 6 strains produced on blood agar, large, round, moist, rather flat, green colonies, 2-4 mm. in diameter, with regular edges, which had a tendency to become confluent. The colonies often showed umbilication after longer incubation. The green discoloration was only under the colony. After 24 hours' incubation and 24 hours' refrigeration, a narrow, very slight hemolytic area was seen around the edge of the colony and a similar zone just inside the colony, giving the appearance of three rings. The hemolysis corresponds to the alpha type of Smith and Brown.[24] Plates were made according to Brown's[25] method: 5% blood agar (12 c c) was inoculated with a 24-hour broth culture and poured into a Petri dish, 9 cm. in diameter. After 48 hours' incubation and 24 hours' refrigeration the colonies appeared biconvex, the deep colonies being about 0.5 mm. in diameter, with a somewhat greenish discoloration and partial hemolysis of the blood corpuscles immediately surrounding the colony for about 0.5 mm., and surrounded by a second, clearer, not discolored, partly hemolyzed zone of about the same diameter. When incubated 48 hours and refrigerated, the characteristic appearance seen on the surface of blood-agar plates after 24 hours' incubation was lost.

The same green-producing cocci were isolated in pure culture from the blood, pleural, pericardial and spinal fluids in two cases. In a third case, that of a pregnant woman, the placental and fetal blood were sterile.

Of the 7 strains studied, only 1 was soluble in bile. This bile soluble culture was not agglutinated by pneumococcus serums of types 1, 2 and 3.

[24] Jour. Med. Research, 1915, 13, p. 455.
[25] Monograph No. 9, Rockefeller Inst. for Med. Research, 1919.

All 7 strains fermented glucose, lactose, saccharose and raffinose. Six fermented salicin, 2 inulin and 2 mannite. Hiss' sheep serum water was used and the cultures were incubated one week. The cocci produced little sediment in 1% glucose broth, except one culture.

Morphologically, the organisms were generally pointed diplococci with a capsule. Some were distinctly round, but the shape varied with cultivation. Some cultures produced longer chains than others.

The virulence of these organisms was not tested when first isolated. Two of the 4 strains tested were virulent at the end of 3 months, $1/200$ of a 24-hour broth culture killing a mouse within 24 hours. These two organisms had been transplanted about once a week during the three months.

According to our present method of classification, the bile insoluble strains would be called streptococci. The bile soluble strain, which would be classed as pneumococci of type 4, was otherwise like the insoluble strains. Immunologically, they were found to react alike. Rabbits immunized with the bile insoluble streptococci isolated from sputum and pneumonic lungs in influenza produced opsonins and agglutinins for all of these brain strains. These experiments are discussed later.

Apparently the brain cocci are like the cocci isolated by Mathers and others from influenza and its complications. The colonies closely resemble those of the Str. viridans isolated by Zingher [26] from empyema and from the lung, but the cocci differ in possessing a capsule and in not as a rule growing in long convoluted chains in broth, leaving the fluid clear.

IMMUNITY EXPERIMENTS

As opsonin is the antibody most easily demonstrated for streptococci, and agglutinin the antibody generally used to differentiate pneumococci, observations were made on both these antibodies.

Rabbits were immunized in various ways with different strains of the peculiar green producing cocci from influenza and its complications. At first they were inoculated intravenously about every 4 days with increasing doses of living cocci grown on goat blood-agar slants, the largest dose given being the growth on 4 slants. The rabbits bore the inoculations badly, several dying before immune bodies were demonstrable. Some rabbits were inoculated with killed cocci, at first subcutaneously, later intravenously, and then with living organisms. One rabbit received only killed cocci. For the tests the cocci were transplanted from goat blood-agar to 1% glucose broth and incubated at 24, or 48 hours, if necessary, for growth.

[26] Jour. Am. Med. Assn., 1918, 71, p. 451; 1919, 72, p. 1020.

The opsonic tests were made as follows: At first the serums were used unheated and undiluted, or diluted 1:4 with normal salt solution, and then equal parts of washed human leukocytes and bacterial suspensions were added. It was sometimes necessary to dilute the broth culture suspension if the growth was profuse. Later the point of opsonic extinction of the serums was determined; the results of the two methods were similar. The specimens were incubated at 37 C. for 15 minutes, smears stained with carbol thionin, 50 polymorphonuclear leukocytes counted, and the number taking part in phagocytosis noted.

Later the normal and immune rabbit serum was first heated for one-half hour at 56 C. to destroy the thermolabile element, and the serums then diluted to the point of opsonic extinction, the mixtures of serum, leukocytes and cocci then being incubated for 25 minutes. The results were on the whole the same as with unheated serum. It is important to note that heated and unheated normal serum as a rule contained practically no opsonins at 1:3 for these cocci.

Agglutination was studied by mixing equal parts of serum and broth culture in capillary pipets, incubating at 37 C. for 2 hours and refrigerating 20 hours when the results were read macroscopically (Lister).

The antibodies were produced slowly. Three subcutaneous injections of large numbers of killed organisms (the growth on 4-8 blood-agar slants) produced no agglutination in most instances and not much opsonin. Some rabbits so injected died after receiving a small number of living cocci. Agglutinins as a rule were produced several weeks later than the opsonins, never in high dilutions and generally in much lower dilutions than the opsonins. A few strains agglutinated spontaneously and therefore could not be used in the agglutination tests though suitable for the opsonin determinations. The strains differed in their power to produce agglutinins, and in some rabbits these antibodies appeared earlier than in others. The apparent ready response on the part of the rabbit with opsonins and slow response with agglutinins is in accord with my results with influenza serum which gave marked increase in opsonins for the cocci while no agglutination could be demonstrated.

The serum of the immune rabbits 1 and 2 (table 1) which was tested undiluted or diluted 1:4 caused marked phagocytosis of the influenza cocci — an average of six times more phagocytosis than normal rabbit serum. The serums of the other rabbits which were heated and diluted opsonified the homologous coccus in dilutions as high as 1:11,200; the weakest serum gave phagocytosis with the homologous strain at 1:60. The average dilution at which phagocytosis ceased for heterologous strains was between 1:60 and 1:120. Normal serum, as a rule, showed no opsonins for the strains at a dilution of 1:3, the dilution reached by the addition to the serum of leukocytes and bacterial suspension.

TABLE 1

OPSONINS AND AGGLUTININS IN THE SERUM OF RABBITS IMMUNIZED WITH THE PECULIAR GREEN PRODUCING STREPTOCOCCI FROM INFLUENZA

Serums	Cocci: Percentage of Peculiar Green Producing Influenza Cocci for which the Serum Showed Definite Increase in Opsonin and Agglutinin	Cocci: Control Tests with Green Producing Streptococci from Sources Other than Influenza, Pneumococci of All Types, Hemolytic Streptococci
Serum 1. Rabbit immunized with coccus from sputum at onset of attack of uncomplicated influenza; coccus not soluble in bile, not agglutinated by pneumococcus serum		
Opsonin	87%	0%
Agglutinin	93%	0%
Serum 2. Rabbit immunized with serum from influenza-pneumonia; bile insoluble, not agglutinated by pneumococcus serum		
Opsonin	90%	0%
Agglutinin	90%	0%
Serum 3. Rabbits immunized with coccus from influenza-pneumonia; bile insoluble, not agglutinated by pneumococcus serum		
Opsonin	76%	0%
Agglutinin	78%	0%
Serum 4. Rabbit immunized with coccus from sputum in influenza-pneumonia; bile insoluble, not agglutinated by pneumococcus serum		
Opsonin	82%	0%
Agglutinin	94%	0%
Serum 5. Rabbit immunized with coccus from influenza-pneumonia; bile insoluble, not agglutinated by pneumococcus serum		
Opsonin	90%	0%
Agglutinin	83%	0%
Serum 6. Rabbit immunized with coccus of brain of case of influenza-pneumonia; bile insoluble, not agglutinated by pneumococcus serum type 2		
Opsonin	85%	0%
Agglutinin	83%	8%
Serum 7. Rabbit immunized with coccus from influenza-pneumonia; slowly soluble in bile, agglutinated by pneumococcus serum type 3		
Opsonin	93%	0%
Agglutinin	87%	0%

Of the strains used to immunize the rabbits, 1, 2, 3, 5 and 7 were isolated at Camp Meade; 4 and 6 in Chicago. Strain 2 was isolated after death from the lung and strain 7 from the blood of the same patient.

Serum 6 agglutinated a strain of pneumococcus, type 2, at a dilution of 1 to 10.

Agglutination was marked with immune rabbit serum at 1 : 2, but generally no agglutination was observed above 1 : 20, except with the homologous organisms, and then no agglutination was observed above 1 : 320. One rabbit agglutinated its own organisms at 1 : 10 only. Normal rabbit serum did not agglutinate the influenza strains except one which, after long cultivation, was agglutinated at 1 : 80.

The serum of rabbits 1 and 2 (table 1) were tested with the 34 influenza cocci and 13 strains of cocci from other sources (pneumococci of types 1, 2, 3 and 4; hemolytic streptococci from bronchopneumonia and empyema; and Str. viridans from measles, rubella and bronchitis). The serums of rabbits 3, 4, 5, 6 and 7 (table 1) were tested with 20 influenza cocci and the same strains from other sources. All these immune serums showed a marked increase in opsonins and agglutinins for 86% of the influenza strains. The negative results were obtained with some of the bile soluble strains (pneumococci of types 2 and 4) from Camp Grant. The immune serums showed no increase in opsonins or agglutinins for the cocci from sources other than influenza except that the serum of rabbit 6 agglutinated a pneumococcus of type 2 at a dilution of 1:10. The serum of rabbit 7 immunized with a coccus agglutinated by a pneumococcus type 3 serum, did not agglutinate noninfluenzal pneumococci of type 3.

The results show that the serum of rabbits, immunized with certain green-producing cocci from influenza and its complications, contained opsonins and agglutinins for the influenza strains, whether soluble or insoluble in bile, and whether belonging to the pneumococcus groups or not. Hence, the results indicate that we are dealing with a group of cocci which are closely related immunologically, although certain strains differ in their bile solubility and agglutinability by pneumococcus serums.

Major Fennel of the Army Medical School kindly sent me a large number of strains of pneumococci of type 4 and of Str. viridans isolated from influenza and other sources. The majority of influenza strains were isolated late in the epidemic. With the exception of two strains isolated from spontaneous pneumonias in monkeys, they did not produce colonies similar to those produced by the Mathers coccus and other peculiar green-producing cocci from influenza. No antibodies could be demonstrated for these strains with the 5 immune serums tested, except in these instances: opsonification at a dilution of 1:2 occurred with one influenza strain from Camp Meade and one immune serum; agglutination at 1:2 was demonstrated with two serums and one monkey strain and another Camp Meade influenzal strain. These three strains were type 4 pneumococci. The influenzal history of the two Camp Meade strains is not definite. These results suggest that the strains isolated at the onset and height of the epidemic differed from those isolated later.

ABSORPTION EXPERIMENTS

Absorption experiments were made to determine whether the agglutination of the allied organisms was due to partial or minor agglutinins. Serum 1 was absorbed with the homologous and four closely related influenzal coccus strains and by pneumococci of types 1 and 2. Killed organisms were suspended in the serum which was incubated for 2 hours, refrigerated for 24 hours, then centrifugated and the supernatant fluid tested. This process was repeated three times when the serum was found no longer to agglutinate the homologous coccus. Absorption with the homologous influenza coccus not only removed the agglutinins for that organism, but also for the 4 closely allied cocci. Absorption with each of the 4 allied influenza cocci, bile insoluble and bile soluble, also absorbed the agglutinins for the homologous coccus as well as for the allied strains, but absorption with pneumococci of types 1 and 2, not of influenzal origin, failed to remove either the agglutinins for the homologous organisms or for the allied strains. These results indicate that these green-producing cocci from influenza and its complications form a group of immunologically closely related organisms.

COMMENT

The experiments I have described indicate that certain green-producing influenzal cocci are closely related to both pneumococcus and Str. viridans. The bile insolubility of most of these strains and the sugar reactions relate them to streptococci. However, inulin fermentation by these cocci varies. The cocci obtained by Mathers, Rosenow, Howell and Anderson, and Jordan generally did not ferment inulin. Nuzum says his cultures varied a good deal in inulin fermentation. My cultures also varied in this respect. The frequency of lanceolate shape and capsule formation and the type of colony point to their relation to pneumococci. The bile solubility or slow solubility of some of the influenza cocci and the agglutinability of some strains by pneumococcus serums also speak for their close relationship to the pneumococcus. It may be of interest in this connection to refer to certain observations showing that bile-insoluble cocci may be agglutinated by pneumococcus serums and that agglutination with pneumococcus serums is not always specific.

Thus Sutton and Sevier[27] described a Streptococcus mucosus, which was bile insoluble, and morphologically unlike type 3 pneumococcus, but was agglutinated by type 3 serum. During the recent influenza epidemic, Keegan[10] and his co-workers found that some of the fixed pneumococcus types, identified by agglutination, did not show a distinct bile solubility. Mathers[28] and Clough[29] each observed pneumococci which agglutinated equally with types 1 and 2 serums. Blake[30] encountered occasional strains of pneumococci which agglutinated in type 3 serum, and which did not show well developed mucoid characteristics and could not be distinguished culturally from other types of pneumococci. He mentions that there is a small number of strains of pneumococci belonging to type 4 which agglutinate in all 3 types of antipneumococcus serum. In her study of type 4 pneumococci Olmstead[31] observed that groups F and G were agglutinated by both type 4 and type 2 serum. She considers that some members of these groups serve as connecting links between type 2 and type 4, but owing to a closer relationship with the latter they should be classed as of type 4. Recently Clough[32] described 9 strains, three not completely dissolved by bile, which were agglutinated with antipneumococcus serum of types 1, 2 and 3. One strain showed a mutation while under observation. On isolation it had the cultural reactions of a typical pneumococcus and the phagocytic and agglutinative reaction of an atypical type 2 strain. After cultivation it was agglutinated by antipneumococcus serum types 1, 2 and 3 and became bile insoluble, did not ferment inulin and caused precipitation in glucose ascitic fluid agar. She suggests that these pneumococci reacting with all 3 types of antipneumococcus serums may represent primitive, relatively undifferentiated forms from which fixed types may arise. It consequently may be possible that the influenza cocci which I am considering and which have both pneumococcus and streptococcus characteristics form a group between these two forms of cocci.

It does not seem possible to determine definitely the etiologic relation of the peculiar green-producing cocci to influenza and its complications. At Camp Meade the Mathers coccus was the prevailing organism during the onset and height of the epidemic, being present in 87% of the sputums examined. It was the organism which appeared with the onset of influenza—Pfeiffer's bacillus having been present in the respiratory diseases for several weeks previous. The Pfeiffer bacillus was found in 58% of the influenzal sputum cultures. In Chicago, Jordan found this coccus present in a few more cases (66%) than the Pfeiffer bacillus (64%). When present, it was always found in the early days of the attack, and was more closely associated with

[27] Johns Hopkins Hosp. Bull., 1917, 28, p. 315.
[28] Jour. Infect. Dis., 1915, 17, p. 514.
[29] Bull. Johns Hopkins Hosp., 1917, 28, p. 306.
[30] Jour. Exper. Med., 1917, 26, p. 67.
[31] Jour. Immunol., 1917, 2, p. 425.
[32] Jour. Exper. Med., 1919, 30, p. 123.

pneumonia cases than the Pfeiffer bacillus. However, Jordan found the coccus present in colds and tonsillitis in about the same proportion of cases as in influenza, while Pfeiffer's bacillus was found in only 14%. Rosenow also observed this peculiar streptococcus in and about Rochester, Minn., at the very beginning of the epidemic of influenza. K. F. Meyer found the same coccus (personal communication) in 85% of the cases of influenza during the epidemic in California.

My experiments and those of Rosenow and of Howell and Anderson showed that the serum of convalescent influenza and influenzal pneumonia patients contained definite, specific opsonins, agglutinins and complement fixation bodies for these streptococci, which indicates that this coccus played at least some part in the reactions in the epidemic and also that it was of wider distribution than commonly recognized. Unfortunately, human or monkey inoculations and preventive vaccination with this coccus alone were not made during the epidemic.

SUMMARY

Various investigators isolated peculiar green-producing cocci with the characteristics of both pneumococcus and streptococcus, from influenza and its complications, during the onset and at the height of the recent epidemic. This coccus is oftener lanceolate than round, generally it possesses a capsule, and produces large, moist green colonies on blood-agar plates. It is, as a rule, insoluble in bile, and rarely ferments inulin.

I have isolated this coccus from the edematous brain in influenzal bronchopneumonia, and generally in pure culture. In no instance was the Pfeiffer bacillus cultivated from the brain.

The serum of rabbits immunized with strains of this coccus from influenza and its complications contained opsonins and agglutinins for other similar, bile-insoluble influenzal cocci, and also for certain influenzal cocci, which were bile soluble and agglutinable by antipneumococcus serums. These results indicate that the green producing influenzal cocci form a group, the members of which are closely related immunologically.

The results of absorption experiments with reference to agglutinins also suggest that we are dealing with a group of closely allied organisms. Immune rabbit serum treated with the homologous influenza coccus lost its agglutinins for the homologous coccus and for allied influenza cocci. Absorption with allied influenza organisms also removed the immune bodies for the homologous coccus as well as for the closely related cocci, but absorption with pneumococci of types 1 and 2 not of influenzal origin, did not remove the agglutinin for the influenza cocci.

THE FERMENTATION OF POLYSACCHARIDS BY BACILLUS AEROGENES

R. L. Laybourn

From the Department of Bacteriology and Hygiene, Iowa State College, Ames, Iowa

From recent work on the coli-like bacteria it is agreed that they may be divided into two subgroups which are differentiated by the Voges-Proskauer or methyl red reactions. These two groups are quite well correlated with habitat. The B. coli group (Voges-Proskauer negative — methyl red positive) is characteristically of fecal origin, whereas the B. aerogenes-cloaca group (Voges-Proskauer positive — methyl red negative) is relatively infrequent in feces, but predominates in the soil and on grains. B. aerogenes, although rarely found in the feces as voided, is a common inhabitant of the upper part of the intestinal tract of man. Under certain conditions it may constitute a considerable portion of the coli-like bacteria of a stool. It thus becomes of some practical significance to differentiate the B. aerogenes of intestinal origin from the B. aerogenes found in soil and on grain. Rogers pointed out that the fermentation of adonitol may be employed for this purpose with a high degree of reliability. It was thought that a study of the fermentation of the polysaccharids from different sources, particularly glycogens from vegetable and animal sources might possibly be of value in differentiating fecal from nonfecal types of B. aerogenes.

Historical

In 1883 Wortman was led to believe that starch could be decomposed by bacteria, and he observed that if starch was prepared and allowed to ferment spontaneously an organism which he termed Bacterium termo predominated. This work led him to infer that many bacteria produce an enzyme which shows the properties of diastase. He also observed that various starches were not broken down with equal celerity and suggested that this is due to differences in specific gravity.

Durham (1901) states that members of the B. lactis-aerogenes group may be separated from other coli-like bacteria by their ability to ferment starch and inulin, and thinks that they may be separated into three groups by their action on these substances. Some ferment starch and inulin with gas and acid production, others starch alone and still others inulin alone.

F. A. Baldwin (1917), in a preliminary report of work on the colon group, employing the Bergey and Deehan classification, finds that many forms may be differentiated by the differences in their action on corn and potato starch.

Received for publication Jan. 16, 1920.

Johnson and Levine observed that the B. aerogenes types decomposed corn starch quite readily. About 18% of their strains formed acetyl-methyl-carbinol whereas the others apparently did not, indicating the possibility of differentiation within the group.

It is difficult to review the literature on starch fermentation by bacteria because it is very rarely stated what starch was employed. The number of recorded instances in which starches from different sources were used is negligible.

EXPERIMENTAL

Sources of cultures.—In the initial experiments, 117 strains were employed, including 49 of the B. aerogenes type which were starch fermenters and 68 different varieties of B. coli and B. cloacae; the latter being regarded as starch nonfermenters. It was observed that the strains of B. coli and B. cloacae did not ferment any of the polysaccharids employed with acid and gas production and will therefore not be discussed further.

TABLE 1

AMONG THE 49 B. AEROGENES STRAINS INCLUDED

Soil	13
Sewage	6
American Museum of Natural History	12
Grains (furnished by L. A. Rogers)	3
Lederle Laboratories	1
University of Toronto (originally from the Pasteur Institute, Paris)	1
Isolated from virus hogs, Iowa State College	8
American Museum (marked B. mucosus-capsulatus)	2
Chicago University (B. mucosus-capsulatus)	1
Northwestern Medical School (B. mucosus-capsulatus)	1
University of Toronto (B. pneumoniae-Friedländer)	1

Except as indicated the original sources of these strains were not known.

Medium.—The medium used was made up as follows: A solution of 1% Witte's peptone and 0.5% dipotassium phosphate in distilled water was prepared, flasked and autoclaved. A quantity sufficient for the entire work was made up at one time.

Preparation of Test Substances. — Eight hundred c c of the dipotassium phosphate-peptone solution were brought to a boil and while heating 5 gm. of the test substance were thoroughly mixed in 200 c c of the cold medium and added slowly to the 800 c c of the boiling medium. The mixture was then boiled for ten minutes and the loss of weight made up with distilled water. This gave a medium containing 0.5% of the test substance. The medium was then placed in Durham fermentation tubes, autoclaved for 10 minutes at 10 lbs. pressure and quickly chilled with cold water. When prepared in this manner there was no evidence of the presence of reducing sugars when tested with Fehling's solution.

The following test substances were used:

Starches.—Arrowroot-Post Natal (*Maranta sp.*)
Arrowroot-St. Vincent's (*Maranta sp.*)
Barley (*Hordeum sativum Jess.*)
Bean (*Phaseolus sp.*)
Buckwheat (*Fagopyrum esculentum*)
Canna (*Canna edulis Edw.* and other species)
Corn (*Zea Mays L.*)

Ginger (*Zingiber officinalis Roscoe*)
Lentil (*Lens esculenta Moench*)
Oat (*Avena sativa L.*)
Pea (*Pisum sativum L.*)
Potato (*Solanum tuberosum L.*)
Rice (*Oryza sativa L.*)
Rye (*Secale cereale L.*)
Sago (*Cycas sp.*)
Tapioca (*Manihot utilissima Pohl*)
Wheat (*Triticum sativum Lam.*)

These starches were all "Lilly's Authentic Starches," prepared by the Eli Lilly Co. They were given a careful microscopic examination and appeared to be pure.

Inulin.—Merck's Inulin-Kiliani was used.

Glycogen.—Horse glycogen, from the liver of a normal horse, was prepared by Pflüger's method as given by Plimmer. Polyporus (*Polyporus rulphureus*) was used as an example of a plant glycogen. The latter specimen was prepared by the Chemical Section of the Agricultural Experiment Station through the courtesy of Dr. Dox.

Hemicellulose.—Hemicellulose from date seeds was used.

Incubation.—Incubation was at 37.5 C. for one week. For the first 3 days the tubes were looked over each day, and those that did not show gas were shaken to insure the entrance of the organisms into the gas tubes.

Records.—At the end of three days a preliminary record of gas production was made. At the end of a week the final records were made, consisting of the approximate percent. of gas produced and the reaction to methyl red.

Results.—About half of the cultures were tested for their reaction to phenolphthalein. The hydrogen-ion concentration was such that all were acid or neutral to phenolphthalein.

Fehling's solution and Barfoed's reagent were used in testing for reducing sugars. None of the tubes tested showed the presence of reducing sugars.

The Voges-Proskauer reaction was also tried on half of the strains and was found to be uniformly negative.

Forty-six strains produced gas from all the starches studied. Of the three organisms remaining, a B. aerogenes isolated from virus hog failed to form gas from bean and ginger starch, a B. pneumoniae Friedländer culture from the U. S. Hygienic Laboratory, failed to produce gas from lentil, oat and wheat starch, and the Roger's strain produced small amounts of gas from corn, tapioca and wheat starch only.

Only three organisms produced gas from inulin. These included two strains of B. aerogenes from soil and the culture of B. lactis-aerogenes from the University of Toronto.

Three organisms (all B. aerogenes types from soil) produced gas from the two glycogens. Two of the three inulin fermenters were included in this group of organisms. The glycogen fermenters produced gas from all the starches.

Twenty organisms produced gas from dulcitol. Eight of these were indol negative and twelve indol positive. As reported by Johnson and Levine, there appeared to be no correlation between the fermentation of dulcitol and indol production.

None of the organisms used produced gas from date seed hemicellulose.

DISCUSSION

Gas Production.—It was observed that if an organism fermented one starch it usually fermented all the starches tested. Of the 49 strains studied there were only 3 that did not conform to this rule, and these 3 did not seem to be interrelated with reference to the starches from which they produced gas. This peculiar behavior of a few of the strains toward starch is difficult to explain.

A study of starch from the chemical and physical standpoint has led to the belief that it is not a uniform compound, but exists in many isomeric and polymeric forms in different plants. Reichert, in discussing stereochemistry and some of its applications, says:

(1) That it is theoretically possible for a complex compound, such as starch or hemoglobin, to exist in a countless number of stereoisomeric forms; (2) that the slightest alteration in the configuration or arrangement of the component units of a molecule may give rise to a change of properties that may be profound, and sometimes of a predictable character; (3) that stereochemistry is inseparably associated with the problems of nutrition, species, disease, heredity and the innumerable manifestations of protoplasmic activity which in the aggregate constitute life.

Fischer emphasizes the fact that stereoisomeric substances often show a greater differentiation in their properties than is usually observed in related isomers.

Isomeric substances, such as the carbohydrates, are unique in their fermentation reactions in that each one requires a specific enzyme to bring about its decomposition. One enzyme is often capable of breaking down all the members of a group which do not bear an isomeric relation to each other. The fats, for example, while differing widely in molecular weight, belong to a homologous series, and one enzyme, lipase, can cause the decomposition of all the members of the group. Fischer believes that it is necessary for an enzyme to have a complementary configuration in order to bring about the decomposition of a compound. To use his analogy, the enzyme must be adjusted to the substance, much as the key is adjusted to the lock.

A brief glance at the literature is sufficient to show that bacteria that are quite closely related show wide differences in the enzymes produced and in the consequent fermentations.

The fact that an organism which ferments one starch usually ferments all the others would indicate that the same enzyme is capable of breaking down all of them and that the starches are polymers. Another point of view would be that the organism produced a multiplicity of enzymes.

Acid Production.—The most striking thing noted in this work was that although organisms fermented all the starches with gas production there was a very marked difference in the hydrogen-ion concentration produced with different starches. The following table summarizes the reactions to methyl red of the organisms with the starches which they fermented. It was not possible, at the time this work was being done, to repeat the experiments in the case of a few contaminated cultures. There are, therefore, several differences in the total number of fermentations of the several starches recorded in this table.

TABLE 2
REACTIONS TO METHYL RED OF ORGANISMS AND STARCHES THEY FERMENTED

Starches	Acid	Neutral	Alkaline
Arrowroot P. N.	15	5	29
Arrowroot S. V.	16	14	19
Barley	10	5	33
Bean	10	5	34
Buckwheat	8	2	39
Canna	22	4	21
Corn	13	6	30
Ginger	3	4	41
Lentil	7	3	38
Oat	0	2	46
Pea	17	7	25
Potato	19	3	27
Rice	4	5	29
Rye	14	5	30
Sago	20	6	23
Tapioca	20	5	24
Wheat	12	6	31

The differences in reaction with the same organism on different starches and with different organisms on the same starch were so varied that correlation tables seemed of no practical value for the differentiation of strains.

These differences are of considerable interest, at least from the theoretical standpoint. It is customary to say that when a starch is decomposed that it has been hydrolyzed, and it is usually assumed that the decomposition has taken place through a number of stages; i. e., erythrodextrin, achroadextrin, maltose and glucose. In bacterial fermentations the glucose is broken down with the liberation of acid, gas and other end products usually observed. In this group of organisms we are dealing with strains which assimilate glucose with the production of acetyl-methyl-carbinol and in a concentration of 0.5% glucose give an alkaline reaction to methyl red. It was shown by Levine, Weldin and Johnson that with a concentration of 1.0% glucose the reaction to methyl red becomes alkaline after 3 days at 37 C. If it is assumed that all the starch is hydrolyzed to glucose the maximum concentration would be 0.556% glucose, a concentration at which all the B. aerogenes strains would give an alkaline reaction after seven days at 37 C. The fact that in many instances these organisms produced an acid or neutral reaction seems to indicate that the starches are not utilized as glucose. If the starches are first reduced to glucose before utilization we should expect to find the same end products as when glucose is used directly.

It is generally recognized and accepted that B. aerogenes characteristically produces acetyl-methyl-carbinol from glucose. This was the case with the cultures used in this study. Of the 25 strains tested for acetyl-methyl-carbinol from starch fermentation not a single strain was positive, which again indicates that the decomposition of starch probably did not progress to the glucose stage before assimilation by the bacteria.

In no instance was there any evidence of a reducing sugar when tested with Fehling's solution or Barfoed's reagent. This may be explained on the assumption that (1) no reducing sugar was formed, or (2) reducing sugar was produced in small quantities and quickly utilized. If the latter were true, we would expect to find the same end-products as when glucose is used directly. The findings tend to show that in the decomposition of a starch by bacteria there is some metabolic process going on which is quite at variance with accepted ideas. An investigation of what really takes place under these conditions will, at least, be of considerable theoretical interest.

SUMMARY

B. aerogenes usually ferments starches of widely different origins.

The results obtained tend to show that B. aerogenes does not hydrolyze starch through the usual series of compounds and eventually utilize it as glucose.

The difference in the amount of gas and the final reaction produced when a given strain of B. aerogenes ferments starches from different sources indicates that there is some difference in the composition of starches from different sources.

Starches do not appear to be of value in the differentiation of strains of B. aerogenes derived from fecal and nonfecal sources.

EXPERIMENTS ON IMMUNIZATION WITH PSEUDOBLACKLEG PELLETS

T. P. Haslam and O. M. Franklin

From Kansas State Agricultural College, Manhattan, Kans.

In a previous report[1] it was shown that a certain brand of commercial blackleg vaccine made in the pellet form consisted wholly or in large part of an organism somewhat similar, but distinctly different from B. chauvei, and which we called the bacillus of pseudoblackleg, pending the determination of its exact classification. The same peculiarity in the same make of vaccine has recently been observed by Muriel Robertson,[2] and the organism classified by her as B. oedematis-maligni Koch. At the time of our first report similar observations of Theobald Smith[3] in 1905 unfortunately were not known to us. Smith states that the strain of blackleg sent him by one manufacturer of blackleg vaccine differed from typical blackleg in gas formula, gas formation from lactose, odor, and action on milk, and concludes: "It may be possible that the one factory uses as backleg vaccine a wide-spread, spore-forming, pathogenic bacillus, belonging to the group of malignant oedema."

Because so many of these pseudoblackleg pellets were used by the farmers and stock men in the United States, in the vaccination of calves against blackleg, further experiments were undertaken to determine whether these pellets possessed any ability to immunize calves against blackleg.

The plan of the experiment was to vaccinate one group of calves with the commercial pseudoblackleg pellets, and a second group with pellets prepared in our laboratories from blackleg virus secured from naturally occurring cases of blackleg. Both groups of calves were given as nearly as possible the same number of treatments, and the original plan of the experiment called for the pellets prepared from naturally occurring blackleg virus to be of the same virulence to guinea-pigs as the commercial pellets. After two vaccinations all calves were tested for immunity against blackleg by receiving a dose of blackleg virus derived from natural cases of blackleg.

The pellets of the blackleg vaccine under investigation were purchased in the open market, and used within the period of potency as indicated by the expiration date stamped on the package. These pellets will subsequently be

Received for publication Feb. 16, 1920.

[1] Jour. Infect. Dis., 1916, 19, p. 408.

[2] Jour. Path. and Bacteriol., 1916, 20, p. 327.

[3] Zeitsch. f. Infektionskr. d. Haust., 1906, 1, p. 26.

referred to as "commercial pellets," and the pellets prepared by us from the blackleg virus as "laboratory pellets." Part of the commercial pellets were of the grade known as "single vaccine," and part were of a stronger grade known as "second double vaccine." The single vaccine was of such virulence that a dose of one pellet killed 90% of the guinea-pigs inoculated. The double vaccine was usually fatal to guinea-pigs in doses of one-half a pellet. This was a higher virulence than the laboratory pellets possessed, although only tissue showing pronounced lesions of blackleg was used in preparing the laboratory pellets, and the period of attenuation was reduced to 80 C. for two hours. The laboratory pellets lost virulence rapidly with age, and therefore were usually made and tested immediately before each treatment. The commercial pellets did not seem to lose virulence during the course of the experiment.

The virus used as a test dose in these experiments was in part obtained from natural cases of blackleg and in part from calves killed by inoculation with such virus. In order to be sure that the natural cases of blackleg were genuine blackleg, in each case the causative organism was isolated and identified as B. chauvaei. In addition to the cultural reactions, the virus was further tested against blackleg serum. The serum employed was either that of Foth, or Leclainche and Valle. Guinea-pigs were given an injection of antiblackleg serum and 24 hours later were injected with several lethal doses of the blackleg virus to be tested. If the serum treated guinea-pigs survived the virus injection, and the virus check pigs died, the cultural identification of the active principle of the virus as B. chauvaei was considered confirmed.

The size of test dose used in determining immunity of the vaccinated calves was given careful consideration, as it was desired to use a test dose that would produce blackleg in the checks with considerable regularity and without using a larger dose of virus than was necessary. A dose of virus that will kill 50% of the virus check calves is satisfactory, provided one works with a considerable number of animals. Blackleg virus strong enough to kill guinea-pigs in doses of 2 or 3 mg., will kill calves with fair regularity in doses of 1 gm. As the dried virus loses strength rather rapidly, the test dose used in these experiments was not always lethal to guinea-pigs in 3 mg. doses.

The data in regard to the immunization and immunity test on calves follow. This experiment was not done all at once but 7 groups of calves were vaccinated during a period of 9 months, and as nearly as possible half of the calves used at any one time were vaccinated with commercial pellets, and half with laboratory pellets. Each calf received two treatments before being tested for immunity. Sixteen calves were vaccinated with commercial pellets. For their first vaccination 6 of the calves received 1 pellet each of the grade known as double, 5 received 2 pellets each of this grade, while 5 received only 1 pellet of the grade known as single. Measured in terms of lethal doses for a guinea-pig, the pellets given in the first vaccination had a virulence varying between 1 and 4. No ill effects were noted on any of the calves following this vaccination. The second immunization vaccination was given from 11-19 days later. For the second vaccination, the vaccine of the grade known as double was used, and from 2-5 pellets were given, three pellets being the usual dose. The virulence of the vaccine dose used varied between 4 and 10 guinea-pig lethal doses. None of the calves developed any symptoms or disturbance after vaccination. The test for immunity was made about 3 weeks after the second vaccination, though in some instances the time was as short as 16 days, and in one instance as long as 68 days. The time interval did not appear to influence the results. One gram of blackleg virus was used as the dose in testing for immunity. Of the 16 calves so tested, 8 died of blackleg. As a check on the virus, 8 untreated calves were inoculated with 1 gm. of blackleg virus, and 4 died of blackleg. When this is compared with the results obtained on the calves vaccinated with the commercial pellets, it is evident that no appreciable immunity against blackleg had been given the calves by the commercial pellets. That these calves would have received protection against blackleg had the commercial pellets consisted of attenuated blackleg virus is shown by the results with the laboratory pellets. Eleven calves were vaccinated with laboratory pellets and later tested for immunity against blackleg virus. For the first vaccination with laboratory pellets 6 of the calves received 1 pellet, 3 received ½ pellet, while 2 received 2 pellets each. The laboratory pellets had a virulence of one lethal dose for a guinea-pig per pellet. No symptoms developed following this vaccination except in the calves receiving 2 pellets. One of these died of vaccination blackleg, and the other was off feed. The second vaccination was given from 11-14 days later, the usual dose being 3 pellets of the same virulence as given. In a few instances 4 or 5 pellets were given. Of the 10 calves vaccinated, 4 showed no symptoms, 5 developed slight swellings at the point of inoculation, and 1 died of vaccination blackleg. The surviving 9 calves of this group were tested for immunity from 12-33 days later by inoculation with 1 gm. of blackleg virus. All withstood the immunity test.

It should be cautioned that the immunization of calves in actual practice cannot safely be carried out with such a strong vaccine as was used in this experiment. It is of interest to note that at the same time this experiment was carried out, calves on farms in the vicinity of Manhattan were vaccinated with laboratory pellets prepared as for immunization in this experiment, but not quite so virulent. Forty-one calves were vaccinated with 1 pellet having a virulence of from ½-1 guinea-pig lethal dose. Of the 41 calves, 4 died from vaccination blackleg. The susceptibility of calves varies so greatly that a large margin of safety must be maintained when administering spore containing vaccines.

CONCLUSIONS

One half of the calves treated with pseudoblackleg commercial pellets succumbed to a 1 gm. test dose of blackleg virus.

All calves treated with true blackleg laboratory pellets were immune against a 1 gm. test dose of blackleg virus.

One half of the nontreated calves succumbed to a 1 gm. dose of blackleg virus.

The pseudoblackleg commercial pellets did not immunize calves against blackleg under conditions in which true blackleg vaccine produced immunity without exception.

THE DIFFERENTIATION OF THE PARATYPHOID-ENTERITIDIS GROUP

VII. IRREGULAR AND VARIABLE STRAINS

Edwin O. Jordan

From the Department of Hygiene and Bacteriology, University of Chicago

While the majority of the strains of the paratyphoid-enteritidis group that I have had under observation during the past six years have given, whenever tested, uniform cultural and agglutination reactions, others have shown considerable irregularity and variability. Since these observations may throw light on the interrelationships of the subgroups and help to explain the frequent discordant statements in the literature, the history of some of these variable strains is here recorded.

No. 10.—This culture came to me originally (in 1913) from the collection of the American Museum of Natural History where it had been sent from the Hygienic Laboratory of the U. S. Public Health Service in Washington, D. C. It was isolated from human blood in a case of paratyphoid fever and was considered a para B type. When it was first received by me it gave irregular cultural and agglutinative reactions. Sometimes dulcite was fermented, sometimes not; sometimes milk would remain acid for a week or more and sometimes it would turn alkaline within a few days. In other respects its reactions were inconstant. On Nov. 3, 1913, it failed to agglutinate in a 1:250 dilution with a para B serum (strain 2, titer 1:4,000) while on April 26, 1914, a positive agglutination of 1:1,000 was observed with fresh serum from the same rabbit (strain 2, titer 1:4,000). The culture was plated on plain agar and on endo medium and the colonies were apparently all alike. Twelve colonies were picked from Endo medium to plain agar slants and from these in 24 hours inoculated into litmus milk. Four strains produced alkali (like typical para B) within 4 days, the other 8 at 4 days were more acid than the control. One of the acid cultures (5) began to change about this time and in 7 days was more alkaline than the control. In 14 days one other (10-9) had become alkaline. In 18 days the remaining 6 acid strains had begun to change and were like the control and at the end of 31 days all were more alkaline than the control.

Two of the strains showing early alkalinity (10-8, 10-11) did not ferment dulcitol, but two of the acid strains (10-3, 10-6) produced acid and gas in 3 days (not in 48 hours). The latter in their slow attack of dulcitol as their behavior in milk, resemble the typical paratyphoid strains

One of the strains producing early alkalinity in milk (10-10) was selected for the stock culture of this organism and transferred in the usual way with the other cultures. After two years it was plated and twelve colonies picked

Received for publication Feb. 11, 1920.

from the plate. All were alike in their behavior toward milk (early alkalinity), xylose (acid, but no gas) and galactose (acid, but no gas), thus showing that the strain had bred true and possessed stable characters.

TABLE 1

SHOWING CHARACTERS OF 12 STRAINS PICKED AT RANDOM FROM PLATINGS OF TEST-TUBE CULTURE

	Milk				Dulcitol*		Xylose*		Sorbitol*		Galactose*		Agglutination†	
	4 Days	7 Days	14 Days	31 Days	24 Hours	10 Days	24 Hours	10 Days	24 Hours	10 Days	24 Hours	10 Days	Para B (12)	Para A (4)
10-1	a	a	a	alk	0	a+	0	0	+a	+a	+a	+a	0	+
10-2	a	a	a	alk	0	a+	0	0	+a	+a	+a	+a	?	?
10-3	a	a	a	alk	0	a	0	0	+a	+a	0	+a	0	+
10-4	a	a	a	alk	0	a+	0	0	+a	+a	+a	+a	0	+
10-5	a	alk	alk	alk	0	0	a	a	a	a	a	a	+	0
10-6	a	a	a	alk	0	a+	0	0	+a	+a	+a	+a	0	+
10-7	a	a	a	alk	0	a+	0	0	+a	+a	+a	+a	0	+
10-8	alk	alk	alk	alk	0	0	a	a	a	a	a	a	+	0
10-9	a	a	alk	alk	0	a	0	0	+a	+a	+a	+a	0	+
10-10	alk	alk	alk	alk	0	0	a	a	a	a	a	a	+	0
10-11	alk	alk	alk	alk	0	a	a	a	a	a	a	a	+	0
10-12	alk	alk	alk	alk	0	0	a	a	a	a	a	a	?	?

* Gas production is indicated by the + sign.

† To save space only the final results are given here, although all strains were tested in various dilutions from 1:250 up to the titer limit (paratyphoid B 12 = 1:2,000; paratyphoid A 4 = 1:5,000). Only perfectly definite agglutination affinities are recorded; two strains, 10-2 and 10-12, gave doubtful results. The strain 10-5 showed the most unmistakable relation to the paratyphoid B type, but in no instance was the agglutination reaction as marked as with the homologous strains or with other strains belonging definitely to paratyphoid B or paratyphoid A groups.

No. 66.—This culture was received in October, 1913, from Dr. C. J. Hunt, labeled "B paratyphoid B. Stock strain from University of Pennsylvania, obtained by them from Cushing, Boston." From this notation it was thought possibly to be the strain isolated by Cushing in 1900 from a rib abscess and designated by him "Bacillus O."[1] It cannot, however, be definitely determined that this is the original Cushing strain. Cultural descendents of bacillus O seem to have given aberrant results. At the time when it was first isolated it produced alkali in milk rather slowly (not until after 8 days) and was agglutinated by a "hog cholera" serum. Buxton[2] a little later noted that bacillus O turns litmus milk faintly blue in 10 days and remarks that this strain is "somewhat erratic." Proescher and Roddy,[3] working with what was apparently this same strain some years afterward, state that "the results obtained by Cushing are remarkable in that we find it impossible to repeat them. A complete examination of this bacillus made with the greatest of care, and employing all the known means of identification, described in another part of this work, prove the organism isolated by Cushing, and named 'bacillus O,' to be a typical paratyphoid A bacillus; whereas his result would put it in the paratyphoid B group."

In my hands this culture, No. 66, has given results during a period of six years that place it definitely with the suipestifer group. The milk reaction is of the unmistakable para B suipestifer-enteritidis type. Dulcitol fermentation is either absent or much delayed. Eight out of 30 colonies picked from agar plates to agar slants and after 24 hours' incubation inoculated into dulcite

[1] Bull. Johns Hopkins Hosp., 1900, 11, p. 156.
[2] Jour. Med. Research, 1902, 3, p. 201.
[3] Archives of Int. Med., 1910, 5, p. 263.

all gave gas and acid in 15 days, but none within 48 hours. The remaining 22 were negative in 15 days. Only one of the 30 had produced gas in arabinose at the end of 15 days. All the agglutination tests have indicated a relationship to the suipestifer type. The following example will suffice.

TABLE 2

SERUM PARATYPHOID B 12 ABSORBED WITH B. SUIPESTIFER 167

Strain	250	500	1,000	2,000	5,000	10,000	20,000
12 before absorption.......	+++	+++	+++	+++	++	++	+
12 after absorption.........	++	++	++	+	+	tr	0
202 before absorption.......	+++	++	++	++	+	tr	0
202 after absorption.........	++	++	+	tr	tr	0	0
66 before absorption.......	+++	++	++	+	tr	0	0
66 after absorption.........	0	0	0	0	0		

Other absorption experiments made at different times have given similar results. Whatever the original source and history of this culture, therefore, there is no doubt that it is a suipestifer and not a paratyphosus B type. In the absence of a definite pedigreed history, however, it is not absolutely certain that No. 66 is a descendent of Cushing's bacillus O isolated in 1900.

No. 47.—This strain, originally isolated in 1911 from the feces of a water-borne case of paratyphoid,[4] gave constant reactions for some time after it was first received (1913), but in about a year began to show some irregularity in dulcitol fermentation. On plating, two types from apparently similar Endo medium colonies were found, one fermenting dulcitol rapidly in 24 hours, the other not fermenting until after 4-5 days and in some instances not within 15 days. The slow dulcitol fermenters also attacked arabinose tardily or not at all. Agglutinative as well as cultural differences were observed.

TABLE 3

AGGLUTINATIONS OF TWO TYPES OF STRAIN 47 WITH TYPICAL PARATYPHOSUS B (12) SERUM

	250	500	1,000	2,000	5,000	10,000	20,000
12............................	+++	++	++	++	++	+	0
47_1 (fails to ferment dulcite within 15 days)..........	+++	++	++	+	tr	0	0
47_3 (ferments dulcite with gas production within 24 hours)................	+++	+++	+++	++	++	+	tr

The rapid dulcitol fermenters agglutinated with paratyphosus B serum in higher dilutions than the nonfermenters. This suggests a splitting off from strain No. 47 of a type akin to B. suipestifer. The rapid dulcitol fermenters bred true and showed stable characters (100 colonies) 4 years later.

Nos. 169 and 175.—These two strains were isolated in 1915 from the lungs of two "virus hogs" at the hog cholera serum plant, Ames, Iowa. Both when first received showed the fermentative and agglutinative characters of what I have called the B. suipestifer type.[4] The change that occurred in No. 169 has been previously described.[1] I have only to add that a few months later No. 175 altered in exactly the same way so that now both cultures possess the characteristics of the paratyphosus B type.

[4] Jour. Infect. Dis., 1917, 20, p. 457.

No. 179.—When first isolated by Robinson,[5] this strain was recorded as failing to ferment dulcitol and in giving permanent acidity in litmus milk. Since coming into my hands it has produced acid and gas in dulcitol within 24 hours and has turned litmus milk alkaline in five days. No variation has been noticed in two years.

No. 134.—This is the atypical strain isolated by Dorset in 1899 from the spleen of a pig[6] dead of acute hog cholera. It was kindly sent to me in May, 1914, by Dr. Dorset with the memorandum that it had "recently been tested out on the various laboratory mediums and found to have the same characteristics described in the enclosed reprint." It has shown no deviation from the original culture since coming into my hands. In addition to the fermentation reactions recorded by Dorset (glucose = acid, no gas, lactose = 0, saccharose = 0), I have found that the other carbohydrate reactions correspond exactly to those of the typical suipestifer[4] save that in no case is gas produced (sorbitol, maltose, mannitol, galactose, xylose, rhamnose = acid; salicin = 0). Neither dulcitol nor arabinose is attacked within 15 days Its agglutinative reactions are typically those of B. suipestifer as determined by the absorption test.[4] This organism seems to be essentially similar to the nongas-producing strain of the hog cholera bacillus isolated by Tenbroeck from an old laboratory culture.[7]

No. 205.—This strain was kindly sent me in June, 1916, by Dr. J. G. Cumming labeled "B. enteritidis VII. Isolated Dec., 1914, by S. G. from stool of calf during epidemic of diarrhea in the dairy; agglutination 1 : 10,000. Typical sugar reactions." The organism has been typical in all respects save that arabinose is usually not fermented at all and dulcitol is attacked very slowly; in this respect it differs from all the other B. enteritidis strains I have had under observation and bears the same relation culturally to them that B. suipestifer bears to B. paratyphoid B. Its agglutinative reactions, however, show no divergence whatever from the other members of the B. enteritidis group.

No. 48.—This culture was originally isolated from feces and was received by me in 1913. It was sent as the A type and its cultural characteristics relate it definitely to this group; it has been so described in an earlier paper.[4] Xylose is not fermented, dulcitol fermentation is slow and arabinose rapid. It is agglutinated by B. paratyphosus A serum in dilution practically to the titer limit. It is, however, also agglutinated with certain B. paratyphosus B serum (from three out of four rabbits tested) to the titer limit. This does not seem to be due to an admixture or splitting off of types, such as observed in No. 10, but rather to a mingling of common agglutinating affinities in the same cell. Twenty-five colonies picked from a plating of this culture showed no deviation in their characters.

Nos. 62, 115, 161, 169, 175.—The origin and history of these strains have been given in an earlier article.[4] The five strains are all of porcine origin and some of these have been carried in laboratory collections under the name of hog cholera bacillus. As I have shown previously, however, they possess the chief characteristics, both cultural and agglutinative, of the B. paratyphosus B type. Similar strains from hog cholera cases have since been described by Krumwiede, Kohn and Valentine,[8] and by Tenbroeck.[9] This interesting group of organisms, although resembling very closely the paratyphosus B type of

[5] Ibid., 1915, 16, p. 448.

[6] Eighteenth Ann. Rept., Bureau of Animal Industry, 1901, p. 566.

[7] Jour. Exper. Med., 1916, 24, p.213.

[8] Jour. Med. Research, 1918, 33, p. 89.

[9] J. Exper. Med., 1918, 28, p. 759.

human origin, differs in some respects. I have elsewhere[10] pointed out their different behaviors in lead acetate agar, and Krumwiede, Kohn and Valentine have called attention to some agglutination differences in the strains they studied. Tenbroeck found that in agglutination experiments the type of clumps formed is different, and that when injected into rabbits such strains produce an immunity to the hog cholera bacillus while B. paratyphosus does not.

The existence of this subdivision of the B. paratyphosus B type, which is of porcine origin and unmistakable relationship to B. suipestifer, adds to the complicating difficulties within the group and has probably been responsible for much of the classificatory confusion in which the paratyphoid-enteritidis group has been so long involved.

A particularly large number of variations and irregularities have been reported for the paratyphoid-enteritidis group. Anaerogenic strains comparable to No. 134 have been found belonging both to the B. paratyphosus B[11] and to the B. suipestifer[12] types. Some of these have been isolated from animal bodies, but others like the strain of B. suipestifer isolated by Tenbroeck[7] and that of B. paratyphosus B, isolated by Loewenthal and Seligmann[13] have apparently developed out of gas-producing strains grown in culture mediums in the laboratory. One member of the group, B. sanguinarium, which is found not uncommonly in epidemics among barnyard fowls (fowl typhoid), ferments characteristically a number of carbohydrates, but in no instance produces gas.[14] Another avian paratyphoid bacillus, B. pullorum, typically produces gas in glucose broth, but anaerogenic strains of this organism have been observed by Rettger and Koser,[14] Smith and Tenbroeck,[14] and Mulsow.[14] Anaerogenic strains themselves sometimes show variation. The strain of B. pullorum received from Smith and Tenbroeck by Krumwiede and Kohn[15] resumed or acquired the ability to ferment glucose. As a rule, however, such variation as has been observed consists in the loss of gas-producing power originally present. No gas-producing strain of B. typhosus or of B. sanguinarium has to my knowledge ever been reported. Acid production in glucose broth is shown without exception by all members of the group.

[10] Jour. Infect. Dis., 1917, 21, p. 571.

[11] Oette, E.: Centralbl. f. Bacteriol., I, O., 1913, 68, p. 1; Wagner, G.: Ibid., 1913, 71, p. 25; Ohno, K.: Ibid., 1914-15, 75, p. 288.

[12] Preisz, H.: Cited by Tenbroeck, Jour. Exper. Med., 1916, 24, p. 213; Bock, F.: Arb. a. d. k. Ges., 1906, 24, p. 238; Graber, K.: Cited by Tenbroeck (Footnotes 7 and 9); Bainbridge, F. A.: Jour. Pathol. and Bacteriol., 1909, 13, p. 443.

[13] Loewenthal and Seligmann: Berl. klin. Wchnschr., 1913, 50, p. 250.

[14] Moore: 12th and 13th Annual Reports, Bur. Animal Ind., U. S. Dept. of Agr., 1895; Rettger: Jour. Med. Research, 1908, 18, p. 227; Rettger and Koser: Ibid., 1917, 35, p. 443; Smith and Tenbroeck: Ibid., 1915, 31, p. 503; Krumwiede and Kohn: Ibid., 1917, 36, p. 509; Mulsow: Jour. Infect. Dis., 1919, 25, p. 135.

[15] Jour. Med. Research, 1917, 36, p. 515.

The fermentation of carbohydrates other than glucose is apparently less profoundly related to fundamental or specific qualities. At all events a very wide range both of variation and of variability exists with respect to the ability to attack certain carbohydrates. In addition to the strains described in this paper a number of similar instances are scattered throughout the literature. While a certain proportion of such cases are doubtless to be attributed to cultural impurity or to mistakes in labeling, there is a residuum that can hardly be explained in this way. Savage [16] notes that one strain ("Hog Cholera Maryland"), which in his tests showed inability to ferment dulcitol, had previously in Morgan's hands produced acid and gas from this carbohydrate. The same strain was received by me in 1902 direct from Prof. Theobald Smith and in my hands has never fermented dulcitol. Dulcitol and arabinose are two carbohydrates that appear to be attacked with considerable irregularity. As shown by the writer in an earlier paper,[4] some strains of porcine origin attack dulcitol, while others fail to show any acid production within 15 days. Variations in avidity for this carbohydrate were also shown by strains of the paratyphosus A type. Arabinose likewise is attacked tardily by some porcine strains, not at all by others. Changes in the fermentative power of certain strains for this carbohydrate have also been noted.

Mulsow [17] has observed some particularly interesting variants with respect to maltose fermentation among strains of the two avian paratyphoid types B. pullorum (ordinarily not fermenting maltose) and B. sanguinarium (ordinarily maltose +). Sorbitol is attacked by some strains of B. sanguinarium and not by others. The mammalian types of paratyphoid bacilli attack both these carbohydrates with much greater constancy, and relatively few instances of variability have been reported. Grote,[18] however, has recorded the appearance in a stock culture of B. paratyphosus of a variant unable to ferment maltose and differing also from the maltose-fermenting stock in the kind of colony formed on Drigalski medium. In the course of about six months the power of fermenting maltose was slowly acquired.

Agglutination reactions in general are subject to a considerable range of variation, and in the paratyphoid-enteritidis group especially are to be accepted only guardedly as criteria of relationship. Perhaps the most striking case of lack of correlation between agglutination

[16] Report of Medical Officer, Local Gov't. Bd., London, 1909, p. 430.
[17] Jour. Infect. Dis., 1919, 25, p. 135.
[18] Centralbl. f. Bakteriol., I, O., 1913, 70, p. 15.

reactions and cultural characteristics is the close agglutinative relationship of the culturally diverse avian paratyphoid bacilli and B. typhosus.[19] Mulsow has shown further that B. enteritidis and B. abortus equinus also manifest agglutinative affinities to this group. On the other hand, as well known, B. enteritidis and B. paratyphosus B, while agglutinatively distinct, possess the closest cultural similarity. It is interesting that B. sanguinarium and B. pullorum agglutinate in about equal degree with B. typhosus serum, altho the slow rhamnose fermentation of B. sanguinarium would seem to indicate that it is more clearly related to the typhoid bacilli than is B. pullorum.

It is hardly possible to catalog all the variations that have been noted, especially with relation to agglutinative properties. Some observers [20] have recognized the existence of a "Paratyphosus C" type resembling B. paratyphosus B in its cultural characteristics, but differing agglutinatively. I have not been able to secure any cultures of the so-called "C" strains and hence do not know what relation they bear to the types described in the first article of this series. One of the most remarkable changes in agglutinative qualities yet observed has been described by Sobenheim and Seligman.[21] This consisted in the singular behaviour of certain B. paratyphosus B strains which became inagglutinable to B. paratyphosus B serum, and at the same time acquired the property of being agglutinated by B. enteritidis serum. The serum produced, however, by inoculation of these converted strains agglutinated B. paratyphosus B cultures and not B. enteritidis strains. I have not observed this change in the cultures I have had under observation for six years.

Considering all the evidence, there seems no escape from the conclusion that variations both in nature and in artificial test-tube cultures are exceedingly common throughout the paratyphoid-enteritidis group. These variations affect agglutination and fermentation characters, as well as less fundamental qualities. At times a special tendency to variability seems to exist within the confines of a test-tube culture, and a number of varieties are split off from the parent stock. This is well illustrated by culture No. 10 described in this paper. The stimuli leading to such outbreaks of variability are at present practically

[19] Smith and Tenbroeck: Jour. Med. Research, 1915, 31, p. 503; Rettger and Koser (Footnote 14); Krumwiede and Kohn (Footnotes 14 and 15); Mulsow (Footnote 14).

[20] Heinemann, W.: Centralbl. f. Bakteriol., I, O., 1912, 66, p. 211; Mackie, F. P.: Jour. Roy. Army Med. Corps, 1919, 33, p. 154.

[21] Centralbl. f. Bakteriol., Beiheft, 1911, p. 50.

unknown. The conditions under which these epidemics of variability occur suggest the possibility of conjugation phenomena rather than the direct action of environment.

As with higher forms of life, the variations do not often, if ever, overstep certain limits. The ability of the paratyphosus-enteritidis subgroup to attack rhamnose as contrasted with the lack of avidity of B. typhosus for this carbohydrate, the inability of the B. paratyphosus A strains to attack xylose, and the fundamental quality of fermenting glucose possessed by the whole coli-typhoid-paratyphoid group seem rarely subject to variation and are perhaps on this ground to be regarded as more fundamental than agglutinative reactions.

THE LIMITING HYDROGEN-ION CONCENTRATION OF VARIOUS TYPES OF PNEUMOCOCCI

H. M. Jones

From the Department of Pathology and Bacteriology, University of Illinois, College of Medicine, Chicago

The final reaction produced by an organism when grown in a medium containing a utilizable carbohydrate is known as the limiting hydrogen-ion concentration of that organism. In a previous paper [1] it was shown that this reaction varies for a given organism, depending on factors which favor or hinder abundant growth. As the growth of the pneumococcus is markedly influenced by slight changes in environment, it was necessary to establish rather definite conditions under which the final H-ion concentrations were developed.

Glucose broth, with the initial reaction of P_H 7.0, is commonly used in making final H-ion concentration determinations, but in dealing with such delicately growing organisms as the pneumococcus, this medium was found unsuited for the purpose, because of the irregularity with which growth was obtained with some of the strains.

Table 1 shows the wide variations in the final H-ion concentrations of a number of strains of each of the four types of pneumococcus, when such a medium was used.

TABLE 1

Inoculations from Rapidly Growing 24-Hour Blood-Agar Cultures Made Into Broth Containing 1% Peptone, 0.3% Beef Extract, 0.7% NaCl, 1% Glucose, and Having an Initial Reaction of Ph 7.0

Organisms	Viability	Final Ph
1	+	6.6
2	+	5.8
3	+	6.4
4	+	5.8
1 R	+	5.7
2 R	—	7.0
3 R	+	5.6
4 R	+	5.7
1 Vir.	+	6.2
2 Vir.	—	7.0
3 Vir.	+	6.4
4 Vir.	+	6.6
1 Vac.	+	6.0
2 Vac.	+	6.5
3 Vac.	+	5.7
4 Vac.	+	5.6

Received for publication Feb. 9, 1920.

[1] Jones, H. M.: Jour. Infect. Dis., 1920, 26, p. 160.

"Viability" of the organism in table 1 does not imply growth. It was proved by simply plating on blood-agar at the end of the four-day incubation period. The H-ion concentration determinations were made by the hydrogen electrode described elsewhere.[2]

None of the strains developed a greater final concentration than P_H 5.6. Lack of growth macroscopically was no indication of the lack of change in reaction; and visible growth was, likewise, no indication that the P_H had reached its highest possible concentration. To show the effect on the limiting H-ion concentrations, and also in diminishing these wide variations in P_H shown in table 1, contrast the results shown in table 2, in which the same series of organisms were inoculated into broth differing from that used in the previous experiment only in having an initial reaction of P_H 7.6, instead of P_H 7.0.

TABLE 2

INOCULATIONS FROM 24-HOUR BLOOD-AGAR SLANTS MADE INTO 1% GLUCOSE BROTH HAVING AN INITIAL REACTION OF P_H 7.6

Organisms	Viability	Final P_H
1	+	5.2
2	+	5.3
3	+	5.6
4	+	5.4
1 R	+	5.0
2 R	—	7.6
3 R	+	5.1
4 R	+	5.3
1 Vir.	+	5.2
2 Vir.	+	5.2
3 Vir.	+	5.2
4 Vir.	+	5.1
1 Vac.	+	5.4
2 Vac.	+	5.0
3 Vac.	+	5.4
4 Vac.	+	5.2

A surprising difference in the abundance of growth was also noted. The range of the final H-ion concentration of this series was from P_H 5.0 to P_H 5.6, which is about the same range of final concentrations for hemolytic streptococci of virulent type. The hope of utilizing this method for the differentiation of the types of pneumococci from each other, or from the streptococci, was therefore abandoned.

A comparison of tables 1 and 2, however, very clearly shows how the final concentration of the H-ion is affected by the initial concentration. The initial alkaline reaction of P_H 7.6 was very obviously favorable to abundant growth, and abundant growth, in turn, was favorable to final concentrations which were more uniform throughout the series. Lord[3] noted that the final H-ion concentrations for his

[2] Ibid., 1919, 25, p. 262.

[3] Jour. Am. Med. Assn., 1919, 72, p. 1364.

series of pneumococcus strains were approximately within these same limits.

Cullen and Chesney,[4] however, found that "acidification during growth in beef infusion media proceeds until a P_H of about 7.0 is reached. At this point growth stops." The error of their findings is not difficult to explain when it is recalled that they did not add glucose to their medium. That growth does not stop at P_H 7.0 was easily shown by inoculating some of our strains into glucose broth with an initial reaction of P_H 6.8 and making plates of the cultures after one

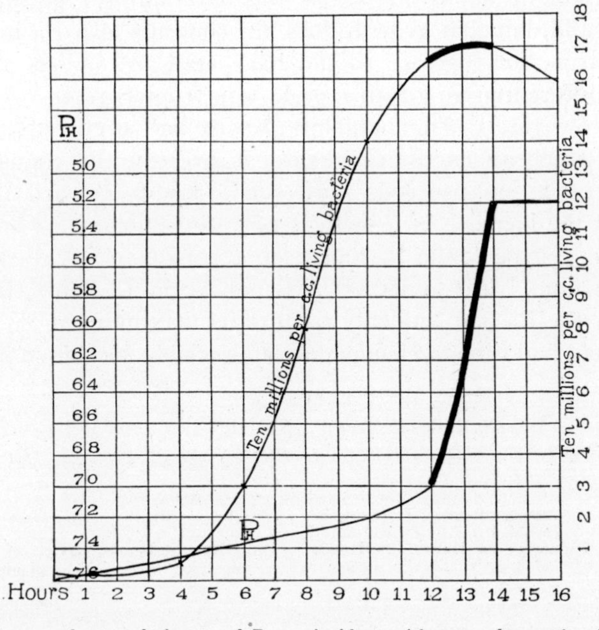

Fig. 1.—Curves of rate of change of P_H, coincident with rate of growth. Note that the greatest period of growth occurs while the reaction is still near neutrality, the interval indicated by light lines; and that the greatest period of sugar utilization occurs after the growth rate slows down — the interval indicated by heavy lines.

hour and again after 24 hours. Strain 3 R, for example, in 24 hours had increased from 24,000 to 52,000,000 viable bacteria per c c of culture. The P_H in the meantime had risen to P_H 5.9.

That their cultures developed an acid reaction in spite of the fact that glucose was not added to the medium, is explained by the fact that beef infusion medium contains considerable quantities of "muscle sugar." The final P_H reported by them would have been higher had

[4] Jour. Exper. Med., 1918, 28, p. 289.

they added more sugar, or lower if they had added a buffer, as disodiumphosphate. To obtain the final H-ion concentration of a given strain of bacteria, which will be reproducible in subsequent determinations, one should use a medium containing carbohydrate in excess of the amount which the given strain can remove from that medium.

A similar oversight is seen in the work of Dernby and Avery [5] who also used a beef infusion medium without addition of glucose. Their final concentrations would have been higher had glucose been added, as doubtless also would their bacterial counts. Their contention, that an initial reaction of about P_H 7.8 is the optimum for getting growth started is valid, but that growth does not continue at a P_H higher than 7.0 is not true, for then we should have here an obvious and simple basis for differentiation of this organism from Streptococcus hemolyticus. However, when abundant growth had occurred in a given culture in which an excess of glucose is present, the change in concentration of H-ion proceeds with such rapidity toward the higher ranges that the increase in growth is not proportionate. For example, in a culture of type 1, the P_H had risen from 7.6 to 7.0, the count had increased from 11,000 to 165,000,000 per c c in 12 hours, but in two hours more the P_H had suddenly risen to its maximum of P_H 5.2, while the count had had time to change only appreciably, as shown in figure 1.

TABLE 3

THE EFFECT OF AN INITIAL REACTION OF P_H 7.0 IN HINDERING THE DEVELOPMENT OF PNEUMOCOCCI INTRODUCED, WITH 2 C C OF PURE BLOOD, INTO 100 C C OF GLUCOSE BROTH

Strain	Glucose Broth Initial P_H 7.0 P_H After 24 Hours	Growth per c c After 24 Hours	2% Blood in Glucose Broth Initial P_H 7.0 P_H After 24 Hours	Growth per c c After 24 Hours
1	6.6	15,000	4.8	800,000,000
2 Vac.	6.5	23,000	4.8	1,200,000,000
4 Vir.	6.6	2,500	5.0	2,000,000,000

This inability of the pneumococcus to grow in a medium of the usual reaction employed in ordinary bacteriologic mediums, namely P_H 7.0, is pronounced in some strains. For example, strains 1 of type 1, 2 Vac. of type 2, and 4 Vir. of type 4, produced no visible growth in such a medium, and, as seen in table 1, only very slight change in the P_H of the medium. The fact that blood cultures in pneumococcic septicemia often fail, seemed probably due to the fact that a broth of this unfavorable reaction may prevent the development of organisms, even though they may have been present in the blood under

[5] Ibid., p. 345.

examination. Accordingly, the effect of two parts of pure blood when introduced into 100 parts of glucose broth of this reaction, was tested, using those strains which grew poorly in glucose broth of P_H 7.0. Incidentally, the addition of the blood was shown to have no measurable effect in changing the reaction of the medium.

The results show that the introduction of 2% of blood is sufficient to cause profuse growth, even at the same reaction, P_H 7.0, at which growth in ordinary glucose broth fails. The experiment was repeated, using ascitic fluid in place of blood. In general, the effect was the same, both as to the abundance of growth, and the higher concentrations of H-ion developed by these strains. Long boiling renders these fluids useless in stimulating the profuse growths which resulted in the experiment described above.

In a previous paper [1] attention was called to the effect which these body fluids have in increasing the tolerance of Streptococcus hemolyticus of virulent type to the toxic ion of hydrogen. In other words, when these fluids are added to glucose broth, which is frequently done to insure growth, such a P_H is then developed that the virulent is made to imitate in P_H the avirulent types of streptococci. Table 3 show that the pneumococcus enjoys, with the streptococcus, this same increase of tolerance to the toxic ion of hydrogen, when these body fluids are added to the medium, which is of importance in connection with the fact that the virulent strains of streptococci are sometimes differentiated with great difficulty from the avirulent strains on the one hand, and the pneumococcus on the other.

No explanation of the action of the body fluids in stimulation of growth and increasing the organism's tolerance to hydrogen-ion, is attempted here, but since strong acidification, long boiling, etc., destroy this unknown "active principle," further search may reveal still other phenomena having "vitamins" as a basis of their explanation.

SUMMARY

The final hydrogen-ion concentration produced by pneumococci of various types when grown in glucose broth varies, with different strains, between P_H 5.0 and 5.6, being indistinguishable in this respect from various strains of Streptococcus hemolyticus of virulent type.

The regularity with which these final hydrogen-ion concentration values can be reproduced depends largely on the initial reaction, ordinary glucose broth of P_H 7.0 being useless for this purpose. None of the strains failed to grow, however, when the initial reaction was set at 7.6.

This failure to grow in broth of P_H 7.0 does not account for the often observed failure to secure growth of the pneumococcus as when blood cultures are being made, since the addition of 2% of whole blood renders the medium of P_H 7.0 even superior to glucose broth of P_H 7.6 in stimulating growth.

A marked increase in tolerance toward the hydrogen-ion is also observed, as is also the case with Streptococcus hemolyticus.

SENSITIZED AND NONSENSITIZED VACCINES IN CHOLERA IMMUNIZATION

Matsuziro Takenouchi

From the Institute for the Research of Infectious Diseases, Imperial University of Tokio

Some clinical observers claim a relative superiority for sensitized vaccine over nonsensitized on the ground that sensitized cholera vaccine causes only slight symptoms when inoculated subcutaneously, while inoculation with nonsensitized vaccine is sometimes followed by local pain, fever and other reactions. If inoculation of sensitized cholera vaccine causes the formation of antibodies that we can trace in vitro, or of some other protecting agencies in the body against cholera bacilli, i. e., is more efficient or just as efficient as that of nonsensitized vaccine, and if the undesirable symptoms following the inoculation of sensitized vaccine are much milder than those following the inoculation of the nonsensitized, the latter obviously should not be used for prophylactic inoculation on human beings.

As early as 1901, Pfeiffer[1] published results obtained by immunization of rabbits with a mixture of cholera bacilli and cholera immune serum, testing fewer animals than we have used and employing as antigen for immunization a material somewhat different from the so-called "sensitized cholera vaccine." S. Yabe[2] reported the results of his experiment on 17 students in the Higher Normal School of Tokio. He noted that the bacteriolytic activity tested in vitro of the serums of 9 students, in whom he had previously (16 days before) injected two times his nonsensitized cholera vaccine subcutaneously for prophylaxis, was much higher than that of the serums of 8 students injected with the same amount of his sensitized cholera vaccine under the same experimental conditions. Later, however, he makes no mention of the valuable results obtained in his experiments on human beings.[3]

In an attempt to determine, if possible, the relative value of sensitized and nonsensitized vaccines in cholera immunization, I made the following experiments.

Preparation of Vaccine

Cholera bacilli were cultivated on ordinary slightly alkaline agar-agar mediums in large tubes, incubated at 36 C. for 18 hours. The bacilli were gathered by means of a large platinum loop into a weighing bottle (avoiding mixing the condensed water as much as possible) and were weighed on a chemical balance.

Received for publication Dec. 6, 1919.

1 Deutsch. med. Wchnschr., 1901, pp. 867 and 891.
2 Tokio Iji Shinshi, 1916, No. 1997, p. 1.
3 Shiga, K., Takano, R., and Yabe, S.: Kitasato Arch. of Exper. Med., 1918, 2, p. 1.

Sensitized Vaccine.—To each 10,000 gm. of cholera bacilli, made into homogeneous emulsion with sterile salt solution of 100 c c or 150 c c, are added 10 c c of sterile inactive anticholera horse serum, the agglutination titer of which is over 20,000. This was stirred with a sterile glass rod to insure thorough mixture. Marked agglutination occurred almost instantaneously. After two hours at 37 C., when agglutinated bacilli had settled almost entirely, the contents were again stirred up and the whole suspension was kept for another two hours at 37 C. It was then subjected to strong centrifugalization, and the mass of bacilli was separated and suspended in 1,000 c c of sterile normal salt solution, to which 0.5% carbolic acid was added. The carbolized emulsion of sensitized germs was placed over night at 37 C. and cultivation tests made to make sure that the vaccine was sterile. For ordinary prophylaxis we used both sensitized and nonsensitized cholera vaccines of the concentration of 2 mg. of bacilli in 1 c c.

Nonsensitized Cholera Vaccine. — This was prepared according to Kolle.[4] Throughout the work we used both kinds of vaccines of the same date for each series of comparative experiments.

To determine the toxicity of each vaccine, guinea-pigs weighing between 150-230 gm. were used. Both kinds of vaccine were injected intraperitoneally or subcutaneously, and the smallest amount causing death within, or nearly within, 24 hours observed. Of the sensitized cholera vaccine, 125-150 mg. injected intraperitoneally, caused death in 12-15 hours, while 15-20 and 18-20 mg. of nonsensitized cholera vaccine caused the death of the test animals in 12-16 and in 20 hours, respectively. Of sensitized vaccine 200-250 mg., injected subcutaneously, caused death of the test animals in 28 hours; 75-100 mg. of nonsensitized cholera vaccine, injected subcutaneously, caused death in 29 hours.

The lethal dose of living cholera bacilli sensitized for two hours at 37 C. and then centrifugalized was found to be 5-10 mg., injected intraperitoneally; this dose proved fatal in 35 hours. Intraperitoneal injection of 0.50-0.75 mg. of living cholera bacilli caused death in 26 hours. Of living cholera bacilli 5-7 mg. injected subcutaneously, caused the death of test animals in 27 hours.

The lethal doses of cholera vaccines varied in accordance with the so-called virulence of the respective cholera strain. For example, the lethal dose of nonsensitized cholera vaccine from strain "Yanagiwara" 1 was found to be 18-20 mg. (the lethal dose of the cholera bacilli being 0.75-1 mg.). The lethal dose of strain "Yanagiwara" 3 was 10-12 mg., while the lethal dose of the cholera bacilli was 0.25 mg., illustrating the observation previously reported that cholera vaccine made from more virulent strains is more toxic than that from less virulent strains.

Some investigators may attribute the marked reduction of toxicity of cholera vaccine by means of sensitization to the "washing" in the course of sensitization. Certainly some of the loss in, or diminution of, bacillary substance may be due to the sensitization and washing (centrifugalization), but it is obviously a mistake to assume that during the process of sensitization of living cholera bacilli, the bacillary substances are diminished to 1/8 or 1/7, reducing the toxicity of sensitized cholera vaccine to 1/8 to 1/7 of that of nonsensitized vaccine.

We noticed that the loss of bacillary substances, owing to sensitization and washing by means of centrifugalization, tested by the nitrogen determination method of Kjeldahl, was not so large as the reduction of toxicity of vaccine examined by animal tests. Some cholera bacilli may escape, or die, or lose

[4] Deutsch. med. Wchnschr., 1897, 1, p. 4.

their toxic substances during sensitization and washing. This loss, however, would account for only a small part of the tremendous difference between the lethal doses of living bacilli sensitized and nonsensitized.

Are toxic properties of the bacillary substances neutralized in the process of sensitization, or does the specific anticholera serum used in the sensitization exert some influence on the bacilli and favorably prepare the way for phagocytosis in vivo?

To determine the protective efficiency of inoculation of cholera vaccine, sensitized and nonsensitized, against cholera infection, guinea-pigs, 150-200 gm., and rabbits were inoculated, both intraperitoneally and subcutaneously, with vaccine. To test the degree of active immunity thus produced, we used principally (1) the infection test and (2) the serum test in vitro of the amount of bacteriolytic substance contained in the serum of the inoculated animals.

In 12 series, using from 3 to 6 animals in each series, 1 c c of 1:100 dilution of cholera vaccine was inoculated intraperitoneally, employing in each series a test dose of twice the lethal dose of cholera bacilli, sensitized and nonsensitized. The infection test was made from 3 to 24 hours after the inoculation, and all the animals survived with the exception of those in series 9; 3 guinea-pigs died when the infection test was made 3 hours after the injection of nonsensitized cholera vaccine. In series 13, in which 5 guinea-pigs were inoculated with nonsensitized cholera vaccine and the test made 3 hours after inoculation, 1 died and 4 survived. In series 14, using sensitized vaccine with the same number of guinea-pigs, 2 survived and 3 died in the same period after the inoculation.

To test the bacteriolytic activity and the agglutination of serum from guinea-pigs previously inoculated with cholera vaccine, sensitized and nonsensitized, two guinea-pigs were inoculated intraperitoneally with 1 c c of 1:100 dilution of sensitized vaccine and tested after 3, 5, 7, 24, 48 and 72 hours. Bacteriolysis in vitro was negative with 0.1 c c of the serum. Using nonsensitized vaccine and testing the guinea-pigs at the same periods, bacteriolysis in vitro was negative with the same amount of serum. Agglutination in all these tests was negative in 1:4 dilution.

No marked difference in the efficiency of inoculation of cholera vaccine of either kind was apparent. It is possible that there may have been some individual variations in resistance against intraperitoneal cholera infection among the guinea-pigs.

Guinea-pigs previously inoculated intraperitoneally with 1 c c of 1:10 dilution of the original vaccines, did not survive infection with three or more than three times the lethal dose of living cholera bacilli administered intraperitoneally 48 hours, 4 days and even 6 days after the vaccine inoculation. In this case we could not see, of course, any difference in the efficiency of either cholera vaccine.

The determination of a suitable or adequate test dose constituted ultimately the hardest part of our experiments. The larger test doses that we used in the standardization of antibacterial serum by means of the infection test, seemed to be too large for our present purpose, because the amount of antibodies in the serum of guinea-pigs, or rather the degree of protecting power in general, after the inoculation of cholera vaccine, is not so abundant as in the case of testing of immune serum. The futility of conducting an infection test of this kind with inadequate or improperly chosen test doses of living cholera bacilli was emphasized in my discussion of the work of S. Yabe.[5]

[5] Tokio Iji Shinshi, 1916, No. 2.

The protective power in animals inoculated against intraperitoneal infection with cholera bacilli of double the lethal dose seems to consist of some agency combined with the bacteriolytic and agglutinating substance in the serum of inoculated animals.

The efficiency of the subcutaneous inoculation of cholera vaccine, sensitized and nonsensitized, on guinea-pigs was observed by making infection tests and determining the bacteriolytic activity of the serum of animals previously inoculated with 1 c c of 1:100 dilution of the original cholera vaccine sensitized and nonsensitized. On a series of 28 animals we noted (1) that the bacteriolytic activity tested in vitro was negative with 0.1 c c of serum of both series of guinea-pigs inoculated with both kinds of vaccine, respectively, even on the tenth day after inoculation; (2) that the agglutination titer of serum of both series is lower than 1:4 dilution; (3) that even on the eighth day after inoculation the animals of both series could not show enough protecting power against the intraperitoneal infection with double the lethal dose of cholera bacilli; (4) that no difference in protecting efficiency of inoculation of sensitized or nonsensitized cholera vaccine against intraperitoneal infection was detected.

Using subcutaneous inoculation of a larger amount of cholera vaccine of both kinds than in the previous experiment, we obtained somewhat better results. A rather marked superiority in protecting power of animals inoculated with nonsensitized cholera vaccine was evident in comparison with that of animals inoculated with the same dose of sensitized cholera vaccine. The higher protecting power of guinea-pigs against the intraperitoneal infection with 1.5-2.5 lethal doses of cholera bacilli was especially marked and could be seen 5 days after subcutaneous inoculation.

In the early stage of immunization by means of subcutaneous inoculation of 1 c c (2 mg.) of cholera vaccine, sensitized as well as nonsensitized, the protecting power is so small that the animals are unable to survive even one lethal dose of cholera bacilli, while in intraperitoneal injections of 1 c c of 1:100 dilution of original vaccine of both kinds, as early as the fifth hour after the inoculation, all animals survive the intraperitoneal injection with double the lethal dose of living cholera bacilli. A test of more than one lethal dose of cholera bacilli is therefore entirely useless, at least in the early stage of immunization of guinea-pigs by subcutaneous inoculation, for the purpose of determining the difference in efficiency of the two types of cholera vaccines.

With a test dose of more than three lethal doses of cholera bacilli, all infection tests were negative even after 9 days of subcutaneous inoculation.[6] In attempting to determine the difference in efficiency of subcutaneous inoculations of cholera vaccines of both kinds by means of infection tests, the test doses, therefore, must not exceed 2.5 lethal dose of cholera bacilli.[5]

Rabbits were inoculated subcutaneously with cholera vaccines to determine the bacteriolytic activity of the serum. Of a 1:30 dilution of the original vaccines, sensitized and nonsensitized, respectively, 1 c c was given subcutaneously to each of the 5 rabbits for the first injection. This was followed after 3 days'

[6] In this connection it may be of some interest to refer to the work of Otto Schöbl and C. S. Panganiban (Philippine Jour. Sc., Manila, 1917, Sec. B, 12, p. 43). In their study on experimental cholera carriers and immunity, there was no apparent shortening of the duration of cholera carriers in guinea-pigs effected by preventive vaccination and vaccine therapy. Guinea-pigs immunized by the subcutaneous administration of graduated doses of suspension of killed cholera vibrios and infected at intervals varying from three to twelve days after the infecting dose, gave positive cultures of cholera vibrios from the gall-bladder, duodenum, ileum and cecum in almost every case.

interval by a second injection of 1 c c of a 1: 15 dilution of the original vaccines. After 7 days a blood sample was taken from the rabbits (1 rabbit died from an unknown cause on the fifth day after the second injection) and the bacteriolytic activity of the separated serum was tested in vitro by the plate method according to Neisser and Wechsberg.

The bacteriolytic activity of the serum from rabbits inoculated subcutaneously with sensitized cholera vaccine is by far weaker than the bacteriolytic activity of serum from rabbits inoculated with nonsensitized cholera vaccine. This result agrees with the result obtained by S. Yabe in his study on 17 students.[2] According to his report the highest bacteriolytic activity of serum from 8 students inoculated with his sensitized cholera vaccine (positive bacteriolysis with 0.00005 c c of serum) coincided with the lowest titer of the serum obtained from 9 students inoculated with his nonsensitized cholera vaccine under the same experimental conditions. He inoculated the students twice subcutaneously for prophylaxis, and on the sixteenth day after the second injection blood samples were taken to determine the bacteriolytic power.

Testing 10 rabbits, 5 inoculated subcutaneously with nonsensitized vaccine and 5 with sensitized vaccine, the agglutinative power of the serum from rabbits inoculated with the nonsensitized vaccine was found generally to be remarkably higher than that of serum from rabbits injected with sensitized vaccine. This is analogous to the result obtained by K. Imai[7] in his investigation on the sensitized typhoid, paratyphoid A and paratyphoid B vaccines.

Though the bacteriolysin alone may not be the principal agency which confers the protecting power on animals inoculated with cholera vaccine, we seem warranted in concluding that the higher bacteriolytic activity may go hand in hand with a greater protecting power for animals. It is therefore probable that the nonsensitized vaccine that causes greater production and appearance of bacteriolytic substance in the blood, when injected subcutaneously in rabbits as well as in human beings (according to S. Yabe), is superior in efficiency to the sensitized vaccine which does not produce as much bacteriolysin in the blood.

CONCLUSIONS

During the process of sensitization, the toxicity of cholera vaccine as tested on guinea-pigs is diminished greatly. This reduction of toxicity is caused not only by the washing, but also by the specific influence of anticholera serum on the toxic substances of cholera bacilli.

Further investigation and observation will determine whether there is a reduction of toxicity of cholera vaccine by sensitization for human beings.

Careful selection of the test dose is a fundamental necessity for the infection tests on guinea-pigs that have been inoculated with cholera vaccines, either intraperitoneally or subcutaneously.

In order to determine the comparative value of sensitized and nonsensitized cholera vaccine on intraperitoneal inoculation, further tests,

[7] Kaigun, Gunidan, 1916, No. 12.

using twice the lethal dose of cholera bacilli within 3-5 hours after the intraperitoneal inoculation, must be employed on guinea-pigs.

Nonsensitized cholera vaccine is markedly superior to sensitized cholera vaccine in protecting power for guinea-pigs inoculated subcutaneously. Nonsensitized cholera vaccine produces more bacteriolytic substance in the blood of rabbits inoculated subcutaneously than sensitized cholera vaccine. S. Yabe observed this same phenomenon in his experiments with cholera vaccines on human beings.

Nonsensitized cholera vaccine, inoculated subcutaneously, is much more effective than the sensitized.

THE ACTION OF LEUKOCYTIC EXTRACTS ON THE PHAGOCYTIC ACTIVITY OF LEUKOCYTES

Ruth Tunnicliff

From the John McCormick Institute for Infectious Diseases, Chicago

A large amount of work has been done experimentally and clinically with leukocyte extracts and, according to Zinsser,[1] there seems to be little question about their having a favorable influence both in experimental infections in animals and in the treatment of human cases, but there has been considerable difficulty in determining the reason for this influence.

Pettersson[2] found that leukocytes and leukocyte extracts possessed distinct bactericidal properties for various strains of proteus, but not for the cholera vibro and typhoid bacillus. Hiss[3] found that extracts of normal rabbit leukocytes had a distinct modifying and curative action in rabbit infections, due chiefly, he thought, to poison-neutralizing or destroying properties. Later Hiss[4] and Zinsser[5] found that distinct precipitates were formed when leukocyte extracts and bacterial extracts were mixed. Their observations tended to show that leukocytic substances exert only slight, if any, bactericidal action and do not of themselves inhibit to any considerable extent the development of bacteria; further that the extracts do not to any marked degree directly increase intraperitoneal phagocytosis. However, they did note that there seemed to be a more rapid accumulation of phagocytes in the peritoneal cavities of guinea-pigs infected with cholera spirilla when leukocytic extracts were injected with the bacteria. Later Zinsser states that "from subsequent experiments it is not impossible, in fact it seems probable, that the protective properties of the leukocyte extracts are attributable, in part at least, to their positively chemotactic effect."

Alexander[6] was the first to note that the injection of leukocyte extracts, prepared according to the method of Hiss and Zinsser, was followed by a marked leukocytosis within 24 hours. Archibald and Moore,[7] using extracts made directly from the blood of normal animals, found that the injection of such extracts into guinea-pigs produced a marked increase in the number of leukocytes in from 2-6 hours, the maximum being reached about 6 hours after the injection, the leukocytosis being more marked than that produced by the injection of nuclein. The increase in leukocytes was in the number of polymorphonuclear cells. Red-staining granules were observed in these cells, increasing in number for about six hours. Zinsser[1] later concludes that he is "inclined

Received for publication Feb. 14, 1920.

[1] Infection and Resistance, 1918.

[2] Centralbl. f. Bakteriol., I, O., 1905, 39, pp. 423 and 613.

[3] Jour. Med. Research, 1908, 19, p. 323.

[4] Ibid., p. 399.

[5] Ibid., p. 411.

[6] Brit. Med. Jour., 1911, 1, p. 355.

[7] Archiv. Int. Med., 1914, 14, p. 120.

to believe at present that the beneficial effects of leukocyte extracts are based on the same principles as that which determines the reactions following the injection of bacterial or any other protein." Zinsser and Tsen,[8] however, found that the injection of leukocytic extract does not arouse as vigorous a leukocytic response as does the injection of bacillary protein, but that on the other hand the leukocytic extract does not induce so severe a leukopenia.

In a previous article I [9] showed that the leukocytes in an aleuronat exudate in rabbits were more actively phagocytic than those in the blood, probably due to their being young cells. The following experiments were made to determine whether the activity of the new leukocytes produced by injection of leukocytic extracts were more actively phagocytic than normal cells.

The extracts were prepared according to the method of Hiss and Zinsser and also that of Archibald and Moore. Later, extracts were kindly furnished by Dr. John W. Anderson, director of the biological department of Squibb and Sons; these extracts were derived from the horse and were made according to the method of Hiss and Zinsser.

Hiss and Zinsser produced a double purulent exudate in the pleural cavities of rabbits by the injection of sterile aleuronat solution. This exudate was centrifuged quickly and the serum decanted. Distilled water in amount equal to that of the fluid poured off was added and the exudates thoroughly emulsified and allowed to stand for a few hours at 37 C. and then at icebox temperature until used. The cell residue as well as the supernatant fluid is injected.

Archibald and Moore used leukocytes directly from the blood of normal animals (horse, dog, or other domestic animal). They found that dog leukocytes produced the highest leukocytosis. I therefore used dog leukocytes. Blood was collected in a 1% sodium citrate solution, and 0.5 of 1% acetic acid was added. The mixture was centrifuged and the supernatant fluid discarded. The sediment was washed several times in salt solution and ground with quartz sand and neutralized. Distilled water was then added in the proportion of 4 parts of water to 1 part of sediment, and the mixture was kept at a temperature of 58 C. for 1 hour and then put in the icebox. The supernatant fluid was decanted and trikresol added.

The phagocytic activity of leukocytes is determined as follows: The leukocytes from rabbits injected with extract and from normal rabbits are collected in 2% sodium citrate solution, centrifuged and washed twice in normal salt solution to remove all trace of serum. To determine the activity of leukocytes it is essential to use suspensions containing approximately the same number of polymorphonuclear leukocytes. Such suspensions are obtained by counting the number of polymorphonuclear leukocytes in each and equalizing them with normal salt solution or by counting the number of cells in the circulating blood and collecting the same amount of blood from each rabbit and then

[8] Jour. Immunol., 1917, 2, p. 247.
[9] Trans. Chicago Path. Soc., 1911, 8, p. 208.

equalizing according to the count. The same serum is used to provide the necessary opsonin in the test of the two kinds of leukocytes. Any organism which is not spontaneously phagocytable may be used, but a virulent organism which is not opsonized by normal serum for normal leukocytes is not suitable. Pneumococci and Strep. viridans were used in my experiments. Equal parts of serum, leukocytic suspension and bacterial suspension, are mixed in bent capillary pipets and incubated 25 minutes. The mixtures are smeared on glass slides and stained. The phagocytic activity of the leukocytes is determined by comparing the number of bacteria taken up by the two sets of leukocytes (cytophagic index). Fifty cells are counted on each slide.

From 2 to 10 c c of the leukocytic extract were injected subcutaneously in 5 rabbits. Two rabbits were injected with rabbit exudate extract, one with dog leukocyte extract, the other rabbits with extracts of horse leukocytes. Leukocyte counts were made before and every two or three hours for six hours after the injection, and then daily until the count returned to normal. The activity of the leukocyte was estimated from time to time. A leukopenia was not observed following the injections, but no counts were made before two hours after the injection of the extract.

The highest leukocyte count as a rule was reached about six hours after the injection, the horse exudate causing a somewhat slower rise than the other exudates. The leukocytosis lasted from one to four days, and the increase was in the number of the polymorphonuclear cells. No change in their staining reaction was observed. The average number of leukocytes in the normal control rabbit was 8,000, and the average highest leukocyte count in the injected rabbit was 15,900. During the height of the leukocytosis the polymorphonuclear cells were found to be from two to four times more actively phagocytic than normal. Repeated injections of extract caused an increase in the number and activity of the leukocytes, but not as a rule greater than that produced by the first injection.

Two rabbits were injected intravenously, one with 7, the other with 3 c c of extract of horse leukocytes. The number of leukocytes in the rabbit receiving 7 c c began to rise in 15 minutes, increasing 8,000 in 30 minutes and 13,200 in one hour. The number returned to normal two hours after the injection. During the height of the leukocytosis the polymorphonuclear cells were three times more active than normal cells. The second rabbit received 3 c c and this produced a slight fall in the number of leukocytes for 30 minutes, followed by a rise of 5,000 in one hour and a rise of 21,500 in two hours. The number of leukocytes returned to normal three hours after the injection. During the height of the leukocytosis the polymorphonuclear cells were eight times more actively phagocytic than normal.

I have not tried to determine whether there is an increased activity of the cells in leukocytosis produced by other proteins.

I have shown [10] that the leukocytes in the leukopenia of measles and influenza are considerably less actively phagocytic than normal cells. Hence it seemed desirable to determine whether the leukocytes in leukopenia could be stimulated to greater activity by the injection of leukocytic extract. Leonard [11] has found that the administration of leukocyte extract in measles and influenza results in an increase in the number of leukocytes. As I was unable to study the activity of leukocytic extract in measles and influenza, leukopenia was produced in rabbits by the subcutaneous injection of benzene and olive oil (1 c c per kilo of weight). After three injections a distinct decrease in the number of leukocytes occurred, and one rabbit now received three daily subcutaneous injections of 10 c c of extract of horse leukocytes, but without in any way affecting the leukopenia. Another rabbit received simultaneously benzene and leukocytic extract together on three successive days, but the leukopenia was not prevented. The leukopenia produced by benzene is, of course, not comparable with that produced by infection, and observations must be made in cases of infection with leukopenia to determine definitely whether leukocytic extracts can then increase the phagocytic activity of leukocytes.

SUMMARY

The results of the experiments show that the subcutaneous injection of leukocytic extract in rabbits produces an appreciable increase in the number of leukocytes in the circulating blood lasting from one to four days. The leukocytes set free by the extract possess considerably more phagocytic power than normal leukocytes. While the intravenous injection of leukocytic extract produces a more rapid rise in the number and activity of the leukocytes, the duration is shorter than that produced by subcutaneous injection. Leukocytic extract appears to exert no influence on the leukopenia produced by benzene.

[10] Jour. Infect. Dis., 1912, 11, p. 474; Jour. Am. Med. Assn., 1918, 71, p. 1733.
[11] Jour. of Med. Soc. N. J., 1919, 16, p. 354.

ACID PRODUCTION BY STREPTOCOCCUS VIRIDANS IN MEDIUMS OF DIFFERENT HYDROGEN-ION CONCENTRATION

LINWOOD G. GRACE AND FLORENCE HIGHBERGER

From the Research Institute of the National Dental Association, Cleveland, Ohio

That the reaction of culture mediums is important is a mere reiteration of a statement found in every textbook on bacteriology. As to just how important it is we are only beginning to realize. Various reports have been made as to the optimum reaction for different organisms. It is quite probable, however, that much work will have to be done before it can be stated just what this is, for each known organism or group of organisms, with any degree of certainty.

In the literature we find numerous references to the initial reaction of given mediums used for the cultivation of the streptococcus. A bulletin from the Army Medical School suggests P_H 7.6 to P_H 7.8 for both the hemolytic and viridans varieties. Norton [1] says he uses agar with a P_H value of 8.1 as a basis for blood agar and obtains excellent results in growing both the streptococcus and pneumococcus. Avery and Cullen [2] used medium having an initial reaction of P_H 7.6 to P_H 7.8.

Since our work involves study of Strep. viridans, we determined to make an effort to find out whether a medium of one reaction was superior to that of another for growing this particular organism. In our experiments we assumed that the rate of acid production was a fair index of the rate of growth and vitality. It may be that the reaction which favors the most rapid growth will not produce an organism with the maximum degree of virulence. Such, indeed, seems to be the case with the diphtheria bacillus, as Bunker [3] found that the most rapid growth of the diphtheria bacillus occurs in a medium having an initial reaction between P_H 7.0 and P_H 7.5, while the greatest toxin production takes place in a medium having a reaction of P_H 7.8 to P_H 8.2.

We made four different tests, using cultures which varied in age from 14 up to 48 hours. Two different kinds of broth were used. The basis of both was beef extract (Liebig's) 0.3%; peptone (Difco brand), 1%; sodium chlorid,

Received for publication Feb. 1, 1920.

[1] Am. Jour. Public Health, 1919, 9, p. 190.
[2] Jour. Exper. Med., 1919, 29, p. 215.
[3] Jour. Bacteriol., 1919, 4, p. 379.

0.5%. This was made up and autoclaved at 20 pounds' pressure for 15 minutes. It was then divided into 2 parts. To one was added 1% glucose and to the other 5% ascites fluid and 0.2% glucose. Each of these was again divided into 5 parts and the parts given initial reactions of P_H 6.4, P_H 6.8, P_H 7.2, P_H 7.6 and P_H 8. We had then, practically, 10 different batches of broth. These were autoclaved at 15 pounds' pressure for 15 minutes, the reaction readjusted, filtered, tubed and autoclaved.

The ascites fluid used was first prepared by rendering it alkaline by adding 2.5% of a 40% sodium hydroxid solution and autoclaving it for 15 minutes at 15 pounds' pressure. It was then stored in the icebox until ready for use.[4]

In the experiment the simplified colorimetric method of determining the H-ion concentration as suggested by Barnett and Chapman[5] and somewhat elaborated by Norton[1] was used. Although this method is probably not suited for the most exact work, we believe it sufficiently accurate for adjusting the reactions of mediums. Checks made by the electrometric method have shown an error not exceeding 0.06.

Our results would seem to indicate that growth will take place in medium having a P_H value anywhere between 6.4 and 8.0. The index in this was that sufficient acid was produced in all the cultures in 24 hours to bring about the maximum color change in bromthymol blue. Further, all the tubes presented the typical appearance which indicates a growth, and subcultures all grew out in 24 hours.

There is an indication, however, that growth was distinctly retarded in medium which had a reaction more alkaline than P_H 7.6, and further, that the most rapid growth was obtained in medium which had an initial reaction of P_H 6.8.

The following is a detail of the procedure in one experiment, together with a table of the results. The others were all carried out in the same way, the only variation being the age of the culture used. This varied within the limits above given. As near as we could tell, the results were the same except that when using an older culture the acid production and the accompanying changes in the appearance of the medium will not take place quite as rapidly as it will with a younger one. The organism used was isolated from the root of a tooth, the apex of which had been the seat of infection.

One hundred c c of the 5% ascites broth, having an initial reaction of P_H 7.2, was inoculated and incubated 14 hours at 37 C. This was used for inoculating the test tube. The medium to be tested was given the different desired reactions, put in tubes—10 c c to a tube—and autoclaved at 15 pounds for 15 minutes. Five-tenths c c of the broth culture was introduced into each tube and all placed in the incubator at 37 C. At intervals one tube from each concentration was removed from the incubator and the reaction noted. The

[4] Report in press.

[5] Jour. Am. Med. Assn., 1918, 70, p. 1062.

reaction immediately after inoculating was also noted to serve as a control. A set of uninoculated tubes was also incubated and the reactions noted after 25 hours. The reason for using separate tubes instead of having the medium in bulk and taking out the amount to be tested each time was to avoid any chance of contamination. Numerous checks have served to show that the reaction of one tube is practically the reaction of all the tubes of that concentration and composition at that time. This, of course, is as it should be since each tube contained the same amount of medium and each was inoculated with an equal amount of the culture. We made no attempt to determine the P_H value after it became more acid than P_H 6.3 except to note whether it would bring about the maximum color change in bromthymol blue. This would indicate a higher degree of acidity than P_H 6.3. In this experiment we were concerned only with the rate of acid production and were making no effort to determine the final H-ion concentration.

Ascites broth having an initial reaction of P_H 6.8 reached this end point after 6 hours' incubation while glucose broth of the same concentration reached the same point after 7 hours' incubation. The broth having an initial reaction of P_H 6.4, of course, closely approximated this. But since a comparative slight addition of acid would be sufficient to bring this medium to the end point one would expect that if an equal degree of acid had been produced in each tube, those of a P_H value of 6.4 would reach the end point first. With the ascites broth this was not the case. It was with the glucose broth, but there is not sufficient difference to justify such an assumption. When comparing the broth of concentration P_H 6.8 with those of a more alkaline reaction, it will be noticed that there is a difference of from 3-6 hours in the time required to reach the end point. In the case of ascites broth, P_H 8, there was no appreciable acid production until after 12 hours' incubation.

The gross appearance of the tubes corresponded to the rise in P_H value, that is, as the tubes became more acid they also became more turbid.

Although nearly all textbooks, when describing cultural characteristics of various organisms, speak of the turbidity or cloudiness and the formation of precipitates in liquid mediums, the reason for such reactions and just what they indicate is not made clear. Although the student is told that such changes in the appearance of mediums indicate that bacteria are present, he is not always told why their presence produces such a change.

Kendall[6] dismisses the matter by saying that visible changes in the appearance of broth cultures incidental to the development of bacteria are not of great importance, and mentions the fact that they consist essentially of turbidity, sediment and occasionally a ring or pellicle.

It is a significant fact, however, that all bacteria do alter the physical appearance of fluid mediums, and that this fact is always referred to in some way. So important is it that in the fabrication of

[6] Bacteriology, General, Pathological and Intestinal, 1916.

fluid mediums, clearness is insisted on whenever possible in order that these changes may be the more readily detected.

Like all other living organisms, the metabolic processes of bacteria may be divided into two phases, anabolism and catabolism. In the case of bacteria the catabolic phase predominates.

Any alteration in the composition or appearance of mediums due to anabolic processes are so slight that they can be disregarded. During the first few hours after inoculation the anabolic phase may go on quite rapidly and a slight cloudiness may result in fluid mediums, due chiefly to the rapid increase in the number of bacterial cells.

This phase is rapidly succeeded by the catabolic one and then the greater changes, due to the breaking down of the various constituents of the mediums, take place, and with it the accompanying changes in the physical appearance are noted.

Without going into great detail, since the details have been ably set forth by many, these catabolic changes are divided into two main groups: those that have to do with the breaking down of proteins and those that are concerned in the splitting up of sugars.

All bacteria do not possess the power to do both, nor can all bacteria split up both proteids and sugars to the same extent. The resultant end products produced by different types of organisms have been studied and used as an aid in identification.

One of the principal end products resulting from the activity of both proteolytic and sugar splitting enzymes is an acid in one form or another. Not only will this acid alter the reaction of the medium, but it will often precipitate substances that were held in solution; for example, phosphates. These precipitates will be the principal factor in the change from a clear to a cloudy medium. Some of the end products are only slightly soluble, and as they are formed they appear as precipitates or suspensions.

All of these changes are important and indicate that an organism is present. The changes are not only due to the presence of myriads of bacterial cells, but also to alterations in the composition of the medium resulting from bacterial metabolism. Eventually the organism may die, due either to the exhaustion of the available food supply or to the liberation of so much in the way of decomposition products that the environment is no longer favorable to its existence.

An analogous change is often noted when adjusting the reaction of mediums. If the medium is too alkaline it becomes necessary to add acid, usually normal hydrochloric, to bring it to the proper point. The addition of such an acid always throws down a precipitate, either at once or on heating. This precipitate can, of course, be filtered out. It is reasonable to suppose that acid produced as the result of bacterial metabolism would also bring about such a change.

It is a significant fact that in the experiment herein described, the typical indications of a vigorous growth, such as cloudiness and the formation of a precipitate, only appeared as the degree of acidity approached P_H 6.3. Not until they reached this point would a mere inspection of the tubes reveal the presence of a culture. Control tubes of uninoculated medium which were incubated with these cultures did not show any such changes.

TABLE 1

RESULTS OF EXPERIMENTS

Original Reaction before Final Tubing and Autoclaving	Reaction just before Inoculating	Reaction just after Inoculating	Reaction after 3 Hours' Incubation	Reaction after 6 Hours' Incubation	Reaction after 7 Hours' Incubation	Reaction after 8 Hours' Incubation	Reaction after 9 Hours' Incubation	Reaction after 12 Hours' Incubation	Reaction after 25 Hours' Incubation	Reaction of Uninoculated Tubes after 25 Hours' Incubation
	P_H	P_H	P_H	P_H	P_H	P_H	P_H	P_H	P_H	P_H
5% ascites, 0.2% glucose, P_H 6.4	6.4	6.4	6.4	6.3	6.3—	...	...	...	...	6.4
5% ascites, 0.2% glucose, P_H 6.8	6.8	6.7	6.6	6.3—	...	...	...	...	...	6.6
5% ascites, 0.2% glucose, P_H 7.2	7.3	7.3	7.3	6.7	6.6	6.4	6.4	6.3—	...	7.3
5% ascites, 0.2% glucose. P_H 7.6	7.6	7.6	7.4	7.2	6.9	6.6	6.3	6.3—	...	7.6
5% ascites, 0.2% glucose, P_H 8.0	8.0	8.0	8.0	7.8	7.8	7.8	7.8	7.8	6.3—	8.0
1% glucose.............. P_H 6.4	6.4	6.4	6.4	6.3—	...	...	...	...	...	6.4
1% glucose.............. P_H 6.8	6.7	6.6	6.7	6.3	6.3—	...	...	...	...	6.6
1% glucose.............. P_H 7.2	7.0	7.0	6.6	6.4	6.3	6.3	6.3—	...	...	7.0
1% glucose.............. P_H 7.6	7.4	7.4	7.4	6.8	6.8	6.4	6.3	6.3—	...	7.4
1% glucose.............. P_H 8.0	7.4	7.4	7.4	6.8	6.9	6.6	6.4	6.3—	...	7.4

P_H 6.3— is used to indicate the maximum color change in bromthymol blue.

The chief source of acid production in our medium is the glucose content. It is shown by Avery and Cullen [2] that the amount of glucose, at least in concentrations between 0.5% and 1.5%, does not influence the final H-ion concentration or to any appreciable extent the rate of acid production. According to their experiment, too, very little acid is produced in a plain or sugar-free broth. The slight increase in acidity which they do show might easily be due to the final sterilization and in no way to the action of bacteria. They do not speak of any control which covers this point.

Our own experiments show a somewhat greater amount of acid produced in plain broth. We inoculated several series of 10 tubes each with a Streptococcus viridans and incubated them for 6 days. The P_H value of the broth just before inoculating was between 7.1 and 7.3. At the end of this time the reaction in all tubes was P_H 6.6. Control tubes of uninoculated medium incubated for the same length of time showed no change in reaction. This broth was made from beef extract and was reasonably free of sugar. It was not made absolutely so by fermenting with B. coli, however.

CONCLUSIONS

While there may not be a great deal to choose between P_H 6.4 and P_H 7.6, a broth given an initial reaction of P_H 6.8 will favor a more rapid growth, while a broth having a reaction more alkaline than P_H 7.6 will distinctly retard growth. Between the 5% ascites, 0.2% glucose broth and the 1% glucose broth there appears to be no appreciable difference when growing a pure culture.

VARIATIONS IN THE HYDROGEN-ION CONCENTRATION IN UNINOCULATED CULTURE MEDIUM

LINWOOD G. GRACE AND FLORENCE HIGHBERGER

From the Research Institute of the National Dental Association, Cleveland, Ohio

Within the last few years, the methods of adjusting the reaction of bacteriologic culture mediums have undergone considerable change. Titrating, using phenolphthalein as an indicator, has been shown to be almost as inaccurate as the older method of using litmus. A faint shade of pink was considered the neutrality point, but was difficult for even experienced workers to determine accurately this point. Further, it was almost impossible for one worker to duplicate another's results. It is possible that many discrepancies found in the results of different investigators may be due to this fact.

The newer method of adjusting the reaction by determining the hydrogen-ion concentration more nearly approaches the ideal than anything yet advanced and is fast finding its way into all bacteriologic laboratories. By this method the reactions of different batches of mediums can be more carefully controlled. So much has been written concerning this method and its advantages that any lengthy discussion would be mere repetition.

By comparing the titratable acidity as determined with phenolphthalein with the P_H value, Norton[1] and others have shown the wide variations possible in different batches of mediums when the older method was used, although it was apparently made and titrated in the same way. Carrying out the same thought along different lines Ayers, Johnson and Davis[2] found that titratable acidity, as a measure of the fermentative activity of an organism, is influenced so much by the nature and buffer content of the culture medium that this method should be supplanted by the determination of the hydrogen-ion concentration. Fennel and Fisher[3] found that it was only after using the hydrogen-ion determination method in making up their mediums that they obtained a luxuriant growth of pneumococci with any degree of consistency. Strong[4] speaks of the unsatisfactory results obtained by titrating mediums and suggests a simplified method for adjusting the reaction, based on the H-ion determination.

While making a study of the rate of acid production by Strep. viridans[5] some interesting facts concerning the broth used were brought to light.

Received for publication Feb. 1, 1920.

[1] Am. Jour. Pub. Health, 1919, 9, p. 190.
[2] Jour. Infect. Dis., 1918, 23, p. 290.
[3] Ibid., 1919, 25, p. 444.
[4] Jour. Am. Med. Assn., 1919, 72, p. 413.
[5] Jour. Inf. Dis., 1920, 26, p. 451.

Briefly, our experiment was this. The same strain of Strep. viridans was grown simultaneously in broth, the composition of which was the same, but the initial reaction was varied between P_H 6.4 and P_H 8.0. We then made observations on the rate of acid production with the idea of determining the reaction which favored most rapid growth.

The medium used had the following composition: Beef extract (Liebig's), 0.3%; peptone (Difco), 1%; NaCl, 0.5%; glucose, 1%. The batch was divided into 5 parts which were given the reactions of P_H 6.4, P_H 6.8, P_H 7.2, P_H 7.6 and P_H 8.0, respectively, and then autoclaved at 15 pounds' pressure for 15 minutes. The reaction was then readjusted, the mediums filtered, tubed and again autoclaved at 15 pounds' pressure for 15 minutes.

The reaction was adjusted by the simplified colorimetric method of determining the H-ion concentration as suggested by Barnett and Chapman[6] and somewhat elaborated by Norton.[1]

This procedure for making up mediums is the one usually followed, it being assumed that the change produced in the reaction by the final autoclaving would be so slight as to be disregarded.

For the experiment in question we felt, however, that it was necessary to have an exact knowledge of the H-ion concentration of the medium just before it was inoculated. Careful tests were accordingly made to determine this. We also kept uninoculated tubes of the various reactions in the incubator and noted their reaction at the conclusion of the experiment. These control tests brought out the fact that the reaction was not as stable as we had once supposed. Not only would the final autoclaving produce a change, but the reactions also varied from day to day.

In an effort to determine whether there were any consistent changes or whether the reaction would finally reach an equilibrium, we carried out four tests.

Batches of the medium were made up at different times, under conditions as nearly identical as we could make them, according to the procedure given. Some of the tubes of each reaction were put in the incubator at 37 C., some in the icebox and some allowed to stand at room temperature. Each day the P_H value of one tube from each batch was tested. Numerous checks served to show that the reaction of one tube was practically the same as that of others of that same set at that particular time.

[6] Ibid., 1918, 70, p. 1064.

TABLE 1

RESULTS FROM ONE TEST

1% Glucose Broth				Medium Stored in Tubes								Medium Stored in Flasks							
Initial Reaction Given Mediums	Reaction after First Autoclaving	Reaction after Final Autoclaving	*	Reaction after Standing One Day	Second Day	Fourth Day	Sixth Day	Seventh Day	Eighth Day	Ninth Day	Tenth Day	First Day	Second Day	Fourth Day	Sixth Day	Seventh Day	Eighth Day	Ninth Day	Tenth Dyy
P_H6.4	P_H6.4	P_H6.4	R.	P_H6.4	P_H6.4	P_H6.4	P_H6.4	P_H6.4	P_H6.4	P_H6.4	P_H6.4	P_H6.4	P_H6.4	P_H6.4	P_H6.4	P_H6.4	P_H6.4	P_H6.4	P_H6.3
			Inc.	6.4	6.3	6.3	6.4	6.4	6.4	7.2	6.3	6.4	6.4	6.4	6.4	6.4	6.4	6.4	6.4
			I.B.	6.4	6.6	6.4	6.5	6.4	6.4	6.4	6.6	6.4	6.4	6.4	6.4	6.4	6.4	6.4	6.4
6.8	6.8	6.6	R.	6.8	6.8	6.8	6.8	7.2	6.5	6.6	6.8	6.8	6.8	6.8	6.8	6.6	6.6	6.6	6.6
			Inc.	6.6	6.8	6.8	6.6	6.6	6.6	6.4	6.8	6.8	6.8	6.8	6.8	6.6			
			I.B.	6.8	6.8	6.8	6.8	7.2	6.6	7.0	6.8	6.8	6.8	6.8	6.8	6.6	6.6	6.6	6.6
7.2	7.0	7.2	R.	6.6	6.3	6.3	6.3	6.3	6.4	6.4	6.5	7.1	7.2	7.0	7.0	7.0	7.0	7.0	7.2
			Inc.	6.6	6.3	6.3	6.5	6.4	6.4	6.4	6.3	6.9	6.9	6.9	6.9	6.5	6.9	6.9	6.9
			I.B.	6.5	6.4	6.3	6.3	6.4	6.4	6.3	6.3	7.1	7.2	7.0	7.0	7.0	7.0	7.0	6.9
7.6	7.2	7.3	R.	7.4	7.4	7.4	7.4	7.4	7.3	7.4	7.3	7.2	7.2	7.3	7.2	7.0	7.0	7.2	7.0
			Inc.	7.4	7.4	7.3	7.4	7.4	7.3	7.4	7.3	7.3	7.0	7.0	7.0	6.6	6.9	6.9	6.9
			I.B.	7.4	7.5	7.4	7.4	7.4	7.3	7.4	7.3	7.3	7.2	7.3	7.2	7.0	7.0	7.2	7.0
8.0	7.8	8.0	R.	7.0	7.0	7.7	7.8	7.8	7.6	7.7	7.7	8.0	7.6	7.6	7.8	7.4	7.7	7.7	7.6
			Inc.	8.0	8.0	7.7	7.8	7.8	7.6	7.7	7.7	8.0	7.6	7.6	7.8	7.3			
			I.B.	8.0	8.0	7.7	7.8	1.8	7.6	7.7	7.3	8.0	7.6	7.6	7.8	7.4	7.7	7.7	7.6

* R. = room temperature. Inc. = incubator, 37 C. I.B. = icebox.

A part of the same medium was put in flasks and kept under similar conditions in the incubator, in the icebox and at room temperature. Each day a definite amount was removed by sterile pipets and the reaction noted.

One experiment was continued for 7 days, two for 10 and one for 13 days. Table 1 gives the results obtained in one test. It shows how the reaction varied, although when compared with results obtained in the other tests there was nothing consistent about these changes. Table 2 gives the limits of change under various conditions and is taken from all the experiments.

TABLE 2

LIMITS OF CHANGE UNDER VARIOUS CONDITIONS FROM ALL EXPERIMENTS

Initial reaction given medium	P_H6.4	P_H6.8	P_H7.2	P_H7.6	P_H8.0
Limits of variation produced by autoclaving	6.3-6.9	6.6-7.2	6.9-7.4	7.2-7.8	7.4-8.0
Limits of variation in tubes at room temp.	6.4-6.8	6.5-7.2	6.3-7.2	7.1-7.9	7.6-8.0
Limits of variation in tubes in incubator	6.4-6.7	6.6-6.8	6.3-7.2	7.2-7.6	7.4-8.0
Limits of variation in tubes in icebox	6.4-6.7	6.6-7.2	6.3-7.2	7.1-7.6	7.3-8.0
Limits of variation in flasks at room temp.	6.3-6.3	6.6-7.2	7.0-7.2	7.0-7.6	7.4-8.0
Limits of variation in flasks in incubator	6.3-6.6	6.6-6.9	6.5-7.2	6.6-7.6	7.3-8.0
Limits of variation in flasks in icebox	6.3-6.6	6.6-6.9	6.9-7.4	7.3-7.6	7.4-8.0

As a final test, a batch of plain broth was treated in the same way with the results shown in table 3. While there was some variation in the reaction it will be noted that it is not nearly so great as was observed in the glucose broth. Presumably, therefore, the resulting acid formed by the breaking up of the glucose is the chief factor responsible for these changes. Amino acids formed from the peptone may also be a contributing factor.

We checked our work carefully in order that the charge of faulty technic would not be made to account for these variations. Every care was used in the preparation of the medium. The flasks and tubes were cleaned before using by boiling in soap suds, rinsing in ammonia water, then in tap water and finally in distilled water. In order to assure the constancy of the values of the colorimetric standards, checks were made by the electrometric method. These checks showed an error not exceeding 0.06.

A preliminary report of the findings was sent to a number of bacteriologic laboratories with a request that we be advised whether any similar observations had been made. Although we received a large number of replies, only a few offered any explanations or had noted such changes.

It was suggested by Professor F. G. Novy that storage of medium in tubes must lead to change, partly because of solution of alkali from the glass, partly because of absorption of CO_2 and also perhaps because of slow hydrolysis.

TABLE 3

RESULTS OF FINAL TEST WITH PLAIN BROTH

Plain Broth			Medium Stored in Tubes						Medium Stored in Flasks				
Initial Reaction Given Medium	Reaction after First Autoclaving	Reaction after Final Autoclaving	*	Reaction after Standing Two Days	Third Day	Fifth Day	Sixth Day	Seventh Day	Second Day	Third Day	Fifth Day	Sixth Day	Seventh Day
			R.	PH 6.6	PH 6.4	PH 6.4	PH 6.4	PH 6.4	PH 6.5	PH 6.4	PH 6.4	PH 6.4	PH 6.4
PH 6.4	PH 6.4	PH 6.4	Inc.		6.4	6.4	6.4	6.4		6.4	6.4	6.4	6.4
			I.B.	6.6	6.4	6.4	6.4	6.4	6.5	6.4	6.4	6.4	6.4
			R.	7.2	7.1	7.2	7.4	7.3	7.2	7.4	7.2	7.1	7.2
6.8	6.9	7.2	Inc.		7.1	7.2	7.2	7.2		7.4	7.2	7.1	7.2
			I.B.	7.4	7.1	7.2	7.4	7.3	7.2	7.4	7.2	7.1	7.2
			R.	7.5	7.4	7.5	7.5	7.5	7.5	7.5	7.4	7.4	7.4
7.2	7.5	7.5	Inc.		7.4	7.5	7.5	7.5		7.5	7.4	7.4	7.4
			I.B.	7.5	7.4	7.5	7.5	7.5	7.5	7.5	7.4	7.4	7.4
			R.	8.0	7.9	7.8	7.6	7.8	7.9	7.8	7.8	7.6	7.7
7.6	7.6	8.0	Inc.		7.9	7.8	7.6	7.8		7.8	7.8	7.6	7.7
			I.B.	8.0	7.9	7.8	7.8	7.8	7.9	7.8	7.8	7.9	7.7
			R.	8.0	8.0	8.0	8.0	8.0	8.0	8.0	8.0	8.0	8.0
8.0	8.0	8.0	Inc.		8.0	8.0	8.0	8.0		8.0	8.0	8.0	8.0
			I.B.	8.0	8.0	8.0	7.8	8.0	8.0	8.0	8.0	8.0	8.0

* R. = room temperature. Inc. = incubator, 37 C. I.B. = icebox.

Such also was the opinion of Colonel F. F. Russell of the Army Medical School at Washington where observations similar to the above had been made. In his communication Colonel Russell states that changes toward the acid side have usually been attributed to the sterilization and subsequent to the absorption of CO_2. They have observed that tubes which are flamed and ampules which are sealed with a blast lamp take up an appreciable amount of CO_2, with a change in the P_H value of several tenths. Dr. F. P. Gay advised us that similar, although not identical, observations had been made at the University of California. It seems that variations were noted only in medium which was given an initial alkaline reaction.

It is probable, of course, that these changes have always occurred in mediums without our being aware of the fact. Most bacteria will grow over a very wide range. When grown in mediums they bring about changes in reaction until a final end point is reached. This end point seems to be pretty definite for certain types of organisms and has been used as a means of identification. Clark [7] discusses the diagnostic value of the final H-ion concentration in differentiating cultures of B. coli. Ayers,[8] Ayers, Johnson and Davis,[2] and Avery and Cullen [9] have all contributed to our knowledge of the end point reached by different varieties of streptococci.

As to just how important the initial reaction given culture mediums is, we are only beginning to find out, and it is quite probable that much work will have to be done before an optimum can be definitely established for each known organism or group of organisms.

As the latter question assumes greater significance, so will it grow to be more important to have a definite knowledge of the reaction of the medium just before it is inoculated. The variations that occur independent of the activities of bacteria must also be taken into account when making such studies.

It is possible that the simple method of adding normal acid or alkali solutions to mediums to give them the required degree of acidity or alkalinity may have to undergo some modifications.

[7] Jour. Biol. Chem., 1915, 22, p. 87.
[8] Jour. Bacteriol., 1916, 1, p. 84.
[9] Jour. Exper. Med., 1919, 29, p. 215.

INFLUENZA STUDIES

I. IMMUNITY IN INFLUENZA *

Edwin O. Jordan and W. B. Sharp

Opinion has long been at variance with respect to the degree and duration of immunity conferred by an attack of influenza. Some observers have asserted that one attack imparts little or no protection against subsequent attacks. Parsons [1] cites the medical officer of health of Ulverston as having had the disease in 1857, again in 1890 and three times in 1891. Squire [2] declares that second attacks are observed frequently when one epidemic succeeds another: "Not only is one attack not protective against a recurrence, but it seems to me rather to predispose to it." Other opinions to the same effect are quoted by Parsons [1] and by Leichtenstern.[3]

On the other hand, the belief has been expressed [4] that the relatively low attack rate in elderly persons observed in 1918 was due to an immunity acquired in 1889-1890. Unfortunately for the latter view, the age incidence of the disease seems to have been the same in 1889-1890 and in earlier epidemics as it was in 1918, although the intervals between successive epidemics have been of different length. The case rate per 1,000 population in 1918 in the age group 60-70 was apparently much lower than the case rate in the age group 35-45 [5] in spite of the fact that the members of both of these groups were exposed, presumably in equal degree, in the 1889-1890 epidemic.

Much confusion doubtless has been introduced into discussions of immunity to influenza by the impossibility of making a definite diagnosis. Since influenza cannot even now be identified with certainty either clinically or bacterially, recognition of a genuine second attack is necessarily conjectural. One of us has described two cases of supposed second attacks following soon after the first attack, in which it

Received for publication March 1, 1920.

* This is one of a series of studies carried out in connection with the Influenza Commission established and financially aided by the Metropolitan Life Insurance Company of New York. Part of the expense of these studies has been met by a grant from the University of Chicago.

1 Report to Local Government Board, 1893, p. 51.

2 Lancet, 1890, 1.

3 Influenza: Nothnagel's Specielle Path. u. Ther., 1896, 4, p. 54.

4 Jour. Am. Med. Assn., 1918, 71, p. 1595.

5 Frost, W. H., and Sydenstricker, E.: Public Health Reports, March 14, 1919.

is a plausible assumption that influenza-like symptoms were caused by infection with a micro-organism differing from that responsible for the primary attack of true influenza.[6] Perhaps a considerable proportion of so-called relapses may be explained in this way. Evidence supposed to be obtained from the presence or absence of the Pfeiffer bacillus [7] is certainly not convincing since this organism is found in a considerable proportion of normal throats as well as in several diseases, such as whooping-cough and measles, in which it can hardly be the primary exciting cause.

The question of immunity can probably be best approached in connection with cases occurring in successive waves of the disease separated by months or years. Aside from the opinions of individual physicians based on personal experience little information is available. Exact numerical data hardly exist. One of the few definite instances in the literature is given by Parsons and refers to the experience in the Industrial Schools at Swinton near Manchester. In March, 1890, 171 of 589 children had influenza. In 1891, when a second epidemic occurred, there were in the schools 449 children who had been there at the time of the first epidemic. Four cases (2.6%) occurred among the 150 who had had influenza in 1890, and 17 (5.7%) among the 299 who had escaped the first visitation. The existence of a slight degree of immunity has been inferred from these figures, but the numbers dealt with are too small to carry conviction.

The successive waves of influenza in 1918-1920 have given some opportunity to study the question of immunity. At the San Quentin prison in California it was observed that men who entered the prison after the April (1918) epidemic were attacked in later outbreaks in the same year "in greater numbers than those who had come before, although there were more of the latter than the former." [8] Italian observers have reported that when certain hospitals and asylums were visited by influenza inmates who had previously suffered an attack were exempt.[9] Ovazza,[10] however, notes that a number of persons who had had influenza in the spring of 1918 contracted it anew in the fall, although the return cases were strikingly mild and always free from complications.

[6] Jordan, E. O.: Jour. Infect. Dis., 1919, 25, p. 28.
[7] Thalman: Archiv. f. Hyg., 1913, 79-80, p. 142.
[8] Stanley, L. L.: Public Health Reports, May 9, 1919, p. 996.
[9] Scoccia: Policlinico, 1918, 25, p. 1249; abstr. in Jour. Am. Med. Assn., 1919, 72, p. 529. Folcioni: Policlinico, 1919, 26, p. 133; abstr. Jour. Am. Med. Assn., 1919, 72, p. 1039.
[10] Policlinico, 1919, 26, p. 271; abstr. Jour. Am. Med. Assn., 1919, 72, p. 1335.

In Spain it was observed that towns that were spared at the first invasion, such as Barcelona, suffered most at the second invasion.[11] It was thought, too, that the incidence of the disease in the barracks indicated the existence of same degree of immunity among the soldiers who had had the disease in the spring.[11] Joltain and Banfle[12] record the instance of a troop of soldiers from Indo-China nearly all of whom had the disease lightly in the spring of 1918. When the disease reappeared in October it spared this troop completely, while troops and civilians in the vicinity developed it.

The following observations, on about 6,000 men of approximately the same age living in barrack organization in the vicinity of Chicago, are offered as a contribution to this question.

Great Lakes Naval Training Station.—Through the courtesy of the post commandant we have been enabled to make inquiry concerning the influenzal history of the recruits at the Great Lakes Naval Training Station during and following the outbreak in January, 1920. The post strength is about 5,500 to 6,000 men. Most of them are young recruits, averaging perhaps 20 to 21 years of age. Nearly all had been home during the 1918 influenza epidemic, and with rare exceptions do not appear to have received vaccine against respiratory infection.

The 1920 epidemic of influenza broke out in January, the first cases coming to the hospital January 12. The origin of the outbreak is uncertain. In the Radio School, the first organization affected, were regiments that had just arrived from the Norfolk Station and many other men returning from furloughs.

This year's influenza epidemic at the Station is considered similar in practically all respects to that of last year. The symptoms were the same, though perhaps of less average severity. We studied twenty cases in detail. Coming on with a mild chill or chilly sensation, the temperature rose to somewhere between 100 and 105 F., usually between 102 and 104. It frequently became normal in a day or so and remained normal, but sometimes an irregular, low-grade fever continued for several days. Most of the patients had a headache — often frontal — sometimes severe. Half of them had general aching, backache and other symptoms. Practically all coughed, and many

[11] Jour. Am. Med. Assn., 1919, 72, p. 665.

[12] Bull. de la Soc. méd. d. hôp., 1918, 42, p. 991; abstr. Jour. Am. Med. Assn., 1919, 72, p. 529.

raised a little sputum. The throat often became irritated or slightly sore. Those seen during the fever were flushed; pneumonia patients only were cyanosed. The throat appeared normal or generally hyperemic. Rhinitis was rare. Acute infections of the nose, accessory sinuses, tonsils, etc., were not found. The pulse was somewhat slower than the degree of fever led one to expect. The leukocyte count varied from 4,800 to 15,000. Throat cultures from tonsil and nasopharynx swabs were positive for hemolytic streptococcus and Pfeiffer's bacillus in nearly all cases and for other organisms less frequently.

With the cordial cooperation of the post authorities we were able to have a few brief, simple questions put to approximately 4,000 men at the post and the results recorded on typewritten forms.

The men's statement regarding previous influenza was accepted whenever the attack was said to have occurred during the influenza period of 1918-1919, i. e., in September, October, November, December, January, February and March. The great majority were reported for the period of September to December. Only a few cases were reported as occurring in March, and perhaps these actually occurred somewhat earlier than the men recalled. A few cases were accepted as influenza when reported as occurring in Europe during July and August, 1918.

The possibility that various noninfluenzal affections might have been diagnosed as influenza during the 1918-1919 period was tested by closer questioning of a few hundred men. Patients at the main hospital who gave a positive history during that period (September to March) in nearly all cases remembered typical influenza symptoms: fever, aching and other symptoms, with cough and without much sore throat, occurring in the midst of local epidemics. We are convinced that most of these patients knew whether they had had actual influenza. It seems probable that the same is true of the men throughout the post area.

Table 1 indicates the number of men who had influenza previously and again in 1920, the number that had influenza previously but not in 1920, the number that did not have influenza previously but did in 1920, and the number that had not been attacked at all. Those listed as doubtful gave a history of influenza occurring at a time, in most cases, when the disease was not prevalent. A few company reports that did not differentiate between 1918 and 1920 attacks are not included; the reports of 662 men were thus discarded.

From table 1 it appears that of 3,905 men who gave a clear history, 1,112 had had influenza in 1918-1919 (28.5% incidence), and 881 were attacked in 1920 (22.6%).

Of the 1,112 who had had influenza, 236, or 21.2%, had a repeated attack in 1920, while of 2,793 who had not had a previous attack, 645, or 23.1%, were attacked in 1920.

TABLE 1

INCIDENCE OF INFLUENZA IN 1918 AND 1920 AMONG THE MEN AT THE GREAT LAKES TRAINING STATION IN JANUARY, 1920

	Influenza in 1918-1919, Also in 1920	Influenza in 1918-1919, Not in 1920	No Attack in 1918-1919, Influenza in 1920	No History of Influenza	Doubtful History
Hospital	113	7	264	9	7
Aviation	81	421	217	993	95
Radio	11	163	71	469	30
Signal	2	10	7	26	3
16th Regiment	20	127	40	232	16
13th Regiment	4	38	11	94	9
3rd Regiment	5	110	35	325	21
Total	236	876	645	2,148	181

Table 2 is to be read as in the Great Lakes series:

TABLE 2

INCIDENCE OF INFLUENZA IN 1918 AND 1920 AMONG THE MEN AT CAMP GRANT, ROCKFORD, ILLINOIS, IN JANUARY, 1920

	Influenza in 1918-1919, Also in 1920	Influenza in 1918-1919, Not in 1920	No Attack in 1918-1919, Influenza in 1920	No History of Influenza	Doubtful History
Headquarters Troop, 6th Division	2	11	5	25	1
318th Engineers	5	35	10	154	9
3d Field Artillery	4	46	10	162	10
78th Field Artillery	1	11	6	126	4
11th Field Artillery	13	60	48	285	15
Provisional Recruit Company	1	38	4	175	27
6th Ammunition Train	0	0	2	5	1
6th Field Signal Battalion	0	5	5	41	4
52d Infantry	4	9	9	102	4
53d Infantry	0	5	12	60	2
54th Infantry	0	7	3	78	2
16th Machine Gun Battalion	1	3	2	20	0
17th Machine Gun Battalion	1	1	1	26	0
18th Machine Gun Battalion	0	5	1	30	0
Medical Detachment, Camp Hosp.	12	21	30	79	5
Motor Transport Corps	3	11	6	108	9
Quartermaster Corps	13	26	52	225	7
Cooks and Bakers	1	7	6	44	2
Remount Depot	0	21	8	85	8
Stockade	0	7	7	25	4
	61	229	227	1,855	114

Camp Grant, Rockford, Ill.—The 1920 influenza epidemic at Camp Grant, Rockford, Ill., was somewhat less severe than that at Great Lakes. It occurred at about the same time, reaching its height on Jan. 12, 1920. The age and previous history of the men were very similar to those at Great Lakes. Many were recruits, but some had returned from overseas service.

The camp surgeon kindly undertook to have the men report any history of influenza before 1920, with place, month and year of attacks. We have accepted the histories of the reported cases that occurred during the 1918-1919 epidemic period, as outlined above for the Great Lakes series. Discards were made for various errors of record covering 676 men.

Table 2 shows that of 2,472 men at Camp Grant, 390, or 15.8%, had influenza in 1918-1919, and 288, or 11.7%, in 1920. Official figures on the 1920 epidemic up to the time of our census showed 471 cases among 4,400 men, or 10.7%. Of the 390 men with previous influenza history, 61, or 15.6%, had a repeated attack, while of 2,082 without previous history of influenza, 227, or 10.9%, were attacked in 1920.

SUMMARY

Influenza epidemics broke out about Jan. 12, 1920, at the Great Lakes Naval Station containing perhaps 5,500 or 6,000 men, and in Camp Grant containing perhaps 4,400 men. In each post a census was taken in order to divide the men into the groups of those attacked and those not attacked in the 1918-1919 epidemic, and to determine the number in each group attacked in the recent epidemics. The results are:

TABLE 3

INFLUENZA ATTACK RATE IN JANUARY, 1920, IN MEN WITH AND WITHOUT PREVIOUS INFLUENZA HISTORY

	Number Giving Definite History	Number that Had Influenza in January, 1920	Percentage Attacked in January, 1920
Great Lakes			
Number that had influenza, 1918-1919	1,112	236	21.2
No history of influenza	2,793	645	23.1
Camp Grant			
Number that had influenza, 1918-1919	390	61	15.6
No history of influenza	2,082	227	10.9
Totals			
Number that had influenza, 1918-1919	1,502	297	19.8
No history of influenza	4,875	872	17.9

These results indicate that no marked immunity to influenza exists 12 to 15 months after a previous attack. They do not show that some degree of immunity may not obtain at an earlier period.

STUDIES IN INFLUENZA AND PNEUMONIA

STUDY V. OBSERVATIONS ON THE BACTERIOLOGY AND CERTAIN CLINICAL FEATURES OF INFLUENZA AND INFLUENZAL PNEUMONIA

E. C. Rosenow

Division of Experimental Bacteriology, The Mayo Foundation, Rochester, Minnesota.

The bacteriologic studies of the epidemic of influenza of 1889-1890,[13] of lesser outbreaks prior to the pandemic of 1918,[15] and the preliminary studies of the pandemic by others have shown that while influenza bacilli occur commonly the organisms of the pneumococcus-streptococcus group are constantly associated with this disease. In the course of my studies on this group of organisms and the diseases due to them I have been impressed repeatedly by the marked changes they undergo at times, particularly in infecting powers and immunologic reactions. In some instances these changes appeared to be true mutations.[25] It was thought possible that the peculiar picture presented in influenza, such as the marked prostration, cyanosis, leukopenia, and its almost simultaneous appearance over wide areas might be due to variants or mutation forms of organisms commonly present in the respiratory tract of man. Accordingly, as the epidemic reached Rochester a comprehensive plan of study, taking into consideration this possibility, was determined on. The results obtained form the basis of the series of experiments that I report. Preliminary statements, including a description of the somewhat peculiar green-producing streptococcus isolated quite constantly,[22] of immunologic studies,[24] and of the extraordinary invasive power of the streptococci from influenza on intratracheal application,[23] have been published.

In this paper are recorded the more important bacteriologic findings obtained throughout the four epidemic waves of influenza which occurred in Rochester during the autumn and winter of 1918-1919, and these findings correlated with certain clinical features of the disease.

The epidemic of 1918 began in Rochester during the latter part of September. An emergency hospital was opened and when this became inadequate certain parts of other hospitals were set aside for the care of influenza patients. The source of the material studied was, in the main, from patients admitted to these hospitals, most of whom had come to the Mayo Clinic for the treatment of some other condition or to accompany patients. A large number of cultures, however, were made from persons residing permanently in Rochester who had contracted influenza. A large proportion of the first group came long distances from widely separated communities, and many developed symptoms before or soon after their arrival. Some no doubt were infected en route or before leaving home; hence, the cases studied represent a heterogeneous group and the findings accordingly may be regarded as quite representative of the epidemic.

TECHNIC

Cultures were made from throat swabs prepared in the usual manner, from sputum, anterior nares, lung exudate, trachea and bronchi, peritracheal lymph gland, pleural fluid, the blood after death, and in some instances, from the blood during life. The sputum was collected in sterile, wide-mouthed glass vials and taken to the laboratory while fresh. Cultures were made on the surface of blood-agar plates directly or after washing in sodium chlorid solution, and into tall columns of dextrose broth, dextrose-brain broth or dextrose-blood broth. Owing to the mucoid and serous character of the sputum in influenza washing the sputum was quite unsatisfactory since it led to too great a dilution and hence the plates were made routinely by spreading a rather large amount of the unwashed sputum (about 0.1 c c) directly over the plates by means of triangular-shaped spreaders made from flat nicrome wire. The material was spread over the whole surface of the plate, part of the plate was heavily, and part lightly inoculated. The plates were incubated twenty-four hours at from 33 to 35 C. and then read. If influenza bacilli were not present the plates were incubated for an additional twenty-four or forty-eight hours. The air in the incubator was kept saturated with moisture by means of an open dish of water and by reducing the amount of ventilation to the minimum. The results of the cultures on the plates were recorded according to the numerical scale of 1 to 4; 1 indicating from 1 to 10 colonies; 2 from 11 to 100 colonies; 3 from 101 to 1,000 colonies and 4, 1,000 colonies and above, of the different bacteria. After death material was collected in sterile pipets by the pathologist in charge and brought directly to the laboratory for examination. The cultures of this material were made in the same manner as those from the sputum. Smears from throat and sputum during life, and of material after death were made, stained for bacteria and examined, in some cases in order to check the results of the cultures, and to study the proportion and character of the cells and their behavior toward the bacteria present. In order to check the results of cultures and direct examination of the exudate still further, and to determine which of the bacteria nearly always present had the greatest invasive powers in influenza, the sputum and exudates of some of the cases were injected intraperitoneally and intratracheally into guinea-pigs and intraperitoneally into white mice. Smears and cultures of the peritoneal or lung exudate and blood of these animals were made according to the method just described.

At first plain agar, made from beef extract and peptone, to which 5 per cent. of defibrinated human blood was added, was used, but since influenza bacilli were not detected on these plates, the so-called "hormone" or "vitamine" agar was substituted. The medium was carefully titrated to + 0.6 per cent. to phenolphthalein, and cleared by the use of a centrifugal machine. Usually, however, it was slightly opalescent from fat which was not wholly removed from the meat. One and seven-tenths per cent. agar was added instead of from 2 to 2.5 per cent. as is usually done. To this medium, cooled to about 60 C. approximately 4 per cent. of defibrinated human blood was added before it was poured into the plate. The plates were not usually incubated previously so that the surface of the agar was not hard and dry, but soft and moist. The advantages of this medium over the plain agar medium for growing influenza bacilli were striking. Large numbers of typical influenza bacillus colonies developed from the sputum of patients when few or none had been detected previously on plain-blood agar. In order to make sure that the lack of growth of bacilli on the plain blood-agar used previously was not due to their absence, but to a difference in the medium, parallel cultures on the two mediums were made of the sputum of 8 cases of typical influenza occurring at the outset of the first wave. All hormone-blood-agar plates showed countless numbers of influenza bacilli which grew in symbiosis with the green-producing streptococcus or pneumococcus, hemolytic streptococcus, and staphylococcus colonies, whereas the plain blood-agar plates showed few or no colonies of influenza bacilli. The colonies were usually found in the heavily inoculated part of the plate and surrounding colonies of green-producing streptococci and staphylococci, but were found also in other parts of the plate. Cultures from throats of some of these patients yielded similar results although influenza bacilli were present in larger numbers. Because of these findings, this medium was adopted for routine platings throughout the study. During the latter part of the work the special mediums for the isolation of influenza bacilli such as Avery's oleate agar [1] and of "chocolate" blood-agar plates were also used.

RESULTS

Cultures were made of the sputum or from the exudate of the throat of 571 patients with influenza or influenzal pneumonia during life, of the lung exudate, peribronchial lymph glands, or the blood after death in 107 cases. In 309 of the group of 571 and in 65 of the 107, both the clinical history and pathologic findings left no doubt as to the diagnosis. In the remaining 262 cases complete histories were not available for final analysis, but the diagnosis of influenza or influenzal pneumonia was made by the physician in charge at the time of the attack. The findings after death in 42 of these were clearly those of influenza, and since the bacteriologic findings in all were similar to those in the undoubted cases the diagnosis of influenza may be considered quite accurate.

TABLE 1

Result of Cultures of Material from Influenza and Influenzal Pneumonia

Bacteria	Material Cultured, Blood-Agar Plates					
	Sputum During Life (571 Cases)			Lung Exudate after Death (107 Cases)		
	Predominating or in Pure Culture, Percentage	Not in Predominating Numbers, Percentage	Total Percentage	Predominating or in Pure Culture, Percentage	Not in Predominating Numbers Percentage	Total Percentage
Green-producing streptococci or pneumococci	41	54	95	18	37	55
Hemolytic streptococci	9	29	38	23	54	77
Staphylococci	17	55	72	10	40	50
Bacillus influenzae	5	8	13	0	5	5
Micrococcus catarrhalis	0	6	6	0	3	3
Bacillus mucosus	0.8	1	1.8	4	7	11
Bacillus coli	0	0.8	0.8	3	15	18

The results obtained are summarized in Table 1. The figures giving the number of instances in which the various bacteria were found are omitted from the table and only those indicating the percentage are given, thus making direct comparisons readily possible. Fractions of a per cent. below 0.5 are dropped, to those 0.5 or above, one is added. The tabulations shown represent cases and not specimens. In many cases the sputum was cultured repeatedly during the course of the initial influenzal attack and during the influenzal pneumonia which followed. The figures in the first and fourth columns indicate the percentage incidence in which the different bacteria were present in predominating numbers or in pure culture; in the second and fifth columns the percentage incidence in which the bacteria were present, but not in predominating numbers; and in the third and sixth columns the total percentage incidence to the occurrence of the different bacteria in the sputum and lung exudate respectively.

Green-producing streptococci (some of which fermented inulin) were isolated from the sputum in predominating numbers or in pure culture in 41 per cent., and not in predominating numbers in 54 per cent., a total of 96 per cent. of the 571 cases studied; they were isolated from the lung exudate after death in predominating numbers or in pure culture in 18 per cent., and in smaller numbers in 37 per cent., a total of 55 per cent. of the 107 cases in which necropsies were made. Hemolytic streptococci occurred in the sputum in predominating numbers or in pure culture in 9 per cent., and not in predominating numbers in 29 per cent., a total of 38 per cent. of the cases studied during life; they occurred in the lung exudate in predominating numbers or in pure culture in 23 per cent., and not in predominating numbers in 54 per cent., a total of 77 per cent. of the cases after death. Staphylococci were isolated in varying numbers from the sputum in 72 per cent. and from the lung exudate in 50 per cent. of the cases. The influenza bacillus was isolated from the sputum in 13 per cent., and in predominating numbers in 5 per cent.; it was isolated from the lung exudate in 5 per cent. of the cases, never in predominating numbers. Micrococcus catarrhalis was found in the sputum in 6 per cent., and in the lung exudate in 3 per cent. of the cases, always in small numbers. The Bacillus mucosus was found in the sputum in 1.8 per cent., and in the lung exudate in 11 per cent. The colon bacillus occurred in the sputum in 0.8 per cent., and in the lung exudate in 18 per cent. of the cases.

The figures represent only in a general way the relative importance of a series of different types of bacteria isolated during life and after death. Thus the incidence of staphylococcus in predominating numbers in the sputum in 17 per cent. of the cases should not be taken to mean that this organism was the cause of the attack in this percentage of cases, because in many only one or two cultures were made, often late in the disease when staphylococci had become relatively numerous. The lowering in total incidence of green-producing streptococci of from 96 per cent. in the sputum to 55 per cent. in the lung exudate, and the increase in incidence of hemolytic streptococci of from 38 per cent. in the sputum to 77 per cent. in the lung exudate may be regarded as expressing roughly the importance of these two types of streptococci as causes of death in influenzal infection. Instances occurred in which the bloody fluid from the lungs of patients who died from acute hemorrhagic edema showed large numbers of green-producing streptococci or hemolytic streptococci in pure culture, as well as mixtures of these two types of streptococci. Cultures made from throats of patients who could not raise sputum at the onset of the attack and in some as controls of sputum cultures, showed similar results to those obtained from the sputum. Throat cultures at the beginning of influenza often showed large numbers of the green-producing colonies, in pure or almost pure form.

The number of colonies of the different bacteria which developed on the blood-agar plates was recorded according to the numerical scale of 1 to 4. It was thought worth while to determine the figure expressing the average incidence by days of the three main varieties of bacteria (green-producing streptococci, hemolytic streptococci, and staphylococci) which were isolated in influenza and in influenzal pneumonia throughout the four epidemic waves. This was done by adding the figures representing the number of colonies of each organism and dividing this sum by the total number of specimens of sputum cultivated on the different days. There was no noteworthy difference in the average incidence of the various bacteria for influenza and for the first five days of influenzal pneumonia; hence these cases are considered together. The number of green-producing streptococci averaged highest each day for the first five days, the average figures being 3.7, 3.4, 3.6, 3.6 and 3.4, respectively. The average figures for the first five days for staphylococci were 2.0, 2.4, 2.2, 3.0 and 2.4. The average figures for hemolytic streptococci were 1.2, 1.6, 1.8, 1.7, and 2. In numbers staphylococci occupied the middle position and hemolytic streptococci the lowest position, but there was a tendency to an average increase in staphylococci and hemolytic streptococci during the later stages of the disease. The figures representing the average incidence of the different bacteria after the fifth day varied between wide limits. Thus the figures expressing the average increase of green-producing streptococci occupied the middle position on the sixth, seventh, eighth, tenth, and eleventh days; hemolytic streptococci, the lowest position on the sixth, seventh, eighth, tenth and eleventh days, the highest position on the ninth and twelfth days; staphylococci, the highest position on the sixth, seventh, eighth, tenth, and eleventh days, and the middle position on the ninth day. It becomes apparent, therefore, that the time in the attack when the cultures are made must be considered in order properly to interpret their meaning.

Marked variations in the type of bacterial flora were often noted at different stages of the disease during life and after death, and at different periods in the epidemic waves. In almost all instances of undoubted cases of influenza green-producing streptococci, together with a variable number of staphylococci or Micrococcus catarrhalis were the predominating flora at the outset of the influenzal attack throughout the epidemic waves. In most of the patients who recovered without developing pneumonia and in many who developed nonfatal or fatal attacks of pneumonia during the earlier part of the waves, this flora persisted. Later in the epidemic waves, however, there was a tendency for the green-producing streptococci to be displaced by hemolytic streptococci. This tendency to an increase in hemolytic streptococci in the later stages of the disease was noted especially in the patients who succumbed to the infection. Thus, in 21 fatal cases in which repeated cultures were made of the sputum during life and in which the lung exudate was cultured after death, green-producing streptococci predominated in the sputum during life in 16, and hemolytic streptococci in 5, while in these same cases hemolytic streptococci predominated in 11, and green-producing streptococci in 10, in the lung exudate after death. There was a shifting, therefore, from a predominant green-producing streptococcal flora to a hemolytic streptococcal flora in 6 of these fatal cases. The sputum usually became bloody as this occurred; the blood count showed no noteworthy change. The interval from the time of the sputum cultures to the time of the lung culture in these 6 cases was 1, 2, 4, 12, 12, and 4 days, respectively, or an average of 5.8 days. In some of the patients who recovered, on the other hand, the green-producing streptococcal flora again became predominant as the symptoms disappeared. This shifting of bacterial flora occurred both in cases of influenza without demonstrable lesions in the lung, as well as in influenzal pneumonia, but it occurred more often in the latter condition. The lack of agreement in the flora was noted not infrequently in cultures from the blood, from the lung, and from the pleural and other exudates after death. At times this occurred simultaneously in groups of patients who contracted the disease at about the same time. The blood after death proved to be sterile in about one-third of the cases cultured, and in the others green-producing streptococci or hemolytic streptococci alone or with staphylococci were isolated in about an equal number of cases. Green-producing streptococci were, at times, found in pure culture in the blood when the lung and other exudates showed few or no green-producing streptococci, but hemolytic streptococci with or without staphylococci. The cases which showed empyema usually yielded a predominating number of hemolytic streptococci.

The lack of agreement in the type of streptococcus colonies isolated from material after death, as noted in some cases, is well illustrated in the cultures from a case of fulminating influenzal bronchopneumonia and ulcerative laryngitis. The necropsy was performed soon after death. Cultures from the larynx, bronchial tubes and lung exudate showed large numbers of moist, spreading, slightly hemolyzing streptococci, a few typical hemolytic streptococcus colonies, and a moderate number of staphylococci, while blood-agar-plate cultures from dextrose broth inoculated with the blood from the heart showed pure growth of moist, spreading, nonhemolyzing green-producing colonies of streptococci. The morphology and character of the colony of the slightly hemolyzing streptococci and the green-producing streptococci from the blood were identical. In another case of influenzal bronchopneumonia with huge right and slight left empyema and beginning pericarditis, the cultures showed large numbers of hemolyzing streptococci and staphylococci from the pneumonia, a few hemolyzing streptococci and staphylococci from the left pleura, staphylococci from the pericardium, and larger numbers of green-producing streptococci and a few staphylococci in the pus from the right pleural cavity.

Staphylococci were rarely found in large numbers in the sputum early in the disease, but there was in general a tendency to an increase in the numbers of these organisms during the later stages, especially of influenzal pneumonia. In many instances the green-producing streptococcal flora noted at the outset when the sputum was mucoid in character was later partially or wholly displaced by staphylococcal flora, as the sputum became more purulent in character. This occurred especially during the later stages of the epidemic waves and in groups of patients who became ill at about the same time. Usually no particular change was noted in the patient's condition as staphylococci became more numerous in the sputum. Staphylococci were often found in predominating numbers or in pure culture in the pus from abscesses in bronchopneumonic areas in cases in which hemolytic or green-producing streptococci were the predominating organism in the pneumonic exudate remote from these abscesses. In such instances it was impossible to evaluate the exact rôle played by these organisms. In some cases, however, there could be little doubt that they were the cause of death just as was the case in the series of staphylococcal pneumonia that developed during the influenza epidemic at Camp Jackson, as reported by Chickering and Park.[6] In these there was a rapid change for the worse in the patient's condition as the staphylococci appeared in large numbers in the sputum and as the sputum became bloody, although purulent in character. The leukocyte count remained at about the same level or became lower as death occurred from acute hemorrhagic edema, or acute bronchopneumonia in from one to three days. The lung exudate after death showed enormous numbers of micrococci in groups in smears and staphylococci in enormous number usually in pure or in almost pure form in cultures. The freshly isolated organisms from some of these cases were found to be extremely virulent for animals. Intratracheal injection into guinea-pigs produced violent symptoms associated with leukopenia, and frequently death occurred from acute hemorrhagic bronchopneumonia, hemorrhagic edema, and voluminous lungs. The picture in these animals was quite different from that following injection of freshly isolated strains of staphylococcus from furunculosis, and from the abscesses in the lungs of some patients who died later. In the latter, symptoms were slight or absent, leukocytosis developed, recovery was the rule, and while areas of bronchopneumonia were found acute hemorrhagic edema never developed.

Influenza bacilli were isolated from the sputum in large numbers only during the early part of the first wave and almost not at all after that. These organisms were present in only a small number of cases after death, and when found were always in small numbers. That the absence of this organism in the cultures was due to their absence in the material cultured and not to their inability to grow on the medium used is certain. The medium which we used throughout the different waves was found quite efficient for cultivating this organism from swabs of the nasopharynx of influenza patients and from normal persons by Dr. Williams and Dr. Hatfield, working in our laboratory during the fourth wave. It is true, however, that cultures made at the same time on the special mediums which they used for isolating influenza bacilli showed this organism in a somewhat higher percentage of cases. We were especially interested in whether or not influenza bacilli were present in the exudate of the lower respiratory tract, the point of chief attack, but cultures of sputum at this time again showed influenza bacilli in only a few cases, and in these in small numbers. Smears of the sputum, lung exudate, and tracheal mucus failed to show influenza bacilli when they were absent in cultures.

The results of the injection into animals (mice and guinea-pigs) of the sputum and lung exudate directly or of the primary mass culture in dextrose-blood broth served as an additional check on the cultures, for it was thought that growth of influenza bacilli, if of great significance in the production of symptoms in the disease in our cases, might occur in animals known to be susceptible to these organisms. Moreover, it was thought that a fairly accurate knowledge of the degree of invasive power of the different bacteria might be obtained in this way. A study was, therefore, made of the relative numbers of the different bacteria in the sputum and primary cultures in dextrose broth of sputum which was injected into animals and their relative numbers from the peritoneal and lung exudates of the animals that died. Sixty-eight animals succumbed to the intraperitoneal or intratracheal injection of sputum or of primary cultures from sputum and from lung exudate. Green-producing streptococci were the predominant organisms in the material injected in 68 per cent. of the animals, while after death this organism predominated in the blood, peritoneal or lung exudate in 78 per cent. of the animals. In most of the others hemolytic streptococci, and in a few, staphylococci, were the predominating organisms. Influenza bacilli were not isolated in a single instance, notwithstanding the fact that some of the specimens of sputum injected contained this organism in large numbers. The blood-agar plates made from the peritoneal exudate usually showed a mixture of streptococci and staphylococci in about the same proportions as in the material injected, while the blood nearly always contained pure cultures of streptococci, usually of the green-producing variety. In some animals, however, striking deviations from this rule occurred. Staphylococcus colonies in varying numbers often developed from the peritoneal exudate when the blood-agar plate from the material injected showed only streptococcus colonies. In some instances green-producing streptococci were isolated from the blood of these animals in pure culture, or together with hemolyzing streptococci when pure cultures of hemolyzing streptococci were injected, and vice versa. These findings were noted also when the cultures injected were derived from single widely separated colonies and at the same time in series of animals including several species.

The respiratory infections were of quite different types during several weeks prior to the occurrence of the first epidemic wave, at the height of the waves, as the waves subsided, and for several weeks following. Prior to the first severe outbreak mild attacks of pharyngitis and bronchitis with little fever and with slight or no constitutional symptoms occurred. Cultures from these cases showed a green-producing streptococcal flora in the sputum and throat. At the height of the epidemics, especially the first wave, marked prostration, cyanosis and leukopenia, high fever, and marked tendency to lung involvement with slight injection of pharynx and tonsils dominated the picture. Deaths from acute hemorrhagic edema were relatively common. As the waves subsided the symptoms became less marked, leukopenia was less persistent, deaths from respiratory involvement occurred later, and the lung showed relatively more true consolidation, but symptoms referable to infection of the nose and throat were more pronounced. In such cases it was often difficult to make the diagnosis, and cultures in some showed hemolyzing streptococci from the beginning of the attack. Still later well marked pharyngitis, often associated with follicular tonsillitis, absence of leukopenia or even leukocytosis, became prevalent. Involvement of the lung was now rare and deaths from pneumonia no longer occurred. Cultures from the throat and tonsils of patients in the latter condition showed hemolytic streptococci to be the chief organism.

The technic of making the cultures was uniform throughout the four waves, and the results were recorded according to the scale of 1 to 4, thus affording opportunity to study the changes in the character of the colonies of the different species and changes in their relative numbers as the epidemic waves appeared and disappeared. Each of the four epidemic waves studied ran its course in about six weeks, and the crest was reached in about two weeks; accordingly the results of sputum cultures from cases of influenza and influenzal pneumonia, and the fatal cases, were arranged into three groups of two weeks each, and the average of the three main types of bacteria (green-producing streptococci, hemolyzing streptococci, and staphylococci) determined. The first period comprised the first two weeks, the second the third and fourth weeks, and the third the fifth and sixth weeks of the four waves. The figures representing the average incidence of green-producing streptococci for the three periods of the four waves were 2.6, 2.3 and 2.7; for hemolyzing streptococcus 1.1, 1.4, and 1.4; and for staphylococci 1.8, 2.1, and 2.4, respectively. According to these figures it is evident that the green-producing streptococcus in the sputum averaged the highest throughout the epidemic waves, and that the hemolyzing streptococcus and staphylococcus while comparatively few early in the epidemic became relatively more numerous as the waves subsided. In the case of cultures after death the figures representing the average for green-producing streptococci for the three periods were 1.5, 2.6 and 1.0, for hemolyzing streptococcus 1.1, 1.7 and 2.5, and for staphylococcus 1.1, 1.1 and 2.1, respectively. According to these figures, the green-producing streptococcus was the chief cause of death during the first four weeks of the waves, and the hemolyzing streptococcus and staphylococcus during the fifth and sixth weeks, or as the waves were subsiding.

Morphology, Cultural Characteristics and Fermentative Powers of the Streptococci from Influenza

Green-Producing Streptococci. — The somewhat peculiar green-producing streptococcus isolated during the first wave has been described (Study 1). The further results, throughout the subsequent waves, have in the main corroborated the earlier findings, although greater differences in cultural characteristics have been noted than were at first apparent. From a study of a large number of cases we have found green-producing streptococci, including pneumococci, to be the most common organism present in influenzal infection. The strains when first isolated usually produced rather moist, spreading, non-adherent greenish colonies on blood-agar plates and a diffuse cloud in glucose broth. Smears of young cultures from these mediums showed gram-positive oval shaped diplococci of quite uniform size, singly, in pairs, and usually in fairly long chains. These were of about the size of pneumococci and were often indistinguishable from them, although chain formation was usually more marked and the capsule less distinct. Smears from older cultures, especially in the deeper layers of tall columns of glucose-brain broth, often showed diplococci of extreme variations in size and shape. During the first wave the colonies were quite moist, usually resembling type III pneumococci, although less mucoid in character; in the subsequent outbreaks, especially during the later stages, they were usually not so moist and were often indistinguishable from pneumococcus colonies. The more moist spreading type of colonies, some resembling Pneumococcus mucosus, were isolated, however, during these waves in some instances. This was true particularly early in each wave, in severe cases occurring in groups of persons who contracted influenza soon after arriving in Rochester, and who came from the same locality, as well as in individual families residing in Rochester and in the surrounding country. The chief distinguishing characteristics of these strains as of those in the first wave, however, were their marked and peculiar invasive power on intratracheal injection. As the

TABLE 2

THE VARIABILITY IN FERMENTATIVE POWER OF GREEN-PRODUCING STREPTOCOCCI FROM INFLUENZA

Date of Test	Strain	Dextrose	Lactose	Maltose	Saccharose	Raffinose	Mannite	Salicin	Inulin	Control
9/25/18	2539.6	+4	+4	+4	+4	+4	0	+4	0	0
3/ 6/19	2539.8	+3	+2	+2	+4	+4	+	+2	0	0
3/ 4/19	2341.17	+3	+3	+3	+4	+4	0	+3	+	0
12/30/19	2341.20	+2	0	+	+	0	0	0	0	0
3/ 3/19	2347.12	+3	+3	+2	+4	+4	+	+	+	0
11/14/19	2347.23	+3	+3	+4	+3	0	0	0	0	0
3/ 3/19	2349.12	+3	+3	+3	+4	+4	0	+2	+2	0
11/14/19	2349.18	+4	+3	+4	+3	0	0	0	0	0
3/ 6/19	2531.8	+3	+2½	+3	+4	+	0	0	+2	0
11/ 4/19	2531.12	+3	+3	+3	0	0	0	0	0	0
3/ 6/19	2532.0	+3	+3	+3	+4	+4	0	+3	+2	0
11/ 4/19	2532.8	+3	0	+2	+2	+	+3	+3	0	0
3/15/19	2620.3	+3	0	+3	+4	0	0	+4	0	0
3/15/19	2620.3	+2	+	+2	+4	0	0	+3	0	0
3/10/19	2724.8	+3	+2	+2	+4	+4	0	0	0	0
11/18/19	2724.11	+	+3	+3	+3	0	0	0	0	0
3/12/19	2789.4	+3	+3	+2	+4	0	0	0	0	0
12/17/19	2789.8	+3	+	+2	+2	0	0	0	0	0
3/12/19	2748.8	+3	+3	+3	+3	+4	0	+3	0	0
5/ 8/19	2748.10	0	+	+2	+3	+4	0	+	+3	0
11/22/19	2748.11	+3	+	+2	+	0	0	0	0	0
3/12/19	2762.6	+3	+3	+	+4	+4	0	+4	+3	0
11/22/19	2762.8	+	+3	+2	+	+2	+2	0	0	0
3/12/19	2763.6	+3	+3	+3	+3	+4	+2	+4	0	0
10/22/19	2763.14	+4	+	+3	+	0	0	0	0	0
11/22/19	2763.9	+3	+3	+2	+	+3	0	+	0	0
3/12/19	2770^2.7	+3	+4	+3	+3	+4	0	+3	0	0
3/12/19	2770^2.7	+3	+3	+3	+3	+4	0	+2	0	0
5/ 8/19	2770^2.9	+2	+2	+2	+4	+4	+	+4	+2	0
3/19/19	2818.6	+3	+3	+3	+4	+4	+4	+3	+3	0
10/22/19	2818.9	+3	+2	+3	+3	+1	+2	+3	0	0
3/26/19	2824.6	+3	+2	+2	+3	+4	0	0	0	0
11/ 6/19	2824.14	+3	+2	+2	+4	0	0	+3	0	0
3/26/19	2825.6	+3	+3	+3	+4	0	0	0	0	0
4/18/19	2825.11	+3	0	0	+2	0	0	+4	+	0
11/10/19	2825.3	+4	+	+3	+4	0	0	0	0	0
4/16/19	3365.2	+3	+3	+3	+4	+4	0	+3	0	0
4/16/19	3365.2	+4	+3	+3	+4	+4	0	+3	+3	0
11/14/19	3365.7	+3	+3	+3	+3	+	0	+	0	0

epidemics subsided and the infections became milder the colonies of green-producing streptococci from sputum became smaller, and less moist, capsule formation was slight or absent, the chains were longer, and growth in glucose broth was more granular or occurred only at the bottom of the tubes. The virulency of these, determined by intraperitoneal injections into mice and intratracheal injections into guinea-pigs was of a lower order. This difference in character of growth was

TABLE 3

THE VARIABILITY IN FERMENTATIVE POWER OF HEMOLYTIC STREPTOCOCCI FROM INFLUENZA

Date of Test	Strain	Dextrose	Lactose	Maltose	Saccharose	Raffinose	Mannite	Salicin	Inulin	Control
3/15/19	2541.3	+3	0	+2	+4	0	0	+3	0	0
12/12/19	2541.6	+3	+2	+3	+3	0	0	+3	0	0
3/15/19	2559.5	+3	0	+	+4	0	0	+4	0	0
12/12/19	2559.8	+4	+2	+3	+3	0	0	+3	0	0
3/ 6/19	2557.14	+3	+3	+2	+4	0	0	+3	0	0
3/ 6/19	2557.14	+3	+3	+3	+4	0	0	+3	0	0
12/16/19	2557.16	+3	+3	+3	+4	0	0	0	0	0
5/ 8/19	2774.10	+2	0	0	+3	0	0	+2	+3	0
12/19/19	2774.13	+3	+2	+3	+4	0	0	0	0	0
3/19/19	2821.6	+4	+2	+3	+4	0	0	+4	0	0
10/23/19	2821.12	+4	+	+3	+	0	0	+2	0	0
3/21/19	2815.6	+3	0	+2	+4	0	0	+	0	0
12/17/19	2815.28	+3	+2	+2	+3	0	0	0	0	0
3/26/19	2826.6	+2	0	+3	+4	0	+4	0	0	0
10/26/19	2826.5	+4	+3	+	+3	+2	+2	0	0	0
3/26/19	2851.3	+3	+2	+4	+3	0	0	+3	0	0
3/26/19	2851.4	+3	+3	+3	+3	0	+4	0	0	0
12/19/19	2851.6	+3	0	+3	+3	0	0	+2	0	0
4/ 8/19	2902.3	+3	+3	+2	+4	0	0	0	0	0
11/24/19	2902.4	+3	+3	+3	+2	0	0	+4	0	0
4/16/19	3358.2	+3	+3	+3	+3	0	+4	+4	0	0
12/22/19	3358.6	+4	+	+2	+	0	+2	+3	0	0
4/29/19	3387^{2}.3	+2	+4	+2	+3	+3	0	+3	0	+
11/14/19	3387^{2}.5	+4	+3	+4	+3	0	0	+4	0	0
4/29/19	3395.5	+2	+4	+3	+3	+4	0	+3	0	0
12/19/19	3395.9	+2	+	+	+	0	0	0	0	0
4/29/19	3398.4	+3	+3	+2	+3	0	+2	+3	0	0
5/24/19	3398^{2}.5	+4	+2	+2	+4	+4	0	+3	0	0
1/ 3/20	3398.7	+2	0	0	+	0	+2	0	0	0

noted in strains isolated directly from the sputum as well as from the animals that succumbed to injections of sputum. Distinct as these differences were in cultural features, immunologic studies (Study III) showed most of them to be identical, especially those isolated early in the attack. In making cultures from the sputum and lung exudate on blood-agar plates small indifferent colonies of streptococci resembling influenza bacilli were frequently noted. This resemblance was often so marked that examination of smears stained with a Gram stain were necessary to differentiate them. These often acquired the power to produce green on blood agar after one or more cultivations in tall tubes of glucose broth. Moreover, colonies which appeared to be transition forms between green-producing and hemolytic streptococci were frequently noted, especially in the sputum of patients as the epidemics were subsiding. After cultivation on artificial mediums the strains often showed marked changes. The colonies became dry, and smaller; and often diffuse growth in glucose broth no longer occurred, but instead a growth with granular sediment resembling Streptococcus viridans. In some instances indifferent colonies developed and in many instances they acquired hemolytic power. This was of all grades from a narrow zone peripheral to an inner green zone to well marked hemolytic zones beginning immediately around the colony.

Hemolytic Streptococci.—The infections of the lung by hemolytic streptococci, as they occurred during the pandemic of influenza usually without empyema, without tonsillitis and without leukocytosis, but with leukopenia, indicated peculiar infecting powers not possessed by hemolytic streptococci found so commonly in normal throats and tonsils in acute follicular tonsillitis, and in the pneumonia empyema epidemic of 1917-1918. This has been found actually to be the case. Strains from the sputum and lung in cases of acute hemorrhagic edema reproduced this condition associated with leukopenia in guinea-pigs on intratracheal injections; whereas strains of hemolytic streptococci from simple pharyngitis caused leukocytosis (reported elsewhere), but never acute hemorrhagic edema of the lung. Culturally, there was often a distinct difference between these strains and those isolated from cases of empyema and the throats of persons suffering from pharyngitis and tonsillitis. The colonies were more moist, less opaque, often spreading in character, quite as the colonies of green-producing streptococci, and the hemolytic zone was not so wide, not so clear, and the margin less sharply defined. Freshly isolated strains from acute cases produced diffuse growth in glucose broth, while hemolytic streptococci from the pus in cases of longer duration like those from other sources, usually grew granular with flocculent sediment. Morphologically, these strains were at times indistinguishable from the green-producing streptococcus, the smears showing elongated diplococci singly and in chains of various lengths. After cultivation on artificial mediums for a time these peculiar properties tended to disappear, in some instances abruptly, and were no longer distinguishable from the hemolytic streptococcus obtained from other sources. In some instances the hemolytic streptococci acquired the power to produce green colonies.

The tendency of the green-producing streptococci to acquire hemolytic powers, and to a lesser degree the tendency of the hemolytic streptococci to acquire the power to produce green colonies was so marked that it was found necessary in agglutination experiments to plate the cultures actually agglutinated in order properly to interpret the results obtained. The tendency of hemolytic streptococci to lose their hemolyzing powers was especially marked in freshly isolated cultures when grown in tall tubes of glucose-brain broth. This frequently occurred in cultures derived from single colonies from plates showing large numbers of the organism in question in pure form. The cultures which were put aside for study were made on blood-agar slants from single colonies, or from a group of colonies well separated from other bacteria. The tendency to mutations in these cultures may best be illustrated by giving the results of subcultures when this point was especially noted. Thus of a total of 623 cultures, green-producing streptococci bred true to type in 348 instances, and hemolytic streptococci in 168, a total of 516. In the remaining 115 cultures, green-producing streptococci yielded hemolytic streptococci in 45 instances, indifferent streptococci in 27, and staphylococcus colonies in 22, while hemolytic streptococci yielded green-producing streptococci in 9 instances, indifferent streptococci in 7, and staphylococci in 5. In most instances the changes in type occurred abruptly, under various conditions, but especially when old cultures on blood-agar and dextrose-brain broth were transferred. The instability of the streptococcus strains from influenza often made it difficult to obtain the proper proportions of the different strains in the vaccine which was used for prophylactic inoculations. The routine procedure consisted of transferring single colonies or a group of colonies of the different bacteria to bottles containing 150 c c of 0.2 per cent. glucose broth, incubating these over night, making smears, plating a loop full, and inoculating about 30 c c with a bulbed pipet into large bottles containing about 3,500 c c of glucose broth. Smears and blood-agar plates were again made of the latter. It frequently happened that while the plating from the small bottles of broth showed pure growths of the type inoculated, the plating from the large bottle often showed a partial or totally changed streptococcus flora, and not infrequently showed staphylococcus colonies as well, in spite of great precautions taken to avoid accidental contamination. Owing to these findings, further studies were made on this point. The findings in Case 3101 and the behavior of the strain isolated will suffice to illustrate results obtained along this line:

Case 3101, a man, aged 32, became sick Feb. 28, 1919, with severe headache, aching all over the body, marked prostration and chilly sensations, but no distinct chill. The next day he was admitted to the hospital with a temperature of 104, pulse 90, and respiration 20. The throat was slightly infected, and moderate dullness and decreased breath sounds over the base of both lungs were found. The temperature ranged between 100 and 104 until March 5. March 6 the temperature was higher and scattered areas of dullness with râles were elicited. March 7 the patient became cyanotic, extremely short of breath, and expectorated large amounts of bloody, frothy material. He grew rapidly worse in spite of venesection (400 c c) and transfusion of 250 c c of convalescent human blood, and died March 8. The leukocyte count on March 3 was 10,600; March 4, 9,000; March 5, 9,500; March 7, 9,100. March 2 and 6 the sputum was mucopurulent and showed large numbers of green-producing streptococci, slightly hemolyzing streptococci, and staphylococci. March 7, the day the patient became worse, the sputum showed no change in flora, but a blood culture yielded a pure growth of hemolytic streptococci. March 8 the sputum contained enormous numbers of hemolytic streptococci and staphylococci, but no longer green-producing streptococci nor slightly hemolyzing streptococci. One guinea-pig was injected with the twenty-four hour primary culture from the blood in glucose-brain broth. The animal was ill for a time and lost 30 gm. in weight, and then recovered. A second guinea-pig was injected March 9 with 2 c c of the glucose-brain broth culture made from a single colony of hemolytic streptococcus on a blood-agar plate inoculated with the culture injected into the first guinea-pig. The plate showed a pure culture of hemolytic streptococcus. The guinea-pig lost in weight, and respirations were increased. It was chloroformed two days after injection and two large areas of consolidation in the right diaphragmatic lobe were found. From these areas pure cultures of green-producing streptococci, but no hemolytic streptococci were obtained. The tube of glucose-brain broth inoculated with the blood, which showed on plating a hemolytic streptococcus in pure form, was placed in the ice chest until September 8, when a glucose-brain-broth culture and a plating on blood-agar were made. The blood-agar plate yielded one colony of hemolytic streptococcus. From this colony a blood-agar plate and a tall tube of glucose-brain broth were inoculated (September 13). The former showed pure cultures of hemolyzing streptococci. The latter developed abundant growth, but the tube was not opened until November 28, at which time two blood-agar plates were made; both showed many colonies of hemolyzing streptococci as well as green-producing streptococci. From this plate single hemolyzing and green colonies well separated from other colonies were inoculated December 1 into one tube of glucose-brain broth each. Both tubes developed abundant diffuse growth, and platings on blood-agar December 2 showed pure cultures of green-producing streptococci. In both instances intratracheal injection into 3 guinea-pigs of the growth in the tube inoculated with hemolytic streptococcus colonies resulted in the production of acute bronchopneumonia with death of two on the third day while the third animal recovered after three days of illness. Green-producing streptococci were isolated in large numbers from the two that died. Hemolytic streptococci in the tube of glucose-brain broth when fresh were injected intratracheally into one guinea-pig. It developed bronchopneumonia and from the lung lesions pure cultures of green-producing streptococci were isolated. The tube of glucose-brain broth inoculated (September 9) showed diffuse growth, and a blood-agar plate September 10 contained pure culture of typical hemolytic streptococci. A single colony was used to inoculate a blood-agar plate and a tube of glucose-brain broth. The former yielded a pure culture of hemolytic streptococci; a plating of the latter September 13 also showed a pure culture of the hemolytic streptococcus, but a plating made November 28, after incubation at 35 C. since September 9 showed countless numbers of indifferent colonies of streptococci and moderate numbers of slightly hemolytic streptococci. The tube of glucose-brain broth inoculated with a single colony September 10 developed diffuse turbidity and September 12 yielded countless hemolytic streptococcus colonies on blood-agar plates. A blood-agar plate made of this same tube November 28 showed countless staphylococcus colonies with no hemolytic or green-producing streptococcus colonies. December 2 intratracheal injection into two guinea-pigs of this culture containing staphylococci caused leukopenia, increased respiration for a time, and death on the eleventh day. There was no lung involvement and the organism was lost. The culture in glucose-brain broth made from a single colony of hemolytic streptococci September 13 was injected intratracheally into one guinea-pig and intraperitoneally into a mouse. The guinea-pig had marked increased respiration for a number of days, and died nineteen days after the injection from interstitial bronchopneumonia. The mouse lived thirteen days, and then died. Cultures of the blood of both yielded hemolytic streptococci.

The infecting power and immunologic conditions of the organisms as changes occurred have been studied extensively. The details of these experiments will be reported elsewhere, but it may be stated that high and peculiar invasive powers of the changed forms have been noted repeatedly, and that as cultural properties changed immunologic reactions usually became different also.

FERMENTATIVE POWERS OF THE STREPTOCOCCI

The fermentative powers of the streptococci over the usual test sugars have been determined in a large number of strains. The method which we have found most efficient and convenient for this study is a modification of the Hiss serum water medium. This modification consists of the Hiss serum water medium with the addition of 0.5 per cent. agar, just sufficient to jell, 1 per cent. of the different test sugars, and Adraid's indicator instead of litmus. The medium is placed in small tubes, 3 inches by 3/8 of an inch, about 2 c c into each tube, and steamed in the usual manner on three successive days. Inoculations are made by stabbing the medium with a loop containing organisms from fresh cultures on blood-agar. The tubes are incubated for seventy-two hours, and then read. Negative reactions can be determined easily since if growth has taken place a streak along the line of inoculation can readily be made out. A negative result is not recorded unless a distinct growth has taken place. The degree of acidity is indicated with one or more + signs according to the depth of red color produced.

Altogether, we have tested the fermentative power of 254 strains of the green-producing streptococci soon after isolation. Of these, 94 per cent. fermented dextrose; 90 per cent. lactose; 93 per cent. maltose; 78 per cent. saccharose; 49 per cent. raffinose; 35 per cent. mannite, 67 per cent. salicin, and 38 per cent. inulin. After cultivation for from six to nine months on blood-agar, 139 strains were again tested. The results in dextrose, lactose, maltose and saccharose were practically the same as with the freshly isolated strains, but the number fermenting raffinose, mannite, salicin and inulin was decidedly less in each, the percentage being 22, 16, 45 and 17, respectively. Tests of the fermentative power of 119 strains of hemolyzing streptococci soon after isolation resulted as follows: 91 per cent. fermented dextrose, 71 per cent. lactose, 87 per cent. maltose, 82 per cent. saccharose, 19 per cent. raffinose, 16 per cent. mannite, 79 per cent. salicin, and 8 per cent. inulin. After prolonged cultivation a general lowering of fermentative powers was noted in 70 strains tested. This was especially marked in the case of lactose and salicin. The instability of these strains as noted on blood-agar and other mediums was noted also with respect to their fermentative powers. The results obtained from a study of a large series of strains by testing each strain on different dates are well illustrated by the summaries in tables 2 and 3. It becomes apparent at once from a study of these tables that a classification of the streptococci, especially the green-producing streptococci, on the basis of their fermentative reactions would have little real meaning, since they frequently acquire or lose, quite without regard to rule, the power to ferment important carbohydrates.

GENERAL DISCUSSION AND SUMMARY

From a bacteriologic study of a large series of cases of influenza and influenzal pneumonia throughout four epidemic waves, green-producing streptococci (including pneumococci) were found to occur more constantly and in larger numbers than any other organisms commonly associated with this disease. This flora predominated alike in the cases of influenza without lung involvement, in those of lung involvement in the initial febrile attack as well as in those in which influenzal pneumonia developed after a quiescent interval following influenza. This was especially true early in the attacks throughout the epidemic waves, and the flora usually persisted and was the chief cause of death during the early part and during the height of the epidemic waves. Moreover, the agglutination experiments with a monovalent immune horse serum have shown that most of the strains isolated early in the disease are immunologically alike, whereas later they become more heterogeneous, just as do the specific strains after cultivation on artificial mediums.

During the latter part of the outbreaks hemolytic streptococci became relatively more numerous, especially late in the disease, and death was often the result of invasion by these organisms. A similar increase in the number of staphylococci occurred, and in some instances these appeared to be the immediate cause of death. The change in the type of the disease and the character of the lesion in the lung, which were noted during each of the epidemic waves, appeared to be due more to a change in the virulence of the organisms than to a change in the type of flora. Thus well marked instances of acute hemorrhagic edema occurred, but almost wholly at the height of the epidemic waves in which each of these organisms was found in pure culture or in mixture in various proportions.

The influenza bacillus was found in the sputum in the early part of the first wave only in a few cases and always in association with streptococci, while throughout the remaining three waves it was isolated only occasionally. The criticism which has been raised by those who believe the influenza bacillus to be the cause of influenza, that the methods used by those who fail to isolate this organism are inadequate, does not apply to this study, because the medium used throughout this study was proved effective for the growth of the influenza bacillus. Special mediums were employed during the latter part of the study, smears failed to show the organism, and influenza bacilli were not found in the animals injected directly with sputum and lung exudate. Hence it is certain that in the majority of cases studied this organism played little or no rôle in the production of symptoms. Its presence in large numbers in some cases in the early part of the first wave and its almost complete absence in sputum and lung exudates subsequently indicate that the difference in the frequency of isolation of this organism by various workers is in general, as emphasized by

MacCallum and others, a measure of its prevalence in the particular epidemics studied, and that many epidemics of typical influenza occur that are not due to this organism. Moreover, when found it is usually associated with organisms of the pneumococcus-streptococcus group (Park, Williams, Dick and Murray).

The finding of a preponderance of the pneumococcus-streptococcus group of organisms reported herewith is in accord with the results obtained by the pneumonia unit at Camp Lewis, by Blanton and Irons, Friedlander, McCord, Sladen and Wheeler, Stone and Swift, Jordan, Hirsch and McKinney, Dunn, and many others.

It has been demonstrated repeatedly in this study that the peculiar infecting power of streptococci from influenza does not depend on their power to ferment certain carbohydrates, and that the fermentation reactions are variable. Hence the difference in the relative number of instances in which green-producing streptococci, hemolytic streptococci, or Group 4, or even type pneumococci were isolated by the different workers during the pandemic does not necessarily mean that the different strains did not have the infecting power peculiar to influenza, just as has been found to be the case in our hands. A striking example in support of this idea occurred at Camp Grant in which type II pneumococci of extreme virulency were found to be the cause not of lobar pneumonia, but of acute bronchopneumonia typical of influenza during an extremely fatal epidemic as described by Hirsch and McKinney.

The changes observed in morphology, cultural characteristics, fermentative and immunologic reactions in the green-producing streptococci indicate that the organism described by the English observers and designated by them as diplostreptococcus, the green-producing streptococcus found by Mathers as described by Tunnicliff, the diplococcus epidemicus described by Bernhardt and by Segale, the diplococcus mucosus described by Stephan, and the pleomorphic streptococcus described by Wiesner in influenza, are identical with the green-producing streptococcus isolated in this study, or modifications thereof. Moreover, the marked changes or true mutations that have occurred in the culture tube under controlled conditions indicate that the change in the bacterial flora at different stages of the disease in the individual and in the epidemic waves may not always be the result of superimposed infections from the upper respiratory tract as is now generally believed.

BIBLIOGRAPHY

[1] Avery, O. T.: A Selective Medium for B. Influenzae Oleate-Hemoglobin-Agar, Jour. Am. Med. Assn., 1918, lxxi, 2050-2051.

[2] Bernhardt, G.: Zur Aetiologie der Grippe von 1918, Med. Klin., 1918, xiv, 683-685.

[3] Blanton, W. B. and Irons, E. E.: A Recent Epidemic of Acute Respiratory Infection at Camp Custer, Mich., Jour. Am. Med. Assn., 1918, lxxi, 1988-1991.

[4] Brem, W. V., Bolling, G. E. and Casper, E. J.: Pandemic "Influenza" and Secondary Pneumonia at Camp Fremont, California, Jour. Am. Med. Assn., 1918, lxxi, 2138-2144.

[5] Camp Lewis Pneumonia Unit: The Relation of Bronchopneumonia to Influenza, Jour. Am. Med. Assn., 1919, lxxii, 268-269.

[6] Chickering, H. T. and Park, J. H.: Staphylococcus aureus Pneumonia, Jour. Am. Med. Assn., 1919, lxxii, 617-626.

[7] Dunn, A. D.: Observations on an Epidemic of Bronchopneumonia in Omaha, Jour. Am. Med. Assn., 1918, lxxi, 2128-2130.

[8] Friedlander, A., McCord, C. P., Sladen, F. J., and Wheeler, G. W.: The Epidemic of Influenza at Camp Sherman, Ohio, Jour. Am. Med. Assn., 1918, lxxi, 1652-1656.

[9] Goodpasture, E. W.: The Significance of Certain Pulmonary Lesions in Relation to the Etiology of Influenza, Am. Jour. Med. Sc., 1919, clviii, 863-870.

[10] Hirsch, E. F. and McKinney, M.: An Epidemic of Pneumococcus Bronchopneumonia, Jour. Infect. Dis., 1919, xxiv, 594-617.

[11] Influenza Committee of the Advisory Board to the D. G. M. S., France: A Report on the Influenza Epidemic in the British Armies in France, 1918, Brit. Med. Jour., 1918, ii, 505-509.

[12] Jordan, E. O.: Observations on the Bacteriology of Influenza, Jour. Infect. Dis., 1919, xxv, 28-40.

[13] Kinsella, R. A.: The Bacteriology of Epidemic Influenza and Pneumonia, Jour. Am. Med. Assn., 1919, lxxii, 717-720.

[14] MacCallum, W. G.: Pathology of the Pneumonia Following Influenza, Jour. Am. Med. Assn., 1919, lxxii, 720-723.

[15] Mathers, G.: The Bacteriology of Acute Epidemic Respiratory Infections Commonly Called Influenza, Jour. Infect. Dis., 1917, xxi, 1-8.

[16] Medalia, L. S.: Influenza Epidemic at Camp MacArthur: Etiology, Bacteriology, Pathology, and Specific Therapy, Boston Med. and Surg. Jour., 1919, clxxx, 323-330.

[17] Neufeld, F., and Papamarku, P.: Zur Bakteriologie der diesjährigen Influenzaepidemic, Deutsch. med. Wchnschr., 1918, ii, 1181.

[18] Nuzum, J. W., Pilot, I., Stangl, F. H., and Bonar, B. E.: Pandemic Influenza and Pneumonia in a Large Civil Hospital, Jour. Am. Med. Assn., 1918, lxxi, 1562-1565.

[19] Park, W. H.: Bacteriology of Recent Pandemic of Influenza and Complicating Infections, Jour. Am. Med. Assn., 1919, lxxiii, 318-321.

[20] Park, W. H.: The Bacteriology of Influenza and Its Complications, Med. Rec., 1919, xcvi, 215.

[21] Potter, A. C.: Bacteriology of the Present Epidemic of Influenza, Journal-Lancet, 1918, xxxviii, 708-709.

[22] Rosenow, E. C.: Prophylactic Inoculation Against Respiratory Infections, Jour. Am. Med. Assn., 1919, lxxii, 31-34.

[23] Rosenow, E. C.: Studies in Influenza and Pneumonia. II. The Experimental Production of Symptoms and Lesions Simulating Those of Influenza with Streptococci Isolated During the Present Pandemic, Jour. Am. Med. Assn., 1919, lxxii, 1604-1608.

[24] Rosenow, E. C.: Studies in Influenza and Pneumonia. III. The Occurrence of a Pandemic Strain of Streptococcus During the Pandemic of Influenza, Jour. Am. Med. Assn., 1919, lxxii, 1608-1609.

[25] Rosenow, E. C.: Transmutations Within the Streptococcus-Pneumococcus Group, Jour. Inf. Dis., 1914, xiv, 1-32.

[26] Segale, M.: Azione dei filtrati di "Str. pandemicus" in rapporto alla dottrina della filtrabilita del virus grippale, Policlinico, 1919, xxvi, 289-290.

[27] Stephan, R.: Ueber einen neuen Infektionserreger bei epidemischer Influenza, München. med. Wchnschr., 1917, lxiv, 257-260.

[28] Stone, W. J., and Swift, G. W.: Influenza and Influenzal Pneumonia at Ft. Riley, Kansas, from Sept. 15 to Nov. 1, 1918, Jour. Am. Med. Assn., 1919, lxxii, 487-493.

29. Tunnicliff, Ruth: Phagocytic Experiments in Influenza, Jour. Am. Med. Assn., 1918, lxxi, 1733-1734.

[30] Wiesner, R. R.: Streptococcus pleomorphus und die sogenannte Spanische Grippe, Wien. klin. Wchnschr., 1918, xxxi, 1101-1104.

[31] Williams, Anna W.: The Etiology of "Influenza," Proc. New York Path. Soc., 1918, xviii, 83-90.

STUDIES IN INFLUENZA AND PNEUMONIA

VI. THE LEUKOCYTIC REACTION IN INFLUENZA AND INFLUENZAL PNEUMONIA

E. C. Rosenow

Division of Experimental Bacteriology, The Mayo Foundation, Rochester, Minnesota.

Leukopenia, or absence of leukocytosis, has come to be regarded as an important aid in the diagnosis of influenza, and a persistent leukopenia as of bad prognostic import. The cause of the leukopenia has been the subject of much speculation. It is thought by many observers that an unknown virus produces the initial leukopenia, and that this virus interferes with the leukocytic response when secondary infection by streptococci or pneumococci is believed to occur as pneumonia develops.

No matter what the cause of influenza may be, the absence of leukocytosis is a striking phenomenon. The exact leukocytic reaction, however, throughout the initial influenzal attack and in influenzal pneumonia in fatal and nonfatal infections has not been determined, nor has a systematic study of the leukocytic reaction in animals been made following injections of the different species of bacteria that are so commonly isolated in influenza. It was therefore thought worth while to determine the leukocytic curves in the spontaneous disease and in experimental animals in which the dosage and type of organism introduced could be accurately controlled and might throw light on the question as to the cause of leukopenia in influenzal infection and determine more accurately the prognostic significance of the lack of leukocytic reaction in this disease.

In figure 1 the curves indicate the average leukocyte counts by days in influenza and influenzal pneumonia in man, and experimental influenzal pneumonia in guinea-pigs, according to fatal and nonfatal infection. There were no deaths from influenza without lung involvement among the cases included in part 1 of figure 1. The dotted line represents the count in the cases in which fatal attacks of influenzal pneumonia later developed. The average count for the first six days in influenza was about 6,500, and was approximately the same in the fatal

Received for publication Feb. 28, 1920.

and nonfatal cases. From the seventh to the tenth day the count rose somewhat in the patients who recovered, while it dropped in those who later developed influenzal pneumonia from which they succumbed. It will be noted that, contrary to the general belief, the average leukocyte count when influenzal pneumonia developed was no higher than during the initial influenzal attack. The count in the nonfatal infections then gradually rose, while in the fatal infections it rose for two days and then gradually declined. This finding is in accord with that of Haase

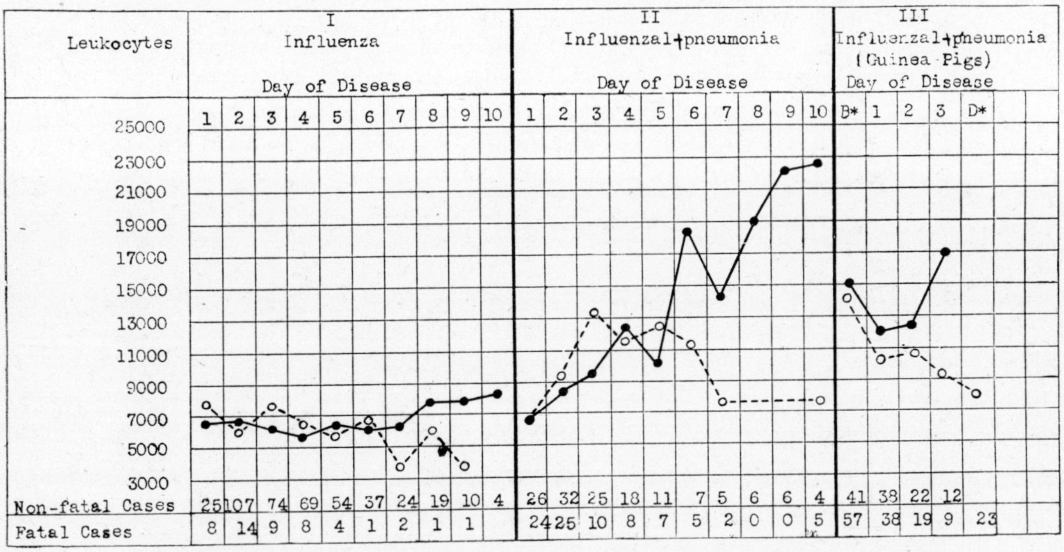

Fig. 1.—Average leukocyte count by days in influenza and influenzal pneumonia in guinea-pigs according to fatal and nonfatal infection. —denotes the average leukocyte count in nonfatal infection; — — average leukocyte count in fatal infection; * B, before injection; * D, after death.

and Wohlrabe [1] who also found that there is a tendency of the leukocyte count to rise in the later stages of influenza and influenzal pneumonia.

Marked individual differences were noted in the leukocytic response in guinea-pigs following injection of bacteria from patients with influenza. If a series of animals was injected with the same dose of a given strain, nearly all showed a drop in the number of leukocytes; the drop in some was slight, in others it was marked, and occasionally an animal showed leukocytosis. There was no definite relation between

[1] Haase, N., and Wohlrabe: Ueber das Blutbild bei Influenza, Deutsche. med. Wchnschr., 1918, 44, p. 1383.

the mortality rate and the initial leukopenia, but a persistently low count occurred more often in the fatal infections. In part III of figure 1 the average leukocyte count by days in nonfatal infections shows a decided drop for two days following injection and then a rise, while in the fatal infections there was a progressive diminution. These curves are believed to be accurately representative, since they include, as indicated, the average of a large series of animals and correspond roughly with the curves in the spontaneous disease. The leukocyte count in apparently normal guinea-pigs varies greatly, but counts made repeatedly show that it tends to remain at a given level

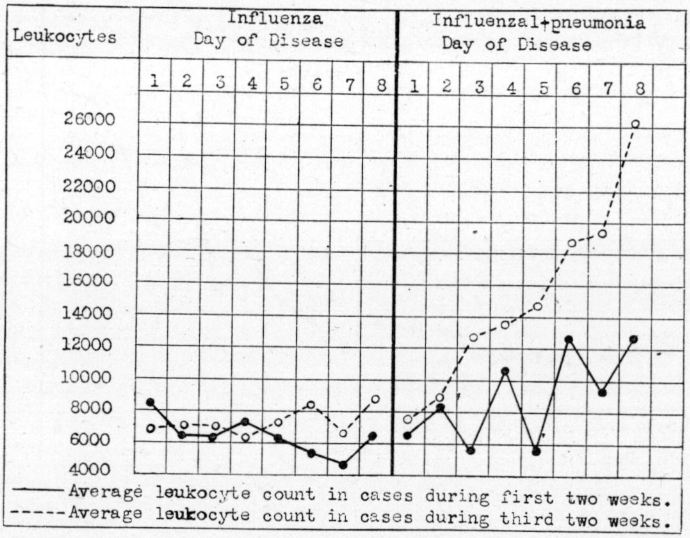

Fig. 2.—Average leukocyte count by days according to time in epidemic waves.

over a period of some days. The injections were made in various ways with sputum, primary cultures, exudates and pure cultures of green-producing streptococci from the sputum or lungs in undoubted cases of influenzal infection.

It has been our observation that the most typical cases of influenza and the highest mortality rate occurred at the height of epidemic waves. It was thought worth while, therefore, to group the cases with leukocyte counts according to the time in epidemic waves (figure 2), and to learn whether the average leukocyte count might not be lower in the cases at the height of epidemic waves as compared with that in the cases as the epidemic waves subsided. It was found that each of the four waves of influenza that occurred in Rochester during the fall of 1918 and winter and spring of 1919 ran its course in about six weeks, and that the crest of the wave was reached in about two weeks in each. Each wave was therefore arbitrarily divided into two-week periods for study. The average counts by days of patients developing influenza and influenzal pneumonia during the first two weeks and the third two weeks were determined and traced in figure 2. The average count for the first five days of the influenzal attack in the two groups was about the same; after that the count was decidedly lower in the group contracting the disease during the first two weeks of each wave than during the third two weeks. The average count during influenzal pneumonia was about the same during the first two days and no higher than at the outset of influenza, but after that the rise in leukocytes was decidedly less during the first two weeks than during the third two weeks of each wave. The mortality rate in the first two weeks was definitely higher than in the third two weeks.

In table 1 are given the leukocytic reaction and other findings in guinea-pigs injected with material, first, from patients showing marked leukopenia, and second, from patients showing no reduction or a moderate increase in the leukocyte count. It will be seen that the average leukocyte count in the five patients (table 1, part I) showing leukopenia was 4,340. Two of these died. Four had influenzal bronchopneumonia, and one (case 2,981) showed symptoms of intestinal influenza. All of the 19 animals injected with material from this group of patients showed reduction in the leukocyte count on the day after injection. In some instances this was very marked (P 961, P 981, P 1,069), while in others it was relatively slight. The average diminution in the leukocyte count was 58%. The average reduction 48 hours after injection was 36%. The reduction occurred over a wide range of dosage, 0.1 c c to 1.5 c c. It followed subcutaneous as well as intratracheal injections of green-producing streptococci isolated from the throat, sputum, lungs, blood, and stool. The cultures of streptococci injected were in the first to the fourth generation, and some were derived from single green colonies on blood-agar plates. Injection of a filtrate of a fresh culture of green-producing streptococci also showed reduction in leukocytes (P 996, P 997). This is in accord with the findings following injection of other filtrates (table 2). The mortality in this group of animals was 47%. The reduction in leukocytes twenty-

TABLE 1

LEUKOCYTIC REACTION IN GUINEA-PIGS FOLLOWING INJECTION OF MATERIAL FROM INFLUENZA AND INFLUENZAL PNEUMONIA

I. Cases Showing Marked Leukopenia

			Guinea-Pigs Injected								
				Material Injected			Leukocyte Count				
Number	Leukocyte Count	Result	Number	Dose in c c	Organisms in Glucose Broth Culture or Sputum	Culture Generation	Place	Before Injection	Twenty-Four Hours after Injection	Forty-Eight Hours after Injection	Findings
			P951	1.5	Hemolytic streptococcus, throat	3	Trachea	26,000	21,000	19,200	Marked increased respiration; subnormal temperature; death sixth day from bronchopneumonia; acute peritonitis apparently secondary to colitis; green streptococci from blood
			P955	1.5	Green streptococcus, throat	2	Trachea	16,000	11,000	17,000	Sick; marked increase in respiration for two days; weight from 450 gm. to 320 gm.; recovered
			P959	0.1	Sputum, green streptococcus	0	Trachea	16,400	6,200	19,000	Fever; increased respiration for three days; recovered
			P961	1.5	Green streptococcus, throat	2	Subcutaneous tissue	10,400	2,400	1,600	Fever; increased respiration for two days; weight from 420 gm. to 320 gm.: death fourth day of bronchopneumonia and hemorrhagic edema; green streptococci from blood, lung, and uterus
			P971	1.5	Green streptococcus, lung	1	Trachea	11,000	9,000	27,000	Fever for two days; recovered
2,800	2,800	Death	P973	1.5	Green streptococcus, blood	1	Trachea	17,600	10,600	25,000	Remained well
			P981	1.5	Green streptococcus, blood	2	Trachea	8,000	2,000	6,200	Respirations slightly increased for two days; recovered
			P983	1.5	Green streptococcus, blood	3	Trachea	8,500	4,600	5,400	Increased respiration for a time, then better; death on eighteenth day from marked lesions in stomach and throughout intestinal wall; green-producing streptococci and B. coli from blood, uterus, stomach, and intestinal contents
			P984	1.5	Green streptococcus, blood	2	Trachea	8,800	4,400	9,600	Respirations increased for several days
			P993	1.0	Green streptococcus, blood	3	Subcutaneous tissue	26,000	12,000	9,200	Subnormal temperature; death in 48 hours; emphysema (13 c c), edema and hemorrhage of lungs; subcutaneous cellulitis; countless green streptococci
			P994	1.5	Green streptococcus, blood	2	Trachea	6,800	4,800	15,200	Subnormal temperature; death on seventh day from bronchopneumonia
			P995	1.5	Green streptococcus, blood	2	Trachea	9,600	6,200	14,400	Increased respiration for a few days, then better; death from bronchopneumonia eighteenth day after injection; hemorrhagic pleuritis, myocardial degeneration; countless green streptococci
			P996	1.5	Green streptococcus, blood (filtered)	2	Trachea	11,000	5,000	5,400	Remained well

			P997	1.5	Green streptococcus, blood (filtered)	2	Trachea	15,600	9,800	8,200	Remained well
			P1056	1.5	Green streptococcus, blood	4	Trachea	12,000	6,600	5,000	Increase in temperature and respiration for three days; recovered
2,770	3,800	Death	P870	0.1	Green streptococcus, sputum	1	Trachea	17,000	8,900	5,800	Diffuse coalescing bronchopneumonia; death on seventh day from hemorrhagic pleuritis; green streptococci from blood, lung, and pleura
2,873	6,200	Recovery	P1069	1.5	Green streptococcus, sputum	2	Trachea	11,600	4,200	......	No noteworthy symptoms
2,981	5,400	Recovery	P1174	1.5	Green streptococcus, sputum	2	Trachea	18,000	6,800	9,400	Increased respiration for two days; recovered
3,208	3,500	Recovery	P1261	1.5	Green streptococcus, stool	1	Trachea	11,800	7,000	5,800	Death in 48 hours; diffuse coalescing bronchopneumonia and acute myocardial degeneration; large number of green streptococci from blood, lung, pleural and peritoneal fluid
Average	4 340	....	....	.....	....	.....	....	18,000	7,500	11.570	Total: 19 animals injected; 9 died

II. Cases Showing No Reduction or Moderate Increase in Leukocyte Count

2,616	9,300	Death	P755	3.0	Green streptococcus, lung	0	Peritoneal cavity	15,000	12,000	9,400	Recovered
2,619	7,700	Recovery	P749	0.3	Sputum, green streptococcus	0	Peritoneal cavity	5,600	10,800	6,600	Recovered
			P750	0.3	Sputum, green streptococcus	0	Peritoneal cavity	14,400	4,600	......	Increased respiration; expiratory difficulty; relieved with epinephrin; death 48 hours after injection; emphysema; hemorrhagic edema; bronchopneumonia; serofibrinous peritonitis; green streptococci from blood and peritoneal fluid
2,620	11,100	Recovery	P752	0.3	Sputum, green streptococcus	0	Peritoneal cavity	25,500	20,500	6,800	Recovered
2,621	14,500	Recovery	P751	0.3	Sputum, green streptococcus	0	Peritoneal cavity	6,600	12,750	15,300	Recovered
2,798	12,500	Recovery	P957	1.5	Hemolytic streptococcus	2	Trachea	16,000	19,000	16,500	Increased respiration; death sixth day from hemorrhagic pleuritis; countless numbers of green streptococci in pleural fluid and lung
			P1109	5.0	Hemolytic streptococcus	2	Stomach	12,000	7,400	......	Remained well
2,887	11,000	Death	P1110	2.0	Hemolytic streptococcus	2	Trachea	7,600	6,000	11,200	Increased temperature and respiration rate for two days; recovered
3,206	11,300	Recovery	P1258	1.5	Primary culture, sputum, green streptococcus	1	Trachea	11,000	12,000	......	Death in 24 hours from acute hemorrhagic edema and hemorrhagic pleuritis; pleural fluid, lung, and blood showed countless numbers of staphylococci
3,207	13.000	Recovery	P1260	1.5	Primary culture, sputum, green streptococcus	1	Trachea	11.200	10,800	......	Death fourteenth day from bronchopneumonia due to green streptococcus
Average	11.300	....	....	.....	....	.....	....	12,490	11.580	10.960	Total: 10 animals injected; 4 died

four hours after injection was practically the same in the fatal and non-fatal infections, whereas forty-eight hours after injection the leukocyte count was usually lower in the animals that died as a result of the injection than in those that recovered (P 961, P 983, P 870, P 1,261).

Injections were made of material from 8 patients with undoubted influenza but who showed no reduction, or even a slight increase, in leukocytes at the time the animal experiments were performed (table 1, part II). The symptoms of these patients were the same as of those in the former group, although not so severe. The average leukocyte count was 11,300; two of these patients died. Four of the patients had influenza without lung findings, and 4 influenzal pneumonia (1 complicated with empyema) at the time of the animal injections. The leukocyte counts in the 10 animals injected with material from these patients averaged 12,490 the day before injection. Six of the animals showed slight reduction in leukocytes and 4 showed a slight increase twenty-four hours after injection; the total reduction in leukocytes was only 9%. The total average reduction of leukocytes in forty-eight hours after injection was also slight (11%). It is thus evident that injections of material from the patients showing marked leukopenia caused a greater reduction in leukocytes (58%) twenty-four hours after injection than the material (9%) from patients showing little or no reduction.

In table 2 is summarized the incidence of the occurrence of leukopenia, leukocytosis, and no change in the leukocyte count of guinea-pigs following injections of material from patients with influenza (part I), and in a control series with material from sources other than patients with influenza (part II). Injections of sputum, primary cultures from sputum, pure cultures of green-producing streptococci and hemolytic streptococci from patients with influenza were followed by the occurrence of leukopenia in a high percentage of the animals injected and to a lesser degree (33%) following injection of influenza bacilli. Moreover, injection of filtrates from sputum, lung emulsions, and broth cultures likewise was followed by a reduction in leukocytes in 65% of 26 animals injected. The total average of 99 animals in which leukocyte counts were made following injection of material from influenza which showed leukopenia was 57%; leukocytosis, 12%, and no change in the leukocyte count, 29%.

Sharp reductions in leukocyte counts were noted also following injection of staphylococci from the lungs or sputum of patients with influenza. This in some instances was as marked as following the injection of the green-producing streptococcus from the same case. Thus, 2 guinea-pigs were injected intraperitoneally with these strains isolated from single colonies on a blood-agar plate inoculated with the peritoneal fluid of a guinea-pig that died from injection of sputum. The one injected with Staphylococcus aureus showed 9,200 leukocytes before injection; twenty-four hours after injection, 3,200; and forty-

TABLE 2

THE LEUKOCYTIC REACTION IN GUINEA-PIGS INOCULATED WITH MATERIAL FROM PATIENTS WITH INFLUENZA AND FROM OTHER SOURCES

I. Material from Patients with Influenza

Injection	Place of Injection	Animals	Percentage of Animals Showing		
			Leukopenia	Leukocytosis	No Change
Sputum	Trachea	5	80	0	20
Sputum	Peritoneal cavity	5	40	20	40
Primary culture of sputum	Trachea	9	78	11	11
Green-producing streptococci	Trachea	41	46	17	34
Green-producing sterptococci	Peritoneal cavity	4	75	0	25
Hemolytic streptococci	Trachea	6	83	17	0
Influenza bacilli	Trachea	3	33	0	67
Filtrates from lung emulsions and broth cultures	Trachea	26	65	7	27
Total	....	99	57	12	29

II. Material from Sources Other Than Patients with Influenza

Hemolytic streptococci from a patient with simple nasopharyngitis and leukocytosis	Trachea	3	0	67	33
Sputum and cultures of green streptococci from a patient with simple tracheitis, nasopharyngitis and leukocytosis	Trachea	7	29	57	14
Type pneumococci from patients with lobar pneumonia	Trachea	9	11	22	67
Broth (controls)	Trachea	6	16	17	67
Total	....	25	16	36	48

eight hours after injection, 6,000. It died of peritonitis and pancreatitis with moderate emphysema of the lungs, and a few small, localized hemorrhages, with a leukocyte count of 3,240, and large numbers of hemolytic staphylococci in the blood and peritoneal fluid. The one injected with the green-producing streptococcus showed 6,000 leukocytes before injection; twenty-four hours after injection, 4,800, and forty-eight hours after injection, 3,600. This animal also died in three days with serofibrinous peritonitis, beginning pericarditis, acute pancreatitis, and moderate emphysema of the lungs, showing a few small circumscribed hemorrhages and large numbers of green-producing streptococci in pure culture in the blood, together with a moderate number of staphylococcus aureus in the pericardial and peritoneal fluid. The blood-agar plate of the material injected in each of these animals showed pure cultures of staphylococci and green-producing streptococci, respectively.

The percentages following injection of material from sources other than influenza patients are quite different. In this group the first case was that of a patient with a severe attack of nasopharyngitis and sinusitis, in which the throat was extremely red and the tonsils absent, and in which much mucopurulent material, at first tinged with blood, came from the nose and throat. The attack began with marked chilliness, but no distinct chill, and was followed by fever for a number of days and a leukocytosis of 14,000 on the first day. The patient recovered without developing symptoms of infection of the trachea or bronchi. The hemolytic streptococcus in the second culture generation isolated from the throat produced, on intratracheal injection, leukocytosis in 67% of the animals. The patient, it should be noted, developed no symptoms suggesting infection of the trachea or bronchi and the streptococcus caused no deaths on intratracheal application. This finding is in sharp contrast with the results of injection of the hemolytic streptococci from influenza in which leukopenia occurred in 83% and leukocytosis in only 17% of the animals injected, and in which death from hemorrhagic edema, hemorrhagic pleuritis, or bronchopneumonia occurred in a high percentage of animals injected (figure 1).

The results in the second case are also in sharp contrast to those obtained with material from patients with influenza. In this case the patient awoke in the morning with marked soreness in the upper part of the chest and a painful cough by which thick, mucopurulent material was raised. The day following, the cough and soreness in the chest continued and typical symptoms and signs of a nasopharyngitis had developed, with sneezing and abundant mucous discharge associated with redness of the mucous membranes of the nose and throat. There was little general aching, slight fever, and a leukocytosis of 13,500 on the second day. Recovery was practically complete on the fourth day. Intratracheal injections of the sputum and cultures of the green-producing streptococcus in the primary culture from the nasopharynx, and the same organism in the third culture generation isolated from the sputum on the second day was followed by leukocytosis in 57% of the animals. There was leukopenia in 29% and no change in leukocytes in 14%. None of the animals died of acute hemorrhagic pulmonary edema or hemorrhagic pleuritis. Three developed mucopurulent discharge from the nose in which the streptococcus injected was present in large numbers.

The intratracheal application of type pneumococci isolated originally from lobar pneumonia and proved virulent on intraperitoneal injection just prior to intratracheal injection was followed by leukocytosis in 22%, leukopenia in 11%, and no change in the leukocyte count in 67% of the animals injected. The relatively few instances of leukopenia following injection of the cultures from sources other than influenza usually occurred in animals that succumbed from overwhelming infection. Most of the intratracheal injections consisted of broth cultures of the different bacteria. Control injections of broth in the same dosage were followed by temporary leukopenia in 16%, leukocytosis in 17%, and no change in 67% of the animals injected. In the experiments in which filtrates of the cultures were injected the broth and culture filtrates were of the same batch. The occurrence of leukopenia in 65% of the animals injected with filtrates in contrast to 16% of those injected with broth represents roughly the "leukotoxin" formed by the growth of the streptococci in the broth. Filtrates of pneumonic lungs also possessed this power to a marked degree. In most instances 0.2% glucose-broth cultures and filtrates of cultures in this medium were injected. The broth cultures usually developed an acidity to phenolphthalein of from 1.5 to 2.5%. A series of experiments was made in which parallel intratracheal injections of 0.5 c c for each 100 gm. of body weight of cultures of acid reaction were given, and the same cultures injected after neutralization with sodium hydroxid. There was no noteworthy difference in the two sets of animals, in the leukocytic reaction, in the immediate respiratory symptoms, or in the late results from infection. Moreover, the "leukotoxin" or the property in broth culture filtrates which causes leukopenia and the symptoms of anaphylactic shock is not destroyed by heating to 60 C. for thirty minutes. (See experiments with filtrates.)

The degree of leukopenia following intratracheal injection of these cultures was found to be roughly proportional to the severity of respiratory embarrassment in the animals. In the case of extremely toxic cultures, a sharp reduction has been noted within a few hours after intratracheal application, and even after intranasal insufflation. In some instances the reduction in the leukocyte count did not occur for several days and then with the occurrence of death, with voluminous hemorrhagic and edematous lungs showing few leukocytes in the alveolar exudate, due to streptococci, a sharp drop in leukocytes was sometimes noted. On the other hand, in the animals that died late and that showed leukocytosis, the lungs were not so voluminous, the areas of consolidation were more firm, less moist on the cut surface, peribronchial in location, and the alveolar exudate was rich in leukocytes. These animals also often showed purulent bronchitis and tracheitis.

The leukopenia following direct inoculation of sputum was no greater and occurred no oftener than following injection of pure cultures of the streptococci. The latter were usually derived from single colonies and were in the first to the eleventh culture generation. The animals that succumbed following injection of sputum nearly always showed green-producing streptococci, and injection of pure cultures of these produced marked leukopenia often to a greater degree than those in the first animal passage.

This finding indicates that the reduction in leukocytes following injection of the material from patients with influenza may not be due to an unknown virus, but to peculiar properties of the streptococci or other bacteria at hand in this disease. These streptococci have the power by growth in vitro and in vivo to produce a soluble filterable substance. The filtrates from broth cultures and from influenzal lungs and sputum when applied intratracheally in guinea-pigs have the power, among other properties, to cause sharp reduction in leukocytes. The reduction in leukocytes has occurred with regularity only in the animals injected with influenza strains and not following injection of streptococci in like dosage from similar conditions showing leukocytosis, or type pneumococci. The average degree of leukopenia in the animals was roughly proportional to that found in the patients from whom the strains were isolated, and the leukocyte curves in fatal and nonfatal infections in the animals correspond roughly to those noted in the spontaneous disease in man. The conclusion seems warranted, therefore, that the leukopenia in influenzal infection in man may be due to peculiar properties of the bacteria which are now generally regarded as secondary invaders and not to an unknown virus. Moreover, according to our findings, a persistent, marked leukopenia, or an increasing leukopenia in influenza predisposes to influenzal pneumonia and in the latter indicates a bad prognosis.

STUDIES IN INFLUENZA AND PNEUMONIA

VII. A STUDY OF THE EFFECTS FOLLOWING THE INJECTION OF BACTERIA FOUND IN INFLUENZA IN NORMAL THROATS, IN SIMPLE NASOPHARYNGITIS, AND IN LOBAR PNEUMONIA

E. C. ROSENOW

Division of Experimental Bacteriology, The Mayo Foundation, Rochester, Minnesota.

CONTENTS

Introduction.

Technic of intratracheal injection.

Incidence of occurrence of voluminous lungs, hemorrhagic edema or bronchopneumonia, and pleuritis following intraperitoneal and intratracheal injection of sputum, lung and other exudates, and cultures from patients with influenza in relation to mortality.

Protocols of experiments following injection of material from influenza.

Control experiments with cultures from the throats of normal persons during and after the epidemic. The detection of the carrier state.

Control experiments with cultures from throat and sputum of patients with simple nasopharyngitis and tracheitis and with cultures from the nose of normal guinea-pigs.

Control experiments with type pneumococci from lobar pneumonia.

Protocols of cases of influenza and influenzal pneumonia and animal experiments. Similarity in localization of micro-organisms.

Experiments with filtrates of lung emulsions and cultures.

Experiments indicating the transmission of influenzal infection by contact.

Symptoms and gross lesions following intratracheal injection of influenzal material.

Microscopic anatomy of the lungs.

Lesions of the female generative organs and of tissues other than those of the lung.

Experiments on the mechanism of respiratory embarrassment in influenzal pneumonia.

Relation of mortality in guinea-pigs to virulency of the organisms isolated in fatal and nonfatal infection in patients.

General discussion and summary.

INTRODUCTION

It is my purpose to record in this paper the results obtained from the injection in various ways into animals of material obtained from patients with influenza and influenzal pneumonia and from sources other than influenza, to give the important facts in a series of cases of influenza in which the findings in the patients and the results from the injections of animals are correlated, to describe and illustrate the gross and microscopic changes that followed the injection of the bacteria

Received for publication Feb. 23, 1920.

from influenza, and to compare these changes with those noted in influenzal infection as it occurred during the epidemic of 1918 to 1919.

In a previous report [21, 22] it was pointed out that the streptococci from patients with influenza when injected intraperitoneally into mice and guinea-pigs possessed high virulency, that following these injections, lesions of the lungs and pleura occurred frequently, and that the animals often showed respiratory embarrassment during life and voluminous, emphysematous, and sometimes hemorrhagic lungs after death (case *2607*, guinea-pig *737*; table *2*).

These findings in the experiments with streptococci suggested that the direct application of influenzal material to the normal, uninjured mucous membrane of the trachea and bronchi of animals might result in the production of lesions more marked than those following intraperitoneal injection, and should this be true, it might be possible to throw light on the mechanism of infection in this disease, and to compare the lesions obtained under controlled conditions of dosage and type of micro-organism in animals with those in man. The experiments on intraperitoneal injection and many clinical findings such as the relatively immobile, expanded thorax, the wheezing râles, the dyspnea, cyanosis, and leukopenia suggest strongly that influenza may be in part an anaphylactic reaction. The voluminous lung noted so commonly after death is another argument for this view. The guinea-pig, known to respond more like man than any other animal with respect to anaphylactic reactions, was selected as probably the most suitable in which to study the pulmonary and other lesions following the injection of influenzal material.

TECHNIC OF INTRATRACHEAL INJECTION

The technic of intratracheal injection should be such as to make it quite impossible to injure materially the lining of the trachea and bronchi. Discarded ureteral catheters cut at an angle of 45 degrees with margins rounded have been found to fulfill this requirement. The guinea-pig is wrapped in a towel; the head is held in place by the handles of an inverted artery forceps. The mouth is held open by spring wire retractors, and the tongue is depressed by a suitable small instrument. Under a strong reflected light, properly shaded, the catheter is inserted into the larynx with a quick stroke before the contraction of the muscles of the epiglottis can divert the tube into the esophagus. The animal's sharp, quick cough and total inability to use its voice, and the sensation of the catheter's passing the tracheal rings, indicate that it has entered the trachea. The catheters are sterilized by boiling and in order to avoid the possibility of transmitting accidental infection from one guinea-pig to another, a separate, freshly sterilized catheter was used for each animal in this series. Care was exercised to use only healthy, vigorous, and active animals from stock that was free from epidemic disease. At first the dose of culture given was very small, and the results in consequence were too irregular to permit accurate analysis. Later the dose was increased; 0.1 c c of the sputum or exudate and 0.5 c c of the glucose-blood or brain-broth culture for each 100 gm. of body weight were used in the experiments reported unless it is otherwise indicated. The cultures for injection were incubated at from 33-35 C. for from eighteen to twenty-four hours in tall columns of glucose-brain broth or glucose-blood broth. Control cultures of the material injected were always made on blood-agar plates. This was found necessary not only in order to prove the viability of the organisms injected, but also in order to determine the type that had grown in the particular culture. As has been pointed out heretofore,[20] the most important organism found in the sputum in influenza was a gram-positive, often lanceolate diplostreptococcus which produces greenish colonies on blood-agar plates. The colonies are larger, flatter, and more moist than those of Streptococcus viridans, often indistinguishable from pneumococcus colonies. In this report I shall designate this organism, including the strains that ferment inulin, as a "green-producing streptococcus" or "green streptococcus" to distinguish it from Streptococcus viridans.

Control experiments were first made to determine the harmlessness of intratracheal injection of varying amounts of salt solution and sterile broth. All guinea-pigs injected with salt solution (1 with 6 c c; 3 with 3 c c, and 1 with 2.5 c c) remained well. They showed a slight increase in respiration immediately after injection. All were free from symptoms the following day and remained so. Fifteen guinea-pigs were injected with glucose broth, glucose-blood broth, or glucose-brain broth (4 with 3 c c; 3 with 2.5 c c, 7 with 1.5 c c, and 1 with 1 c c). They showed relatively slight respiratory disturbance immediately after injection. Some, especially those injected with meat infusion-peptone-glucose-blood broth, showed mild symptoms of anaphylaxis. They coughed, scratched the nose with their paws; and were irritable for a short time after injection. All were well the day after injection, and all but two remained well subsequently. The one which had been injected with 1.5 c c died thirteen days later from an old bronchopneumonia that showed Bacillus bronchisepticus. The other, which had been injected intratracheally with 3 c c glucose broth, died ten days later with bronchopneumonia and a moderate amount of bloody fluid in the pleural cavities. Cultures from the blood showed a few colonies of green-producing streptococci, and from the pleural fluid, staphylococci and B. bronchisepticus. The culture in glucose-brain broth of the green-producing streptococci from the blood was injected intratracheally in 3 guinea-pigs. Two had slightly increased respirations for two days and then recovered. The other had no symptoms; it was chloroformed three days after injection and showed no lesions. None of the guinea-pigs showed leukopenia. The average leukocyte count before injection was 9,600, twenty-four hours after injection 9,100, and forty-eight hours after injection, 12,200.

Incidence of Occurrence of Voluminous Lungs, Hemorrhagic Edema of Bronchopneumonia, and Pleuritis Following Intraperitoneal and Intratracheal Injection of Sputum, Lung and Other Exudates, and Cultures from Patients with Influenza in Relation to Mortality

The more marked effects of intratracheal injection over intraperitoneal injection of material from patients with influenza became apparent at once. The symptoms of respiratory embarrassment were more pronounced and the lungs more voluminous. In table 1 the average volume and weight of the lung of a series of guinea-pigs injected intratracheally, and of normal guinea-pigs are given (fig. 1). The volume of the lungs in cubic centimeters, as measured by displacement of water for normal guinea-pigs weighing about 350 gm., and killed with chloroform, was 6.5 c c, or approximately one-fiftieth or 2% of the weight of the animals expressed in grams. The average volume of the lungs of guinea-pigs that had died from causes other than pneumonia was found to be about normal. The average weight of the lungs was found to be 3.3 gm., or about 1% of the body weight. It is evident from table 1 that the more toxic or virulent the culture, the more severe the reaction in the lung, and the earlier the death occurred following intratracheal injection, the greater was the volume and weight of the lung. Thus the volume and weight were approximately three and four times the normal in the guinea-pigs dying in two and one-half hours and two days after injection, respectively, and in those that died in three days the average volume of the lung was less than twice that and the weight about two and one-half times that of the average normal.

TABLE 1

RESULTS OF INTRATRACHEAL INSUFFLATION OF CULTURES FROM INFLUENZA AS SHOWN BY VOLUME AND WEIGHT OF LUNGS

	Average Weight of Animals, Gm.	Average Volume of Lungs, C C	Average Weight of Lungs, Gm.
Guinea-pigs living an average* of 2.5 hours	410	19	13
Guinea-pigs living an average of 2 days	390	17	14
Guinea-pigs living an average of 3 days	340	10	8
Normal guinea-pigs (controls)	350	6.5	3.3

* The averages of 6 guinea-pigs in each series are given.

The increase in lung volume was about the same following the injection of sputum, primary culture of sputum, pure cultures of freshly isolated strains of green-producing streptococci, hemolytic streptococci and staphylococci (usually in the second or third generation). The average volume of the lung of a large number of guinea-pigs after intratracheal injection of influenzal material was 15 c c, and after intraperitoneal injection 10 c c; after injection of type pneumococci it was 10 c c and 7 c c, respectively.

From table 2 may be obtained a general picture of the differences in the results obtained in the mortality and incidence of lesions of the lungs in guinea-pigs injected intratracheally and intraperitoneally with material from patients with influenza, with cultures from normal throats during the epidemic and after it had subsided, with type pneumococci, and with sputum and cultures from patients with simple nasopharyngitis and tracheitis. The total average mortality following injection of material from 111 cases of influenza in 192 animals was

TABLE 2

Mortality and Incidence of Lesions of the Lungs in Guinea-Pigs Injected with Material from Influenza; with Cultures from Normal Throats During and After the Epidemic; with Type Pneumococci and with Sputum and Cultures from Patients with Simple Nasopharyngitis and Tracheitis

Material Injected	Place of Injection	Number of Strains	Number of Animals: Injected	Number of Animals: Recovered	Number of Animals: Died	Percentage of Mortality	Percentage Showing: Voluminous Lungs	Percentage Showing: Hemorrhagic Edema or Pneumonia	Pleuritis
Sputum	Trachea	16	17	5	12	70	64	62	54
	Peritoneum	38	48	15	33	68	25	8	14
Primary culture	Trachea	17	31	16	15	48	36	55	15
	Peritoneum	12	13	7	6	46	22	22	11
Green-producing streptococci	Trachea	19	33	17	16	48	73	54	26
	Peritoneum	12	16	7	9	56	58	17	42
Hemolytic streptococci	Trachea	9	17	7	10	59	83	71	44
	Peritoneum	4	6	2	4	67	67	0	0
Staphylococci	Trachea	6	11	5	6	55	71	43	43
Total for influenza (111 cases)		133	192	81	111	58	55	46	28
Primary culture of throats of normal persons during epidemic of influenza	Trachea	4	12	7	5	42	17	17	0
Primary culture of throats of normal persons months after epidemic had disappeared	Trachea	15	15	12	3	20	0	20	0
Type I, II, III, and IV pneumococci from lobar pneumonia	Trachea	14	20	14	6	30	30	35*	35
	Peritoneum	14	18	0	18	100	6	0	28
Sputum and cultures from patients with simple nasopharyngitis and tracheitis	Trachea	2	10	8	2	20	0	20	0

* Lobar pneumonia.

58%. The total average incidence of voluminous lungs was 55%; of hemorrhagic edema or bronchopneumonia, 46%, and of pleuritis, 28%. The killing power of the influenza strains was only slightly lower when they were applied to the normal mucous membrane of the trachea and bronchi than when they were injected intraperitoneally. The results of control experiments with type pneumococci were quite different in this respect; their killing power was 100% on intraperitoneal injection, whereas only 30% of the animals died following intratracheal injections of the same dose. The average incidence and the degree of lesions of the lung and pleura were higher, as would be expected, following intratracheal injection than following intraperitoneal injection.

The property in these strains which caused symptoms resembling anaphylaxis, voluminous lungs with acute hemorrhagic edema of lungs and leukopenia, and the general virulency, tended to disappear promptly on artificial cultivation, especially if the organisms were cultivated under aerobic conditions. To illustrate:

The volume of the lungs in 2 guinea-pigs was 20 and 12 c c, respectively (average 16 c c), following injection of the primary culture from the blood of a patient with influenza containing a pure culture of the green-producing streptococcus while that in 2 guinea-pigs injected with the same strain in glucose broth after one plating on blood agar was 12 and 10 c c (average 11 c c), and the hemorrhage and edema of the lung were much less marked. Different strains differed markedly in the loss of this power, depending to some extent on the method of cultivation. Aerobic cultivation on blood agar destroyed these peculiar properties rapidly, while by rapid transfers of glucose-brain broth from tube to tube they might be retained for many generations. The typical picture has followed injection of strains in the eleventh culture generation. The tendency of some of the strains to localize and produce a certain type of lesion was striking, often corresponding to the type of lesions found in the patient. Thus, in a case of death from hemorrhagic edema of the lung with pseudolobar pneumonia and hemorrhagic pleuritis (case 2800), the cultures from the throat in the first and second culture generation produced hemorrhagic edema of the lung and hemorrhagic pleuritis in two guinea-pigs injected into the trachea (g. pigs 947 and 956), and in one injected into the stomach (g. pig 948). The same strain injected about three months later when in the sixth subculture had lost much of its virulency, but it still localized in the same manner and produced bronchopneumonia with localized abscesses in the lung and adhesive pleuritis resulting in perforative peritonitis (g. pig 1311).

Experiments with Lung and Other Exudates.—During the course of the experiments the effects of injecting directly the lung exudates of patients and of lung emulsions, peritoneal, and pleural exudates from animals was also studied. Contrary to expectations, the symptoms and lesions following direct injection were less acute than those following injection of the cultures made from these exudates and following the injection of sputum and cultures of streptococci from the sputum and throat. The mortality following direct intratracheal injection of the exudates from 16 cases into 19 guinea-pigs was only 42% as compared, for example, with a mortality of 70% following injection of sputum. The mortality in the 19 guinea-pigs was almost wholly due to injection of peritoneal and lung exudates in guinea-pigs dead from injection of sputum or cultures. Most of the animals that died showed bronchopneumonia, and only a few acute hemorrhagic edema. This relatively low mortality was not due to a lesser number of viable organisms injected because plate cultures often showed a larger number of living bacteria than were present in the sputum or cultures. Under the conditions of a more forced experiment, intraperitoneal injection, the mortality in 11 guinea-pigs injected with 11 strains was higher (64%). Moreover, the theory that these bacteria when soaked in blood or lung exudate tend to lose their bite, as it were, when applied to the normal pulmonary epithelium is further borne out by the fact that the virulency and incidence of acute hemorrhagic edema were higher following injection of cultures from the sputum and throat than of cultures from the blood. Thus, in one case (case 2,800) the mortality following intratracheal injection of the throat and sputum strains was 64%, while following injection of the strain isolated from the blood it was 33%.

Intratracheal Injections of Influenza Bacilli. — Recently isolated strains from the throats of 5 undoubted cases of influenza — 4 in the second, and 1 in the sixth culture generation — were injected intratracheally into 5 guinea-pigs. The dose was 0.5 c c for each 100 gm. body weight of a dense salt suspension from rich growths on chocolate blood agar. The amount of culture injected ranged from the growth of from 1-5 slants. In 3, leukocyte counts were made; 1 of these showed a drop from 12,000 before injection to 6,800 twenty-four hours after injection and 8,000 seventy-two hours after injection. The others showed no change in the leukocyte count. All the animals recovered. Besides slightly increased respiration immediately after injection there was no noticeable effect, and all the animals seemed quite well without increased respiration or rise in temperature 24 hours after injection. The virulency of 2 of these strains was proved in a mouse. Injection of 0.4 c c of a mixture of 3 of the strains killed the mouse in 24 hours. The animal showed enormous subcutaneous hemorrhages in the right groin adjacent to the point of the intraperitoneal injection, and there were hyperemia of lungs and a number of subpleural hemorrhages, but no gross evidence of peritonitis. The cultures from blood and peritoneal fluid on chocolate and blood-agar plates yielded countless numbers of influenza bacilli. In connection with these experiments with pure cultures of influenza bacilli should be considered the fact that intraperitoneal injections of sputum into mice and intraperitoneal and intratracheal injections into guinea-pigs were never followed by invasion by influenza bacilli as determined by cultures, direct examination of smears, and microscopic examination of

TABLE 3

PREDOMINATING ORGANISM IN SPUTUM AND PRIMARY CULTURES FROM SPUTUM INJECTED IN ANIMALS AND FOUND IN THE ANIMALS THAT DIED

Material Injected	Place of Injection	Incidence of Predominating Organism in							
		Material Injected				Animals That Died			
		Strains	Green-producing Streptococci, per Cent.	Hemolytic Streptococci, per Cent.	Staphylococci, per Cent.	Animals Cultured	Green-producing Streptococci, per Cent.	Hemolytic Streptococci, per Cent.	Staphylococci, per Cent.
Sputum	Trachea or peritoneum of guinea-pigs	54	71	20	9	29	81	4	15
Primary culture from sputum	Trachea or peritoneum of guinea-pigs	29	59	24	17	22	73	14	13
Sputum	Peritoneum of mice	19	69	21	10	17	82	12	6
Total............	....	102	68	20	12	68	78	9	13

sections stained for influenza bacilli as recommended by MacCallum.[17] In some of the sputums thus injected large numbers of influenza bacilli were demonstrated in smears and by cultures before injection. Thus in the lung of the guinea-pig shown in figures 5, 10 and 11 the sputum injected contained large numbers of influenza bacilli, but they were absent in the peritoneal exudate, blood and lung tissue. The invasive power of freshly isolated influenza bacilli (virulent to mice on intraperitoneal injection) and of those in the sputum itself when applied to the tracheal mucous membrane in guinea-pigs was found to be slight as compared with the invasive power of the streptococci. It is possible that tracheal injection of adapted strains or those whose virulency is enhanced by animal passage through intraperitoneal injection might acquire the power to invade the lung and produce bronchopneumonia and possibly hemorrhagic edema of the lungs.

The Comparative Invasive Power of the Bacteria from Patients with Influenza. — The high invasive power of the green-producing streptococcus became apparent early in the work. We have determined which of the different bacteria occurred in predominating number in the sputums injected into guinea-pigs and mice and in the primary cultures from sputum injected into guinea-pigs, and also in exudates and blood of the animals that died as a result of the injections. In table 3 is given the percentage of incidence of the predominating organisms. It will be noted that the green-producing streptococcus was the predominating organism in the material injected in each group of experiments and, what is more significant, it was the predominating organism in a higher percentage of the animals after death, whereas the reverse was true of hemolytic streptococci and staphylococci. The relative importance of these three organisms in influenza might be said to be indicated roughly by the figures in the last line of table 3.

Protocols of Experiments Following Injection of Material from Influenza

Guinea-pig 846, weighing 420 gm., was injected intraperitoneally Dec. 28, 1918, with 2.5 c c of glucose-broth culture of the green-producing streptococcus from the blood of G. pig 828, which had been injected with the sputum from case 2,749. December 29 the animal was found dead. Marked hemorrhagic serofibrinous peritonitis, moderate distention and congestion of the lungs (11 c c), a large number of large and small subpleural hemorrhages, and beginning pleuritis were found. The pleura contained 3 c c of turbid, blood-tinged, chocolate-colored fluid. A moderate amount of bloody, frothy fluid escaped from the cut surface of the lungs. The uterus contained several hemorrhagic areas marking placental attachment. The cultures from the blood, pleural fluid, peritoneal fluid, and placental site showed many green-producing streptococci.

Guinea-pig 981, weighing 470 gm., was injected Jan. 16, 1919, intratracheally with 1.5 c c of the glucose-broth culture of the green-producing streptococcus in the second culture generation isolated from the blood in case 2,800. The white blood count before injection was 8,000; the temperature 102.2 F. January 17 the animal appeared less active than normal and the respirations were slightly increased. The leukocyte count was 2,000 and the temperature 103.2 January 18 the animal was more active, but the respirations were still slightly increased. The leukocyte count was 6,200, the temperature 102.8. January 19 the animal appeared quite well. The respirations were normal, the leukocyte count was 12,200, and the temperature 102.4. The animal made a complete recovery; when it was chloroformed January 24 it showed no lesions. The cultures from the blood and lung remained sterile.

Guinea-pig 995, weighing 470 gm., had injected into the trachea, Jan. 18, 1919, 1.5 c c of the glucose-broth culture of the green-producing streptococcus in the second culture generation isolated from the blood of case 2,800. The white blood count before injection was 9,200, the temperature 102.4. There were moderate symptoms of dyspnea immediately following injection. January 19 the animal appeared quite well but the respirations were definitely increased. The leukocyte count was 6,200, the temperature 103. January 20 the respirations were slightly increased, the leukocyte count was 14,400, the temperature 103. January 25 the animal appeared well. February 24 at 7:30 a. m. the animal appeared ill. The respirations were markedly increased and difficult. The animal when taken from the cage and placed on a table had a typical attack resembling anaphylactic shock with bronchial spasm. At noon the respirations were exceedingly rapid and the animal appeared to be very sick; at 4 p. m. it was found dead. The white blood count was 12,800. There was a large amount of bloody, turbid fluid in both pleural cavities; the right contained a moderate amount of adherent, partially organizing fibrin. The lungs were collapsed and the intermediate lobe was completely consolidated, grayish-red, and covered with a film of fibrin. There were several thickened areas in the mucous membrane of the uterus indicating a resorption of fetuses. The ovaries were normal. The heart muscle was grayish-red. Cultures from the blood and pleura showed green-producing streptococci.

Guinea-pig 1335, weighing 420 gm., was injected intratracheally, May 15, 1919, at 9:50 a. m. with 1.5 c c of glucose-acacia-broth culture of staphylococcus in the sixth subculture from case 2,623. At 10:15 a. m. respirations were rapid, difficult and irregular. There were repeated attacks bordering on bronchial spasm, expiration was forced and prolonged, and the animal was weak. At 10:30 a. m. the respirations were extremely difficult. The animal coughed violently at intervals making desperate efforts with each expiration, and during one of these violent efforts it ran about aimlessly with blood spurting from its nose and mouth; it fell on its side and died with its head in a pool of frothy blood. The lung was found greatly distended (20 c c) and hemorrhagic and edematous throughout. Sections showed marked distention of alveoli and destruction of the epithelium lining the alveoli and of the endothelium of the capillaries. In areas dissolution was so marked as to make it quite impossible to distinguish the alveolar boundaries.

Guinea-pig 956, weighing 280 gm., was injected intratracheally, Jan. 13, 1919, with 1.5 c c of glucose-brain-broth culture of the green-producing streptococcus from a single colony on a blood-agar plate inoculated with the swab from case 2,800. January 14 the animal was very ill; respirations were rapid and difficult. The fur was rough and the animal was restless and irritable. It died at noon. The lungs were markedly distended (15 c c). Both diaphragmatic lobes were dark and mottled. The cut surfaces everywhere were extremely moist and a large amount of bloody, frothy fluid exuded. The other lobes showed smaller areas of hemorrhagic edema. The alveoli were extremely distended, in places almost to the point of rupturing. The peribronchial glands were edematous. The trachea and bronchi were extremely hyperemic and contained a large amount of bloody, frothy fluid. There was a moderate amount of slightly turbid, blood-tinged fluid in the pleural and pericardial sacs. The mucous membrane of the nose was hyperemic. The suprarenals were swollen and there was cloudy swelling of the kidneys. The mucous membrane of the uterus was markedly hyperemic throughout and showed three hemorrhagic areas marking placental attachments. The vagina contained a moderate amount of bloody mucus. Cultures from the blood showed one colony of green-producing streptococci; from the lung and hemorrhagic areas of the mucous membranes of the uterus, large numbers of green-producing streptococci; from the spleen, kidney, liver, and suprarenals, no growth. In sections of the lung were noted marked dilatation of alveoli, marked desquamation of the epithelial lining of bronchi, and marked edema and hemorrhage in the alveoli with little cellular infiltration (fig. 13 b). The Gram stain showed enormous numbers of streptococci distributed particularly along the alveolar walls (fig. 14 c).

Guinea-pig 947, weighing 400 gm., had injected into the trachea, Jan. 10, 1919, 11 a. m., 1.5 c c glucose-brain-broth culture from the throat swab of case 2,800. At 6 p. m. the respirations were rapid and shallow; the voice was weak and the animal appeared sick. January 13 at 7:30 a. m. the animal was found dead. There was a large amount of hemorrhagic, dark colored fluid in the pleural cavities, containing practically no fibrin. The pleura was rough and covered with a thin fibrinous film, and the lung was compressed by the hemorrhagic fluid in the pleural cavities. The right diaphragmatic and intermediate lobes were extremely wet and edematous on the cut surface. A large amount of bloody, frothy fluid escaped. Portions of the diaphragmatic lobe barely floated in water. The mucous membranes of the bronchi, trachea, and nose were extremely hyperemic and covered with a bloody, frothy fluid. The uterus contained four hemorrhagic areas marking placental attachments. A moderate amount of bloody mucus was found in the uterus and vagina. The stomach was distended with gas rich in carbon dioxid, and showed marked postmortem digestion of the mucous membrane. The cultures from the blood showed a small number of colonies of Staphylococcus aureus and hemolytic streptococci; from the lung, pleura, pericardial fluid, and uterus, large numbers of hemolytic streptococci and staphylococci, and a few from the kidney, liver, and suprarenals. Sections of the lung showed extreme interstitial edema and hemorrhage with marked disintegration of the cells lining the alveoli. The gram stain showed enormous numbers of gram-positive diplococci in the pleura and subpleural spaces in the interstitial tissues and around the blood vessels (fig. 20 a and b).

Guinea-pig 948, weighing 300 gm., was injected intragastrically, Jan. 10, 1919, with 1.5 c c of the glucose-brain-broth culture from the throat of case 2,800. January 13 it appeared to be quite well. January 15 it appeared to be quite well, but was less active and sat humped up. January 19 it sat humped up with ruffled fur, with a dry crust about the nostrils, markedly increased respirations, labored and forced expirations and dilated chest. It had lost 40 gm. in weight. January 20 at 8 a. m. the breathing was rapid and difficult and the animal very much weaker. At noon when it was found dead, it weighed 250 gm. The thorax was distended with a large amount of chocolate-colored fluid (15 c c); there were marked pleuritis with loose fibrinous adhesions throughout and a thin layer covering the pleura. The peribronchial lymph glands were much enlarged and edematous; the lungs were collapsed, but hemorrhagic, and showed areas of bronchopneumonia with white necrotic spots in the intermediate lobe. The pancreas was edematous, the spleen enlarged, and the myocardium gray. No lesions in the stomach or intestinal tract were demonstrable. Cultures from the blood showed green-producing streptococci; those from the pleural fluid, green-producing streptococci and staphylococci.

Guinea-pig 1311, weighing 320 gm., was injected intratracheally, March 25, 1919, with 0.2 c c of the glucose-brain-broth culture from the throat swab from case 2,800 in the sixth subculture. March 26 and 28 the animal's respiration was increased but otherwise it appeared well. April 15 it was found dead and showed three circumscribed areas of necrosis with softening in the left diaphragmatic lobe. The pleura over each of these areas was bound down by organizing adhesions. One area over the diaphragmatic lobe showed localized hemorrhages and fibrinous deposit on the peritoneal side of the diaphragm, undoubtedly the source of the serofibrinous peritonitis. One area of consolidation in the right cardiac lobe occupying one third of its volume showed recent diffuse consolidation. The white necrotic areas on the cut surface were wedge-shaped and resembled infarcts; the urinary bladder contained a number of circumscribed hemorrhages in the mucosa; but no other lesions were noteworthy. Cultures from the blood, lung, peritoneal and pleural fluids showed green-producing streptococci.

Guinea-pig 1030, weighing 400 gm., was injected intratracheally, Jan. 22, 1919, with 1.5 c c of the lung emulsion from case 2835. The leukocyte count before injection was 10,200; twenty-four hours after injection it was 7,800, and the animal appeared quite well. February 3 the animal was chloroformed. It showed one large grayish-red area of consolidation posteriorly in the left diaphragmatic lobe and one area of consolidation which was dark red and edematous, and a localized necrotic, wedge-shaped, adherent area over the right diaphragmatic lobe.

The experiments cited in detail are representative of a much larger series. Examples of mild effects, mild early effects and severe late effects and marked progressive symptoms from the time of injection are given following injection of pure cultures of the green-producing streptococcus in the first to the sixth subculture, staphylococcus in the sixth subculture, and of a lung emulsion.

CONTROL EXPERIMENTS WITH CULTURES FROM THE THROATS OF NORMAL PERSONS DURING AND AFTER THE EPIDEMIC. THE DETECTION OF THE CARRIER STATE

The occurrence of voluminous lung, hemorrhagic edema, and bronchopneumonia associated with leukopenia following intratracheal injection of the influenza strains was a striking picture. It was thought that intratracheal injection of primary mass cultures from throats of normal persons might detect carriers of the influenza streptococcus. Two sets of experiments were done, one on persons in an institution during the prevalence in the disease in epidemic proportions, the other four months later when influenza had entirely subsided. In the former set, 12 guinea-pigs were injected with cultures from 4 patients. Seven of the guinea-pigs recovered and 5 died, a mortality of 42% (table 2). In 2 cases the animal injections were without apparent effects; in one, the 2 pigs injected died in three and four days, respectively, of bronchopneumonia without leukopenia. The lungs were only slightly enlarged (average volume 10 c c), and quite dry on the cut surface; the exudate was highly cellular. After death green-producing streptococci, or pneumococci, and staphylococci were isolated from the lung in large numbers. The streptococci were not agglutinated by the monovalent serum. The results in the fourth case were in sharp contrast. The 3 guinea-pigs and 1 mouse which were injected died. One pig and the mouse were injected subcutaneously, the other animals intratracheally. The 3 guinea-pigs showed a sharp drop in leukocytes. Death in all was due to green-producing streptococci (which were agglutinated by the monovalent serum) and staphylococci. The average leukocyte count before injection was 14,000, while twenty-four hours after injection it was 4,260, a loss of 64%. The two animals injected intratracheally showed voluminous hemorrhagic lungs.

Guinea-pig 1004, weighing 350 gm., was injected intratracheally Jan. 19, 1919, with 1.5 c c of the glucose broth culture from the throat of a normal person who had been exposed to influenza (case 2839). The leukocyte count was 13,000. January 20 the leukocyte count was 4,200, and there was marked shortness of breath and difficult breathing. January 21 at 4 p. m. the animal was found dead, with its head lying in a pool of hemorrhagic fluid. The white blood count was 2,600. The lung was distended, very heavy (14 c c and 12 gm.) and almost completely filled with a frothy hemorrhagic fluid. There was little evidence of consolidation. The peribronchial lymph glands were hemorrhagic and edematous. A thin fibrinous film covered the posterior aspect of the lung. Cultures from the blood, lung, suprarenals, and liver showed staphylococci and green-producing streptococci; those from the kidney and spleen were negative.

The experiments with cultures from normal persons months after the epidemic had subsided consisted of the intratracheal injection of 15 guinea-pigs with cultures from the throats of 15 persons. Of these animals, 12 recovered without developing noteworthy symptoms and 3 (20%) died (table 2). None of these animals showed the violent respiratory embarrassment noted in the animals following injection of the influenza strains. The lung picture after death was quite different than that following injection of the influenza strains. The animals died in one, two and five days, respectively, of green-producing streptococci or pneumococci in the two former, and of Bacillus mucosus in the third. The lungs averaged 8.5 c c in volume. The hemorrhages and consolidation were situated immediately around the bronchi and the consolidated areas were relatively dry on the cut surface, and the exudate highly cellular in character, as noted in the following experiment:

Guinea-pig 1364, weighing 280 gm., was injected intratracheally July 24, 1919, with 1.5 c c of the glucose brain-broth culture from the throat of a normal person (case 3515). July 25 the respirations were decidedly increased. At 4:30 p. m. it was found dead. The thorax was not distended. The pleural cavities were free from fluid; the lungs were only slightly distended (9 c c). There were areas in the diaphragmatic lobes of hemorrhage and beginning infiltration. The cultures from the blood were negative; cultures from the lung showed green-producing streptococci.

CONTROL EXPERIMENTS WITH CULTURES FROM THROATS AND SPUTUM OF PATIENTS WITH SIMPLE NASOPHARYNGITIS AND TRACHEITIS AND WITH CULTURES FROM THE NOSE OF NORMAL GUINEA-PIGS

In some cases there was a marked parallelism between the findings in the patient and in the animals injected (case 2798). Hence it was thought worth while to inject the sputum and cultures from patients with simple nasopharyngitis and tracheitis long after the epidemic had subsided and compare the results with those obtained following injection of the strains from influenza. The results are summarized in table 2. Thus, of 10 animals injected from cultures from 2 cases, 2 died (20%), both of bronchopneumonia. None showed marked respiratory embarrassment resembling anaphylaxis, and none died of hemorrhagic edema. Both of the patients showed leukocytosis, and leukocytosis was the rule in the animals injected.

In order still further to control the results of the experiments on intratracheal injections and to make sure that the bacteria of the upper respiratory tract might not be carried into the lung with the catheter, a series of guinea-pigs were injected with the cultures from freshly isolated strains of the green-producing streptococci normally present in the nose in some guinea-pigs.

The strains isolated from the nose of 2 guinea-pigs were each injected in the usual dose into the trachea of 2 guinea-pigs. The leukocyte count from the guinea-pig in which the culture was made was normal and remained so following injection of sterile broth. The 4 guinea-pigs injected were well the day after injection and remained so for a month thereafter. None of the animals showed leukopenia. All showed a slight rise in leukocyte count the day after injection, and only one a moderate reduction forty-eight hours after injection. The average leukocyte count before injection was 12,550, twenty-four hours after injection, 14,750, and forty-eight hours after injection, 10,200. It is thus apparent that the chance of carrying infection from the upper respiratory tract through the trachea is extremely slight, not even occurring when large doses of the normal flora of the upper respiratory tract are introduced.

CONTROL EXPERIMENTS WITH TYPE PNEUMOCOCCI FROM LOBAR PNEUMONIA

In order that a correct standard for comparison might be had in evaluating the results of the experiments in influenza, it was considered necessary not only to inject animals with type pneumococci, but also with strains having at least the same killing power, when injected intraperitoneally, dose for dose, as had the strains from influenza. The virulency of the strains were first determined for mice. Twelve strains * of the various types were injected intraperitoneally into 13 mice, the dose ranging from 0.8 to 1.0 c c of glucose-blood or glucose brain-broth culture. All died of peritonitis. The blood and peritoneal fluid in all showed large numbers of pneumococci, the latter often a few colonies of staphylococcus in addition. These 12 strains freshly isolated from the blood, and 2 other recently isolated strains, 14 in all, were then injected intraperitoneally and intratracheally into guinea-pigs. The doses in both were the same and varied from 0.3 to 3 c c of twenty-four-hour glucose brain broth cultures; the usual dose in these, as in the animals injected with the influenza strains, was 0.5 c c for each 100 gm. of body weight. The weight of the guinea-pigs ranged from 320 to 400 gm., the average being 330 gm. Intraperitoneal injections were made in 18 guinea-pigs with the 14 different strains of type pneumococci, 6 with 6 strains of type 1; 5 with 3 strains of type II; 6 with 4 strains of type III, and 1 with 1 strain of group IV. Eleven of the animals died on the first day and 7 on the second day after injection, a mortality of 100% (table 2). The blood and peritoneal exudate showed large or countless numbers of pneumococcus colonies in all these animals. The peritoneal exudate in most instances and the blood in some instances yielded in addition a small and variable number of staphylococcus colonies. The volume of the lungs ranged from 4 to 9 c c, averaging 7 c c. Noteworthy lesions in the lungs were absent in all. A few showed small hemorrhages. A beginning pleuritis was noted in 5.

* For the strains of pneumococci used in these experiments I am indebted to Dr. Rufus J. Cole of the Hospital of the Rockefeller Institute for Medical Research and Dr. Augustus Wadsworth of the New York State Board of Health.

Successful intratracheal injections were as follows: 7 guinea-pigs with 5 strains of type I; 4 with 3 strains of type II; 5 with 4 strains of type III, and 4 with 2 strains of group IV pneumococcus, a total of 14 strains and 20 animals (table 2). Respiratory embarrassment immediately after injection and the following day was relatively slight as compared with animals injected with the influenza strains. In 7 of those that recovered no noticeable increase in respiratory rate or illness could be detected the day after injection. Five of the others showed increased respiration and rise in temperature for a day or two, and then recovered. Two showed marked increased respiration for 4 days and when improving, on the fifth and sixth day, respectively, were chloroformed. The findings in the former are illustrated in the experiment in guinea-pig 1,450. The other showed a resolving pneumonia with a few pneumococci in the blood and lung exudate. The 6 animals that died (one each injected with types I, II and III, and 3 of group IV pneumococci) showed with one exception progressive increase in respiration rate until death. The one that did not, died eight days later with a resolving pneumonia. The respirations in the 3 that died within five days after injection were extremely rapid, the nostrils remained free from exudate, there was no bleeding from the nose, the animals were quiet, and the breathing was generally free and easy. The picture was thus in sharp contrast to that noted in guinea-pigs that died following intratracheal injection of the highly virulent influenza strains. The tendency to the production of leukopenia following injection of type pneumococci even in fatal infection was far less than that following injection of the influenza strains, occurring respectively in 11 and 57% of the animals injected. The lungs were moderately distended, but smaller than those observed following the injection of influenza strains. The consolidation usually involved whole lobes or was sharply outlined (fig. 4). The pleura overlying the consolidated area was opaque and rough, the consolidated areas, even in the stage of red hepatization, were less edematous than in the influenzal lungs, and the areas showing gray hepatization were uniformly dry and granular. Extensive gray hepatization was noted as early as forty-eight hours after injection. Sections in the early stages showed many red cells and moderate leukocyte infiltration in the alveoli. Later diffuse alveolar infiltration with leukocytes and fibrin occurred with a few red blood corpuscles and little edema. The bronchial and alveolar epithelium showed comparatively little damage (figs. 18a and 19b). The pneumococci were found diffusely distributed in large

Derivation of Three Filtrates and the Results Following Their Injection

Sputum from case of influenza (Case 2749)
Subcutaneous
Guinea-Pig 828
Subcutaneous edema; emphysema of lungs; hemorrhagic endometritis
Green-producing streptococcus from uterus

↓

Intratracheal
Guinea-Pig 851
Emphysema of lung; hemorrhagic edema; bronchopneumonia
Filtrate of pneumonia lung
(Filtrate 3)

↓

Intratracheal

Guinea-Pig 909
Emphysema; rhinitis; sinusitis; edema of lung; endometritis

Guinea-Pig 908
Rhinitis; bronchitis; marked emphysema; hemorrhagic edema
Filtrate of pneumonia lung
(Filtrate 4)

(After incubation 48 hours in glucose brain broth)
Guinea-Pig 918
Hemorrhagic pleuritis; edema of lungs; mediastinitis

(After incubation 48 hours in tissue broth)
Guinea-Pig 921
Emphysema; hemorrhagic edema; bronchopneumonia; rhinitis; sinusitis; tracheitis; bronchitis; myositis; endometritis

(After incubation) 48 hours in tissue broth)
Guinea-Pig 926
Remained well

Filtrate 4 ↓

Intratracheal

Guinea-Pig 930
Death in 10 minutes from emphysema and hemorrhage of lung

Guinea-Pig 931
Increased respiration for several days; recovery

Guinea-Pig 933
Increased respiration for several days; recovery

Guinea-Pig 934
Increased respiration for several days; recovery

(After heating at 60 C. 30 minutes)
Guinea-Pig 929
Immediate symptoms of anaphylactic shock; recovery

(After heating at 60 C. 30 minutes)
Guinea-Pig 932
Immediate symptoms of anaphylactic shock; recovery

↓

Intravenous
Guinea-Pig 844
Emphysema; hemorrhagic edema; bronchopneumonia; pancreatitis; endometritis; abortion
Green-producing streptococcus from pancreas

↓

Intratracheal
Emphysema; hemorrhagic edema; bronchopneumonia; endometritis; abortion
Filtrate of pneumonic lung
(Filtrate 2)

↓

Intratracheal

Guinea-Pig 882
Pseudolobar pneumonia; abortion

Guinea-Pig 888
Emphysema; pleuritis; bronchopneumonia

Guinea-Pig 919
Remained well

Guinea-Pig 923
Adhesive pleuritis; healing; bronchopneumonia

numbers throughout the exudate and showed little tendency toward peripheral aggregation along the alveolar lining, and the perivascular and subpleural spaces (fig. 18b). There was no distinct difference in the exudate in animals injected with the different type strains. The findings in two experiments will suffice to illustrate:

Guinea-pig 1031, weighing 400 gm., was injected intratracheally, Jan. 22, 1919, with 1.5 c c of glucose-broth cultures of pneumococcus group IV after one (intraperitoneal) animal passage. The temperature before injection was 102.4 F., and the white blood count was 13,200. The following day the animal appeared quite well. The temperature was 99.6 and the white blood count was 18,600. January 24 the animal was found dead. The white blood count was 17,500. Most of the right lung was consolidated, uniformly grayish-red, firm in consistency, and quite dry on the cut surface. A number of smaller areas of consolidation were found in the left lung. The cut surface everywhere was fairly dry and nowhere could edematous fluid be made to drip from it. Emphysema was moderate. The total volume of the lungs was 10 c c. The cultures from the blood and lungs showed large numbers of green-producing pneumococci.

Guinea-pig 1448, weighing 380 gm., was injected intratracheally, Oct. 21, 1918, with 1.5 c c of glucose-blood-broth culture of pneumococcus type II (Strain 3625). October 22 the respirations were extremely rapid and the animal sat quietly. October 23 it was dead. A moderate amount of slightly turbid fluid was found in both pleural cavities. The lungs were moderately distended (14 c c) and weighed 10 gm. The right diaphragmatic lobe was quite uniformly gray and completely consolidated; it was dry and granular on the cut surface. A number of smaller areas of hemorrhage with decided consolidation were found chiefly around the bronchi in the left diaphragmatic and right cardiac lobes. There were marked myocardial degeneration and cloudy swelling of the kidneys, but the uterus and other organs were normal. Cultures from the blood yielded many pneumococcus colonies. Sections of the lung showed moderate distention of alveoli, absence of necrosis of alveolar epithelium and capillaries, and marked, highly cellular leukocytic infiltration of the alveoli in which large numbers of diplococci were distributed throughout the exudate with little tendency of the bacteria to be distributed along the alveolar epithelial lining (figs. 18 and 19 b).

PROTOCOLS OF CASES OF INFLUENZA AND INFLUENZAL PNEUMONIA AND ANIMAL EXPERIMENTS. SIMILARITY OF LOCALIZATION OF MICRO-ORGANISMS

Case 2607, a middle-aged woman developed pneumonia during an influenzal attack and died. The sputum obtained Nov. 21, 1918, was bloody; smears showed large numbers of gram-positive, lanceolate diplococci, gram-positive cocci, and small gram-negative bacilli of irregular size resembling influenza bacilli, and large numbers of gram-positive diplococci, at times in chains within epithelial cells. Blood-agar plates showed large numbers of colonies of green-producing streptococci and influenza bacilli. The sputum (0.3 c c) was injected intraperitoneally November 21, into Guinea-pig 737. November 22 at 8 a. m. the animal appeared to be ill, was irritable and short of breath. At noon it was worse. The respirations were greatly increased and it had repeated choking spells resembling anaphylactic shock. At 8 p. m. it was found dead, and was examined at once. A small amount of turbid fluid without fibrin was found in the peritoneal and pleural cavities. The lungs were distended (13 c c), hyperemic and edematous, and showed numerous small hemorrhages and a number of large subpleural hemorrhages posteriorly in the left diaphragmatic lobe (fig. 5). In cultures from the blood were a few green-producing streptococci; the hemorrhagic area in the lung and peritoneal fluid contained large numbers of green-producing streptococci in pure culture. No influenza bacilli were found in smears from the peritoneal fluid. Sections of the lung showed marked congestion of interalveolar capillaries, marked hemorrhage in the alveoli, and desquamation and necrosis of the alveolar epithelial cells in varying degree. Many alveoli and terminal bronchi were greatly dilated; others appeared to be collapsed. The larger bronchi were constricted and their lumen contained numerous red blood corpuscles and desquamated alveolar epithelium; the mucous membrane lay in great folds. The hemorrhagic areas were usually situated around bronchi and beneath the pleura. In the latter position they were often triangular in shape with the base toward the pleura. At no place was there marked leukocytic infiltration (fig. 10). Prolonged study of sections stained by Gram-Weigert and by the combination of Goodpasture and Weigert stains recommended by MacCallum showed an interesting distribution of the bacteria. None were found within capillaries and larger blood vessels. A few were found in the areas of hemorrhage in the alveoli, but by far the largest number were found, as shown in figure 11, just outside the capillary in the interstitial tissue of the alveolar wall (a), along the alveolar lining beneath the desquamated epithelium (b), in the epithelial cells showing poorly stained nuclei, but still in place lining the alveoli showing hemorrhage (c), and in the degenerated, desquamating alveolar epithelial cells (d).

The streptococcus from the peritoneal fluid in this guinea-pig in the third culture generation was injected intraperitoneally into another guinea-pig. It died in twenty-four hours with turbid hemorrhagic fluid in the peritoneal cavity and numerous hemorrhages in a large part of the secum, especially surrounding the lymph follicles, and hemorrhages in Peyer's patches, but with no lesions of the lung. Intraperitoneal injections of the sputum in 3 other normal guinea-pigs was followed by the death of all in from three to ten days. The animal that died in 3 days was found to have emphysema, hemorrhages and edema of the lungs. The others showed no lesions of the lung. Two guinea-pigs injected two weeks previously with the sputum from other cases of influenza recovered.

The points of particular interest in these experiments are the marked affinity of the streptococcus in the sputum for the epithelium of the alveoli of the lung (fig. 11), the noninvasive power of the influenza bacilli found in the sputum, the hemorrhages in the intestine in the second animal passage, and the acquired immunity in the two guinea-pigs previously injected with sputum from other cases of influenza.

Case 2769, Miss M. J., aged 38, came for examination on account of chronic loseness of bowels and loss of weight and strength. Her condition was found to be due to pancreatic insufficiency. The patient contracted influenza Dec. 16, 1918; developed symptoms and signs of bronchopneumonia December 22, and died December 28. The looseness of bowels was worse throughout the influenzal attack. At necropsy were found "a resolving 'lobar' pneumonia, seropurulent pleuritis (1,500 c c), of the right side, chronic parenchymatous and interstitial pancreatitis, and fatty degeneration of kidneys."

Cultures from the lung after death and pus from the right pleura showed many hemolytic streptococci and a few staphylococci. The primary culture in glucose broth from the lung was injected intratracheally into one guinea-pig and intraperitoneally into another. The guinea-pig (Guinea-pig 875) injected intratracheally died nineteen days after injection from hemorrhagic and purulent pleuritis, pericarditis and myocardial degeneration (fig. 7). The animal injected intraperitoneally died after twenty-four hours. It had diffuse peritonitis, extreme hyperemia of the large and small intestines, swollen lymph follicles throughout the intestinal tract, and numerous hemorrhages in the lower two thirds of the small intestine and in the cecum. The contents of the small intestine consisted chiefly of bloody mucus. The duodenum, stomach, and suprarenals were normal. The lungs were emphysematous (11 c c), and showed moderate edema and a number of small hemorrhages. The pleural cavity contained a small amount of hemorrhagic fluid. Cultures from the blood, peritoneal fluid, and intestinal contents showed hemolytic streptococci and staphylococci. The pleural exudate (1 c c) was injected directly into the trachea of a guinea-pig. It aborted four days later and died with marked leukopenia, increased respirations, voluminous lungs (17 c c), marked hemorrhagic pleuritis, hemorrhagic bronchopneumonia and lesions in the psoas muscles. Large numbers of green-producing streptococci were isolated from the lung, pleural fluid, and uterus but none from the spleen, liver, suprarenals and cervix. The culture from the peritoneal exudate was injected intravenously into a rabbit and one guinea-pig, and intratracheally into one guinea-pig. The rabbit died the day following injection with extreme distention of the abdomen due to a large amount of gas (rich in carbon dioxid) in the small intestines. The small and large intestines contained a large amount of mucus. The intestinal contents were liquid or semisolid throughout. The intestinal wall was opaque, but there were no hemorrhages. Six sharply circumscribed hemorrhages were found in the mucous membrane of the cardiac end of the stomach; in the medulla of the kidneys were a few embolic hemorrhagic areas. The myocardium was markedly degenerated. Cultures from the blood showed a large number of hemolytic streptococci and staphylococci. The guinea-pig injected intravenously died five days later. It showed two small areas of bronchopneumonia, swollen Peyer's patches and solitary lymph follicles, a large amount of mucus in the intestines, absence of food in the stomach, but a large amount of turbid mucus showing many gram-positive diplococci, edematous and hemorrhagic mesenteric lymph glands, marked hyperemia of the uterus, turbid mucus in both uterine horns, numerous small hemorrhages in the mucous membrane of the uterus and cecum, and focal lesions in the medulla of the kidney. Cultures from the blood showed one colony; cultures from the pneumonic areas, countless numbers, and from the mucus from the left horn of the uterus, a moderate number of staphylococcus colonies.

The guinea-pig injected intratracheally died six days later. It had voluminous lungs (15 c c), bronchopneumonia and edema of the right and left caudal lobes, hemorrhagic tracheobronchial lymph glands, purulent material in the nostrils, purulent bronchitis and tracheitis, a hemorrhagic fetus in the vagina and one still attached to the uterus; focal lesions in the medulla of the kidneys; and edematous mucous membranes of the pelvis of the kidneys. Cultures from the pneumonic lung and blood showed green-producing streptococci and staphylococci.

The striking features in the animal experiments in this case was the tendency to produce, in addition to the characteristic lung lesions and pleuritis in the first animal passage, lesions of the intestinal tract and medulla of the kidney in the second animal passage.

Case 2770, Mr. S. M., aged 33, was admitted to the isolation hospital Dec. 24, 1918, complaining of severe weakness, backache, aching all over, extreme nervousness and severe cough. These symptoms had begun two days previously. The leukocyte count the day of admission was 3,800. The temperature was 103 F., pulse 118, respirations 28. The patient grew progressively worse, the temperature ranging between 103 and 105. December 26 evidence of involvement of the lungs became apparent. Cyanosis and dyspnea increased as evidence of a rapid filling of the lungs appeared and the patient died December 28, forty-eight hours after the first signs of pneumonia had developed. Necropsy showed voluminous lungs, pseudolobar pneumonia associated with marked hemorrhagic edema involving all lobes, a large accumulation of bloody, turbid fluid in the left thorax (900 c c) and intense hemorrhagic bronchitis. In cultures made from the sputum December 26 were enormous numbers of green-producing streptococci and a few staphylococci; in the lung exudate and blood after death were many green-producing streptococci and staphylococci.

The primary culture in glucose broth from the blood of this patient was injected into the trachea of 3 guinea-pigs in doses of 0.1 c c, 1 c c and 2.5 c c, respectively. The one receiving only 0.1 c c had moderately increased respirations for several hours, then appeared quite well for four days, when the respirations again became rapid and the animal died six days after injection with a moderate amount of hemorrhagic turbid fluid in the pleural cavity, moderate distention of the lung (12 c c) with almost complete consolidation of the left anterior and cardiac lobes. The cut surface of the consolidated areas was mottled grayish-red and edematous between the areas of denser consolidations and necrosis. Cultures from the blood showed green-producing streptococci in pure culture; those from the lung and pleural fluid, green-producing streptococci and staphylococci. The leukocyte count was 17,000 before injection, 8,960 four hours after injection, and 5,200 the following day. The animal injected with 1 c c died in five days after having aborted. It showed acute diffuse peritonitis clearly secondary to infection in the uterus which passed through the left tube, voluminous lung (15 c c), hemorrhagic bronchopneumonia, pleuritis, and marked maxillary sinusitis, tracheitis, and bronchitis. The animal injected with 2.5 c c died in four and one-half hours. It had extreme difficulty in breathing and frequent paroxysms resembling anaphylactic shock; it was found with its head in a pool of hemorrhagic edema fluid. The lungs were voluminous (20 c c), hemorrhagic, and edematous throughout. The trachea, bronchi, and nostrils were filled with hemorrhagic frothy fluid.

The glucose-brain-broth culture of green-producing streptococcus derived from a single colony on the blood-agar plate from the blood in this case was injected into 3 guinea-pigs; all received 1 c c intratracheally. One of these had had an intraperitoneal injection of a primary culture from the sputum in another case of influenza 10 days previously. It showed no symptoms the day after injection and remained well subsequently. One of the others died the day after injection with leukopenia, voluminous lung (12 c c), marked hemorrhagic edema and bronchopneumonia, edematous peribronchial lymph glands, and a moderate amount of fluid in the pleural cavity. The third died in 3 days of hemorrhagic bronchopneumonia, tracheitis, and sinusitis. Both of these showed green-producing streptococci in the blood and green-producing streptococci and a few staphylococci in the lung and pleural fluid. The glucose-brain-broth culture injected into these 3 guinea-pigs was subcultured rapidly in duplicate from tube to tube of glucose-brain broth, and cultures made from one to three times a day. In the eleventh subcultures 2 guinea-pigs were injected intratracheally with 1 c c and 1.5 c c, respectively, of the two cultures.

Both were found dead the following day. The blood-agar plates of the culture injected showed a pure culture of staphylococci and smears showed the absence of streptococci. The lungs in both were hemorrhagic and edematous but were compressed (5 c c) by a huge accumulation of chocolate-colored fluid in the pleural cavities (20 c c in each). Both had hemorrhagic placental masses in the uterus; several were detached and being expelled (fig. 9). Sections of both showed large numbers of staphylococci throughout the lungs, especially beneath the pleura, and no streptococci. Cultures from the blood of both showed staphylococci; from the lung, pleural fluid, and hemorrhagic placental masses, large numbers of staphylococci and a few colonies of green-producing streptococci; and from the liver, kidney, and ovaries a small number of staphylococci. The symptoms in the guinea-pig (Guinea-pig 940) injected with 1.5 c c were noted for nine hours prior to death. Respiratory embarrassment at first consisted chiefly of difficulty in expiration; later breathing became easier but exceedingly rapid as from a filling thorax. The animal was examined immediately after death in order to note the condition of the uterus. Violent waves of uterine contraction continued for some minutes. One of the placental masses was partially detached; all were hemorrhagic. The hemorrhagic pleural fluid was immediately injected into the trachea of another guinea-pig, which showed moderately increased respirations immediately after injection, seemed well the following day and remained so for twenty-six days, when it was chloroformed. The pericardial sac was thickened and distended with bloody fluid. The peribronchial and mediastinal lymph glands were edematous and much enlarged. The pleura and lungs were normal. Cultures from the pericardial fluid and lymph glands showed staphylococci.

The points of special interest in the experiments in this case are the high virulency of the strain isolated from the blood, the tendency to produce the same type of lesions over a wide range of dosage, the immunity induced by a previous injection of a culture from influenzal sputum, the extreme contractions of the uterus, and the marked infectiousness of the culture, showing what seems must be considered as a mutation of green-producing streptococcus into staphylococcus.

Case 2787, a man, aged 59, had influenzal pneumonia and pleuritis from which he made a slow recovery. There was little expectoration. A diagnostic puncture of the chest was made Jan. 8, 1919. A small amount of turbid, bloody fluid was aspirated which showed countless numbers of colonies of hemolytic streptococci in pure culture. A suspension in salt solution of one-thirtieth and one-third of the primary growth on a blood-agar plate was injected into the trachea of 2 guinea-pigs, respectively. The former had increased respirations for several days and then recovered; the latter had increased respirations for several days and died two weeks later of abscess and gangrene of the right diaphragmatic lobe, pericarditis, and pleuritis. The pericardium was markedly thickened and distended with gelatinous organizing, fibrinous exudate. The pleural cavity contained a large amount of foul smelling pus communicating with the abscess (fig. 8). Cultures from the blood showed no growth; the pericardial fluid showed staphylococci, the pleural fluid, staphylococci and gram-negative bacilli.

Case 2798, Mr. E. C. B., aged 26, was admitted to the isolation hospital Jan. 7, 1919. He had been taken ill seven days before with cough, general malaise, sore throat, and chills, but he did not ache severely. The temperature on admission was 103 F., but it dropped to normal the following day. The leukocyte count January 8 was 11,400; January 10, 12,500, and January 11, 14,300. The patient had a moderately severe cough in which he raised mucopurulent sputum. No definite chest signs could be detected on physical examination, but the roentgen-ray examination on the day of admission showed slight bronchial infiltration in the left lung, and January 14 a small area of infiltration in the right middle lobe. The patient was discharged from the hospital January 14, after the temperature had been normal for 5 days, although the cough persisted. January 16, he was again admitted to the hospital complaining of a sharp, severe pain in the right lower chest aggravated by breathing, of malaise, and of feeling weak generally. At this time he had fever for five days; he developed outspoken signs of pleuritis over the right side of the chest, and pleural thickening over this area was manifested by roentgen examination January 26. The sputum obtained January 11 showed countless numbers of colonies of hemolytic streptococci, a few green colonies of streptococci, small indifferent colonies of influenza bacilli, and a number of staphylococci.

The culture in glucose brain broth from a single colony of hemolytic streptococcus (which yielded a pure culture of green-producing streptococci on blood-agar plates) was injected into the trachea of Guinea-pig 957, January 13. The leukocyte count was 16,000 and the temperature 102.4 F. The following day the animal seemed ill, respirations were rapid, the temperature was 97 and the leukocyte count was 19,000. On the second day the symptoms were about the same, the temperature was 103.6, and the leukocyte count was 16,500. January 16 the temperature was 102.8, the leukocyte count was 16,500. January 16 the temperature was 102.8, the leukocyte count was 17,000, the respirations were definitely increased, and the animal appeared sick. January 19 it was found dead. The pleural cavity was distended with a large amount of bloody, chocolate-colored fluid, partially walled off in pockets with fibrinous adhesions, and partially obliterated by fibrinous adhesions, and the visceral and parietal pleura and the pericardium were covered with a thick layer of fibrinous material (fig. 7). The lungs were moderately distended (14 c c), moist and edematous on the cut surface, but consolidation was limited to several small areas. Cultures from the blood, pleural fluid, and lung showed a large number of green-producing streptococci and some staphylococci; from the spleen and kidney, a number of green-producing streptococci, and from the liver and suprarenal, no growth.

The attack in this case of influenza was atypical; there was no reduction in leukocytes, and the attack occurred during a quiescent interval between two epidemic waves. The point of special interest is the fact that the findings in the animal injected with a culture from the sputum paralleled the findings in the patient quite accurately in that leukopenia did not occur; the lung lesions were slight, and the involvement of the pleura was the marked lesion.

Case 2809, M. D., a little girl, aged 3, was admitted to the isolation hospital Jan. 8, 1919, in a weak condition with a temperature of 103.4 F., pulse 152, respirations 32, moderate cyanosis, and a severe cough. She had been taken sick that day, and was running a typical course of influenza without apparent lung involvement. The temperature ranged between 101 and 102 degrees for four days, becoming normal on the fifth day. The throat was moderately red; the tonsils were normal, the tongue coated. The day after admission it was noted that the vulva was inflamed and that pus was discharging from the vagina. The condition yielded promptly to irrigations and douching with a weak solution of potassium permanganate. January 12 smears of the vaginal discharge showed a moderate number of leukocytes, many gram-positive, lanceolate diplococci, often in short chains, gram-negative bacilli, some resembling Bacillus coli and many smaller gram-negative bacilli resembling Bacillus influenzae. Blood-agar plates showed a large number of green-producing streptococci, a moderate number of colonies of colon bacilli, and many small colonies resembling Bacillus influenzae. The colonies of the latter were most numerous and the growth more luxuriant immediately surrounding the colonies of the streptococci. Smears of these small indifferent colonies showed gram-positive and gram-negative small bacilli or short-chained diplococci. A subculture on a blood-agar plate of a single colony of the green-producing streptococcus, including some of the small indifferent colonies, yielded pure growth of green colonies of streptococci; of four single colonies resembling Bacillus influenzae no growth was obtained, whereas subcultures from a group of these colonies yielded countless numbers of influenza bacillus-like colonies and a moderate number of green streptococcus colonies. Subcultures in two bottles of glucose-blood broth from the groups of isolated Bacillus influenzae colonies, well separated from green colonies of streptococci, yielded countless numbers of streptococci, blood-agar plates from these showing countless colonies of green-producing streptococci.

The primary culture in glucose brain broth from the vaginal swab was injected into the trachea of 2 guinea-pigs. Both pigs died within twenty-four hours of markedly dilated lungs filled with acute hemorrhagic edema fluid; both developed marked leukopenia, abortion with hemorrhage in the uterus, and both showed gram-positive diplococci in sections of the hemorrhagic edematous areas in the lung (fig. 17). A pure culture of the green-producing streptococcus in glucose brain broth in the second generation was injected into the trachea of 2 guinea-pigs. The female died within forty-eight hours with marked reduction in leukocytes, massive hemorrhagic bronchopneumonia, edematous mucous membrane of the uterus, cervix and vagina, hemorrhages in the cervix and upper portion of the vagina, and a large amount of turbid mucus in the vagina. Smears from mucus in the vault of the vagina showed a moderate number of gram-positive diplococci and a few large gram-negative bacilli. The male recovered and showed moderate reduction in leukocytes; he had fever for several days, but no other noteworthy symptoms.

The streptococcus isolated in this case, in addition to causing characteristic lesions of the lungs, showed marked affinity for the uterus and vagina; it was agglutinated specifically by the monovalent antistreptococcus serum.

Case 3171, Mr. P. H. L., aged 30, was taken with headache, severe aching all over and chilliness Feb. 26, 1919. He felt so sick that he was obliged to go to bed. After resting for a number of days he felt better, but March 2, after a hearty meal, he developed high fever, cough, and a headache with sweating. The following day cyanosis, rapid respirations, crepitant râles and bronchial breathing over the left lower lobe were noted. The next day numerous moist râles were heard over the right lower lobe, and the respirations were labored. The sputum became serous, bloody, and frothy March 5, and the patient died March 6. At necropsy marked bilateral hemorrhagic pneumonia of the greater portion of both lungs and marked hemorrhagic tracheo-broncho-bronchiolitis were found. Histologic examination of the lungs showed marked congestion of the alveoli which were filled with edematous exudate containing few cells.

Cultures from the mucopurulent material in the larynx, trachea, and bronchi showed numerous spreading, slightly hemolyzing streptococci, a moderate number of staphylococci, and hemolytic streptococci. Cultures from the pleural fluid showed a large number of green-producing streptococci and from the glucose broth inoculated with the blood, green-producing streptococci. The primary culture in glucose broth was injected into the trachea of male G. pig

1249. The respirations the following day were extremely rapid and labored, the animal appeared ill, and was found dead the next day. The lungs were huge, 26 c c, and extremely heavy, 21 gm. A large amount of bloody, edematous fluid ran from the cut surface. The whole left lung appeared uniformly consolidated, and most of the right lung showed irregular areas of consolidation, emphysema, and hemorrhagic edema (fig. 3). There were no other lesions. Cultures from the blood, lung, and spleen showed many large, moist, spreading, green colonies of streptococci.

The primary culture in glucose broth from bronchial exudate was injected intraperitoneally into a mouse and into the trachea of a female guinea-pig. The mouse died of peritonitis within twenty-four hours. The guinea-pig died of hemorrhagic bronchopneumonia, hemorrhagic pleuritis, and a hemorrhagic infection of three fetuses with abortion, in forty-eight hours. The cultures showed large numbers of colonies of typical hemolytic streptococci and a moderate number of staphylococci. The primary culture of the pleural fluid was injected into a male guinea-pig. It appeared ill the following day and sat humped up; its hair was rough, and the voice was hoarse. It gradually improved during the following four days and remained well.

The results in this case, in addition to the production of the characteristic lung and uterine lesions, are of interest because of the bacteriologic findings in the blood, pleural fluid and the lung exudate, and in showing changes in the character of these organisms as they were passed through animals, the green-producing streptococcus from the blood acquiring the property of producing large, spreading, moist, green colonies, and the spreading, slightly hemolyzing streptococcus from the bronchial exudate becoming a typical hemolytic streptococcus.

Case 3175, Mrs. C. S., aged 24, was operated on March 1, 1919, on account of recurring attacks of appendicitis which were considered sufficiently serious to warrant operation for the removal of the appendix even though she was four months pregnant. The patient did well for five days and then developed fever, cough, dyspnea, mucopurulent and bloody sputum, rapidly progressing pneumonia, and pleuritis of the right side. She aborted on the seventh day after the operation and died from acute pulmonary edema on the eighth. Necropsy was refused. The sputum obtained March 7 was purulent and chocolate colored. The blood-agar plate showed countless numbers of staphylococci.

The human fetus (male) was brought to the laboratory while fresh; the membranes had not ruptured. The trunk measured 10 cm. in length. There was marked edema in the anterior cervical region surrounding the trachea and in the left abdominal rectus muscle. The left pleural cavity was free from fluid; the right contained a large amount of turbid hemorrhagic fluid fully 5 c c. The pericardial sac contained a small amount of turbid fluid free from blood. Blood-agar plate cultures from the brain, intestinal contents, pericardial fluid, and edema fluid from the subcutaneous tissue remained sterile. Glucose brain-broth cultures of hemorrhagic fluid from the right pleural cavity, pericardial fluid, and subcutaneous edema fluid showed short-chained streptococci and staphylococci. Sections of brain, kidneys, suprarenals, liver, and spleen showed no noteworthy lesions and no bacteria. Sections of the right lung showed a moderate number of diplococci in the pleura and subpleura of the right side (fig. 22).

The sputum containing streptococci in addition to staphylococci was injected into the trachea of 3 female guinea-pigs. All died within twenty-four hours from hemorrhagic edema of the lung, and hemorrhagic pleuritis, and all aborted.

Two showed interstitial pulmonary emphysema, one in the form of pleural blebs only, the other in frothy fluid in the pleural cavity due to rupture of one of these blebs. Cultures from all yielded staphylococci and streptococci. In order to determine the infecting power of the staphylococcus, the culture in glucose blood broth from a single colony was injected into the trachea of another female guinea-pig. It died within twenty-four hours from hemorrhagic edema, hemorrhagic pleuritis, and abortion, and showed staphylococci in the blood and pleural fluid in pure culture. Sections of the lung of one of these pigs showed the characteristic hemorrhagic edema with slight cellular infiltration and large numbers of streptococci and staphylococci in the lung (fig. 21).

A large white and gray cat (cat 24), with advanced pregnancy, a leukocyte count of 11,600 and a temperature of 101.4 F., was injected in the trachea March 17, 1919, with 4 c c of glucose-blood-broth culture of streptococcus in the second culture from one of the guinea-pigs. March 18 the temperature was 101.4, the white count 6,600, and the animal appeared well. March 19 and 20 it appeared quite well but refused food, and the temperature was 102.2. March 21, 12 m., it was found in labor; one kitten was born. By 6 p. m. 4 kittens had been born; all were alive and appeared nearly full-time size. March 22 the cat and kittens appeared well, but the cat refused food; the kittens nursed. March 23, one kitten was found dead; the cat refused food and appeared sick. March 24, another kitten was found dead, and a third was sick. The cat was worse, refused food, the respirations had increased, and a vaginal discharge of bloody pus had developed. March 25 the third kitten was dead and the fourth was in a dying condition. The cat, which was so weak that she was just able to stand, and had a marked diarrhea and a temperature of 104, was chloroformed. The uterus showed large numbers of small submucous hemorrhages; the mucous membrane was swollen in places, necrotic, and covered with a thick layer of chocolate-colored pus. The liver showed marked fatty degeneration, the kidneys, acute nephritis. Smears from the uterine exudate contained many staphylococci and streptococci. In cultures from the uterus were countless numbers of colonies of staphylococci and green-producing streptococci and number of spreading gram-negative bacilli; from the blood, liver and spleen, a few colonies of staphylococci and streptococci; from the suprarenal and kidney, no growth. Sections of the uterus showed a thick layer of leukocytes covering the endometrium, containing enormous numbers of staphylococci and streptococci. Fetus 1 showed no lesions. Cultures from the blood showed large numbers of stphylococci and a few green streptococci. Fetus 2 was accidentally discarded by the animal keeper. Fetus 3 showed 5,800 leukocytes in the blood and a small amount of blood-tinged pleural fluid, staphylococci, and a few green streptococci in the blood and pleural fluid, together with a spreading gram-negative bacillus. Sections of the lung showed gram-positive diplococci in the subpleural space duplicating the findings in the human fetus (fig. 22). Fetus 4 showed no gross lesions, but the same organisms in blood and urine as in fetus 3.

The points of particular interest in this case are the invasion of the fetus with lesions of the pleura caused by the organisms found in the sputum, the production of marked lesions in the lung and pleura, including interstitial emphysema of the lung in guinea-pigs, the marked affinity for the placenta, the invasion with the production of pleural lesions of the fetuses in the cat, and the sensitiveness of the streptococcus to oxygen.

The findings in the patients and the results obtained in each case reported herewith in detail are quite accurately representative of the findings of the whole series studied. I have purposely included one case (case 2787) in which leukopenia was absent and in which the diagnosis of influenza was doubtful because the results in the animal injected paralleled so accurately the findings in the patient. The points noted which deserve special emphasis are the marked affinity of the streptococci for the epithelium of the lung, even after intraperitoneal injection (fig. 11), the occurrence of characteristic lesions of the lung and pleura, the frequent involvement of the uterus resulting in abortion, and the very great similarity of the results obtained in the animals and the findings in cases 2769, 2770, 2787, 2798, 2809 and 3175. The findings in the little girl who developed vaginitis during her influenzal attack leave little doubt that the vaginal discharge was the result of localization and infection by the streptococcus in the uterus and vagina. The localization of the streptococcus in the pleura of the fetus (fig. 22) of the pregnant patient (case 3175), and in the pleura of the fetuses in the pregnant cat injected into the trachea with the sputum of this case, when absent in other tissues, may be regarded as elective localization of bacteria of high order. On the basis of these findings a study of the tissues of fetuses and of the new-born said to have contracted influenza in utero should be undertaken, since the micro-organism found in the affected tissues under these conditions may be considered responsible for the production of the lesions, and thus add materially to our knowledge of the etiology of influenza.

EXPERIMENTS WITH FILTRATES OF LUNG EMULSIONS AND CULTURES

After it was noted that intratracheal application of the bacteria from patients with influenza had marked effect it was thought that this method of injection might prove valuable in studying the effects of filtrates of material from influenza. Exceedingly small forms of diplococci were frequently seen in smears of sputum, in throat swabs, and in cultures from influenza, especially in deep tubes of glucose brain broth. It was thought possible that the preformed toxic products in filtrates of cultures and lung emulsions might injure the respiratory epithelium and thus facilitate growth of the few organisms which might pass through the filter, and, since the lung appeared to be the point of predilection of these organisms, growth might occur when cultures were introduced in this manner even though control cultures on artificial mediums were negative. Moreover, valuable light might be thrown on the question of the presence or absence of a filtrable virus in this disease. I wish here to summarize the experiments done along this line. The filtrates studied were from sputum obtained, early in the course of the disease, from the lungs of dead animals, with the characteristic picture following injection of sputum or cultures from sputum, and from cultures from the sputum during life and from the blood and lung exudate after death of patients who had died from influenza.

Berkefeld N filters, Mandler filters, and dense unglazed porcelain filters were used. The filtrates from the lungs were obtained by making an approximately 10% emulsion of the pneumonic or hemorrhagic lung tissue in salt solution, centrifuging it fractionally, and filtering the opalescent fluid by the aid of a partial vacuum obtained with a water suction pump. The cultures of influenzal material in the tall tubes of broth were incubated twenty-four to seventy-two hours and filtered without centrifugation. The efficiency of the filters used was controlled with Bacillus prodigiosus, and they were found to remove these small organisms in every instance. Cultures from the filtrates were made on blood agar, and in deep tubes of glucose brain broth and in tissue broth. The brain, which weighed approximately 1.5 gm., was added to each tall tube of glucose broth before autoclaving; the tissue (rabbit kidney) was added in a sterile manner to meat infusion broth sterilized by the fractional method. The inoculations in these mediums were made with at least 0.5 c c of the filtrate. The tubes were incubated at 33 to 35 C. for a week before they were discarded. Altogether, 15 filtrates have been made and studied. The cultures on blood agar were negative in all. Those in broth remained free from growth in 13, while 2 (filtrates 6 and 7) yielded definite growths. In the former, filtration was slow; in the latter, rapid. In 4 of the broth cultures clouding was distinct, but smears and subcultures were negative.

The animal experiments consisted of intratracheal injection of the usual dose of the filtrate itself, of the "negative" cultures in the broth, and in some instances of the respective culture and lung emulsion as controls. Altogether, 42 guinea-pigs were injected intratracheally, 30 with the filtrate directly, and 12 with the "negative" cultures from filtrates. Of these, 13 died; 10 were anesthetized for examination, and 19 recovered. The immediate symptoms following injection of the filtrates were indistinguishable from those following injection of the cultures. Death from fatal infections occurred somewhat later following injection of the filtrates than following injection of the corresponding cultures or emulsions. The lesions were similar. Emphysema, hemorrhage and edema of the lung, with coalescing areas of lobular pneumonia and hemorrhagic pleuritis, were striking features. Microscopically dilated alveoli filled with blood and edema fluid with marked desquamation and destruction of the epithelium of the alveoli and bronchi with relatively slight leukocytic infiltration formed the dominant picture. Of the cultures from the 13 guinea-pigs that died, 8 showed green-producing streptococci as the predominating organism, 2 showed Bacillus bronchisepticus in addition, 1 Bacillus coli, and in 1 the cultures remained negative; cultures were not made from 1 guinea-pig. In the 2 that showed Bacillus bronchisepticus an old pneumonia, easily distinguished from the hemorrhagic lesions due to the injection, was present. Sections of the lungs showed gram-positive diplococci which were most numerous along the alveolar wall. The 10 anesthetized animals had the usual immediate symptoms, increased respirations for from two to three days. Two were anesthetized while the symptoms were severe and progressing. The findings in these were similar to those in the animals that died (guinea-pig 882, guinea-pig 885). The lungs of the rest were only slightly emphysematous; hemorrhagic edema with little infiltration in relatively small areas in the lung was noted in most of the animals. The cultures in these showed green-producing streptococci in 3, no growth in 6, and in 1 the cultures were contaminated accidentally. Symptoms in those that recovered were either absent the day after injection or consisted of increased respirations, lessened activity, and ruffled fur for several days.

Six animals were injected with heated filtrates; all showed the usual immediate symptoms of anaphylactic shock, somewhat less severe but otherwise comparable with the symptoms in animals injected with the corresponding unheated filtrate. They had no symptoms subsequently and all remained well.

Leukocyte counts were made in 26 animals injected with filtrates. In 17 a marked or decided drop in leukocytes occurred, in 2 a slight drop, while in 7 no noteworthy change occurred. None showed leukocytosis. The leukopenia was usually present twenty-four and forty-eight hours after injection, after which return to normal occurred in the animals that recovered; in those that died it usually persisted, and sometimes the count became progressively lower until death (guinea-pig 888). The drop was not usually as marked as that following injection of cultures.

Leukopenia occurred following injection of filtrates from sputum, from lung emulsions, and from broth cultures of freshly isolated strains. Heating to 60 C. for thirty minutes and to the boiling point for ten minutes was found not to destroy the substance causing a diminution in leukocytes, nor did heating destroy the property causing immediate symptoms of anaphylactic shock.

Two filtrates that produced marked effects in animals on intratracheal injection were injected subcutaneously into 3 persons in doses of 4 c c for one, and 5 c c for each of the other two. All developed only slight local reaction and none fever or constitutional reaction. One person's throat was swabbed with a mixture of 2 filtrates, one prepared from the lung, and the other from a culture from the blood of case 2800. No symptoms followed. These filtrates (5 c c) were also injected subcutaneously in each of two persons. No symptoms occurred other than a negligible local reaction.

The results following injection of 3 filtrates (filtrates 2, 3 and 4) in a series of animals, and the derivation of the strain from which they were prepared, are summarized in the tabulation. Two guinea-pigs (guinea-pigs 908 and 909) injected with the fresh filtrate and the 2 (guinea-pigs 918 and 921) injected with the "negative" culture in glucose brain broth developed the characteristic symptoms and findings; 1 (guinea-pig 926) injected with the fresh filtrate remained well. The filtrate from the pneumonic lung of one of these (guinea-pig 908) was injected intratracheally while fresh into 4 guinea-pigs (guinea-pigs 930, 931, 933 and 934), and after being heated to 60 C. for thirty minutes was injected in 2 guinea-pigs (guinea-pigs 929 and 932). All showed decided immediate symptoms and 1 died in ten minutes of anaphylactic shock. Three of the rest had increased respirations for several days and then recovered, while the other 2 showed no symptoms. The filtrate from the pneumonic lung of guinea-pig 874 was injected into the trachea of 4 guinea-pigs (guinea-pigs 882, 888, 919 and 923). Three developed symptoms and died. The usual findings were noted.

Green-producing streptococci in pure culture, or together with staphylococci, were isolated from the characteristic lesions in all that died. Injection of the corresponding cultures into other guinea-pigs was followed by very similar lesions (to be reported elsewhere). The parallelism was so striking that the mortality in the third animal passage (filtrate 3) was higher than in the fourth animal passage (filtrates 2 and 4). Sections of the lungs showed all the characteristic features peculiar to the influenza strains, including the localization of the streptococci. From the filtrate experiments it may be concluded that the green-producing streptococci from influenza in cultures and lung exudate may pass through filters through which Bacillus prodigiosus will not pass, and that they can multiply and grow when injected into the trachea of guinea-pigs, even though cultures remain negative.

Four protocols are given as illustrations:

Guinea-pig 921, weighing 260 gm., was injected intratracheally Jan. 6, 1919, with 1.5 c c of negative culture of the Berkefeld filtrate of the lung emulsion of Guinea-pig 851 (filtrate 3, see tabulation). January 7 the blood-agar plate from the nose made before injection showed a moderate number of colonies of Bacillus coli and staphylococci. January 8 the animal seemed ill and respirations were increased. January 9 and 10 there was marked increase in respirations and the animal seemed sick. January 11 it was found dead. The lungs were found moderately distended; their total volume was 9 c c. The diaphragmatic lobes were firm and heavy. The left lobe contained a whitish area of consolidation 1 by 0.5 cm.) along the margin surrounded by large areas of hemorrhage and edema. The cut surface of the lung was moist and a large amount of bloody fluid escaped. The peribronchial lymph glands were edematous. The uterus was small but showed a circumscribed area containing numerous punctate hemorrhages. On the flat muscles on the inner aspect of both thighs were numerous small whitish necrotic areas. The kidneys showed marked cloudy swelling. The left nostril and the corresponding sinus were filled with mucopus. The mucous membrane of the nose, trachea, and bronchi was edematous and congested. January 13 blood-agar plate cultures from the blood, the areas of consolidation, and edema fluid of the lung, the kidney, and mucus from the right and left horns of the uterus, contained large numbers of streptococci; emulsons of the muscles with lesions, contained 70 green colonies of streptococci; and the emulsions of the normal muscle, contained no streptococci.

Guinea-pig 908, weighing 350 gm., was injected intratracheally Jan. 4, 1919, with 1 c c of Berkefeld filtrate from Guinea-pig 851 (filtrate 3). The nostrils were dry at the time the cultures from the nose were made. January 5, at 11 a. m., the animal appeared to be quite well with slight increase in respiration. At 1 p. m. it suffered from a brief attack of shortness of breath and paroxysms of coughing; the voice was clear. At 5:30 p. m. the animal was hoarse and respirations were definitely increased. A violent attack of shortness of breath followed the making of a second culture from the nose. The blood-agar plate of secretion from the nose made before injection showed a large number of staphylococci and a few green-producing streptococci. January 6 a large number of staphylococci and green-producing streptococci were found in the cultures from the nose made the day after injection. At 9:45 a. m. the animal was short of breath. It had an attack resembling anaphylactic shock; the eyes were watery, the nostrils dry. At 3 p. m. the respirations were rapid and an expiratory grunt had developed. At 8:30 p. m. the animal was very weak; respirations were extremely rapid and difficult, and it often made violent efforts to get its breath. It died in one of these paroxysms. The lungs were found to be extremely distended; their volume was 17 c c and the weight was 14 gm. A large part of both lungs was consolidated. The cut surfaces everywhere were extremely moist; a large amount of bloody, frothy fluid escaped and the trachea and bronchi were filled with a similar fluid. An uninvolved portion of the lung was extremely emphysematous and the alveoli appeared to be at the rupturing point. There were no areas of old lung lesions. The mucous membrane of the nose, the trachea, and the bronchi was hyperemic. The peribronchial lymph glands were edematous. The mucous membrane of the uterus was hyperemic. January 7, blood-agar plate cultures from the blood, kidney, liver, brain, and mucous membrane from the right and left horns of the uterus were sterile; in cultures from the pneumonic lung countless numbers of green colonies of streptococci were found; and from the nose and the mucous membrane of the turbinate bones, countless green colonies of streptococci and a large numbers of staphylococci. Smears from the lung showed large numbers of gram-positive diplococci and those from the nose, gram positive diplococci and staphylococci. No organisms resembling the influenza bacillus were found.

Guinea-pig 888, weighing 490 gm., was injected intratracheally Jan. 3, 1919, with 1.5 c c of the porcelain filtrate of the lung of Guinea-pig 874 (filtrate 2, see tabulation). Before injection the leukocyte count was 10,500. The nostrils were dry when cultures were made. The animal coughed violently several times while being injected and had shortness of breath for 15 minutes following the injection. The temperature rose to 103.4 degrees. January 6, the condition of the animal was about the same although the shortness of breath had increased somewhat. The cultures from the nose showed large numbers of green-producing streptococci and moderate numbers of staphylococci. January 9 the animal was found very weak and short of breath. It acted strangely, constantly pushing its head into the side of the basket or under its mate until it was completely exhausted. At 9 a. m. its temperature was 94; the white count 4,300. At 11 a. m. it died during a violent effort at respiration. The lungs were found distended (14 c c); there was an extensive bronchopneumonia, a mild pleuritis, four hemorrhagic areas, markedly recent placental attachments, one in the right and three in the left horn of the uterus. There was a large amount of turbid mucus in the uterus. January 11 blood-agar plate cultures of the blood were negative; those of the lung showed countless numbers of colonies of streptococci and a few staphylococci.

Guinea-pig 882, weighing 300 gm., was injected intratracheally Jan. 2, 1919, at 10 p. m. with 2 c c of porcelain filtrate of the lung emulsion from Guinea-pig 874 (filtrate 2). Cultures from the nose contained large numbers of staphylococci and diphtheroid bacilli. January 3 at 7:30 a. m. the animal appeared quite well, and without definite shortness of breath. At 11 a. m. there was definite shortness of breath. Much mucus was noted in the left nostril. This was cultivated and was found to contain a large number of green colonies of streptococci and a moderate number of staphylococci. January 4 respiration was increased and the animal had grown thin, weighing 260 gm. January 5 it seemed ill; the nostrils were moist; the temperature was 103.6. It was etherized; the lung was found moderately distended and the left anterior lobe completely consolidated, uniformly grayish-red, and mottled on the cut surface. The consolidated areas were moist and surrounded by hemorrhagic edema. The uterus contained a hemorrhagic area, one in each horn, and bloody mucus in the fundus. In the right horn was found a chocolate-colored, hemorrhagic mass. January 7 blood-agar plate cultures of the blood showed a few green-producing streptococci; of the lung and nose, large numbers of green colonies of streptococci and a moderate number of Staphylococcus aureus; from edematous fluid of the lung, a moderate number of green colonies of streptococci; from the right horn of the uterus moderate numbers of green colonies of streptococci and one of staphylococci. Cultures from the liver and kidney were negative.

Guinea-pig 885, weighing 350 gm., was injected intratracheally Jan. 2, 1919, with 2 c c of Berkefeld filtrate with emulsion of the pneumonic lung of Guinea-pig 869. Cultures taken from the nose before injection showed staphylococci only. January 3 at 7:30 a. m. the animal appeared quite well; there was no apparent shortness of breath; at 11 a. m. the respirations were increased. Smears from the nose showed large numbers of diplococci, often in short chains. January 4 cultures from the nose made twelve hours after injection showed many staphylococci and green colonies of streptococci. The animal appeared sick, coughed and sneezed at intervals; respirations were rapid. January 5 shortness of breath had diminished. The animal was etherized. The lungs were moderately emphysematous (11 c c); one area of consolidation 1 by 0.7 cm. was found in the right diaphragmatic lobe. The pleura was dull over this area. The cut surface was markedly edematous and a large amount of bloody, frothy fluid escaped. A number of smaller areas of consolidation were found in the left diaphragmatic lobe. The peribronchial lymph glands were enlarged and edematous. There was mucopurulent material in the nostril. January 7, blood-agar plate cultures from the blood, liver, kidney and testicle were negative; those from the pneumonic lung showed large numbers of green colonies of streptococci, and those from the nose showed many staphylococci and green colonies of streptococci.

EXPERIMENTS INDICATING THE TRANSMISSION OF INFLUENZAL INFECTION BY CONTACT

The question of the possible transmission of infection by contact in the animals was also studied. Uninjected guinea-pigs and guinea-pigs injected with broth or salt solution were caged with animals inoculated intratracheally with cultures. All of the 8 uninjected pigs, and the 5 injected with salt solution remained well. In 5 of the former and 3 of the latter the nasal mucous membrane was injured with a sterile flexible wire coil when making cultures from the nose. Two of 10 guinea-pigs injected intratracheally as controls with glucose broth became ill with symptoms suggesting respiratory involvement. Both of these animals were caged with guinea-pigs injected with highly virulent cultures. One died in four days from hemorrhagic bronchopneumonia. Cultures from the blood and lung showed countless numbers of green-producing colonies of streptococci. The other died ten days after injection, with a large amount of a bloody fluid in the chest and marked bronchopneumonia. The blood contained green-producing streptococci and the pleural fluid, staphylococci. The green-producing streptococcus from both guinea-pigs was agglutinated specifically by the monovalent serum. It corresponded morphologically and culturally with the streptococci from influenza and neither strain fermented inulin. During the course of these experiments the supply of normal guinea-pigs was large and no epidemic of pneumonia occurred. Examination of those that died spontaneously was made as a further check on the experiments. Five were found with lesions in lungs. These lungs were different in appearance from those that followed injection of the strains from influenza. They were small, the pneumonia process, usually old, was most marked in the anterior lobes instead of the posterior lobes, and the more recent consolidations were ill defined, often resembling atelectatic areas. The cultures from these showed Bacillus bronchisepticus and two showed pneumococci. The latter were not agglutinated by pneumococcus type serums nor by the monovalent serum.

SYMPTOMS AND GROSS LESIONS FOLLOWING INTRATRACHEAL INJECTION OF INFLUENZAL MATERIAL

The more marked effects of intratracheal than of intraperitoneal injection were very apparent. The respiratory embarrassment on intratracheal injection, particularly in the infections that terminate fatally, was often marked immediately after injection and extreme the day following. The thorax was often in full expansion, the eyes had a glazed appearance, lacrimation was frequent, the mucous membranes were cyanotic, the breathing was difficult, rapid, irregular, and chiefly abdominal. The animals were restless and irritable, the fur ruffled. Expiratory efforts were often violent, and recurring coughing and choking spells resembling the bronchial spasm of acute anaphylaxis were common. The degree of respiratory embarrassment in the animals that died within twenty-four or forty-eight hours was found to vary considerably during the hours of observation. There were periods of some minutes when breathing, although rapid, was quite free and easy, and the animals often ate food or drank water. The quiescent intervals were followed by a return of marked difficulty in breathing, during which time, bloody, edematous fluid sometimes escaped from the nostrils. Finally the animals, while perfectly conscious, and bending every effort at breathing, would run about aimlessly with the head extended, often jump out of the basket in violent efforts to get breath, and die with symptoms of acute anaphylactic shock, and in addition with large amounts of hemorrhagic edema fluid escaping from the nostrils. The symptoms in these animals were clearly those of a prolonged anaphylaxis.

The lungs in the animals that died early were always voluminous, dark purplish red, and showed marked hemorrhage and edema with little or no true consolidation. This was true even in those in which the toxicity of the culture killed them in the course of a few hours (figs. 2 and 6), and even following intranasal insufflation. The dark, hemorrhagic and edematous areas often occupied almost the entire lung, but they were always more marked in the posterior lobes. The emphysema was often so extreme that the alveoli were distended to the rupturing point and in some instances rupture was indicated by the finding of subpleural, interstitial emphysema and by the escape of air into the pleural cavity and in the mediastinal and subcutaneous tissues about the chest. The cut surface was extremely wet and large amounts of hemorrhagic edema fluid escaped. The hemorrhagic, edematous areas were often wedge-shaped with the base toward the pleura, or peribronchial. The cyanosis in some of these animals became extreme. The blood was very dark and often remained liquid. In the animals that showed the symptoms described, and that died in two or three days, the lungs were also extremely voluminous and presented the picture of massive pseudolobar pneumonia. At times the consolidation involved almost the entire lung (fig. 3), but although most or all of certain lobes were involved the consolidation was not uniform or complete, but consisted of coalescing areas of lobular pneumonia varying in age and surrounded by areas of hemorrhagic edema. These lungs also contained large amounts of a thin, watery, bloody exudate, and were extremely wet on the cut surface; this was in sharp contrast to the areas of consolidation noted following intratracheal injection of type pneumococci. The smaller bronchi were often found plugged with a bloody exudate, and the mucous membrane of the trachea and larger bronchi was extremely red, and the lumen filled with a blood-tinged froth. These characteristic changes in the lung tended to occur also in the white rat and monkey. A small percentage of the guinea-pigs (about 10%), which showed soon after injection the symptoms of respiratory embarrassment just described, might live for some days with extremely rapid but not difficult breathing, and then die with compressed lungs from hemorrhagic fluid filling the thorax. In these the symptoms of anaphylaxis might be noted at intervals. Usually, however, death seemed to occur from want of air from a rapidly filling thorax. If death in these animals occurred late, the picture was that of hemorrhagic empyema. The fluid in the pleural cavities, whether death occurred early or late, was almost without exception tinged with blood and contained a relatively small amount of fibrin.

Some animals with not very marked symptoms recovered either in a few days or died at a later period. The symptoms of those that recovered usually consisted of a varying degree of increased respirations, of cyanosis of the mucous membrane with evidence of general illness in loss of action and weight, and in fever. The animals sat humped up and with ruffled hair. The drop in leukocytes lasted for from one to three days. When these animals were anesthetized for examination relatively little lung involvement was found, consisting of irregular areas of partial consolidation, often lobular and peribronchial with hemorrhage and edema, while some showed no lung involvement even when examined within four or five days after injection. The tracheobronchial lymph glands were almost constantly found enlarged and markedly edematous on the cut surface.

The animals that died from three to ten days or more after injection usually showed bronchopneumonia of varying extent associated with emphysema and hemorrhagic edema of various degrees of intensity. In some the pneumonia was lobar in distribution, but lobular in character. Some of the animals developed mucopurulent discharge from the nose associated with maxillary sinusitis and marked redness of the nasal mucous membrane. Occasionally after recovery seemed to be complete there was a return of respiratory embarrassment and death occurred from hemorrhagic edema associated with well defined areas of grayish bronchopneumonia. In not a few of these localized abscesses were noted in the areas showing consolidation.

Cultures from the blood of the animals that died within forty-eight hours were usually positive, but the number of colonies was relatively small, while in those that died later the cultures usually remained sterile. The cultures from the lung and pleural exudates were always positive in the animals that died soon after intratracheal injection, but were often negative in the animals anesthetized while recovering. The relative preponderance of the different strains isolated is shown in table 3. In some animals that died in from ten days to two weeks or more after injection, an entirely different picture supervened. In these the respirations became progressively slower as unconsciousness, great weakness, and a tendency to retraction of the head developed. In a few instances the animals appeared mentally deranged. The lungs were usually small, although occasionally there was moderate emphysema and lesions were slight or wholly absent. The brain and cord were soft, the cerebrospinal fluid was clear but increased in amount; the meninges were edematous and congested. Cultures from the brain and cord substance and spinal fluid were usually negative on blood-agar plates, but in some instances yielded green-producing streptococci in tall tubes of glucose brain broth. The blood in these was always sterile.

MICROSCOPIC ANATOMY OF THE LUNGS

The microscopic findings in the lungs of guinea-pigs varied greatly, depending on the method of injection and on how long after injection the animals survived. In those injected intraperitoneally or subcutaneously the lung findings were relatively slight and consisted of localized hemorrhage and edema with a minimal amount of leukocytic infiltration and desquamation of alveolar epithelium. The localization of the streptococci in the tissues about the capillaries and in the swollen and degenerating alveolar epithelial cells in their normal position or about the desquamated cells which showed nuclear degeneration was a striking picture (figs. 10 and 11). But the lungs of the animals injected intratracheally showed the changes that have come to be regarded as more or less characteristic of influenzal pneumonia. They showed marked distention of alveoli and of alveolar ducts with red blood cells, precipitated serum and a varying number of desquamated degenerating epithelial cells often resembling polymorphonuclear leukocytes, almost complete absence of leukocytes in the acute lesions (figs. 12, 16 and 17), and relatively few leukocytes, even in the more advanced stages of consolidation (figs. 13 and 15a). This picture was in sharp contrast to the consolidation due to type pneumococci (fig. 18a) and the consolidations noted occasionally following injection of the bacteria from normal throats. Besides the marked edema and hemorrhage, probably the most striking change noted in the lungs of these animals was the marked and widely disseminated areas showing necrosis of alveolar epithelial cells and interalveolar capillaries (fig. 19a), also a picture in sharp contrast to that noted following injection of type pneumococci (fig. 19b). The latter finding was strikingly similar to that first noted and so clearly described by LeCount in the case of influenzal pneumonia in man. In the experimental animal in which dosage, place of inoculation, and duration of experiment could be controlled, the cause of this necrosis and the resulting hemorrhage and edema has been found to be due to the localization and growth of the micro-organisms in these structures. The number of organisms was often so large that the outline of alveoli and alveolar ducts could readily be made out with the low power in sections stained by Gram-Weigert by means of the dark lines due to huge numbers of streptococci revealed under higher magnifications (figs. 14c, 15b and 16b). This, too, was in sharp contrast to the even distribution of type pneumococci throughout the highly cellular exudate filling the alveoli (fig. 18b) in experiments in lobar pneumonia in the guinea-pig.

The marked edema and dilatation in the perivascular lymph channels noted in many sections was likewise associated with the presence of enormous numbers of Gram-staining diplococci (fig. 20). Moreover, marked hemorrhagic pleuritis was invariably accompanied by the localization and growth of the micro-organisms in enormous numbers in the subpleural lymphatics (figs. 20, 21 and 22).

It has been possible to study the reparative process of the lungs in animals that were recovering from the effects of injections. The striking feature in the cellular reaction throughout was the relatively small part played by polymorphonuclear leukocytes and the large part played by the proliferated fixed tissue cells, probably endothelial leukocytes and the marked proliferation of epithelial cells.

Distinctive features in the gross and microscopic findings were lacking in the lungs of animals that died soon after injection of the various bacteria, green-producing streptococci, hemolytic streptococci, and staphylococci, except that the hemolytic streptococus tended to invade the pleura and produce hemorrhagic empyema more than the green-producing streptococcus. This is in accord with the findings in the lungs of persons dying from influenzal pneumonia, reported by Blanton and Irons. In the animals that lived for a longer period after injection of mixtures staphylococci were isolated in relatively large numbers, and the sections showed staphylococci in larger numbers or in pure form in the localized areas showing marked leukocytic infiltration, and in abscesses when streptococci were the predominating organisms in the larger intervening areas of hemorrhagic edema showing few leukocytes. The tendency of staphylococci to displace the streptococcal flora in the prolonged experiment even when pure cultures of the streptococci had been injected was often a striking feature (case *2787*, fig. 8). These findings in general are in accord with those in human lungs described by Lord,[13] Weichselbaum,[23] Kuskow,[9] and others in previous epidemics of influenza, and by Le Count,[11, 12] MacCallum,[17] Bell,[2] Chickering and Park,[5] Lucke, Wight and Kime,[15] Opie,[18] Lubarsch,[14] Lyon,[16] and others during the recent epidemic.

Altogether, the virulency more than the species of organism injected determined whether hemorrhagic edema with slight leukocytic infiltration, or bronchopneumonia with marked leukocytic infiltration dominated the picture. As a rule, the leukocytic infiltration in the lung occurred more rapidly and to a greater degree in the animals that showed relatively slight leukopenia or even leukocytosis, and in those injected with cultures from patients with mild attacks who had little or no reduction or even a moderate increase in the leukocyte count than in animals injected with strains from cases showing marked leukopenia.

LESIONS OF THE FEMALE GENERATIVE ORGANS AND OF TISSUES OTHER THAN THOSE OF THE LUNG

By far the most important effects or lesions which have been noted outside of the respiratory tract were those of the female generative organs, especially the uterus, and those of the intestinal tract. A consideration of the latter is reserved for a separate paper.

The effect on the female generative organs in influenzal infection is so marked that many authors regard this as of diagnostic importance. The symptoms most commonly encountered are the occurrence of menstruation for the first time in young girls, of intermenstrual hemorrhages in women in whom the menstrual function has been established, its recurrence after the menopause, and the marked tendency to abortions associated with a high mortality rate in pregnant women.

We have injected, altogether, 98 female guinea-pigs, 76 intratracheally and 22 intraperitoneally or subcutaneously with bacteria from influenza. Of these, 61 died as the result of the injection (62%), and 37 either recovered or were anesthetized as recovery appeared likely, or after being caged with males for several months.

A study of the uterus and the other generative organs was made in 75 guinea-pigs, 57 injected into the trachea and 18 intraperitoneally or subcutaneously. Of the 75, 34 were undoubtedly pregnant at the time of injection as shown by examination after death. Only 6 of these showed normal uteri and normal placental masses when examined.

Four were anesthetized, and 2 died in one and eight days, respectively, from the effects of the injection. The cultures from the uterus in 5 were negative; 1 showed a few green-producing streptococci. In the remaining 28 pregnant guinea-pigs the uterus was either found empty with hemorrhagic areas marking the site of placental attachment or it contained one or more detached or attached hemorrhagic placental masses (fig. 9). Cultures from the hemorrhagic placental masses and bloody mucous in the uterus in these often showed exceedingly large numbers of the bacteria injected.

The uterus of the 27 guinea-pigs that died which were not pregnant showed a varying number of hemorrhagic areas in the endometrium. These were usually small in number and the individual hemorrhages relatively small, but in some instances, even in young guinea-pigs, the hemorrhages were more extensive and occurred over wide areas (fig. 9). They almost always occurred in the horns and rarely in the body of the uterus, cervix, or vagina. Lesions of the latter, however, were noted in the guinea-pigs injected with the streptococcus from the vaginal discharge in case 2809. Marked evidence of infection of the mucous membrane was usually limited to the areas marking placental attachment. In these and in the hemorrhagic placental masses, large numbers of the organisms injected were demonstrable in sections. There was a marked difference between the strains with respect to their power to invade the uterus. In some, all animals injected aborted; in others few or none. The affinity for the uterus was particularly marked in the cultures from the patient (case 3175) who aborted. Intratracheal injections of the sputum in a series of female guinea-pigs and a cat were followed by localization in the uterus and abortion in every animal injected.

The effects in the lung associated with marked bronchial spasm and emphysema, the finding in animals of violent contractions in the uterus immediately after death, and in some instances when anesthetized, and the absence of demonstrable infection either in the placental site or the mucous membrane of the uterus in some of the animals injected, are good reasons for the belief that the emptying of the uterus may be due in some instances to the violent contractions of the uterus from the formation and circulation of "anaphylatoxin" and may not always be the result of actual localization of the bacteria at the placental side.

Lesions of the ovary were relatively rare. In some instances, however, one or both were edematous, fully twice the normal size, and in sections evidence of degeneration of cells in the granular layer associated with edema and leukocytic infiltration in the graafian follicles were noted. Lesions in the interstitial tissues of the ovary were not found.

Cultures were made from the sections in the uterine horns in 75 guinea-pigs. In these the amount of material cultivated usually consisted of only one or two drops from the ends of a small pipet. Green-producing streptococci in varying numbers were isolated in pure culture or together with hemolytic streptococci and staphylococci in 28 animals, hemolytic streptococci in 10, and staphylococci in 25.

Altogether, 10 female guinea-pigs were injected with the control cultures, including those from normal throats, from cases of simple nasopharyngitis, and with type pneumococci from lobar pneumonia. Of these 10 were pregnant. Only 3 showed slight lesions of the uterus or placental masses and only 1 aborted. Cultures were made from the uterus in 10. One showed a few colonies of staphylococci; the rest remained sterile. It is thus apparent that the marked affinity for the uterus and the high incidence of abortions in the animals injected with the influenzal strains is not shared by the control strains. When we were dealing with controlled conditions the effects on the female generative organs in the guinea-pig paralleled in so far as is possible those observed in women.

In order to determine whether other effects on the female generative organs might not have occurred following injection of these strains, the female guinea-pigs that survived were mated with males and kept under observation for from two to three months. Only 2 became pregnant, 1 showing 1, the other 2 fetuses. The general health of all these animals appeared to be good. They gained in weight. There was no evidence of disease of the external generative organs either in the males or females and no gross lesions of ovaries, uterus, or vagina in the animals chloroformed to determine the presence or absence of pregnancy. It would appear, therefore, that infection with these microorganisms had a pronounced depressant effect on the female generative mechanism after a recovery in other respects seemed to be complete. On the basis of this experiment a diminution in the birth rate in human beings greater than can be accounted for by the death of women of the child-bearing age might be expected.

The kidneys often showed a marked degree of diffuse, cloudy swelling and less commonly, focal areas of infection situated most often in the medulla; in a few instances these areas seemed to have given rise to pyelitis. Hemorrhages in the mucous membrane of the bladder were rarely noted. The suprarenals were often much swollen and hemorrhagic on the cut surface.

Following intratracheal injection of a few strains, numerous lesions of the muscles occurred, and in a few animals single large, hemorrhagic, edematous, necrotic areas were noted in the abdominal rectus muscle. Lesions of the myocardium occurred not infrequently and consisted usually of a grayish white diffuse degeneration. The ventricles in most of these were of stony hardness and in firm systole.

Lesions of the stomach were rare and occurred almost exclusively in animals that died from overwhelming infection, and consisted almost wholly of small localized hemorrhages with or without superficial ulceration associated with marked distention of the stomach with gas rich in carbon dioxid and marked postmortem digestion of the stomach wall.

General peritonitis following intratracheal injection was noted in 12 guinea-pigs. This occurred usually only when marked pleuritis or empyema was present or when it was otherwise secondary to infection of the uterus and tubes.

EXPERIMENTS ON THE MECHANISM OF RESPIRATORY EMBARRASSMENT IN INFLUENZA

Many findings in influenzal pneumonia, and particularly those in guinea-pigs following injection of bacteria from influenza, suggest strongly that they may be due in part to the formation of "anaphylatoxin," and that the lung picture may be the result of a prolonged anaphylaxis, associated with bronchial spasm. The protective effects of epinephrin and atropin against fatal anaphylactic shock are thoroughly established. It was thought, therefore, that injections of these substances into guinea-pigs having symptoms resembling anaphylaxis might furnish experimental evidence of the nature of the respiratory embarrassment and the use of these substances in treatment.

The effects of subcutaneous injection of epinephrin were studied in 15 guinea-pigs. The dose ranged from 0.02 c c-0.05 c c of a 1:1,000 solution of epinephrin chlorid to each 100 gm. of body weight. Good effects were noted in all but 3 guinea-pigs which showed no improvement; respiratory embarrassment was found to be due either to filling of the pleura or to extensive consolidation of the lung. The improvement, although striking, was always temporary, lasting from one-half to five hours. In a few control experiments in which the same dose of culture was given, life appeared to be prolonged for from one to two days in the animals treated with epinephrin, but in no instances in which recovery took place could it be attributed to the effects of this drug. This would be expected because of the inexhaustible supply of anaphylatoxin causing bronchial spasm due to the multiplication of the bacteria. Protocols illustrate the results obtained.

Guinea-pig 750, weighing 350 gm., was injected intraperitoneally Nov. 25, 1918, at 5:30 p. m. with 0.3 c c of the sputum from case 2620. The white blood count before injection was 14,400. November 26 at 9 a. m. the animal appeared to be sick, the fur was rough, and the respirations were rapid and difficult. The chest appeared to be dilated, and breathing was accomplished chiefly by means of the diaphragm. There was an expiratory rattle in the throat, and the animal's repeated forced efforts at expiration resembled the symptoms of anaphylactic shock. The mucous membrane of the conjunctiva, mouth, and tongue was blue. The leukocyte count was 4,500. At 1 p. m. the condition was unchanged except that respiratory efforts were more labored. A small amount of fluid oozed from the mouth and there was intense cyanosis of the mucous membranes. At 2:30 p. m. the condition was about the same. At this time 0.2 c c of a 1:1,000 solution of epinephrin chlorid were injected subcutaneously. At 2:35 p. m. there was no apparent change in respiration. At 2:45 p. m. the respirations undoubtedly were less labored and the animal appeared to be improved. At 3 p. m. the respirations appeared to be quite normal and the animal appeared to be much improved. At 3:45 p. m. the animal seemed to be comfortable, ate food, and the respirations were only slightly above the normal; cyanosis was absent. At 5:30 p. m. the respiratory difficulty had returned to some extent and the animal had a violent attack resembling anaphylactic shock. November 27, at 8:20 a. m., it was found dead. It showed hemorrhagic serofibrinous peritonitis and moderate emphysema of the lungs (12 c c), and beginning bronchopneumonia associated with marked edema surrounding the consolidated areas. The blood was very dark and had not coagulated. Blood-agar plates of the blood showed a moderate number of green-producing streptococci; from the peritoneal fluid there was a large number in pure culture.

Guinea-pig 965, weighing 360 gm., was injected intratracheally Jan. 14, 1919, at 3 p. m. with 2 c c of the glucose-brain-broth culture of the vaginal swab of case 2809. At 7 p. m. the respirations were extremely rapid and chiefly abdominal, the chest was dilated, the hair ruffled; there was an expiratory grunt, and the animal was restless, appeared uncomfortable, coughed repeatedly, and scratched its nose at intervals; bloody, edematous fluid escaped from the nostrils. At 7:20 p. m. respiratory embarrassment was unchanged. At 7:30 p. m., 0.2 c c of a 1:1,000 solution of epinephrin chlorid were injected subcutaneously. At 7:45 p. m. the picture had completely changed. The respirations were free and easy; the animal walked about, and the discharge of bloody fluid from the nose had ceased. At 11:15 p. m. the respirations were growing more labored; the animal was weak and restless, and breathing was difficult;

there was an expiratory rattle, and the bloody discharge from the nose had returned. At 11:30 p. m. the animal had an attack of severe shortness of breath in which it made violent efforts to breathe, ran around its mate, jumped into the air in a last violent effort at breathing, fell on its side as bloody fluid spurted from the nose and mouth, and died. The lungs were voluminous (22 c c); practically the entire lung was hemorrhagic and filled with hemorrhagic edematous fluid. The peribronchial lymph glands were edematous. A small amount of bloody fluid was found in the pleural cavity and a large subcapsular hemorrhage in the lower pole of the left kidney. Sections of the lung showed marked dilatation of alveoli filled by hemorrhagic edematous fluid, with slight leukocytic infiltration, and large numbers of diplococci in the hemorrhagic areas (figs. 17 a and b).

RELATION OF MORTALITY IN GUINEA-PIGS TO VIRULENCY OF THE ORGANISM ISOLATED IN FATAL AND NONFATAL INFLUENZA IN PATIENTS

If the results obtained in the animals really indicate close etiologic relationship of these streptococci to the disease, the relative mortality in the animals should correspond roughly with that in the patients from whom the material for injection was obtained. During the course of the experiments, the impression was gained that the material from severe or fatal cases is more virulent, producing more severe respiratory embarrassment, more marked hemorrhagic edema, and a higher mortality rate than the material from patients with mild attacks who recovered. It was considered of value, therefore, to determine the mortality in the animals according to whether the material injected was from patients with influenza and influenzal pneumonia who recovered, or from patients with influenza and influenzal pneumonia who died. In table 4 is given the mortality according to the diagnosis made at the time the material injected into animals was obtained and according to whether the patient died or recovered.

The mortality in the animals injected (intratracheally and intraperitoneally) with material from patients with influenza in whom signs of lung involvement were slight or entirely absent at the time of the experiments and who recovered, was about the same (49%) as in patients with influenzal pneumonia who recovered (43%). The 3 persons who had influenza at the time of the experiments and who later died of influenzal pneumonia harbored streptococci which killed the 5 guinea-pigs injected. It should be noted that the mortality in the guinea-pigs injected with material from patients with influenzal pneumonia was 26% lower when the material was taken from patients who recovered than when taken from those who died. In the former it was 43% in 23 guinea-pigs injected with 23 strains; in the latter, 69% in 78 guinea-pigs injected with 39 strains. The average mortality following intratracheal injection of 67 strains in 109 guinea-pigs was

TABLE 4

MORTALITY IN GUINEA-PIGS ACCORDING TO PLACE OF INJECTION AND MATERIAL INJECTED, AND ACCORDING TO DIAGNOSIS AND ULTIMATE RESULT IN PATIENTS FROM WHOM MATERIAL WAS OBTAINED

Place of Injection and Material Injected	Diagnosis at Time of Animal Experiments and Ultimate Result	Number of Strains	Number of Animals			Percentage of Mortality
			Injected	Recovered	Died	
Trachea—sputum, primary culture, green-producing streptococci, hemolytic streptococci, staphylococci	Influenza—recovery.....	32	43	23	21	49
	Influenzal pneumonia—recovery..............	12	11	7	4	36
	Total...............	44	55	30	25	[45]
	Influenza—death........	1	3	0	3	100
	Influenzal pneumonia—death................	22	51	20	31	61
	Total...............	23	54	20	34	[63]
	Total all strains......	67	109	50	59	54
Peritoneum — sputum, primary culture, green-producing streptococci, hemolytic streptococci, staphylococci	Influenza—recovery.....	36	42	21	21	50
	Influenzal pneumonia—recovery............	11	12	6	6	50
	Total...............	47	54	27	27	[50]
	Influenza—death........	2	2	0	2	100
	Influenzal pneumonia—death................	17	27	4	23	85
	Total...............	19	29	4	25	[86]
	Total all strains.......	66	83	31	52	63
Trachea and peritoneum—sputum, primary culture, green-producing streptococci, hemolytic streptococci, staphylococci	Influenza—recovery.....	68	86	44	42	49
	Influenzal pneumonia—recovery............	23	23	13	10	43
	Total...............	91	109	57	52	[48]
	Influenza—death........	3	5	0	5	100
	Influenzal pneumonia—death................	39	78	24	54	69
	Total...............	42	83	24	59	[71]
	Total all strains.......	133	192	81	111	58
Vein—primary culture, green-producing streptococci, hemolytic streptococci	Total all strains.......	9	19	5	14	74
	Grand total (111 cases)	142	211	86	125	59

54%. The average mortality in the 55 animals injected with 44 strains from patients who recovered was 45% in contrast to a mortality of 63% in the 54 guinea-pigs injected with 23 strains from patients who died. The results following intraperitoneal injection were similar.

The average mortality in 83 guinea-pigs injected with 66 strains was only 9% higher, 63%, than following intratracheal injection. The average mortality in 54 guinea-pigs injected with 47 strains from patients who recovered was 50%, in contrast to a mortality of 86% in the 29 guinea-pigs injected with 19 strains from patients who died. A summary of the results following these two methods of injection gives a total average mortality of 58% in 192 guinea-pigs injected with 133 strains from 111 cases, the average mortality in 109 guinea-pigs injected with 91 strains from patients who recovered being 48% in contrast to the mortality of 71% of the 83 guinea-pigs injected with 42 strains from patients who died. The average mortality following intravenous injection of 19 guinea-pigs with 9 strains was 74%. The grand total average mortality in 211 guinea-pigs injected with 142 strains, derived from 111 cases, was 59%.

It would seem from these facts that the virulency of the streptococci in patients who recover is less marked than in patients who die.

GENERAL DISCUSSION AND SUMMARY

The animal experiments that have been carried out heretofore with bacteria isolated quite constantly in influenza, both in 1889 and 1918, have consisted largely of virulency and toxicity tests in which only the usual methods of injection were used, and in which sufficient attention was not directed to the time and method of cultivation before injection. Statements have appeared concerning the high virulency of organisms of the streptococcus group [3, 7] and the ability of influenza bacilli to produce highly toxic products in cultures [19] and a tendency to produce lesions in the lung,[1, 8] but little has been accomplished in the way of reproducing the clinical and pathologic picture of epidemic influenza.

Intratracheal injection has been employed only occasionally in previous studies despite the fact that by this manner of injection of highly virulent pneumococci Lamar and Meltzer [10] have produced the typical picture of lobar pneumonia in the dog, Winternitz and Hirschfelder [24] in the rabbit, Cecil and Blake [4] in the monkey, and Wollstein and Meltzer [25] produced bronchopneumonia in the dog with bacteria isolated from bronchopneumonia in man.

The results of subcutaneous, intraperitoneal and intravenous injections, in my hands, show that the bacteria, particularly green-producing streptococci, isolated quite constantly in epidemic influenza possess high and peculiarly invasive powers. They have a marked tendency to produce leukopenia, to localize electively in the interstitial tissues and epithelial cells of the alveoli and smaller bronchi, and to produce hemorrhage and edema in the lungs, as symptoms of anaphylaxis and emphysema of the lung usually develop. Significant as these facts are, an accurate analysis of the effects of the bacteria and the precise rôle they play in influenza was possible only by the use of methods which simulated more closely the natural conditions, through the application of the bacteria to the normal uninjured epithelium of the lower respiratory tract by the method of intratracheal injection. The guinea-pig was considered the most suitable animal available for this study. Its resistance to streptococcal infection, although higher than that of man, its reaction to bacterial poisons and anaphylaxis are in general quite similar.

There has been much discussion, based chiefly on the results of cultures, with regard to the relative importance of the four main types of bacteria isolated in this disease, green-producing streptococci, including pneumococci, hemolytic streptococci, staphylococci and influenza bacilli. By a combined study of intraperitoneal injection in mice and guinea-pigs and intratracheal injection in guinea-pigs of sputum and lung exudates directly, and of the primary mixed culture of standard dosage a fair knowledge of the degree of the invasive power of these bacteria has been obtained. Invasion by the green-producing streptococcus in pure or almost pure form occurred in most instances even when the bacteria were not present in predominating numbers in the material injected. In some instances invasion by hemolytic streptococci occurred, but usually only when they were present alone or in predominating numbers, and more rarely by staphylococci, but only when they were present in predominating numbers in the material injected. Invasion by influenza bacilli following injection of sputum or lung exudate, which in some instances was proved to contain influenza bacilli, has not occurred in a single experiment. Similar results regarding the relative invasive power of these species have been obtained by injections of pure cultures of each, and again the independent invasive power of influenza bacilli was found to be slight. It should be emphasized that while it was necessary to use rather large doses for routine injections, owing to the relatively high and variable resistance of guinea-pigs and marked variations in invasive powers of the strains, small numbers of the more virulent streptococci sufficed to produce characteristic lesions. They followed intratracheal application of filtrates, intranasal insufflation of particularly virulent cultures and in a few instances through contact infection from guinea-pigs injected with especially virulent cultures.

The effects of intratracheal injection of mixtures of these organisms as they occurred in sputum and primary cultures and of pure cultures of recently isolated strains, varied within wide limits. The animals may be classified in four groups as follows:

Group 1. Animals that showed slight symptoms and then recovered.

Group 2. Animals that showed mild early symptoms and later suffered severe attacks.

Group 3. Animals that showed severe and progressive symptoms of marked lung involvement.

Group 4. Animals that showed extreme and rapidly fatal effects.

Group 1.—The symptoms of the animals in this group were relatively slight, consisting in the main of moderate illness, loss in weight, usually some fever, moderate leukopenia, and slight or moderately increased respirations for a number of days, followed by complete recovery. The animals were found to be immune to subsequent injections of heterologous strains. Those anesthetized for examination showed relatively slight or no lung involvement; the blood was sterile and the lungs were either sterile or contained a few of the organisms injected. These findings may be considered to parallel the clinical findings in patients with relatively mild influenza in whom little or no lung involvement can be demonstrated and in whom relative immunity is conferred as in the animals.

Group 2.—In the animals in this group the initial effects of the injection were more pronounced and lasted longer than those in the animals of group 1. Some of the animals, after apparent recovery, developed severe symptoms of respiratory involvement and died in from one to two days with anaphylactic symptoms, voluminous lungs, and hemorrhagic bronchopneumonia or, more rarely, from hemorrhagic pleuritis. In others the symptoms of respiratory embarrassment progressed more slowly; many of the animals developed rhinitis, and later died from purulent bronchitis and well-defined bronchopneumonia, often with small abscesses, and more rarely from abscess and gangrene, or from emphysema with or without bronchopneumonia. The cultures from the animals that died of relatively acute symptoms in the pneumonic attack usually showed green-producing streptococci, the pneumonic lung showing localized abscesses or abscess, usually staphylococci, or staphylococci and streptococci, and the empyemas usually hemolytic streptococci with or without staphylococci. The findings in this group may be regarded as representative of the findings in the group of patients with the more severe influenzal attacks who later develop influenzal pneumonia or, more rarely, well-defined coalescing bronchopneumonia with slight hemorrhagic edema, but with purulent bronchitis and localized abscesses or a single large abscess, or of empyema with or without bronchopneumonia.

Group 3.—In this group the initial symptoms were severe and usually progressed without intermission until death occurred in from two or three days from an increasing intense cyanosis and respiratory rate or from marked respiratory embarrassment from anaphylactoid symptoms during which in many instances, hemorrhagic edematous fluid escaped from the nose while the animals made violent efforts to breathe. The lungs were huge, in a few cases interstitial emphysema had occurred and extensive consolidation consisting of coalescing areas of pneumonia of different ages and intervening areas of hemorrhagic edema. The blood was dark and remained liquid for a long time. The postmortem and microscopic findings in this group were in every way like those described as typical of acute influenzal pneumonia in man.

Group 4.—In this group extreme dyspnea often occurred almost immediately after injection of highly virulent cultures and their filtrates. The symptoms were quite typical of acute anaphylaxis and many of the animals died while making violent efforts to breathe, as a bloody fluid ran from the nose and mouth. The lungs were huge, a dark purplish red, and hemorrhagic and edematous throughout. The symptoms and postmortem findings resembled very closely those noted in patients who died soon after being taken ill, usually in the initial attack of acute hemorrhagic edema of the lungs before sufficient time had elapsed for the development of extensive consolidation.

The distress from lack of oxygen, the intense cyanosis, and the extreme efforts at respiration of many animals in the latter two groups resembled the picture presented by patients dying from a rapidly filling lung who copiously expectorated a serous, bloody, frothy fluid, and who frequently sat up or left their beds in making violent efforts to breathe as death occurred.

The experiments with the filtrates show that under the proper conditions green-producing streptococci may become sufficiently small to pass through bacterial filters which prevent the passage of Bacillus prodigiosus, and that small numbers of the streptococci, when applied to the normal mucous membrane of the lower respiratory tract, are sufficient to produce the characteristic symptoms and pathologic changes in the lungs of guinea-pigs. Moreover, the results of the experiments with filtrates of cultures, pneumonic lungs, and sputum, and those on the mechanism of respiratory involvement show that the strains from influenza which have high invasive powers also have the power to produce anaphylatoxin in large amount, as measured by intratracheal injection. Many findings in influnza, such as the expanded, hyperresonant, relatively immobile thorax, cyanosis, the sharp leukopenia; the delayed coagulability of the blood, and the voluminous lung appear to be expressions of an anaphylactoid intoxication.

The results obtained following injection of guinea-pigs with influenzal material were so definite and so striking as to rule out quite effectively the possibility of spontaneous infection. However, this possibility was considered throughout the series of experiments. Only vigorous healthy looking pigs were used. No epidemic of pneumonia occurred among the reserve supply. The patchy areas of chronic bronchopneumonia, usually situated in the anterior lobes noted in guinea-pigs, at times were easily differentiated from the acute lesions due to the injections by their appearance and by the fact that cultures in the former condition nearly always showed Bacillus bronchisepticus: Control injections of salt solution and broth were without effect, and finally similar results followed intratracheal injections of influenzal material in other species (rat, rabbit, cat and monkey).

The effects following injection of the control strains of green-producing streptococci, hemolytic streptococci, staphylococci, and type pneumococci in like dosage were quite different. The immediate symptoms were less marked or absent, the mortality rate was much lower, leukopenia rarely occurred, leukocytosis was the rule, respirations while rapid in some instances, were usually free and easy, prolonged anaphylactoid symptoms did not occur, and hemorrhages from nostrils were not observed. The lungs were smaller, the exudate more cellular, the areas of consolidation occurred earlier and were more definitely outlined, and there was either no edema or relatively slight hemorrhagic edema at all times; marked necrosis of alveolar capillaries and epithelium were also absent. The contrast between the gross and microscopic picture of the lung following injections of highly virulent green-producing streptococci from influenza and of type pneumococci was particularly striking. In the former there was huge dilatation of the lung and alveoli, marked desquamation and degeneration of alveolar epithelium, necrosis of alveolar capillaries associated with peripherally placed streptococci in large numbers, and hemorrhage and edema everywhere with relatively slight leukocytic infiltration. In the case of type pneumococci the striking findings were moderate distention of the lung and alveoli with slight degeneration of epithelium and little change in interalveolar capillaries, but with marked diffuse, sharply demarkated, highly cellular exudate filling the alveoli, with the pneumococci diffusely distributed in the exudate, and with little edema.

The occurrence of marked lesions of the lungs, including well-marked pneumonia following injection of pure cultures of staphylococci and the presence of staphylococci in areas of softening in lungs injected with mixtures, and in large numbers in the sputum in some cases, but more particularly in the lung exudate after death, are in accord with the findings of Chickering and Park in Staphylococcus aureus pneumonia; and emphasize anew the importance of the staphylococcus as a cause of death and a factor in the production of lesions in the lung in epidemic influenza.

The theory that influenza and influenzal pneumonia are manifestations of the same infection varying only in degree is supported by these experiments. The bacteriology of the sputum and other exudates in influenza and of the early stages in influenzal pneumonia have been found to be identical. The infecting powers of the strains isolated in these two conditions, particularly of the green-producing streptococci, have been found to be very similar. The mortality in the guinea-pigs injected with strains from influenza is as high as in those injected with strains from patients with influenzal pneumonia who recovered. The mortality in the guinea-pigs was proportionately higher in those injected with material from patients who died than in those injected with material from patients who recovered. The leukocyte curves in the fatal and nonfatal infections in the guinea-pig ran parallel with the leukocyte curves in fatal and nonfatal infections in persos.

From a study of 266 cases of influenza and influenzal pneumonia in which accurate record of the exact onset of the attack was obtainable it was found that 145 patients either had no preceding influenzal attack or developed outspoken signs of pneumonia within three days from the onset of symptoms; 108 became ill with pneumonia after an interval of from four to nine days, and 13 only had an interval ranging from ten to twenty-one days. The number of patients who developed outspoken signs of lung involvement in the initial attack and without a quiescent interval is therefore large, and in general similar to that noted by others. By means of the more refined methods of examination, such as the roentgen ray, the incidence of lung findings in the primary influenzal attack has been greatly increased. Indeed, the manifestations of the disease and the bacteriologic findings in some instances have led good clinicians to regard the so-called complications as the disease itself,[6] and bacteriologists to look on the "secondary invaders" as the cause of sharp outbreaks.[7]

Through a painstaking study of the infecting powers of the streptococci in influenza and influenzal pneumonia throughout several epidemic waves, it has been possible to reproduce in animals, by various methods of injection, but particularly by intratracheal injection, the picture of influenza as seen in man. The symptoms both of influenza and influenzal pneumonia have been closely simulated in these animals as far as possible. Likewise, the gross and microscopic changes which have come to be regarded as quite characteristic of influenzal infection have been reproduced. The same varied picture that often supervenes in the latter stages of influenzal pneumonia in man, such as leukocytosis as evidence of pleural involvement and purulent infection, becomes manifest and the varied pathologic picture in the lung of patients who died late have been noted in guinea-pigs injected intratracheally with these strains. The tendency to involvement of the female generative organs, with a high mortality in pregnancy and a high incidence of abortion, of lesions of the heart, abscess in the rectus muscle, and interstitial emphysema have been noted in the experimental animal quite as they occur in man.

BIBLIOGRAPHY

1. Albert, H., and Kelman, S. R.: Pathogenicity of Bacillus influenzae for laboratory animals, Jour. Infect. Dis., 199, XXV, p. 433.

2. Bell, E. T.: The pathology of the lungs in pneumonia following influenza, Journal-Lancet, 1919, XXXIX, 3.

3. Blanton, W. B., and Irons, E. E.: A recent epidemic of acute respiratory infection at Camp Custer, Michigan, Jour. Am. Med. Assn., 1918, LXXI, 1988.

4. Cecil, R. L., and Blake, F. G.: Active immunity against experimental pneomococcus pneumonia, Jour. Am. Med. Assn., 1919, LXXIII, 715.

5. Chickering, H. T., and Park, J. H., Jr.: Staphylococcus aureus pneumonia, Jour. Am. Med. Assn., 1919, LXXII, 617.

6. Dunn, A. D.: Observations on an epidemic of bronchopneumonia in Omaha, Jour. Am. Med. Assn., 1918, LXXI, 2128.

7. Hirsch, E. F., and McKinney, M.: An epidemic of pneumococcus bronchopneumonia, Jour. Infect. Dis., 1919, XXIV, 594-617.

8. Huntoon, F. M., and Hannum, S.: The rôle of Bacillus influenzae in clinical influenza, Jour. Immunol., 1919, IV, 167-187.

9. Kuskow, N.: Zur pathologischen Anatomie der Grippe, Virchow's Arch., 1895 CXXXIX, 406-458.

10. Lamar, R. V., and Meltzer, S. J.: Experimental pneumonia by intrabronchial insufflation, Jour. Exper. Med., 1912, XV, 133-148.

11. LeCount, E. R.: The pathologic anatomy of influenzal bronchopneumonia, Jour. Am. Med. Assn., 1919, LXXII, 650-652.

12. LeCount, E. R.: Disseminated necrosis of the pulmonary capillaries in influenzal pneumonia, Jour. Am. Med. Assn., 1919, LXXII, 1519-1520.

13. Lord, F. T.: Influenza. In: Osler, Sir W., and McCrae, Sir T.: Modern Medicine, Philadelphia, Febiger, 1913, I, 534-549.

14. Lubarsch: Die anatomischen Befunde, von 14 tödtlich verlaufenden Fällen von Grippe, Berl. klin. Wchnschr., 1918, LV, 771. (Quoted in abstr. of foreign literature compiled by British Medical Research Committee, Jour. Am. Med. Assn., 1918, LXXI, 1573-1579.)

15. Lucke, B., Wright, T.. and Kime, E.: Pathologic anatomy and bacteriology of influenza, Epidemic of autumn, 1918. Arch. Int. Med., 1919, XXIV, 154-237.

16. Lyon, M. W., Jr.: Gross pathology of epidemic influenza at Walter Reed General Hospital, Jour. Am. Med. Assn., 1919, LXXII, 924-929.

17. MacCallum, W. G.: Pathology of pneumonia following influenza, Jour. Am. Med. Assn., 1919, LXXII, 720-721.

18. Opie, E. L., Freeman, A. W., Blake, F. G., Small, J. C., Rivers, T. M.: Pneumonia following influenza (at Camp Pike, Arkansas), Jour. Am Med. Assn., 1919, LXXII, 556-565.

19. Parker, J. T.: The poisons of the influenza bacillus, Jour. Immunol., 1919, IV, 331-357.

20. Rosenow, E. C.: Prophylactic inoculation against respiratory infections during the present pandemic of influenza, Jour. Am. Med. Assn., 1919, LXXII, 31-34.

21. Rosenow, E. C.: Studies in influenza and pneumonia. II. The experimental production of symptoms and lesions simulating those of influenza with streptococci isolated during the present pandemic, Jour. Am. Med. Assn., 1919, LXXII, 1604-1608.

22. Rosenow, E. C.: Studies in influenza and pneumonia. III. The occurrence of a pandemic strain of streptococcus during the pandemic of influenza, Jour. Am. Med. Assn., 1919, LXXII, 1608-1609.

23. Weichselbaum, A.: Bakteriologische und pathologisch-anatomische Untersuchungen über die Influenza und ihre Komplikationen, Wien. med. Bl., 1890, XIII, 83-85.

24. Winternitz, M. C., and Hirschfelder, A. D.: Studies upon experimental pneumonia in rabbits, Jour. Exper. Med., 1913, XVII, 657-678.

25. Wollstein, M., and Meltzer, S. J.: Experimental bronchopneumonia by intrabronchial insufflation, Jour. Exper. Med., 1913, XVI, 126-138.

PLATE I

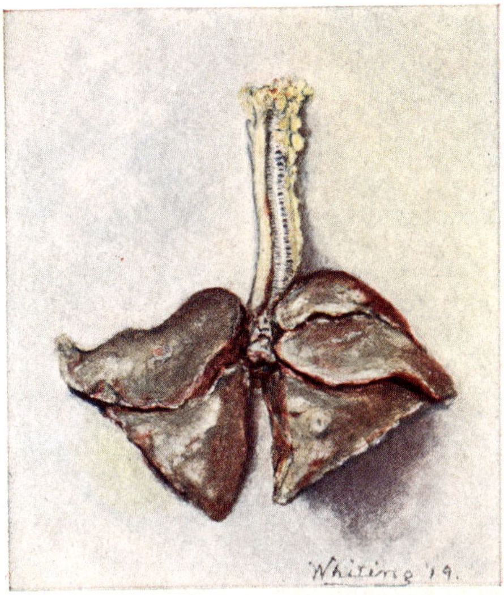

1

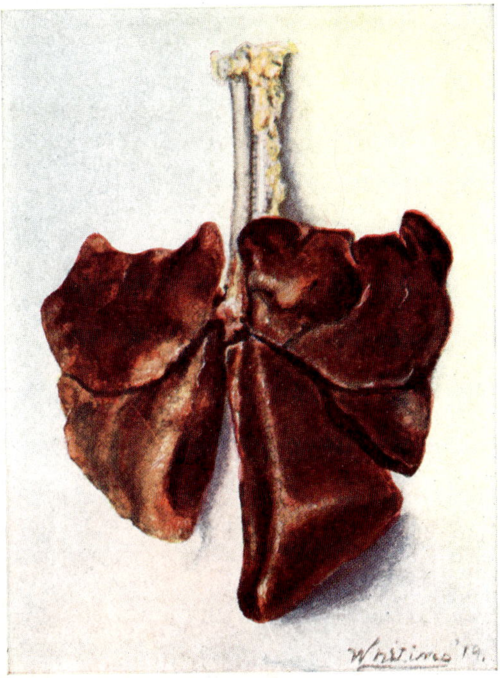

2

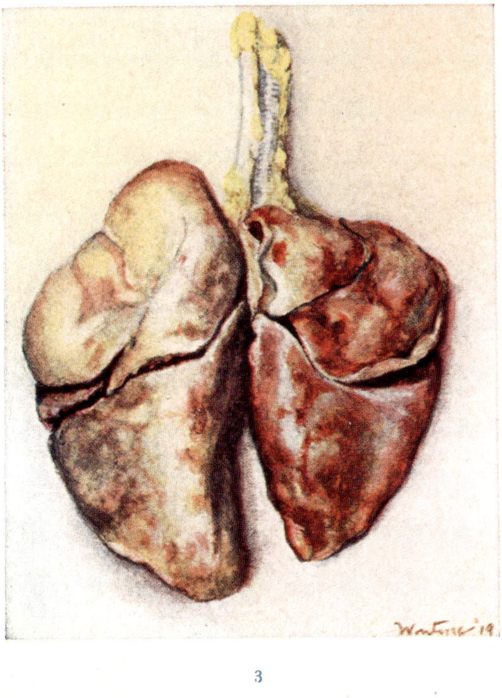

3

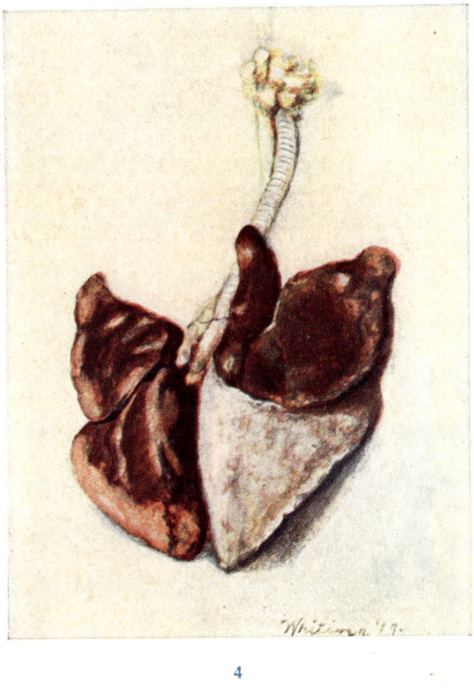

4

Plate II

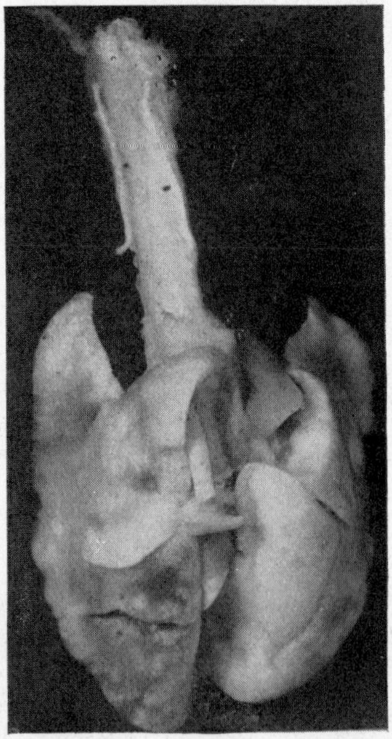

5

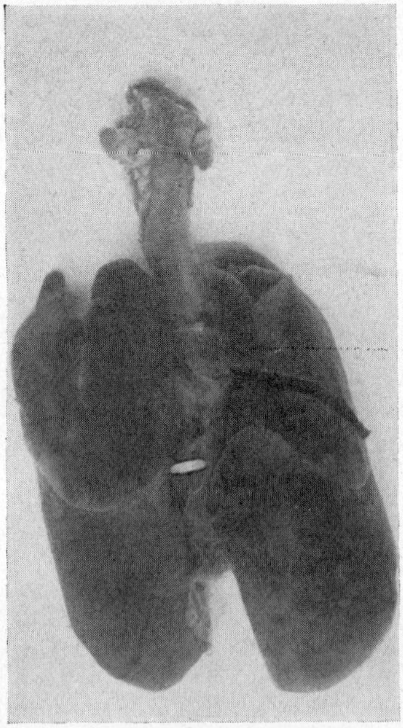

6

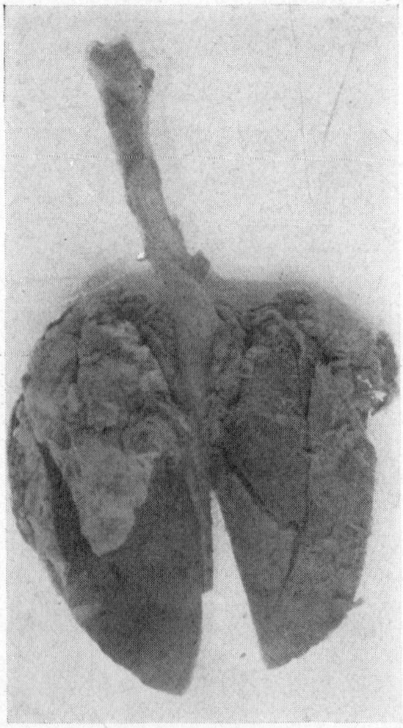

7

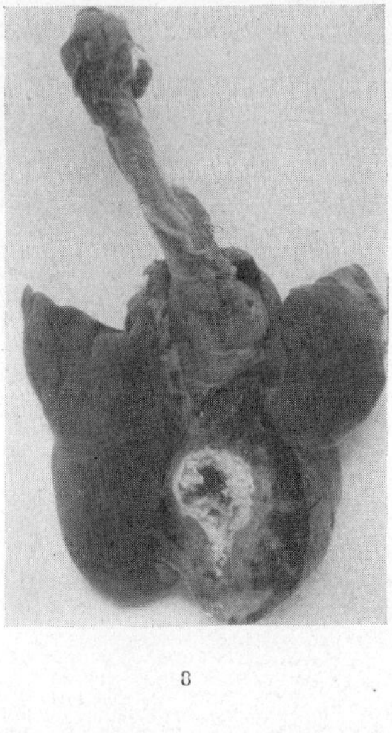

8

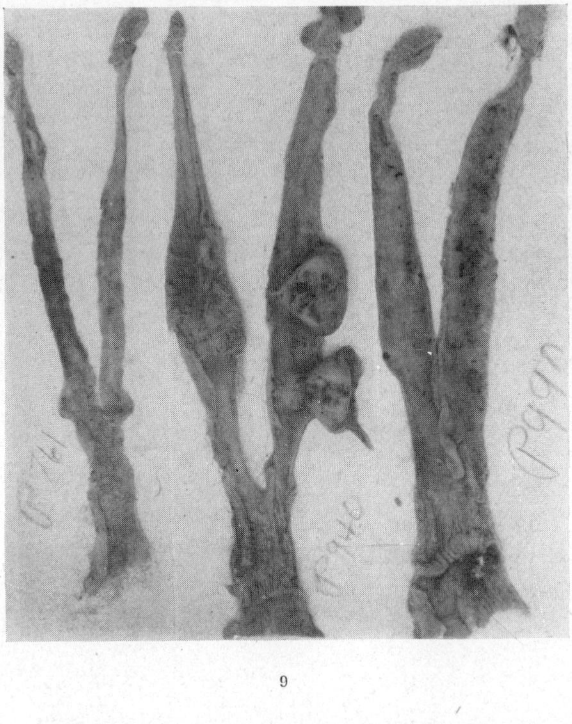

9

PLATE III

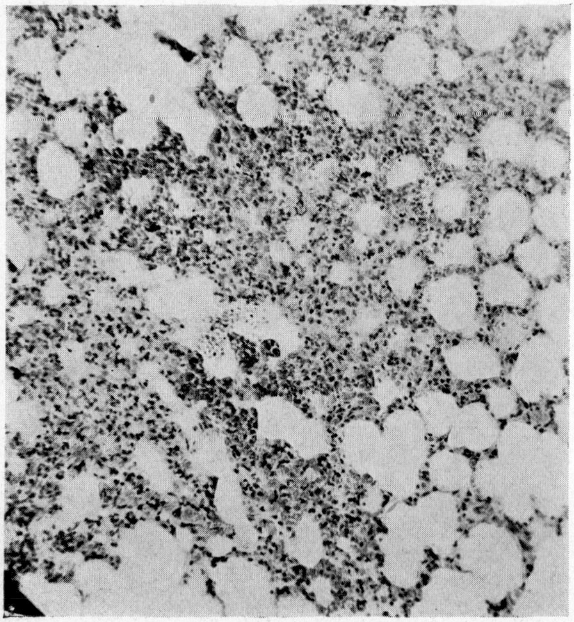

10

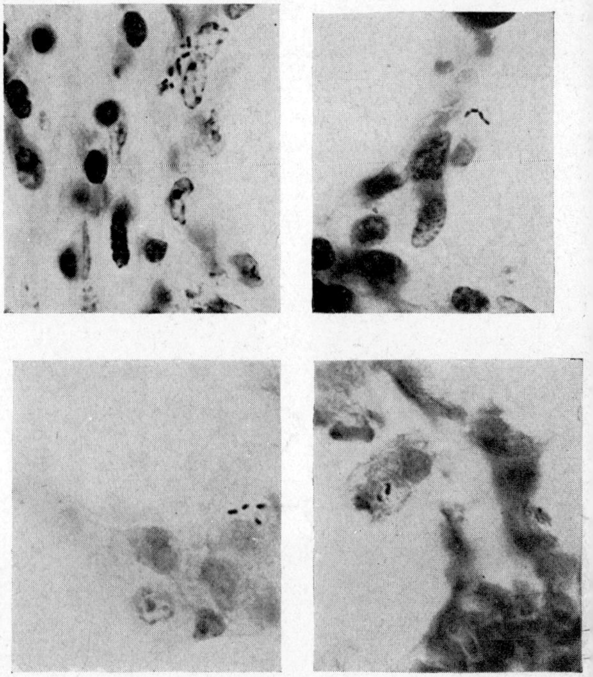

11

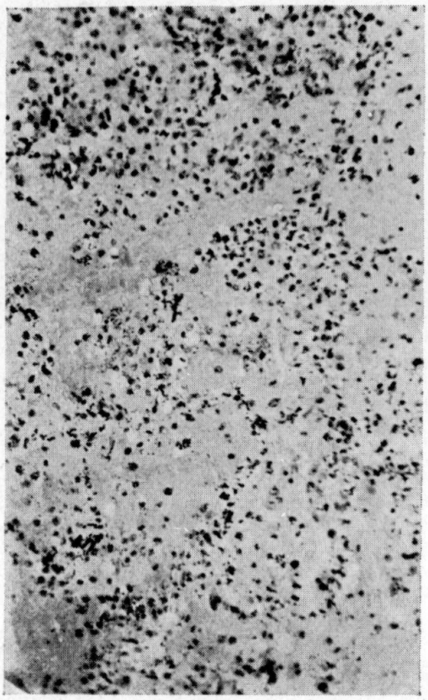

12 (a)

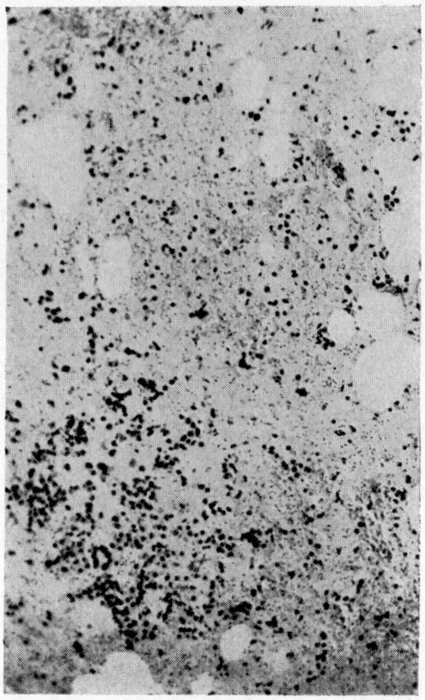

12 (b)

Plate IV

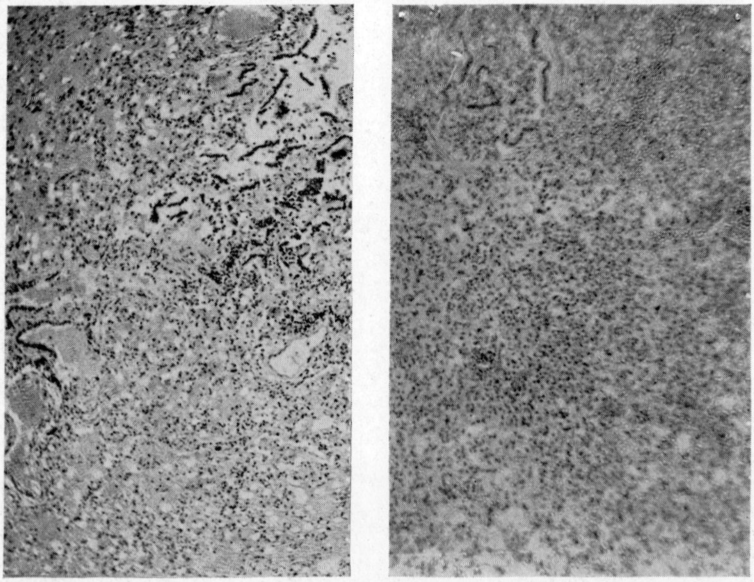

13

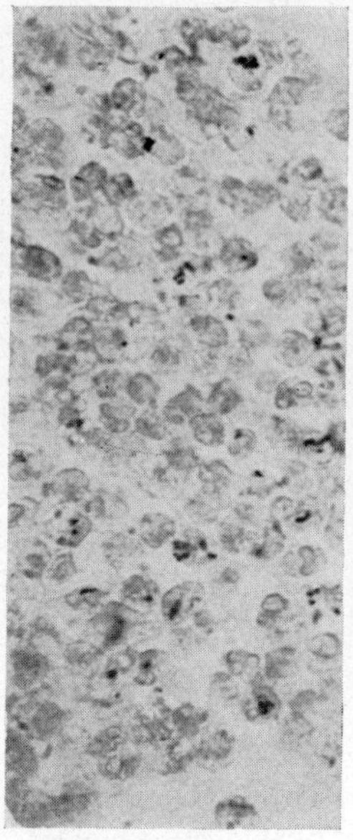

14 (a)

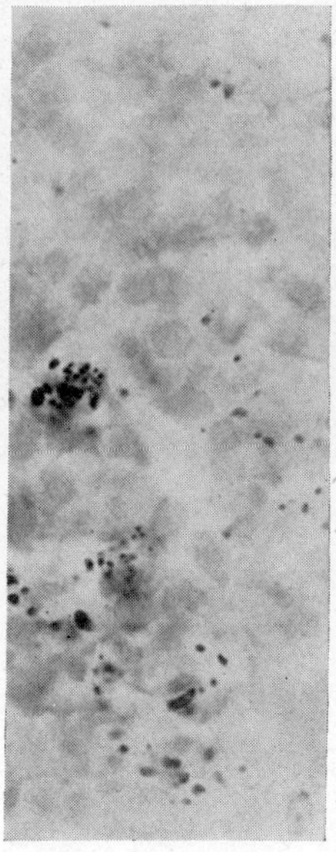

14 (b)

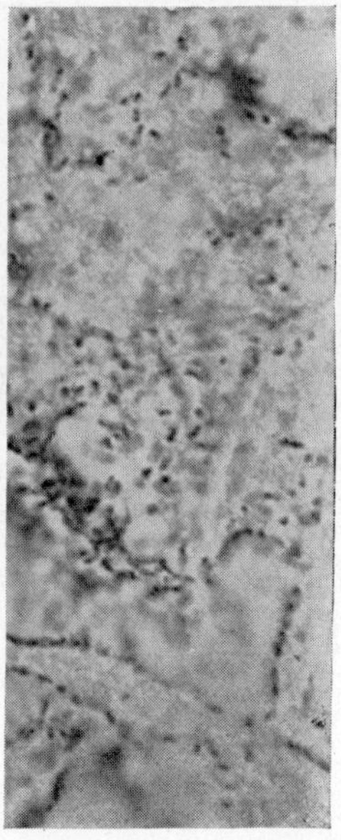

14 (c)

Plate V

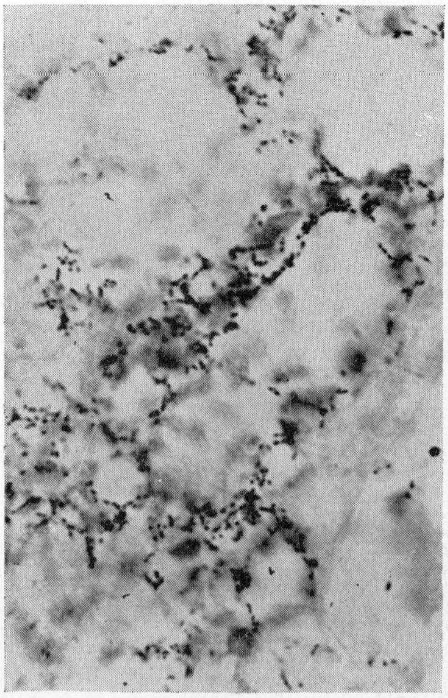

15 (a)

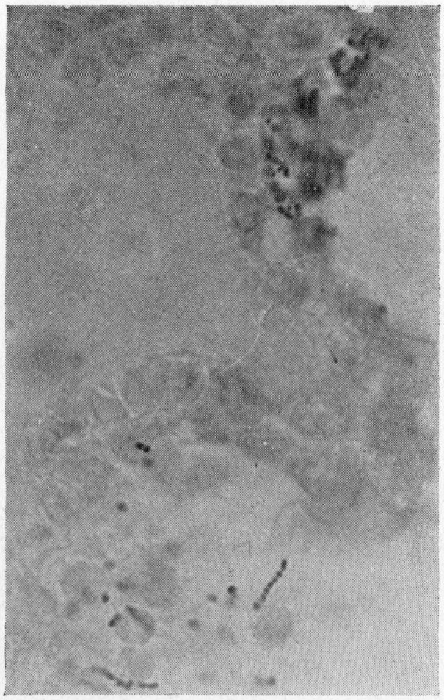

15 (b)

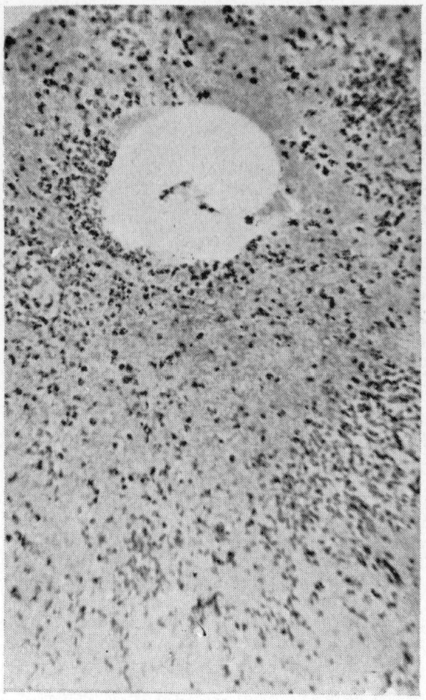

16 (a)

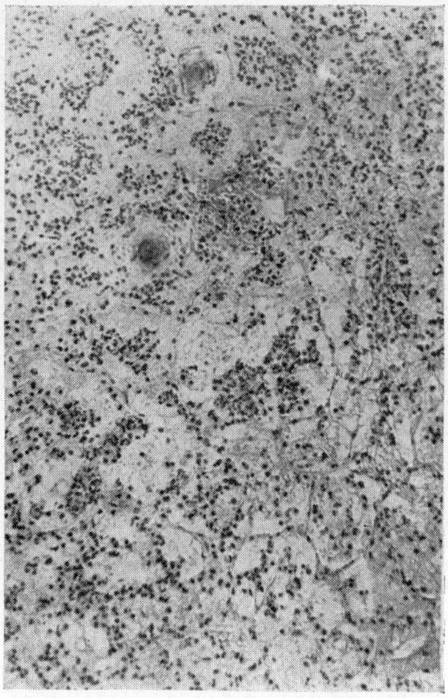

16 (b)

PLATE VI

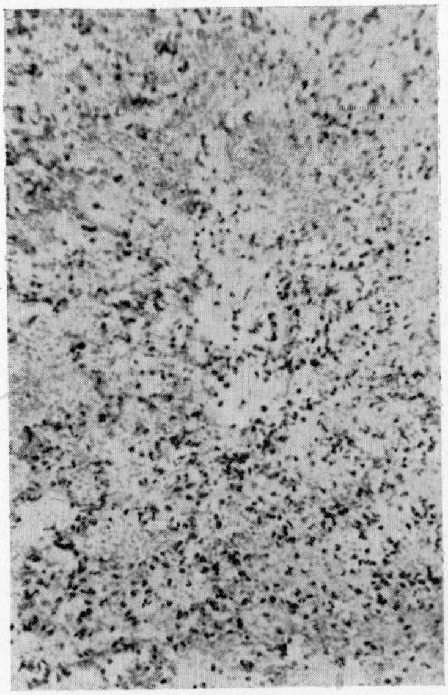

17 (a)

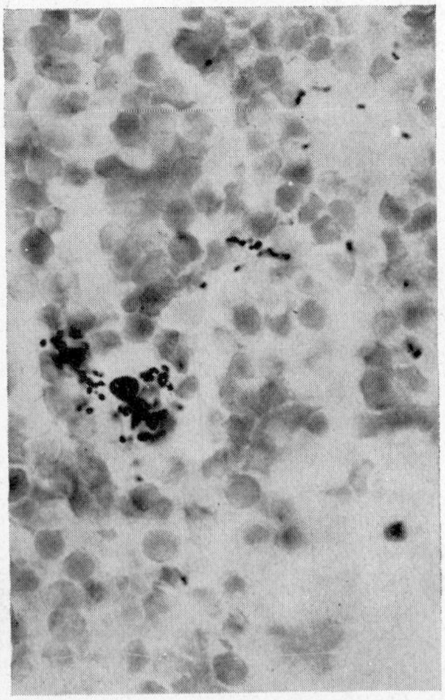

17 (b)

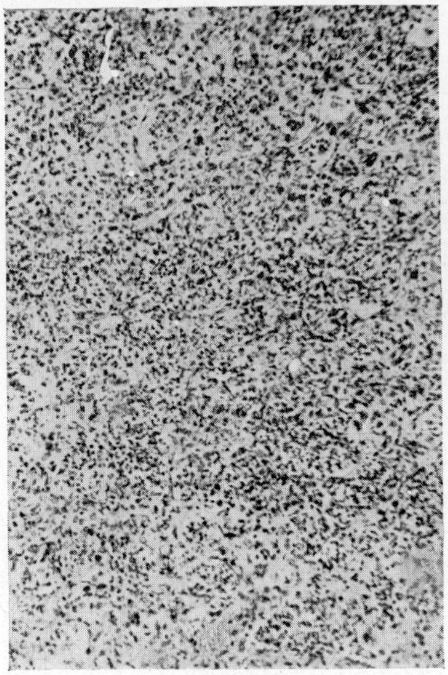

18 (a)

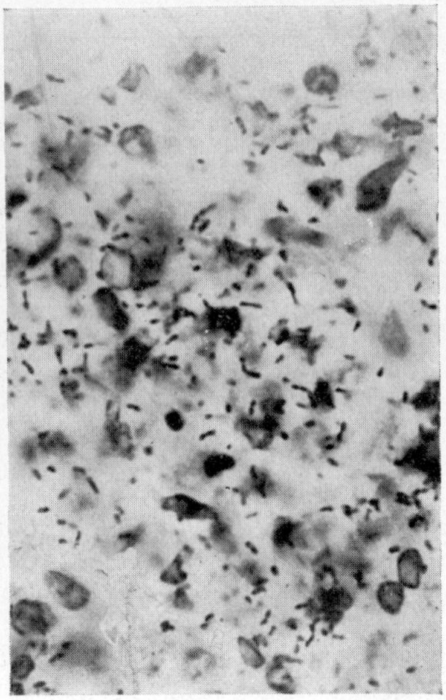

18 (b)

PLATE VII

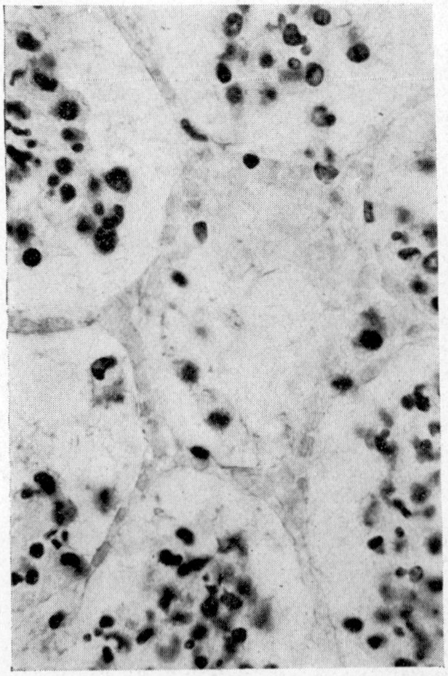

19 (a)

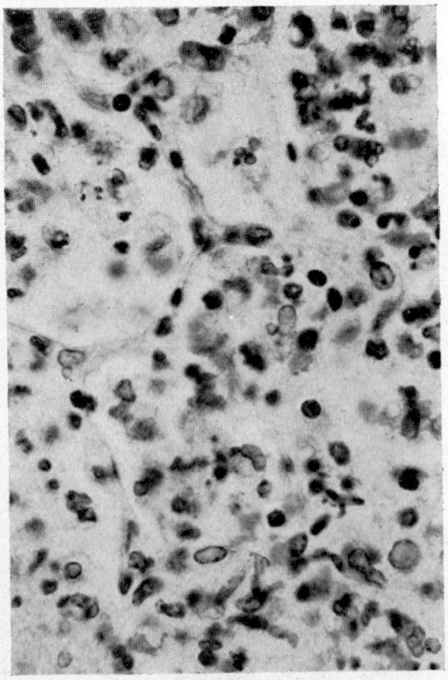

19 (b)

20 (a)

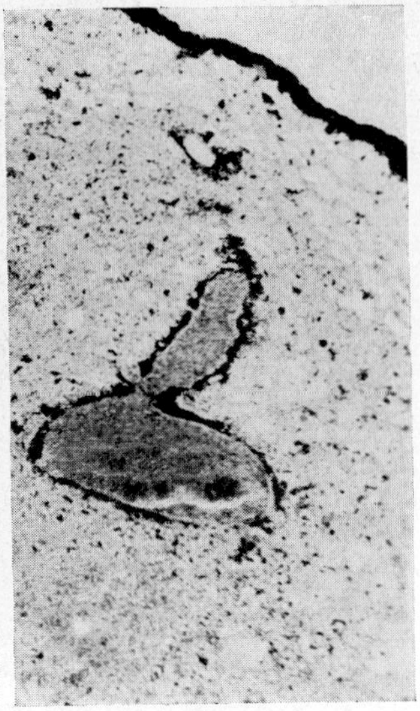

20 (b)

PLATE VIII

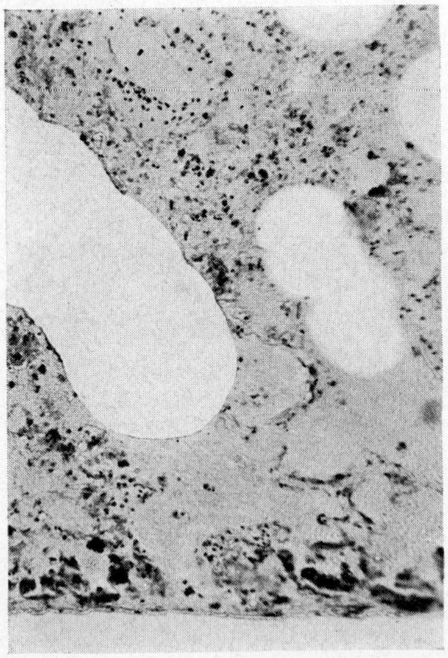

21 (a)

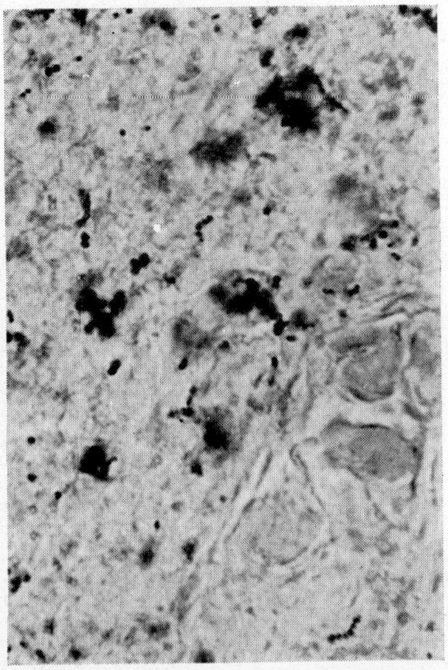

21 (b)

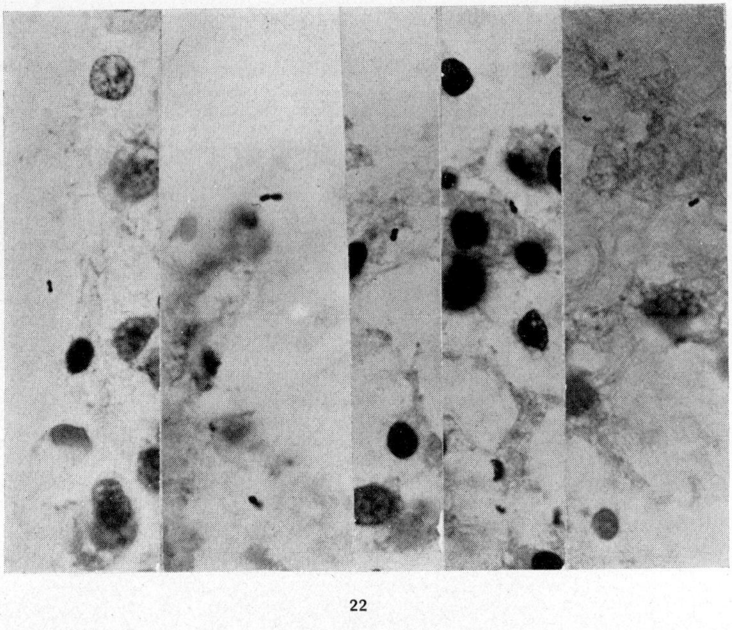

22

Explanation of Plates

Plate 1

Fig. 1.—Lung of normal guinea-pig weighing 350 gm., killed with ether. Total volume of lung 5.5 c c, weight 3.5 gm. (× 1).

Fig. 2.—Lung of guinea-pig 1345, weighing 400 gm., showing acute hemorrhagic edema 2½ hours after intratracheal injection of a culture of green-producing streptococcus from influenza in the fourth culture generation. Total volume of lung 23 c c, weight 18 gm. (× 1).

Fig. 3.—Lung of guinea-pig 1249, weighing 380 gm., showing massive pseudolobar pneumonia 48 hours after intratracheal injecton of the primary culture of green-producing streptococcus from the blood of a fatal case of influenzal pneumonia (case 3171). Total volume of lung 26 c c, weight 21 gm. (× 1).

Fig. 4.—Lung of guinea-pig 1448, showing lobar pneumonia 48 hours after intratracheal injection of type II pneumococcus; total volume of lung 14 c c, weight 12 gm. (× 1).

Plate 2

Fig. 5.—Lung of guinea-pig 737 that died 24 hours after intraperitoneal injection of sputum from case 2607. Note the large size (12 c c) compared with the lung shown in figure 1, and the hemorrhage and edema over the posterior aspect (× 1¼).

Fig. 6.—Lung of guinea-pig 1335 injected intratracheally with culture from sputum (case 2623) 40 minutes before death occurred with symptoms of acute anaphylaxis. Total volume of lung 20 c c. Note the extreme hemorrhage and edema (× 1).

Fig. 7.—Lung of guinea-pig 957 injected 6 days previously with hemolytic streptococci from case 2798. Note the marked thickening of the pleura (× 1).

Fig. 8.—Lung of guinea-pig 944, injected two weeks previously with hemolytic streptococci from case 2787, showing a large gangrenous abscess, numerous small abscesses in the cut surface of the right diaphragmatic lobe and marked pericarditis (× 1).

Fig. 9.—Photograph of uteri of three guinea-pigs, laid open presenting anterior view, illustrating the type of lesions noted in this organ following injection of influenzal material. Note the hemorrhages in the mucous membrane of the left horn of the uterus of guinea-pig 861 and both horns of guinea-pig 990, and their absence in the cervix and vagina, the hemorrhagic fetal masses and the localized edema, and infiltration of the endometrium marking placental attachments in guinea-pig 940 (× 1).

Plate 3

Fig. 10.—Section of the lung of guinea-pig 737, injected intraperitoneally with the sputum of case 2607. Note the marked dilatation of alveoli, congestion of the capllaries, and the alveolar and interstitial edema and hemorrhage. Hematoxylin and eosin (× 100).

Fig. 11.—Sections of the lung of guinea-pig 737, shown in figures 5 and 10; (a) diplococci beneath the epithelial cells in the alveolar wall and just outside of a capillary; (b) chain of diplococci in alveolar wall where epithelial cells have desquamated; (c) diplococci in an epithelial cell in its normal position, but showing disintegration of the nucleus in the wall of an alveolus with hemorrhage; (d) diplococci in desquamating epithelial cell. Gram-Weigert (× 1000).

Fig. 12.—(a) Section of lung of case 2800 showing marked hemorrhagic edema; (b) lung of guinea-pig shown in figure 2 with dilatation of alveoli, marked hemorrhagic edema, and dissolution of parenchymatous cells. Hematoxylin and eosin (× 100).

Plate 4

Fig. 13.—Section of lungs showing (a) hemorrhagic edema with relatively slight cellular infiltration and marked destruction and desquamation of the bronchial epithelium in case 2800, and (b) in guinea-pig 956 twenty-four hours after intratracheal injection of the culture of green-producing streptococcus from a single colony from the throat in this case. Hematoxylin and eosin (× 100).

Fig. 14.—(a) Diplococci in the lung of case 2800 shown in figures 12 and 13; (b) diplococci in the lung of guinea-pig shown in figure 12; (c) diplococci distributed along the alveolar lining of the alveoli in the lung shown in figure 13b.

Plate 5

Fig. 15.—Lung of guinea-pig shown in figure 3; marked hemorrhagic edema, dilatation of the alveoli, desquamation and disintegration of the alveolar epithelium, necrosis of capillary epithelium with relatively slight leukocytic infiltration, and many diplococci lining the alveolar walls; (a) hematoxylin and eosin (× 100); (b) Gram-Weigert (× 800).

Fig. 16.—Lung of monkey 228 injected intratracheally with the emulsion of the hemorrhagic mucous membrane of the stomach in case 2979. Note the hemorrhagic edema, desquamation of the epithelial cells of the alveoli and ductus alveolaris, and the diplococci chiefly along the alveolar lining; (a) hematoxylin and eosin (× 100); (b) Gram-Weigert (× 1000).

Plate 6

Fig. 17.—Section of the lung of guinea-pig 965 injected intratracheally with a culture from the vaginal swab in case 2809. Note the dilatation of the alveoli, the marked edema and hemorrhage, the relatively slight cellular infiltration, and the large number of diplococci in the hemorrhagic and edematous areas; (a) hematoxylin and eosin (× 1000); (b) Gram-Weigert (× 1000).

Fig. 18.—Section of consolidated right diaphragmatic lobe of lung shown in figure 4. Note the marked and uniform cellular, chiefly leukocytic infiltration, relatively slight edema, and the even distribution throughout the alveolar exudate of the pneumococci; (a) hematoxylin and eosin (× 100); (b) Gram-Weigert (× 1000).

Plate 7

Fig. 19. — (a) High power photomicrograph of the lung of guinea-pig 1249 (figures 3 and 15) showing marked dilatation of alveoli, necrosis of capillary endothelium, desquamation and degeneration of the alveolar epithelium, and slight leukocytic iinfiltration. Hematoxylin and eosin (× 500). (b) Section of consolidated lobe of lung of guinea-pig 1448 injected with type II pneumococcus. Note the lesser dilatation of alveoli, the marked leukocytic infiltration, absence of necrosis of endothelial cells lining the alveolar capillaries, and the lesser damage to alveolar epithelium. Hematoxylin and eosin (× 500).

Fig. 20.—Section of lung of guinea-pig 947 injected intratracheally with the primary culture of the throat swab from Case 2800, which died 24 hours after injection with compressed lung from hemorrhagic fluid in the pleural cavities. Note the marked hemorrhage and edema and the poorly staining cells throughout, and the dark areas beneath the pleura and around the large blood vessels. Hematoxylin and eosin (× 50).

Plate 8

Fig. 21.—(a) Section of lung of guinea-pig 1262, injected into the trachea with the sputum of case 3175. There was a moderate amount of turbid hemorrhagic fluid in the pleural sac and a corresponding tendency of the bacteria to localize in the subpleural lymphatics as shown in the dark areas. Note the marked dilatation of the alveolar ducts and the alveoli, and the edema, hemorrhage, and desquamation of cells with relatively slight cellular infiltration throughout. Hematoxylin and eosin (× 100). (b) Diplococci and cocci in hemorrhagic, edematous areas. Gram-Weigert (× 1000).

Fig. 22.—Photomicrograph of diplococci in the edematous and hemorrhagic subpleural space of the pleura of the fetus in case 3175. Gram-Weigert (× 1000).

STUDIES IN INFLUENZA AND PNEUMONIA

STUDY VIII. EXPERIMENTS ON THE ETIOLOGY OF "GASTRO-INTESTINAL" INFLUENZA

E. C. Rosenow

Division of Experimental Bacteriology, The Mayo Foundation, Rochester, Minnesota.

Symptoms of gastro-enteritis, alone or in association with respiratory involvement, have occurred with such regularity during the course of epidemics of influenza and the accompanying prostration has been so pronounced, that a gastro-intestinal type of this disease has come to be quite generally recognized. Kuskow cites cases of his own and of others in which lesions of the gastro-intestinal tract were found, varying from simple enteritis with the swelling of Peyer's patches and hyperplasia of mesenteric lymph glands to severe ulcerative and hemorrhagic gastro-enteritis. Bacteriologic studies, however, are quite lacking; no one has demonstrated bacteria in the lesions, and many regard the severe cases as due to enteritidis-like organisms. The investigations of Sherwood, Downs, and McNaught do not support the latter view since this type of organism was isolated in cases of influenza without symptoms referable to the gastro-intestinal tract and in those with symptoms. I shall report herewith the results of a study of a series of cases of gastro-enteritis, including one fatal case, which occurred during the first two waves of the epidemic of 1918.

The incidence of gastro-enteritis during the first wave was quite high; it was more common in children, but occurred also in adults. The symptoms varied greatly, but prostration and high fever were the striking features. In some instances the symptoms referable to the gastro-intestinal tract occurred without accompanying respiratory involvement; in most instances more than one member of a given family were affected. Cultures from the stools, usually from only one specimen taken at the height of the attack, were made in 15 cases during the first wave. Flakes of bloody mucus were fished out and washed in salt solution and plating on blood-agar made. Varying numbers of green-producing streptococci resembling those from the sputum in influenza were isolated in 9 instances and hemolytic streptococci were isolated in 2. Influenza bacilli were not isolated. Smears from flakes of bloody mucus often showed a large number of gram-positive diplococci resembling those from the sputum. Owing to stress of other work no animal experiments were made at this time. During the second wave opportunity presented itself for the study of one fatal case and one other case in the same family. The findings in detail are:

Case 2979,—A boy aged 3, a patient of Dr. C. T. Granger, after having had symptoms of a slight sore throat for several days, suddenly became ill Feb. 3, 1919, with vomiting, diarrhea, high fever and delirium. The stools showed blood on the first day; this continued and he passed almost pure blood and mucus at times. He grew gradually weaker, vomited blood February 9 and died the following day. Dr. Peters brought the internal viscera to me for examination. The lungs revealed marked hypostatic congestion, moderate edema, but no outspoken areas of consolidation. The stomach contained a moderate amount of dark red, partially clotted, blood. The mucous membrane was covered with chocolate colored blood mixed with mucus. This was removed and numerous small hemorrhages with beginning ulceration, more numerous in the pyloric end, were found. The duodenum was normal. The mucous membrane of the ileum was extensively hyperemic throughout and was covered with mucopurulent bloody material; numerous punctate hemorrhages and in places beginning ulceration were found. The mesenteric lymph glands were edematous and hemorrhagic. The kidneys showed marked cloudy swelling; the spleen and heart were normal. Blood-agar plate cultures of an emulsion of the hemorrhagic mucous membrane of the stomach contained fully 5,000 rather moist, green colonies of bacteria resembling pneumococci and 5 colonies of staphylococci. The emulsion of the mesenteric lymph glands contained 260 colonies of green-producing streptococci, 4 of staphylococci, and a number of colonies of Bacillus coli. Emulsions of the washed intestinal wall revealed 120 colonies of green-producing streptococci, 50 colonies of staphylococci, and 30 colonies of Bacillus coli. Cultures of the spleen were negative. In sections made through the hemorrhagic areas in the ileum were found wedge shaped and diffuse areas of hemorrhage in the mucosa, with only moderate infiltration and edema, and in some instances with superficial ulceration of the mucosa (fig. 1). A large number of gram-positive diplococci were found throughout the hemorrhagic areas, but were most numerous near or on the surface of the ulcerated area (fig. 2 a). The hemorrhagic areas in the stomach showed a similar picture; they contained a large number of gram-positive diplococci. In either case few or no diplococci were demonstrable in the tissues without lesions.

Feb. 12, 1919, the primary culture in dextrose-brain broth of the emulsion of a mesenteric lymph gland was injected, under ether, through a laparotomy incision into the duodenum of one guinea-pig. The leukocyte count was 25,000 before injection. The animal was found dead the following day. Examination revealed 7,200 leukocytes, fibrinous and clotted blood deposit about the point of puncture of the duodenum, a normal intestine above this point, and an extremely hyperemic intestine below. The lumen of the intestine contained a large amount of mucus mixed with chocolate colored blood. The mesenteric lymph glands were edematous. The mucous membrane of the stomach, the uterus, and the cecum was hyperemic and contained a few hemorrhages. The primary culture in glucose-brain broth of the stomach emulsion of the patient was injected in doses varying from 0.1 to 1.5 c c, intratracheally into one monkey and 5 guinea-pigs, and intravenously into one rabbit. The guinea-pig that was given 0.5 c c and the one given 1 c c died in twenty-four hours. Both had hemorrhagic edema of the lungs and hemorrhagic pleuritis; one had marked lesions of the intestine and stomach, the other slight lesions. The other 3 animals were chloroformed for examination the third day. All had bronchopneumonia, one had a large amount of turbid fluid in the pleural cavity, and 2 had lesions of the intestinal tract; cultures from the lung of one of these were agglutinated specifically by the monovalent antistreptococcus serum. One of the guinea-pigs had leukopenia, 1 leukocytosis, and in 2 there was no change in the leukocyte count. The monkey died in twenty-four hours. Examination revealed hemorrhagic edema of the intermediate lobe, marked

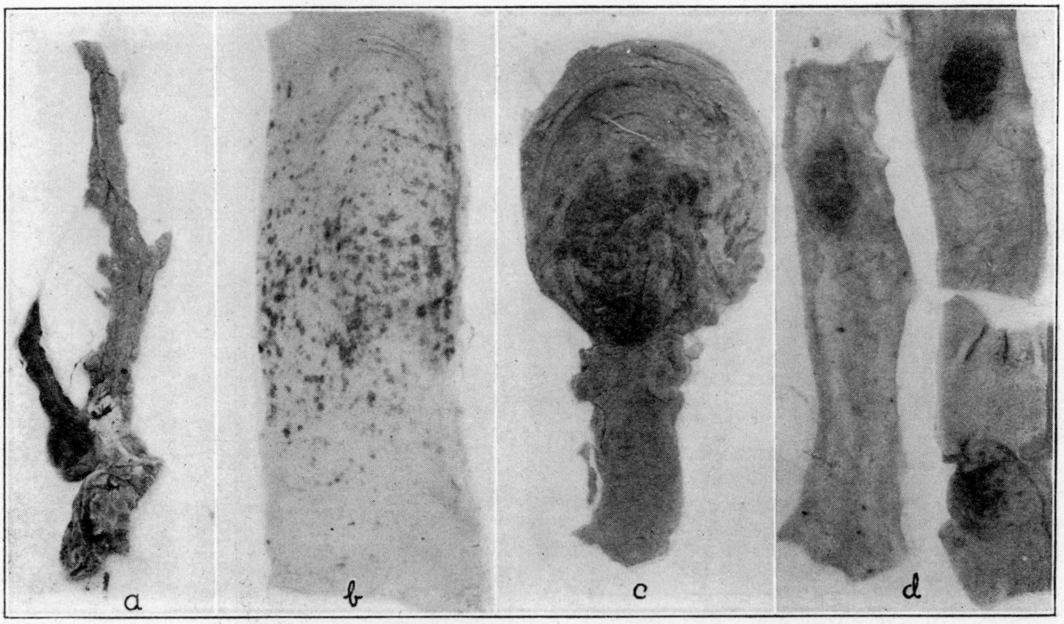

Fig. 1.—Photographs of lesions of the pancreas, intestine, stomach, and Peyer's patches following injection of green-producing streptococcus from influenza. × I.

a. Pancreas of guinea-pig forty-eight hours after intravenous injection of a strain after one animal passage. Note the edema, hemorrhage, and fat necrosis; × I.

b. Ilium of rabbit twenty-four hours after intravenous injection of a strain in the third animal passage. Note the numerous circumscribed hemorrhages in the mucous membrane; × I.

c. Edema and extensive hemorhages in the stomach of a guinea-pig fifteen days after intratracheal injection of a strain in the third subculture; × 0.5.

d. Swelling and hemorrhages of Peyer's patches and the mucous membrane of the duodenum in the ileum and duodenum of rabbit forty-eight hours after intravenous injection of a strain in the fourth animal passage.

distention of the stomach with gas rich in carbon dioxid, edematous and hemorrhagic Peyer's patches and mesenteric lymph glands, and hyperemia and edema of the mucous membrane of the small intestine, especially in the ileum, where it was covered with mucus containing flakes of blood. The leukocyte count dropped from 35,000 before injection to 7,200 after death. The blood contained a moderate number of green-producing streptococci and staphylococci; the upper intestinal contents, a moderate number of staphylococci and green-producing streptococci; the lower intestinal contents, colon bacilli only. Cultures from two mesenteric lymph glands, the kidney, and the peritoneum were negative. Sections of the lower ileum contained subperitoneal hemorrhages and areas of hemorrhage in the mucous membrane showing desquamation of epithelium but no distinct ulceration. A large number of gram-positive diplococci were found in the hemorrhagic areas of the mucous membrane (fig. 3), a smaller number in the subserous hemorrhages, but none in the adjoining normal tissue. The rabbit injected intravenously with the primary

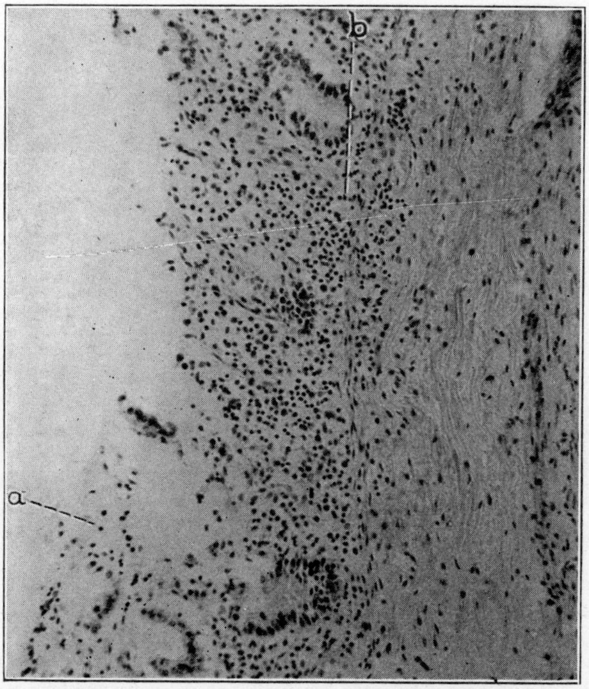

Fig. 2.—Photomicrograph of section of ileum in case 2979. Note the loss of tissue, infiltration by erythrocytes and leukocytes; hematoxylin and eosin, × 100.

culture from the stomach emulsion developed diarrhea and died three days later. Examination revealed two areas of bronchopneumonia posteriorly in the diaphragmatic lobes, hyperemia of the small intestine, swollen Peyer's patches and lymph follicles, much mucus in the intestine, edematous mesenteric glands, embolic lesions in the medulla of the kidney, and a few lesions in the myocardium and skeletal muscles. Cultures from the blood were negative and those from the pneumonic areas in the lung contained green-producing streptococci and staphylococci.

CASE 2981.—A baby girl aged fifteen months, sister of the patient whose case (case 2979) is first recorded, became ill Jan. 9, 1919, with vomiting, high fever (104 F.), and diarrhea six days after her brother had been taken sick. January 11, the child was apathetic, and fussy; the fever and diarrhea continued, and the leukocyte count was 5,400. The skin was dry and without rash, and there was no throat infection; the abdomen was scaphoid; and the stool consisted largely of blood-tinged mucus resembling pus. The diarrhea continued for five days, after which the child gradually recovered. Cultures were made from the tonsils, and from four samples of bloody mucus in the stool. The cultures from the tonsils showed the usual streptococcal flora. The blood-agar plates of the bloody mucus contained countless numbers of Bacillus coli, a few staphylococci, and rather moist, green-producing colonies of streptococci. Three guinea-pigs were injected, one intrarectally, one intratracheally with a salt solution suspension of the bloody mucus, and one with the pure culture of green-producing streptococcus in the second generation. The guinea-pig injected intrarectally appeared well

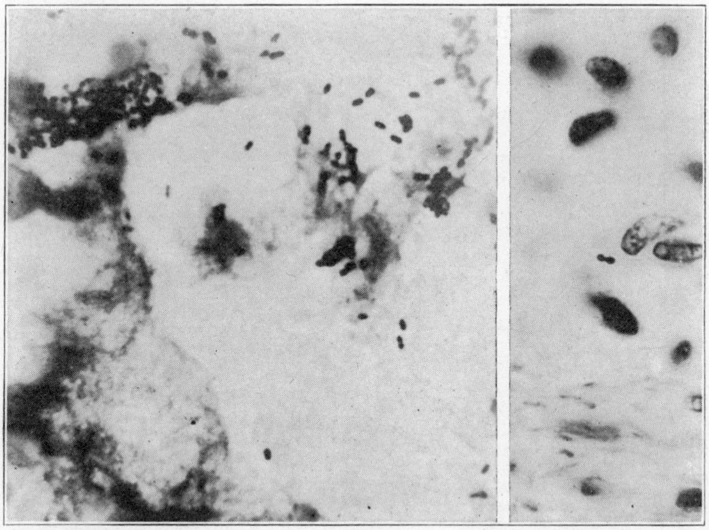

Fig. 3.—Diplococci in ulcerating area shown in figure 2 at a and b.

the following day when it was chloroformed. In the cecum were a large number of small hemorrhages and swollen lymphoid follicles; in the stomach, large circumscribed areas containing small punctate hemorrhages surrounding the cardiac orifice; and in the duodenum a few hemorrhages in the mucous membrane just beyond the pyloric ring. Cultures from the blood, adrenal. spleen, kidney, and liver were negative; staphylococci and green-producing streptococci were produced from the mesenteric and perigastric lymph glands, and from the lung. Sections of the hemorrhagic areas in the duodenum showed marked extravasations of red blood corpuscles, especially in the submucosa in which a large number of diplococci were found. In the guinea-pig injected intratracheally with a suspension the leukocyte count dropped 66 per cent. the following day. The temperature increased 2 degrees, and respirations increased slightly. The animal appeared well four days later when it was chloroformed. The transverse colon and cecum were found to be extremely hyperemic; the intestinal contents contained an abnormal amount of mucus, but otherwise showed no lesions; there was a large subcapsular hemorrhage in the lower pole of the left kidney, consolidation of the upper one-third of the right diaphragmatic lobe, and marked congestion and mucopurulent material in the mucous membrane of the trachea and nose. Cultures from the blood and the uterus were negative; the mucous membrane of the nose and trachea contained a large number of green-producing streptococci and staphylococci. In the guinea-pig injected with the pure culture of the green-producing streptococcus a diminution of 33 per cent. in leukocyte count and a slight increase in respiration occurred the day following the injection. Two days after the injection, when the animal appeared quite well, it was chloroformed. Examination revealed uniform grayish areas of consolidation of the right diaphragmatic lobe, a few hemorrhages in the mucous membrane of the stomach

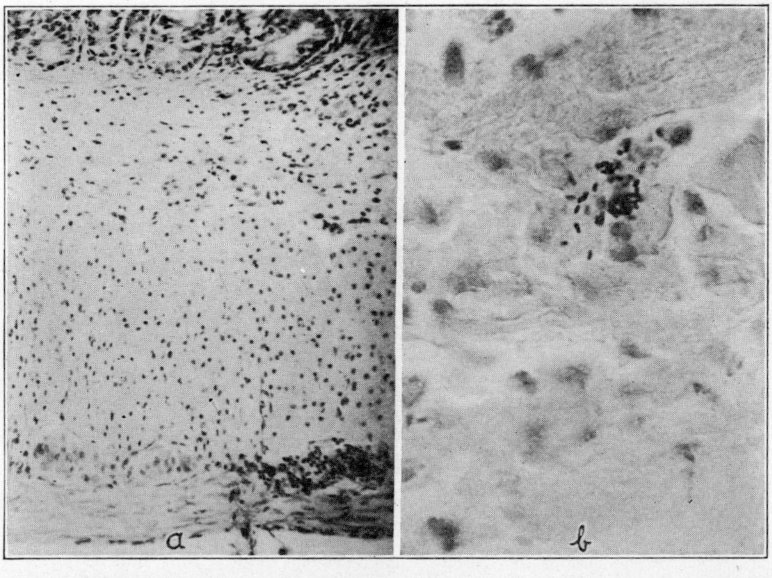

Fig. 4.—Section of the ileum of a guinea-pig injected intrarectally with a suspension of hemorrhagic mucus from the stool in case 2981. Hemorrhage and infiltration and thrombosis of vessel in subperitoneum by leukocytes and by swollen degenerating, desquamated endothelium; gram-positive diplococci in the area of infiltration in the submucosa. a., Hematoxylin and eosin, × 100; b. Gram-Weigert, × 1000.

along the lesser curvature and cardiac end, but no lesions of the intestine. The cultures from the lung contained a moderate number of colonies of staphylococci and green-producing streptococci.

Many green-producing streptococci were isolated from the lesions in the intestines of the patient with the fatal gastro-intestinal infection (case 2979), and from stools in the sister of this patient whose attack was milder and who recovered (case 2981). These attacks occurred at a time when influenza was epidemic in the surrounding community. The organism was present in large numbers in the lesions of the intestines and stomach, and absent in the normal tissues. Injection of the freshly isolated strains from these 2 patients into 14 animals produced well marked lesions in the gastro-intestinal tract, in 12 in which the organism was demonstrable in large number; the lesions were similar to those noted in the patients. In view of these facts there can be no reasonable doubt that this organism was the cause of the gastro-enteritis in these patients. Lesions of the gastro-intestinal tract following injection of streptococci isolated in influenza were noted only occasionally, but they occurred more often after

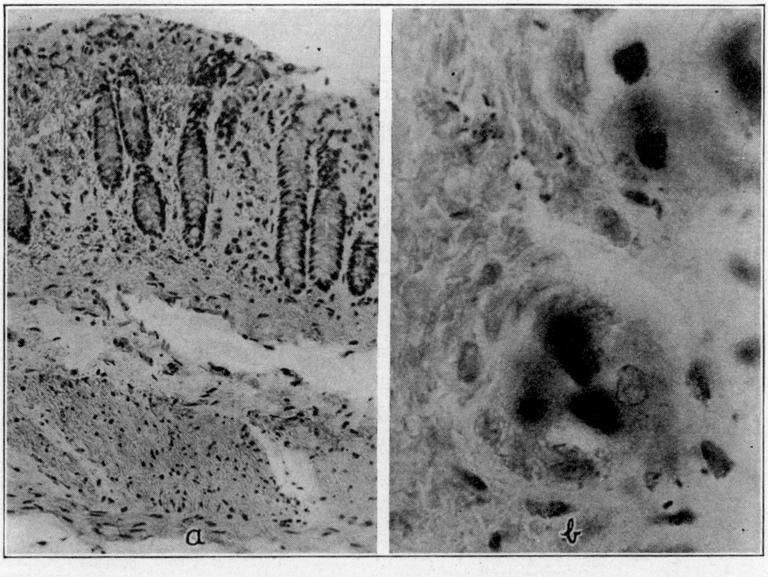

Fig. 5.—Section of transverse colon of a rabbit injected intragastrically with a strain in the fourth animal passage; marked infiltration by red blood corpuscles throughout the mucosa; gram-positive diplococci in the interstitial tissue between the acini. a, Hematoxyln and eosin × 100; b, Gram-Weigert, × 1000.

one or more animal passages. Thus from a series of 176 animals (guinea-pigs, rats, and dogs) injected in various ways with strains from influenza, outspoken hemorrhages of the stomach were noted in 9, hemorrhages or other lesions of the intestines in 12, and hemorrhagic pancreatitis in 5. Cholecystitis did not occur in a single case. The hemorrhages followed injection of the strains as isolated from influenza in 6 instances; the others occurred in animals injected with strains after from one to four animal passages. The lesions of the stomach consisted usually of multiple punctate hemorrhages varying in size, but whether small or large they usually involved considerable areas (fig. 4). Marked edema, and at times necrosis with beginning ulceration of tissue was often associated with the hemorrhages. Post-mortem digestion was often marked. Sections and cultures made in some instances showed that the lesions were the result of localization of streptococci and not due wholly to general toxic effects. Moreover, in nearly all instances the hemorrhage in the stomach occurred only when the virulence was high and when streptococci were isolated from the blood after death. Besides the swelling, hemorrhage, and the edema of Peyer's patches, lymphoid follicles, and mesenteric lymph glands, the most common lesions of the intestinal tract consisted of small but usually numerous hemorrhages of the mucous membrane or submucosa. The hemorrhages were more common in the small intestine but occurred also in the cecum, transverse colon (fig. 4 b), and in one instance in the appendix of a rabbit. The mucous membrane in the area showing hemorrhages was usually covered with a blood tinged mucus. Large amounts of mucus and fluid contents in the intestine were noted in some instances in which the mucous membrane was hyperemic. Peyer's patches and the lymphoid follicles were swollen, but no hemorrhages could be made out. Only a few animals developed outspoken diarrhea. Sections of the intestines through the hemorrhagic areas showed most of the hemorrhages to be in the mucous membrane. The areas were often wedge shaped, with the base toward the lumen, but they extended well into the deeper layers and mucosa, and in some instances into the submucosa. Superficial erosions were noted in some instances, but marked ulcerations were not found. In either case gram-positive diplococci were easily demonstrable throughout the areas, but not in the normal tissues. The diplococci were most numerous near the surface of the hemorrhage, as if the bacteria had been excreted into the lumen of the intestine, but at times they were found in large numbers in the deeper layers of the mucosa. Leukocytic infiltration was quite marked in some instances, and wholly lacking in others. Marked damage to the endothelium of the blood vessels was noted in many sections in, or adjacent to, the areas of hemorrhage and infiltration. In some cases this was evidenced by swelling of the endothelium and irregular staining of the nuclei; in others by the occurrence of masses of desquamated, swollen endothelial cells, with fragmented nuclei, partly or completely plugging the lumina of fair sized vessels. This finding was similar to that of Kuskow in lesions in the intestines in influenza in man. The lesions were particularly common in the vessels in the subperitoneum. More rarely the vessels were filled with leukocytes in which only a few endothelial cells could be found (fig. 4 a). Cultures from the upper intestinal contents, rich in mucus, and of emulsions of washed pieces of hemorrhages from the mucous membrane often yielded a large number of the green-producing streptococci, cultures from the lower respiratory tract usually only colon bacilli. Localization in the intestinal tract rarely occurred following the injection of the hemolytic streptococcus isolated in influenza, but in two instances in which hemorrhages were found, hemolytic streptococci were isolated in large numbers and diplococci were demonstrated in the lesions.

If lesions developed in the pancreas, they were usually severe, and always most marked in the head. They consisted of marked edema, diffuse and circumscribed hemorrhages usually associated with fat necrosis (fig. 4). Sections showed marked separation and degeneration of parenchymatous cells, edema, hemorrhage, and moderate infiltration of interstitial tissue. Some of the capillaries and larger vessels were partially or completely plugged with desquamated and degenerating endothelial cells. Gram stains revealed many diplococci in the thrombosed vessels and throughout the hemorrhagic and edematous areas, but the organisms were not demonstrable in the lumina of vessels and in the tissues, which were unchanged.

The islands of Langerhans were changed little or not at all, and were quite free from bacteria. The lesions noted following the injection after animal passages of strains from cases in which there was no gastro-enteritis, were due to localization of streptococci and not wholly to general toxic effects. They were similar to those noted following injection of the two strains from the cases of gastro-intestinal influenza, similar to those found in persons during the pandemic of 1889 to 1890, and the pandemic of 1918-1919 (Kuskow, Lucke, Wight and Kime). They occurred following intravenous, intraperitoneal, and intratracheal injection, and after introduction into the stomach, duodenum, and lower bowel.

Localization in the gastro-intestinal tract was found to be due largely to peculiar qualities in the streptococci. It occurred in nearly all animals injected with strains from the patients who had similar lesions. It occurred even in different species after injection of some strains isolated from cases of respiratory influenza after one or more animal passages. Thus a strain that produced pancreatitis in a guinea-pig in the second passage produced this condition in the guinea-pig, rat and dog on intravenous injection in the third passage, a property which had disappeared in the fourth passage. The strain from case 2979 was agglutinated specifically by the monovalent antistreptococcus serum from influenza.

The experiments made as a basis of this study suggest that there is a true gastro-intestinal type of influenza and that green-producing streptococci similar to those isolated from the respiratory type of the disease but which tend to localize in the gastro-intestinal tract, are the chief cause. It is not to be concluded, however, that all symptoms in influenza referable to the gastro-intestinal tract are due to localization of bacteria in its mucous membrane. In experiments reported elsewhere [3] it has been shown that the symptoms and findings in influenza are due in part to an anaphylactoid reaction; the severe vomiting and diarrhea noted at the outset of some cases may be an expression of this mechanism.

BIBLIOGRAPHY

1 Kuskow, N.: Zur pathologischen Anatomie der Grippe, Virchows Arch. f. path. Anat. u. Physiol., 1895, cxxxix, 406-458.

2 Lucke, B., Wight, T., and Kime, E.: Pathologic Anatomy and Bacteriology of Influenza, Epidemic of Autumn, 1918, Arch. Int. Med., 1919, xxiv, 154-237.

3 Rosenow, E. C.: Studies in Influenza and Pneumonia. VII. A Study of the Effects Following the Injection of Bacteria Found in Influenza in Normal Throats, in Simple Naso-Pharyngitis, and in Lobar Pneumonia. (This issue, p. 504.)

4 Sherwood, N. P., Downs, C. M. and McNaught, J. B.: Nonlactose Fermenting Organisms from the Feces of Influenza Patients, Jour. Infect. Dis., 1920, xxvi, 16-22.

STUDIES IN INFLUENZA AND PNEUMONIA

IX. CHANGES IN THE GREEN-PRODUCING STREPTOCOCCUS INDUCED BY SUCCESSIVE ANIMAL PASSAGE AND THEIR SIGNIFICANCE IN EPIDEMIC INFLUENZA

E. C. Rosenow

Division of Experimental Bacteriology, The Mayo Foundation, Rochester, Minnesota.

In a previous paper[3] it has been shown that the green-producing streptococcus isolated quite constantly in influenza and early in influenzal pneumonia has peculiar and high invasive powers not possessed by the Streptococcus viridans or pneumococci normally present in the upper respiratory tract. By the intratracheal injection of this organism the findings which have come to be regarded as more or less characteristic of influenza have been reproduced. The severity of reaction, the degree of leukopenia, and the mortality in the animals were roughly proportional to the severity of the symptoms, the degree of leukopenia, and the mortality in the patients from whom the strains were isolated. In this paper I shall report the results obtained in the animals following successive animal passage of this strain, the changes induced in the bacteria, and correlate the findings with those noted in patients at different stages of epidemic waves of influenza.

The changes wrought in the green-producing streptococci by successive intratracheal injections as measured by the leukocyte count and mortality are summarized in table 1. It was found that the leukocyte count made twenty-four hours after injection was quite representative of the total reduction in leukocytes, and hence it is used as a standard for comparison. The average count before injection and twenty-four hours after injection, the percentage of reduction in leukocytes, the percentage of animals developing leukopenia, leukocytosis, or no change in the number of leukocytes, respectively, and the mortality percentage were determined for each series of animals. The reduction in leukocytes, and the percentage of animals showing leukopenia run roughly parallel with the mortality rate; the greater the former two, the greater the latter. The average percentage reduction in leukocytes in the first animal passage was 51, in the second 66, in the third 50, and in the fourth 38. The mortality percentage was

57, 100, 57, and 38, respectively. There were a progressive diminution in the percentage of animals showing leukopenia from 92 to 47, an increase in the animals showing leukocytosis, and no change in leukocytes in from 4 to 25 from the first to the fourth animal passage.

I shall now consider the changes wrought in these strains as evidenced by the character of pulmonary and other lesions in guinea-pigs and by the mortality rate following successive intratracheal application.

The technic employed throughout these experiments was uniform. The dose was 0.5 c c of a twenty-four hour dextrose-brain broth, or

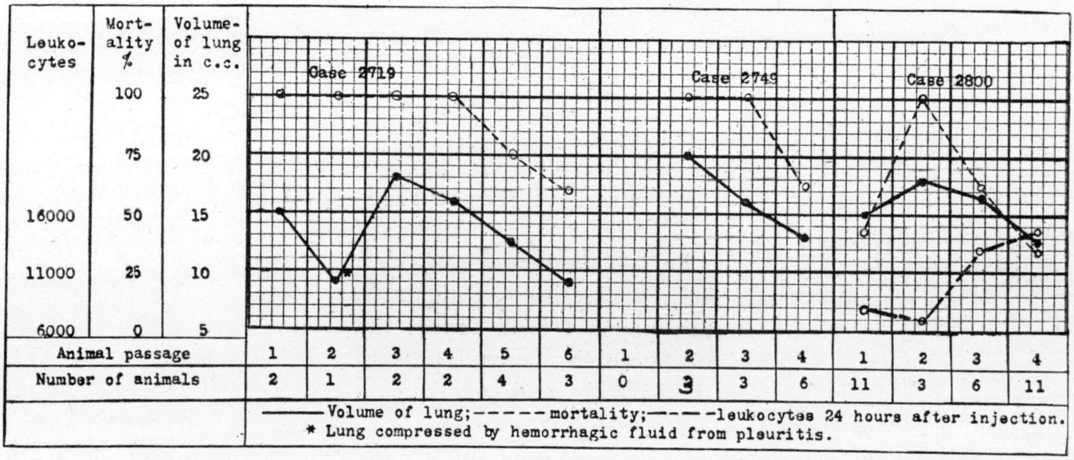

Chart 1.—Volume of lung, mortality and leukocyte count in experimental influenzal pneumonia in guinea-pigs following successive intratracheal injections.

dextrose-blood-broth culture. In order to prove viability and identity of the bacteria injected a plating was made of all cultures which were injected.

The results summarized in chart 1 were obtained from a study of the cases of typical influenza or influenzal pneumonia, and owing to the importance of the findings it is best to consider them separately in some detail.

CASE 2719.—A woman, aged 41, was admitted to the Isolation Hospital Dec. 12, 1918, with a temperature of 103.3, pulse 96, and respiration 31. The patient had been taken sick one week before with headache, backache, aching of the limbs, and fever; this lasted for three or four days, then was less severe until the day before her admission. Examination showed decided cyanosis, moderate dyspnea, scattered râles and areas of dulness, and bronchovesicular breathing over the right lung. Two days later fine râles were heard over both lower lobes and distinct dullness over most of the right lung. December 16, the patient was worse and the right lower lobe was found to be completely consolidated. December 18 the patient became delirious and constantly tried to get out of bed, and at intervals she was markedly cyanotic. In the evening cyanosis grew worse as the respirations became labored and very rapid, and death occurred four hours later.

The white blood count the day after admission was 7,400; no counts were made after that. The sputum December 19 was bloody and

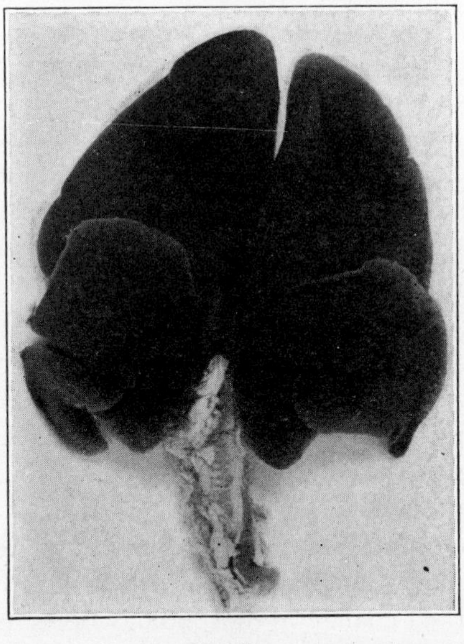

Fig. 1.—Photograph of lung of guinea-pig 853 twenty-four hours after intratracheal injection of green-producing streptococcus from case 2719 in the third animal passage; × 1.

frothy, and the culture showed a large number of characteristic green-producing streptococci and many staphylococci.

The main findings at necropsy were: Lobar pneumonia of the right upper lobe in the gray hepatization stage; bronchopneumonia of the right lower lobe; hemorrhagic edema and edema of the left lower lobe; hypostatic congestion; and emphysema of the left upper lobe. Sections of the lung showed marked congestion, a filling of the alveoli with degenerating red cells, giant cells, degenerating necrotic alveolar epithelial cells in large numbers, and a relatively small number of leukocytes.

The culture from the lung exudate after death contained almost pure growth of the green-producing streptococcus. The washing from a small part of a blood-agar plate was injected intraperitoneally into a guinea-pig; it died in twenty-four hours from peritonitis. The moderately emphysematous lung contained localized hemorrhages and edema. Large numbers of the characteristic streptococcus were found in cultures from the blood and peritoneal fluid. The strain from this animal was used in the successive injection of 20 guinea-pigs; 14 intratracheally and 6 intraperitoneally. The average volume of the lungs and the mortality on successive intratracheal injections are summarized in chart 1. In this series the peritoneal exudate of the first animal was injected directly into the trachea of one guinea-pig (second passage). The culture in dextrose-brain broth from a single colony on a blood-agar plate from the lung of this animal was injected into 2 guinea-pigs (third passage). In the fourth, fifth and sixth passages the primary culture in dextrose-brain broth of the lung of the preceding animal was injected intratracheally.

In order to make sure that the diminution in virulence was not due to cultivation on artificial mediums the emulsion of the lung of one of the sixth passage series was injected directly into the trachea of one guinea-pig. The duration of the successive experiments in animal passages (chart 1) in the animals that furnished the strains for succeeding injections, was one, three, one, one, one, and four days, respectively, or eleven days; the duration of cultivation on artificial mediums between the animal passages was six days, the total seventeen days. Blood-agar plate cultures were made of the exudates of the lung and pleura, the blood, and of the material injected to control the results obtained. No marked change in morphology occurred, but the colonies which at first were quite moist and spreading became smaller and less moist after successive animal passages. None of the strains fermented inulin, nor were they bile soluble. The agglutinating power of the various immune serums, including the monovalent serum, was tested over this strain on isolation, and after one, two, three and four animal passages. It was agglutinated specifically by the monovalent serum for the influenza streptococcus in each of these, but in the fourth passage the strain was less highly differentiated for it was partly agglutinated by type I and type II pneumococcus serums and by antihemolytic streptococcus serum, but to a lesser extent than in the influenza serum. The best measure of the changes which the micro-organism had undergone was found to be its effect on the animals. During the seventeen days of growth differences were noted in the character of the lesions of the lung, and in the mortality.

During the first three animal passages the effects were striking. Intraperitoneal injections were rapidly fatal and the tendency to localize and produce lesions in the lung was marked. The intratracheal injections in the second and third passages were followed by extreme lesions of the lung, consisting of marked exudation of dark hemorrhagic fluid into the alveoli or pleura, and increase in the size of the lung (fig. 1),

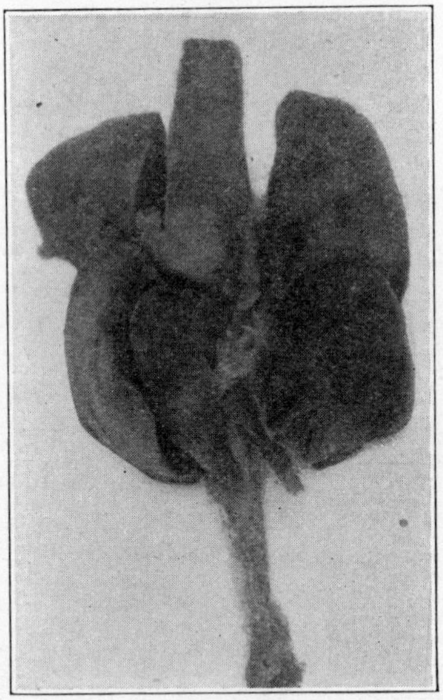

Fig. 2.—Lung of guinea-pig 869 thirty hours after intratracheal injection of the same strain in the fifth animal passage. Note the consolidation of the right diaphragmatic lobe and part of the left diaphragmatic lobe; × 1.

associated with marked degeneration of alveolar epithelium and endothelium (figs. 4 a, 5 a, and 8 a) with relatively slight cellular infiltration and aggregation of large numbers of streptococci along the alveolar lining (figs. 4 b and 5 b). In the fourth passage both guinea-pigs showed relatively less hemorrhagic edema and more leukocytic infiltration. In the fifth passage the difference was striking. In all 4 guinea-pigs well marked areas of consolidation, mostly of lobar distribution, occurred. In 2 this was extremely marked twenty-four (fig. 1) and thirty hours after injection (fig. 2). The consistency of the involved areas was quite firm, the cut surface quite dry, and grayish red, instead of hemorrhagic and edematous as noted in the earlier passages; sections showed marked leukocytic infiltration and relatively slight hemorrhagic edema, and the bacteria were no longer found chiefly along the alveolar lining, but more diffusely distributed throughout the exudate (figs. 6 a and b). In the sixth passage the picture of true pneumonia with no hemorrhagic edema was noted in all of the guinea-pigs injected (fig. 3). Sections showed marked leukocytic infiltration, little hemorrhagic edema, little necrosis of alveolar lining (fig. 8 b) and micro-organisms

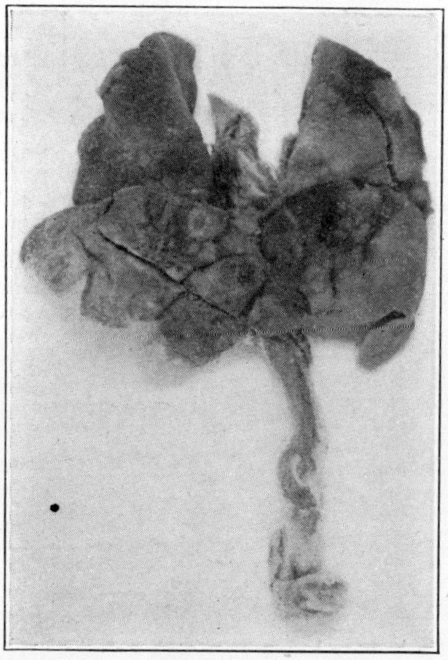

Fig. 3.—Lung of guinea-pig 886 four days after intratracheal injection of the strain in the sixth animal passage. Note the complete grayish consolidation of the left and part of the right diaphragmatic lobe; × 1.

diffusely distributed throughout the exudate (fig. 7). The guinea-pig injected with the lung emulsion from the sixth animal passage developed slightly increased respirations, fever for a few days, and moderate leukocytosis; it then recovered. No pulmonary or other lesions were found when it was chloroformed on the twelfth day. As the gross and microscopic picture of the lung changed from that of a violent destructive reaction with little evidence of response on the part of the host to a less violent reaction in which marked exudation of leukocytes occurred, the volume of the lung and mortality rate decreased. The following experiments are illustrative:

Guinea-pig 820, weighing 370 gm., was injected intratracheally Dec. 23, 1918, with 0.15 c c of a suspension of the peritoneal exudate of a guinea-pig injected intraperitoneally with the sputum from case 2719. December 24 the animal appeared ill. It was short of breath, uncomfortable, made repeated violent efforts at respiration, and coughed violently at intervals. December 26 it was found dead. The pleural cavity contained a moderate amount of bloody turbid fluid. The lungs were only moderately distended (9 c c), and covered with a thin fibrinous film. The left diaphragmatic lobe was large and almost completely consolidated. The areas of consolidation were irregular, and mottled red and gray. Areas of irregular size showing hemorrhagic edema and partial consolidation were found in all the other lobes. The peribronchial lymph glands were edematous and hemorrhagic. The pleural fluid showed many green-producing streptococci; the blood, five colonies of green-producing streptococci; and the pneumonic lung, a large number of green-producing streptococci and a moderate number of staphylococci. In sections of the lung patchy areas of marked leukocytic infiltration were surrounded by areas in which the terminal bronchi were enlarged, the epithelium was desquamated, and the alveoli were greatly distended and completely filled with coagulated serum in which a variable number of red blood corpuscles and relatively few leukocytes were found (fig. 4 a). Exudate in sections stained by the Gram stain showed a large number of diplococci and streptococci which usually were peripherally placed in the alveoli (fig. 4 b). The subpleural and the perivascular lymph channels in areas were completely plugged and distended with gram-positive diplococci and streptococci. In the areas of marked leukocytic infiltration a rather large number of staphylococci were found, whereas in the areas showing hemorrhagic edema, few or none could be demonstrated. Under high power marked nuclear fragmentation and degeneration of epithelial cells and marked necrosis of endothelial cells of the capillaries in the alveoli were observed (fig. 8 a).

Guinea-pig 853, weighing 440 gm., was injected intratracheally Dec. 28, 1918, with 0.5 c c of the dextrose-brain broth culture of the strain isolated from the blood of guinea-pig 820. The animal coughed up immediately a large part of the material injected. December 29 it was found dead. The trachea, larynx, and bronchi were filled with a bloody, frothy fluid. Approximately 5 c c of turbid chocolate colored fluid were found in the pleural cavity. The lungs were voluminous (18 c c), hemorrhagic throughout, and very heavy (fig. 1). The stomach was partially digested and a number of circumscribed areas in the horns of the uterus were congested and swollen. The uterus and vagina contained bloody mucus and the uterine horns a number of submucous hemorrhages. Cultures from the lung, pleural fluid, tracheal mucus, blood, and mucus from the left horn of the uterus showed a large number of the green-producing streptococci. Sections of the lung showed marked dilatation of alveoli and terminal bronchi, extreme congestion of the capillaries and veins, and marked constriction of the larger bronchi which were filled with coagulated serum and blood. There was marked desquamation of the alveolar epithelium and necrosis of the endothelium of the interalveolar capillaries (fig. 5 a). Some areas were slightly infiltrated with leukocytes. The Gram stain showed enormous numbers of diplococci and streptococci. These were especially numerous along the alveolar walls surrounding the bronchi and blood vessels (fig. 5 b). The number of gram-positive diplococci was so large that the outline of the alveoli could be made out readily under the low power of the microscope.

Guinea-pig 869, weighing 330 gm., was injected intratracheally Dec. 31, 1918, with 1 c c of the dextrose-brain broth culture of strain 2719 in the fifth animal passage. January 1 at 1 p. m. the animal was extremely short of breath, it had an expiratory grunt, its hair was ruffled, it was just able to walk, it sat humped up, breathing with all its might, the thorax appeared distended, and the respirations were chiefly abdominal. At 9 p. m. the animal was found dead, the body still warm. The lungs were moderately distended (15 c c); the right lung was almost completely consolidated; the areas of consolidation were quite uniform in consistency and grayish-red. The pleural cavity contained 2 c c of turbid, bloody fluid; the mediastinal lymph glands were edematous and surrounded by bubbles of gas in the mediastinal tissue. One fetus was aborted into the vagina. The area showing its attachment in the left horn of the uterus was hemorrhagic and edematous, and in the right horn was a loosely attached hemorrhagic fetal mass. Other parts of the mucous membrane of the uterus were markedly congested and showed small punctate hemorrhages. Cultures from the blood, liver, spleen, and adrenal were negative; those from the pleural fluid, lung, and the mucous membrane of the uterus and hemorrhagic placenta, showed a large number of green-producing streptococci in pure form. Cultures from the mucous membrane of the nose showed green-producing streptococci and some staphylococci; from the kidney, a few green-producing streptococci. Sections of the consolidated right diaphragmatic lobe presented a very different picture from those in the preceding animals. The alveoli were moderately distended; the epithelial lining only slightly desquamated; the nuclei of these cells and endothelial cells of the capillaries stained normally. The alveoli were filled with a highly cellular exudate consisting largely of polymorphonuclear leukocytes and a relatively small amount of coagulated serum and red blood corpuscles (fig. 6 a). Gram-positive diplococci and streptococci were found in large numbers distributed throughout the alveolar exudate (fig. 6 b).

Guinea-pig 886, weighing 320 gm., was injected intratracheally Jan. 2, 1919, with 1.5 c c of the dextrose-brain-broth culture from the lung of guinea-pig 869. The nostrils, before injection, were dry and clean; cultures from the right nostril showed a large number of indifferent colonies resembling staphylococci. January 3 at 7:30 a. m. the animal appeared quite well, although respirations were definitely increased. At 11 a. m. it appeared well; the respirations were still increased, and cultures from the nose showed a large number of green-producing streptococci and a moderate number of staphylococci. January 4 the nose was wet with a mucopurulent discharge; the weight loss was 50 gm., the respirations were somewhat rapid, and coughing occurred at intervals. January 6, 10 a. m., there was marked crusting about the nostrils almost to the point of causing obstruction, and on removal of the crust, several drops of mucopurulent secretion escaped from the nostril. At 6 p. m. the animal was found dead. The lungs were only slightly distended (9 c c). The left diaphragmatic lobe was completely consolidated and mottled grayish-red; the right diaphragmatic lobe and irregular areas in the right cardiac and apical lobes showed grayish consolidations surrounding the bronchi (fig. 3). The left nostril was plugged with a bloody, mucopurulent material. The right maxillary sinus was filled with bloody pus; the mucous membrane of the nose, trachea, and bronchi was extremely hyperemic. Cultures from the blood were negative. Cultures from the pleura, consolidated areas of the lung, and pus from the nose showed a large number of green-producing streptococci and some staphylococci. Sections of the lung showed slight dilatation of the alveoli, marked cellular leukocytic exudate of quite uniform distribution filling the alveoli completely, with little or no admixture of coagulated serum and blood (fig. 7 a). The epithelial cells lining the terminal bronchi and alveoli, and the endothelial cells of the inter-alveolar capillaries stained quite normally (fig. 8 b). The bacteria were diffusely distributed in large numbers in the alveolar exudate (fig. 7 b).

CASE 2749.—A man, aged 29, a nurse, developed headache, sore throat, severe aching all over, dry cough, and temperature of 100.2, Dec. 16, 1918. The following day his temperature ranged from 102.6 to 103. The headache continued, there were marked backache, soreness through the chest, and a severe cough. December 18 the patient felt weak, perspired, and was chilly at intervals; the ache in the back, soreness in the chest, and the cough were worse. The temperature ranged from 100.6 to 101.8. The cough and soreness in the

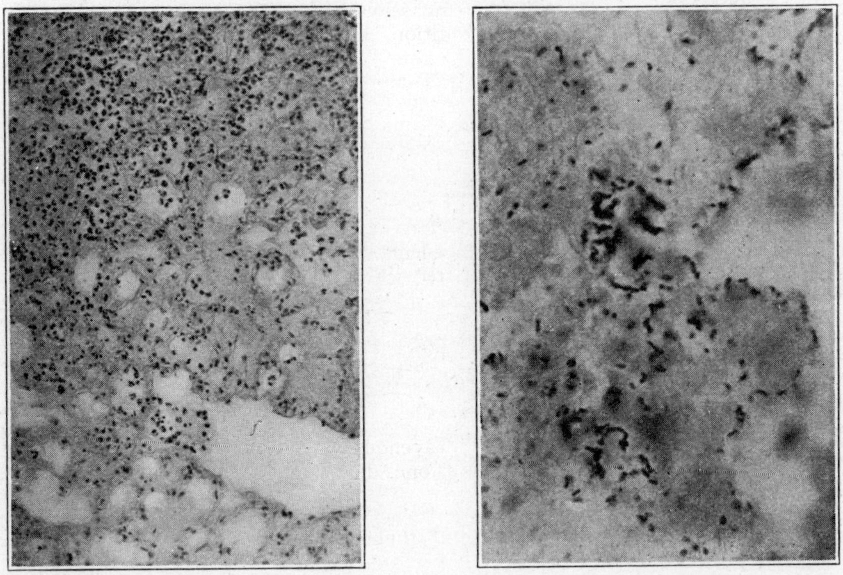

A B

Fig. 4.—Photomicrograph of sections of lung of guinea-pig injected with the green-producing streptococcus from case 2719 after one animal passage. Note the marked edema, hemorrhage, dilatation of terminal bronchi and alveoli, necrosis of cells in alveolar walls and the relatively slight leukocytic infiltration in a, and the distribution of the bacteria along the alveolar wall in b. a. Hematoxylin and eosin; × 100. b. Gram-Weigert; × 500.

chest continued for a week; the nose bled December 22, and a large amount of mucopurulent blood-tinged sputum was raised December 23. This sputum was cultured and injected into animals. The temperature became normal December 23 and the patient made a good but slow recovery. Blood-agar plate cultures from the sputum showed almost pure culture of moist, spreading, green-producing streptococci, a few staphylococci, no hemolytic streptococci, nor influenza bacilli. The sputum, 0.2 c c was injected subcutaneously into a guinea-pig; it died three days later of subcutaneous cellulitis, beginning bronchopneumonia, and hemorrhagic endometritis. Cultures from the blood, lung, and bloody mucus from the uterus, contained a large number of the characteristic green-producing streptococcus colonies. The culture from the uterus was used to inject 7 guinea-pigs, 4 intravenously, and 3 intratracheally, and 2 rats, one subcutaneously, the other intratracheally. All died as a result of the injection. All 4 animals injected intravenously showed moderate emphysema and evidence of localization in the lung, indicated by localized areas of hemorrhage and edema with or without beginning consolidation. The 2 females showed lesions of the mucous membrane of the uterus and both aborted. Two showed, in addition, localization in muscles and myocardium, one acute peritonitis, and one marked hemorrhagic pancreatitis. Cultures from all yielded the organism injected, together with a few staphylococci, and in one a few colonies of hemolytic streptococci developed from the lung and uterus. All 3 guinea-pigs and the rat injected intratracheally died from emphysema of the lungs filled with hemorrhagic bloody fluid, or with bronchopneumonia in various stages of development. The average volume of the lung in the guinea-pigs was 20 c c (chart 1). The rat and 2 of the guinea-pugs showed decided involvment of the pleura in addition to the lung involvement. The only female injected aborted; one of the others showed peritonitis and one hemorrhage and edema of the head of the pancreas. The characteristic streptococcus was isolated from all. The rat injected subcutaneously died in three days from subcutaneous cellulitis, emphysema, and slight hemorrhages of the lung. The green-producing streptococcus was found in the edema fluid and in the bloody mucus in the uterine horns.

The primary culture in dextrose broth from the pancreas, which showed marked swelling and inflammation, was injected intravenously into 2 guinea-pigs and 2 dogs; intratracheally into a guinea-pig and a rat; intraperitoneally into a mouse, and subcutaneously into a rat. All the animals except the dogs died. Both guinea-pigs injected intravenously developed well marked areas of localized bronchopneumonia, and one developed acute hemorrhagic pancreatitis and myocardial degeneration. The dogs were etherized on the fifth day. Lung lesions were absent, but there were lesions in the mucous membrane of the uterus; the one animal that had aborted showed pancreatitis. The green-producing streptococcus was isolated from the mucous membrane of the uterus in both dogs, from the blood of both guinea-pigs, and from the pancreas of the dog showing pancreatitis. The guinea-pig and rat that were injected intratracheally developed marked rhinitis and tracheitis, emphysema of the lung with hemorrhagic edema, and bronchopneumonia. The guinea-pig had endometritis and aborted. The rat injected subcutaneously and the mouse intraperitoneally developed, beside cellulitis and peritonitis, respectively, definite lesions of lung and pleura, from which the organism was isolated.

The primary culture from the hemorrhagic lung of one of the guinea-pigs injected intratracheally in the second animal passage was injected intratracheally into 2 guinea-pigs. Both developed massive bronchopneumonia and purulent bronchitis, and both yielded the organisms in pure cultures. The filtrate from this lung was injected directly intratracheally into 2 guinea-pigs, and after incubation in dextrose-brain broth into 4 guinea-pigs. One of the latter remained well, all the others developed well marked lesions of the lung, quite similar to those in the animals injected with the corresponding culture. The 2 females had endometritis, 3 had rhinitis, sinusitis, tracheitis, and bronchitis, and 1 each had myositis and mediastinitis. Cultures from the lesions and the blood in these yielded the characteristic organism. The details of these and other filtrate experiments have been given elsewhere.

Cultures from 3 of the animals injected with this strain in the third passage were injected intratracheally into 5 guinea-pigs. All developed moderate emphysema and bronchopneumonia of lobar type, 2 developed high grade myocardial degeneration, and 2 marked rhinitis and bronchitis. Two of the females had endometritis. The primary culture in dextrose-brain broth from the pneumonic lung of 2 of the guinea-pigs, third animal passage series, was injected intratracheally into 4 guinea-pigs, and cultures from the uterine horns of the dog that had aborted were injected into 2 guinea-pigs. One of the former and one of the latter recovered after several days of illness. The others died from two to four days after injection. All showed well marked exudative pneumonia, 2 definitely lobar in type with relatively slight hem-

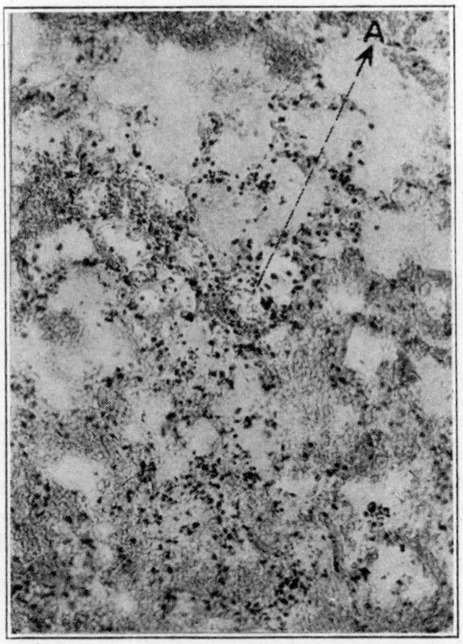

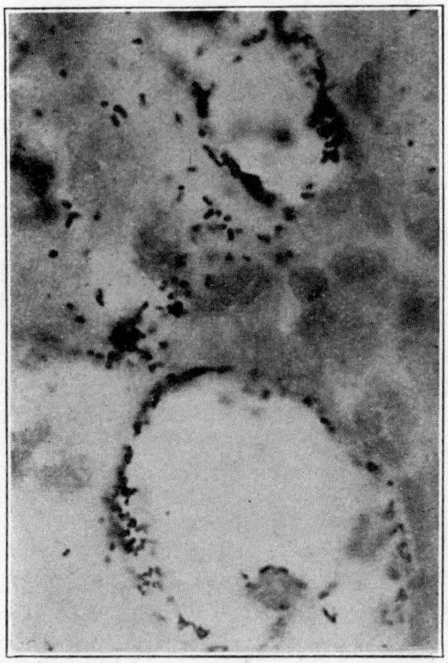

A B

Fig. 5.—Sections of lung of guinea-pig shown in figure 1. Note the marked hemorrhage and edema, the absence of leukocytic infiltration and the marked necrosis of alveolar walls in a, and the peripherally placed streptococci in b. a. Hematoxylin and eosin, × 100. b. Gram-Weigert, × 500.

orrhagic edema, and only moderate emphysema (chart 1). Two of the 3 females had endometritis and myocardial degeneration and 2 had well marked rhinitis, and tracheitis; 1 had hemorrhages in the rectus muscle. The green-producing streptococcus was isolated from all. The filtrate from the lung of 2 of the guinea-pigs (third animal passage series) was injected into the trachea of 12 guinea-pigs. The 2 that were injected with the heated filtrate recovered after severe immediate symptoms of anaphylactic shock, 1 injected with the unheated filtrate died in ten minutes from anaphylactic shock, 6 of the others recovered after severe immediate symptoms, and 3 died. All showed bronchopneumonia; 2 showed marked lesions of the pleura, and 1 aborted. The green-producing streptococcus was isolated from the lesions, and from the uterus of the one that aborted. The curves giving the volume of the lung and the mortality rate (chart 1) represent roughly the effects from the successive injections of this strain. The difference in the symptoms and types of lesions of the lung in the early and in the later animal passages was striking. In the former respiratory embarrassment, hemorrhage, and edema with relatively slight exudation of leukocytes in the lung dominated the picture; in the latter, respiratory embarrassment was less marked; exudative pneumonia, and a relatively slight edema with a greater tendency to involve the upper respiratory tract as well as the pleura, dominated the picture. The greater tendency of leukocytic infiltration was noted even in animals that lived the same length of time. The results on intravenous injection of the organism in the second and third passages, besides showing a tendency to localize in the lung and uterus, showed a marked affinity for the muscle, myocardium, and pancreas; pancreatitis occurred in three species of animals (guinea-pig, dog and rabbit). The lesions in the muscles were focal and hemorrhagic, often occurring in clusters, and often surrounded by edema and hemorrhage. Streptococci were found in large numbers in these lesions and in the pancreas, showing pancreatitis. Altogether 19 animals (guinea-pigs, rats, and mice) were injected with this strain intratracheally, intravenously, intraperitoneally, and subcutaneously, in the first, second, and third animal passages. All succumbed to the effects of the injection. Two of the 6 injected in the fourth passage recovered.

Case 2800.—A woman, aged 24, was admitted to the isolation hospital Jan. 9, 1919, in a very weak condition with a temperature of 104, pulse 120, and respiration 34. The patient had been taken sick six days before with aching of limbs, headache, backache, chills and fever. She complained of pain over the entire chest, and coughed a great deal. The day after admission, her respirations were shallow and labored, she was pale and cyanotic, and the pulse was extremely rapid. A diffuse bronchopneumonia of the right base and bronchial breathing in the area opposite the angle of the scapula on the left side were found. January 12 her condition was very much the same; the chest was in full expansion and respirations were almost wholly diaphragmatic. The symptoms persisted, she grew worse as cyanosis increased and died January 14. The leukocyte count was persistently low, ranging between 1,900 and 3,700.

The chief findings at necropsy were: Bilateral pseudolobar pneumonia; hemorrhagic edema; left hemo-hydro-thorax, 500 c c; and mild acute nephritis. Sections of the lung showed dilatation of alveoli, marked congestion, and alveolar exudate rich in red blood corpuscles, edema fluid, little fibrin, and only a moderate number of leukocytes.

A culture from a throat swab January 12 showed a large number of moist, spreading colonies of green-producing streptococci, many colonies of Staphylococcus aureus, and moist hemolyzing streptococci. Cultures from the blood after death contained green-producing streptococci, hemolyzing streptocci, and staphylococci; and from cultures from the pleural fluid hemolyzing streptococci and staphyloccocci. The history and findings in this case are clearly those of influenza in which well marked lung lesions developed as the symptoms persisted.

The bacteria isolated from the sputum, blood, and lung exudate were a mixture of the organisms most constantly present in influenza. Aside from hemolysis the morphology and type of colony of the green-producing streptococci and hemolyzing streptococci were identical. It was thought worth while to study the effects, including the leukocyte counts, of the injection of mass cultures containing a mixture of these strains, and of pure cultures in a large series of animals in order to note the changes which might occur in the lesions produced following successive animal passage. The effect of intratracheal injections of cultures of the green-producing and hemolytic streptococci or mixtures that occurred in the primary dextrose-brain broth from the blood, and sputum, throat, and lung exudates were very similar. Emphysema of marked grade and hemorrhagic edema with localized areas of peribronchial consolidation of varying size and age dominated the picture. Leukopenia was equally marked regardless of whether the strain was hemolytic or green-producing. The results obtained following successive intratracheal injections of the green-producing streptococci are summarized in

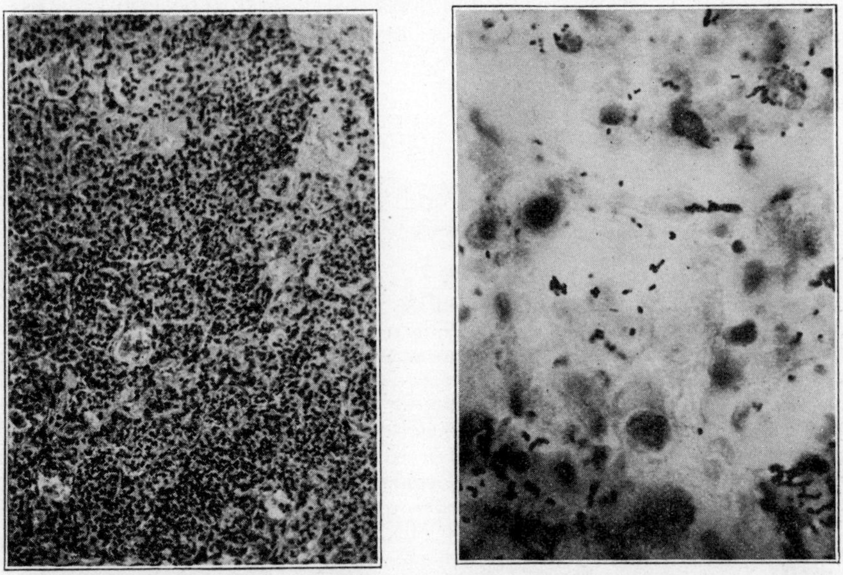

A B

Fig. 6.—Sections of lung shown in figure 2. Note the marked leukocytic infiltration and the slight edema and hemorrhage, and the diffuse distribution of the streptococci in the exudate. a. Hematoxylin and eosin, × 100. b. Gram-Weigert, × 500.

chart 1. In this series of animals the strains used for subsequent injections were first plated on blood-agar. From this subcultures of green-producing streptococci were made in dextrose-brain broth and injected.

It will be noted that during the first and second animal passages, as the volume of lung (severity of reaction) increased, the mortality increased, the drop in leukocytes occurred, and as the volume of lung diminished during the third and fourth passages the mortality and the drop in leukocytes became less marked. The difference in the character of lesions in the lungs was similar to the difference noted between cases 2719 and 2749.

It has been pointed out elsewhere that the green-producing streptococci may acquire typical hemolyzing power (beta type hemolysis), and that the hemolyzing streptococci may acquire the power of producing typical green colonies (alpha type hemolysis). Moreover, a green-producing flora in patients is often displaced by a hemolytic flora and this in turn by a green-producing flora, especially in patients who recover. It was thought worth while to pass the hemolytic streptococcus through a series of guinea-pigs in the same manner as the green-producing streptococcus had been passed, and to observe whether or not the type of lesion produced changed, and whether the streptococcus changed. The primary culture in dextrose-brain broth of the throat swab was injected into the trachea of 6 guinea-pigs and a rat. Two of the guinea-pigs and the rat recovered. Four of the guinea-pigs died from typical lung lesions with or without pleural involvement, and all showed hemolytic streptococci in pure culture, or together with a few staphylococci.

Guinea-pig 947, weighing 400 gm., was injected intratracheally Jan. 12, 1919, 11 a.m., with 1.5 c c dextrose-brain broth culture of the throat swab. A blood-agar plate of the culture injected showed green-producing, hemolytic streptococci, and a few staphylococci. At 6 p.m. the respirations were rapid, the voice was weak, and the animal appeared ill. January 13, 7:30 a.m., the animal was found dead. A large amount of hemolyzed, dark chocolate colored fluid was found in the pleural cavity. The right diaphragmatic and intermediate lobes were large, extremely hemorrhagic and edematous on the cut surface. Both uterine horns contained a moderate amount of blood tinged mucus, and the mucous membrane was hemorrhagic in areas. Cultures from the blood and from the lung and pleural fluid showed a large number of hemolytic streptococci, a smaller number of staphylococci, but no green-producing streptococci; those from the mucus in the left horn of the uterus showed 150 colonies of staphylococci, 9 colonies of hemolytic streptococci, and 21 colonies of green-producing streptococci. The primary culture of the pleural fluid of this animal which yielded hemolytic streptococci and a few staphylococci was then injected into the trachea of another guinea-pig; it died within six hours. The leukocyte count dropped from 15,000 before injection to 3,100 after death. The lungs were huge in size (18 c c) hemorrhagic and edematous throughout, and the pleura contained about 1 c c of hemorrhagic fluid. Cultures from the blood, pleural fluid, and lung exudate showed many moist, spreading colonies of hemolytic streptococci, while those from the liver and kidney showed a few. The dextrose-broth culture from the blood of this guinea-pig was injected into the trachea of 5 guinea-pigs. One recovered and 4 died of hemorrhagic edema and bronchopneumonia, from one to four days after injection; two died with hemorrhagic pleuritis and 2 without. All showed predominating or pure cultures of green-producing streptococci. The findings in the animal whose strain was passed to the next series were similar to those in the others.

Guinea-pig 1043, weighing 480 gm., was injected intratracheally Jan. 23, 1919, with 2 c c of the glucose-broth culture from the blood of the guinea-pig that died six hours after injection. The leukocyte count was 16,800. January 24, 10 a.m., the respiration was extremely rapid, the leukocyte count was 2,200; at 9 p.m. respiration was extremely rapid, the animal was weaker, it made repeated violent efforts at breathing, resembling anaphylactic shock, and had an expiratory grunt. January 25 it was found dead. The pleural cavity contained a moderate amount of bloody chocolate colored fluid. The left diaphragmatic lobe was covered with a fibrinous film. The lung was greatly distended (18 c c) and heavy (17 gm.). A large part of the left lung was consolidated, consisting of coalescing areas of bronchopneumonia, which in places on the cut surface had become grayish and quite dry. Several

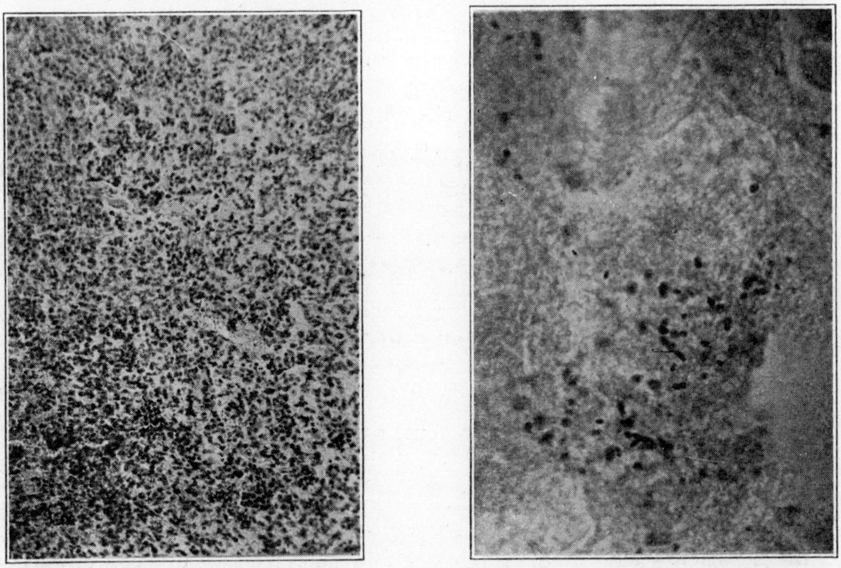

A B

Fig. 7.—Section of lung shown in figure 3. Findings similar to those in figure 6. a. Hematoxylin and eosin, × 100. b. Gram-Weigert, × 500.

similar but smaller areas were found in the right diaphragmatic lobe. Generally the mucous membranes of the nose and trachea were extremely hyperemic and the trachea was filled with a hemorrhagic frothy fluid. A large area (2 by 1.5 cm.) of hemorrage and edema was found in the right rectus muscle of the adominal wall. The involved muscle was friable and ruptured on slight stretching. The leukocyte count of the blood from the heart was 4,400. The myocardium was yellowish gray, the ventricles were in firm contraction, and the auricles dilated. Cultures from the blood, pleural fluid, and lung showed a large number of green-producing streptococci in pure culture, and the liver, adrenal, kidney, brain, and spleen, showed a few. The culture in dextrose broth from the blood after one plating was injected into the trachea of 3 guinea-pigs; 1 of these died of bronchopneumonia in forty-eight hours,

1 recovered, and 1 was chloroformed three days after injection. The third had a moderate amount of bloody fluid in the right pleural cavity, a large wedge-shaped area of grayish consolidation of the right diaphragmatic lobe, and slight emphysema of the lung. The uterus was opaque and contained a moderate amount of mucus. The leukocyte count before injection was 9,400; twenty-four hours after injection 10,400; forty-eight hours after injection 7,200; and after death 8,000. Cultures from the blood were negative; those from the consolidated lung showed large numbers of staphylococci and green-producing streptococci, and the pleural fluid and uterus showed a few green-producing streptococci and staphylococci. This, then, is an example in which a hemolytic streptococcus remained as such throughout two animal passages, but in 4 animals in the third passage it appeared to lose the hemolytic power and to produce green colonies, a property which it retained through the next animal passage. Fifty-three guinea-pigs were injected with cultures of green-producing and hemolytic streptococci isolated from this case and after animal passage. Twenty-three were injected in the first passage, 14 (60%) died; 9 were injected in the second passage, 8 (90%) died; 9 were injected in the third passage, 7 (78%) died; and 14 were injected in the fourth passage, 6 (43%) died.

The average mortality resulting from the animal passage after intratracheal injection of the strains from the 3 cases reported herewith was 57 per cent. of 22 animals injected in the first animal passage, 90 per cent. of 10 animals in the second, 87 per cent. of 16 animals in the third; and 55 per cent. of 22 animals in the fourth. The total mortality, irrespective of the place of injection, ranged as follows: 60 per cent. of the 30 animals injected in the first animal passage, 94 per cent. of the 17 animals in the second, 90 per cent. of the 21 animals in the third, and 52 per cent. of the 19 animals in the fourth passage.

A study of the 3 cases shows clearly that the lesions in the lung in the first few passages resemble very closely those noted in the lungs of the 2 patients who died. They are characterized by marked emphysema, extreme hemorrhage and edema of the lungs (fig. 1), marked evidence of destruction and desquamation of epithelial lining (figs. 3 and 4 a), absence of staining or fragmentation of nuclei of endothelial cells, of capillaries of alveoli (Fig. 8 a), and aggregation of streptococci along the alveolar lining (figs. 3 b and 4 b). Moreover, the relative lack of response, on the part of the host, is evidenced by the slight leukocytic exudation in the lung and the marked reduction of leukocytes in the blood. The symptoms of respiratory embarrassment are often extreme, the mortality rate is high, and death occurs early. After a number of animal passages the picture becomes quite different. The respiratory embarrassment is less violent, the reduction in leukocytes less marked, and the exudation of leukocytes in the lung is the dominant picture (figs. 6 a and 7 a) as hemorrhage and edema become less prominent. The lungs are not so voluminous (figs. 2 and 3). Degeneration and desquamation of the epithelial cells and necrosis of the capillaries are slight (fig. 8 b) and the bacteria are diffusely distributed throughout the exudate instead of along the alveolar lining (figs. 6 b and 7 b). The difference in amount of leukocytic infiltration depends not on the duration of the experiment, but varies with the number of animal passages. The diminution of virulency of these strains from

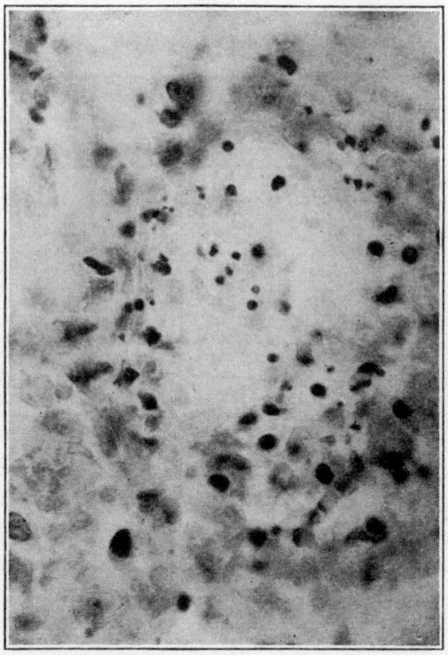

A

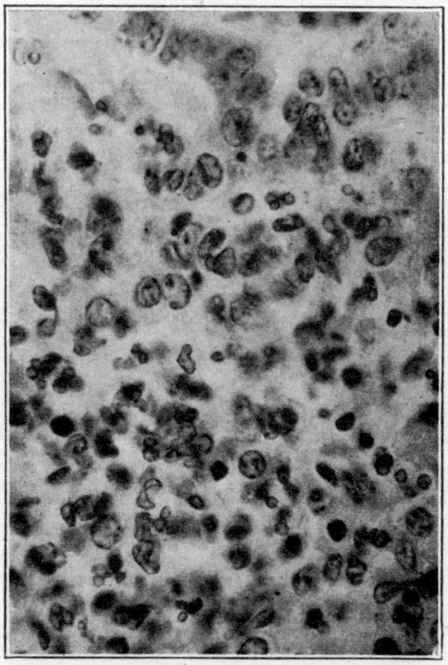

B

Fig. 8.—High-power magnification of sections of lungs shown in figures 4 and 7, illustrating type of lesions obtained during the first few and higher numbers of animal passages. a. Note the marked fragmentation of nuclei of alveolar epithelium and capillaries, the marked hemorrhage and edema, and the almost complete absence of leukocytic infiltration. b. Note the marked leukocytic infiltration and the relatively slight necrosis of cells of alveolar walls. Hematoxylin and eosin, × 500.

cases of influenza as a result of successive intratracheal injections is contrary to the result following successive intraperitoneal injection of strains of the pneumostreptococcus group. The latter method was tested to determine whether the green-producing streptococcus from influenza is peculiar in this respect.

In chart 2 is given a summary of the results of successive intraperitoneal and intratracheal injections of a series of strains of green-producing streptococci from influenza. In the forced experiment on intraperitoneal injection the virulency of the green-producing streptococci increases as that of streptococci and pneumococci from other sources. But when the former micro-organisms are applied successively to the normal mucous membrane of the lower respiratory tract their invasive power increases only during one or two animal passages; it then becomes progressively less during three or four subsequent passages. Most of the strains that were passed through animals were cultivated on artificial mediums for one generation and in one strain

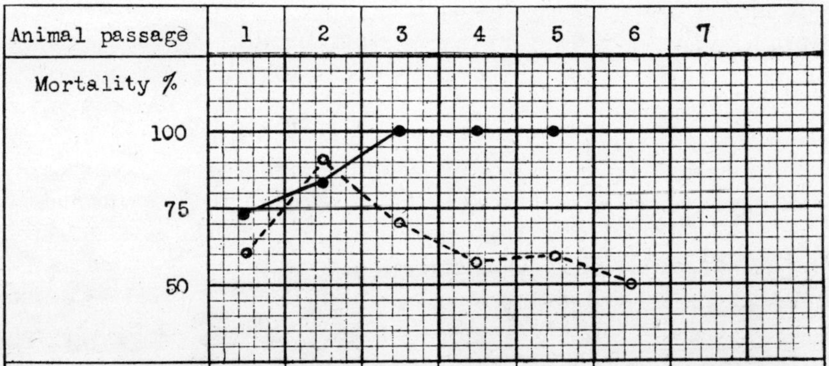

Strains	8	8	6	1	1		Intraperi-
Animals	14	14	8	1	1		toneally
Strains	8	8	6	3	1	1	Intratra-
Animals	14	15	15	12	5	4	cheally

Chart 2.—Mortality in guinea-pigs following successive intraperitoneal and intratracheal injections of streptococci from influenza. The straight line denotes intraperitoneal injection; the broken line denotes intratracheal injection.

(case 2800), for two generations between each passage. In order to make sure that the diminution in invasive power on successive intratracheal application was due to effects exerted on the micro-organism by the body cells or fluids and not due to the culture mediums, control experiments were carried out; emulsions of the consolidated lung were injected directly from animal to animal. The results were similar. The diminution in infecting power was even more rapid than when intervening cultures were injected. This result, contrary to what might be expected, considering what usually happens after direct successive intraperitoneal injections, is in keeping with what has been observed repeatedly when emulsions of lung and pleural fluid from man and from animals are injected directly into the trachea and compared with the results following the injection of the corresponding cultures. The severity of reaction and the mortality following injections of the cultures were greater even when the number of viable bacteria was no larger than that in the exudate. The cells or fluids in the exudate seemed to rob the bacteria of their bite, as it were, a property which they often regained during the growth in suitable artificial mediums. Moreover, in harmony with this idea is the fact that the mortality was higher following the injection of sputum during life than following the injection of the bloody lung exudate after death. During the course of the experiments on intratracheal injection it was also noted that cultures of the green-producing streptococci from the blood and pleural exudate after death in cases of long standing were not so virulent as those from the sputum or throat. Thus in 22 guinea-pigs injected intratracheally with the strains cultured from the sputum of one patient the mortality was 64 per cent., whereas in a series injected with the strains cultured from the blood the mortality was 33 per cent.

Hirsch and McKinney found that the pneumococci at the height of the epidemic at Camp Grant were far more virulent when injected intraperitoneally or intravenously in animals than those isolated as the epidemic was subsiding, and, moreover, the strains isolated from the blood at the height of the epidemic were less virulent than those from the sputum.

EXPERIMENTS SUGGESTING THE OCCURRENCE OF MUTATION IN VIVO

It has been shown elsewhere that marked changes occurred in the bacterial flora in the later stages of influenzal infection, that similar changes often occurred in vitro, and that the new strains or variants were not only virulent on injection in animals, but also tended to produce leukopenia. Following intratracheal injection the changes in the lung closely simulated those of influenzal infection.

Owing to the instability of the streptococci from influenza noted at the onset of this work, we have taken particular pains to observe whether the changes noted in patients and in vitro might occur in the body of the experimental animal. A striking example of the mutation of a hemolytic streptococcus into a green-producing streptococcus simultaneously in a series of guinea-pigs has been detailed in the experiments recorded in case 2800. The lesions produced by the intratracheal injection method resembled closely those observed following injection of the green-producing streptococcus from influenza.

On the other hand, the green-producing streptococcus often appeared to become a hemolytic streptococcus. Thus in case 2749 one of four guinea-pigs injected intravenously with a pure culture of green-producing streptococcus from the blood of a guinea-pig injected subcutaneously with the sputum, showed a moderate number of hemolytic streptococci and Staphylococcus aureus in the pleural fluid, hemorrhagic areas in the lung, hemorrhagic mucus in the uterine horns, and in the pancreas. The pancreas showed a moderate number of green-producing streptococci. The green-producing streptococcus from 2 animals in the second-passage series were injected in various ways into 7 guinea-pigs, 2 rats, 2 dogs, and a mouse. The organism injected was isolated in pure form from all the guinea-pigs, one rat, and one dog. One rat injected subcutaneously yielded a large number of the green-producing streptococci from the blood and subcutaneous tissues, and from the latter a moderate number of Staphylococcus aureus also. The mouse injected intraperitoneally died in forty-eight hours from hemorrhagic peritonitis and pleuritis. The blood and pleural fluid yielded a moderate number of green-producing streptococci, slightly hemolytic streptococci, and Staphylococcus aureus. The one dog which aborted following intravenous injection had a large number of moist spreading hemolytic streptococci, and a moderate number of staphylococci in the bloody mucus of both uterine horns, and the blood yielded a few colonies of green-producing streptococci. The culture in dextrose-brain broth of the hemolytic streptococcus from the uterus, and the green-producing streptococcus from the blood were injected intratracheally into one guinea-pig each. The first animal showed leukopenia for forty-eight hours, then leukocytosis, and died on the third day with distended lungs (17 c c) showing marked exudative pneumonia of pseudolobar type (14 gm.). The lung and pleura yielded green-producing streptococci. The second animal showed a progressive and marked leukopenia and died with similar lung findings the day of injection. Cultures from the blood and kidney showed a few colonies of green-producing streptococci in pure form, while the pneumonic lung and mucus in the right horn of the uterus showed the green-producing streptococci and Staphylococcus aureus.

The results in case 2851 are similar to those observed in others. The patient developed an attack of influenza of ordinary severity, but on the sixth day became suddenly worse and died on the eighth day from acute hemorrhagic edema and bronchopneumonia. The sputum on the second day was mucoid and contained a large number of the green-producing streptococci, a few slightly hemolyzing streptococci, and a few staphylococci. On the seventh day the sputum was blood-tinged but purulent, and showed Staphylococcus aureus in pure form in large number. Permission for necropsy could not be obtained, but a syringe-full of bloody fluid was withdrawn from the left pleural cavity. The blood-agar plate inoculated with this fluid contained a large number of Staphylococcus aureus and a few moist slightly hemolyzing colonies of streptococci. The culture in dextrose-brain broth from a single well isolated colony of the slightly hemolytic streptococcus from the pleural fluid was injected into the tracheas of 3 guinea-pigs. Pure growth of slightly hemolyzing colonies of streptococci was obtained from the blood-agar plate of the culture injected. In all 3 guinea-pigs there was a reduction in leukocytes in from twenty-four to forty-eight hours after injection; the average count before injection was 12,900, twenty-four hours after injection 7,600, and forty-eight hours after injection 8,260. The animals seemed quite well three days after injection, when they were chloroformed. All had bronchopneumonia, and the one female had endometritis with hemorrhagic mucus in both uterine horns. None had pleuritis. In 2 the cultures from the blood were sterile; cultures from the blood of the female contained a few colonies of streptococci. Cultures from the pneumonic lung of all yielded a pure culture of Staphylococcus aureus. The hemorrhagic mucus in the uterine horns yielded Staphylococcus aureus and a few colonies of green-producing streptococci. Cultures from the adrenal, kidney, spleen and liver were sterile.

The culture in dextrose-brain broth from a single well isolated colony of Staphylococcus aureus which showed no streptococci in smears and only staphylococcus colonies on plating was injected intratracheally into a guinea-pig; it died in twenty-four hours from hemorrhagic edema of the lung. The pleural cavity was filled with hemorrhagic fluid, and the visceral pleura was covered with a thin fibrinous film. The leukocyte count of 12,400 before injection dropped to 3,400. Blood-agar-plate cultures from the blood, pleural fluid, lung, kidney and liver showed Staphylococcus aureus in large numbers, those from the adrenal and spleen a few. A few colonies of moist spreading green-producing streptococci in addition to Staphylococcus aureus were isolated from the pleural fluid and lung. A culture in a tall tube of dextrose broth from a single well isolated green-producing colony of the streptococcus from the pleural fluid was made and injected intratracheally into 2 guinea-pigs and intraperitoneally into 1. The latter showed a drop in leukocytes of from 19,000 to 7,600 twenty-four hours after injection, and then recovered. One of the former, a female, died in two days from hemorrhagic edema of the lung, bronchopneumonia, a large amount of hemorrhagic fluid in the pleural cavity, and hemorrhagic endometritis. Cultures from the blood, uterus, lung and pleural fluid revealed a large number of moist spreading green-producing streptococci, and a few Staphylococcus aureus; those from the adrenal, spleen, liver, and brain contained a smaller number of both. The leukocyte count dropped from 6,600 before injection to 2,000 twenty-four hours after injection. No count was made after death. The other pig injected intratracheally had a drop of from 14,200 to 10,000 leukocytes, and increased respiration for a few days; it then seemingly recovered, but died seventeen days after the injection. Serofibrinous pleuritis and peritonitis were found. There were no lesions of the lung. Cultures from the blood remained sterile, while those from the peritoneal exudate contained many colonies of Staphylococcus aureus in pure form. The blood-agar plate made at the time the culture was injected into these animals showed a pure growth of a green-producing streptococcus, and after the same tube was incubated for fifteen days a blood-agar plate showed a moderate number of rather dry green-producing and slightly hemolyzing colonies of streptococci and a large number of colonies of staphylococci.

A dextrose-brain broth culture from a single green-producing colony from the blood of the female guinea-pig that died from hemorrhagic edema and pleuritis was injected into the trachea of one guinea-pig. The leukocyte count dropped from 15,800 to 4,000 in twenty-four hours, respiration was increased moderately for a few days, and the animal then recovered. The strain was lost.

This case is an example of a predominant green-producing streptococcal flora noted early in influenza being replaced by Staphylococcus aureus. Hemorrhagic pleural fluid after death showed a preponderance of the Staphylococcus aureus and a few slightly hemolytic streptococci. A subculture from a single colony of the latter proved only moderately virulent, and in all the guinea-pigs staphylococci only were isolated from the lesions in the lung as recovery seemed assured. The staphylococcus culture from a single colony was extremely virulent. The hemorrhagic lung and pleural fluid yielded, in addition to the staphylococcus, a few colonies of green-producing streptococci. A culture from a single colony of the latter, which showed no staphylococci when injected, yielded staphylococci in both of 2 guinea-pigs as well as in the culture tube after prolonged cultivation. The green-producing strain in the next animal passage produced marked leukopenia, increased respiration for a time, and then was lost as recovery ensued.

In case 2608 the sputum was injected directly intraperitoneally into a guinea-pig. It died from peritonitis. The blood showed the green-producing streptococcus in pure culture; the peritoneal fluid showed this organism and Staphylococcus aureus in moderate number. A well isolated single colony of the former was inoculated into glucose-brain broth. The twenty-four-hour culture was injected intraperitoneally into a guinea-pig. The blood-agar plate of this culture yielded only green-producing streptococci. The guinea-pig died in three days of hemorrhagic fibrinous peritonitis, pericarditis and pancreatitis. The leukocyte count dropped from 6,000 before injection to 4,480 in twenty-four hours, and to 3,600 in forty-eight hours. The cultures from the blood showed a pure growth of green-producing streptococci, whereas the pericardial and peritoneal fluid showed these together with a moderate number of the Staphylococcus aureus. In order to test whether or not the staphylococci found in the pericardial exudate possessed virulency, a culture in dextrose-brain broth from a single colony was injected intraperitoneally into a guinea-pig in the usual dosage (0.5 c c per 100 gm. weight). It died in three days from hemorrhagic peritonitis, with localized areas of hemorrhage and edema in the lungs. The leukocyte counts were 9,200 before injection, 3,200, 6,000, and 3,240, respectively, twenty-four and forty-eight hours later, and after death. Cultures from the peritoneal fluid and blood yielded a pure growth of Staphylococcus aureus.

A summary of a large number of experiments in animals injected with cultures proved to be pure by plate cultures, reveals that apparent mutations occurred in 11 of 75 injected intraperitoneally and intravenously, and in 14 of 73 injected intratracheally.

It is realized that the finding in these animals of bacteria that were not introduced might be interpreted as secondary invasion, if it were not for the fact that these mutation forms develop in the test tube under controlled conditions. Indeed until the pure line requirement and the remote possibility of contamination from the air in the test-tube experiments are met, conclusions with regard to the mutation of streptococci into staphylococci and mutation of influenza bacilli cannot be drawn. However, from a consideration of the precautions which have been taken to exclude accidental contamination, the regularity of its occurrence under certain conditions, and the high virulency of the staphylococci which at times displace the streptococcal flora in fulminating cases of influenzal pneumonia and the high and peculiar virulency of the mutants, the observations are believed worthy of record.

MORTALITY FROM INFLUENZAL INFECTION IN RELATION TO THE RISE AND FALL OF EPIDEMIC WAVES

It has been noted by physicians who have seen many cases of influenza that the attacks were more severe during the height of the epidemic and milder as the epidemic subsided. The mortality statistics of infectious diseases now available are based almost wholly on the number of patients who develop the disease and the number of deaths within a certain number of days, weeks or months. No records of epidemic diseases have come to my notice in which the mortality rate is studied strictly in relation to the time in the epidemic at which the disease was contracted. Owing to the changes noted on successive intratracheal application in the invasive power of streptococci from influenza it was thought worth while to determine the mortality in the patients with influenza admitted to the hospitals according to the period in the epidemic the disease was contracted. In chart 3 each black column represents the number of patients who developed influenza on that day. These columns show that there were four distinct waves and two lesser recrudescences between September, 1918, and April, 1919, and that each wave spent its force in about six weeks. Each wave was divided into three two-week periods, namely, two weeks before and including the day of the crest of the wave, the first two weeks following the crest, and the second two weeks following the crest of the wave. The first row of figures at the bottom of the chart indicates the number of persons with influenza admitted to the hospital in each of these periods. The second row indicates the percentage of deaths from influenzal infection, not during the two weeks, respectively, but during that time or later. In other words, 16 per cent. of the 43 persons contracting influenza during the first two weeks of the first wave ultimately died, 20 per cent. of the 112 persons contracting influenza during the second two weeks died, and 13 per cent. of the 54 persons contracting influenza during the third two weeks died, and so on. By a study of the mortality according to the time the disease was contracted, it was discovered that the highest mortality rate occurred in each of the three main waves in the second two weeks, the time when the largest number of cases developed. It was lower during the first two weeks as the epidemic was on the increase, and in each instance lowest the third two weeks as the wave subsided. The number of cases during the third wave was small and the mortality low; accordingly, the marked rise and fall in mortality did not occur. The slight recrudescence in November also carried with it a low mortality (15 per cent.). The mortality during the recrudescence in April was highest (26 per cent.) when the number of cases was largest (36), and much lower (12 per cent.) as the epidemic disappeared. The curve to the extreme right in the chart represents the average mortality percentage of the four waves, during the three periods of two weeks each, 14, 21 and 12 per cent., respectively.

Besides the change in mortality rate, there was a noticeable difference in the type of the disease during the early part, or the height of each wave, and that found as the wave subsided. The incidence and degree of exudation into the lung was more marked during the middle part of the epidemic. Thus, during the first two weeks of the first wave 24 per cent. of the patients admitted developed pneumonia, during the second two weeks, 30 per cent., and during the third two weeks, 27 per cent. The average percentage incidence of influenzal pneumonia during the four waves for the three biweekly periods was 30 per cent., 37 per cent., and 41 per cent., respectively. The lesions in the lung found at necropsy in our cases as in those of other observers were distinctly different early and late in the waves.

Voluminous lungs with marked hemorrhagic edema and relatively slight true consolidation were the rule at the height of the waves, while exudative pneumonia of the bronchopneumonic type with relatively slight hemorrhage and edema dominated the picture as the waves subsided.

In a previous paper [4] I have shown that the tendency to a persistence of leukopenia in patients contracting the disease late in epidemic waves is less marked than at the height of the waves. In the light of the animal experiments might not this difference as well as the greater tendency to true consolidation of the lung late in the waves be an expression of a diminished virulence on the part of the infecting microorganisms?

In another paper [4] I have shown also that as patients recover from influenza and especially influenzal pneumonia the leukocyte count goes up. Exceptionally this is true also in protracted cases in which the patient dies. This is generally considered to be due to secondary invasion or to a winning fight by the defensive mechanism of the host. The possibility that this is due to changes in the parasite must, in the light of the experiments on successive intratracheal injection, be taken into consideration. Leukocytosis following an initial leukopenia was noted commonly in guinea-pigs injected with sublethal doses of the green-producing streptococcus, and prolonged contact with the body fluids and cells was found to rob these strains of the power to produce leukopenia. The mortality curves in the epidemics studied represent in a general way those noted by others and indicate a rise and a fall of virulency of the infecting micro-organism. The severity of influenza as it passes through smaller groups, such as large families, often shows the same rise and fall.

The difficulties, however, in studying the severity of influenza in sequence in individual families in which quarantine is not strictly observed are obvious. Authentic information regarding the severity of attacks has been obtained, however, in the case of a number of families living in the country. The findings in a family of eleven living in isolation 15 miles from a railroad station are especially instructive in this connection. The date of onset, date of death in the fatal cases, the age of the patients, and the attacks according to severity are arranged chronologically in Chart 4. It will be noted that fifty-three days elapsed from the time the first became ill (September 27) until the last one contracted the disease (November 19). The interval between the groups of cases was about four, twelve, ten, twelve and fifteen days, respectively. The epidemic spent its force in the surrounding community during the same time. The first person to contract the disease had a mild attack, but because he persisted in working, he developed severe symptoms, was in bed with fever for six days, and then recovered. The 3 persons who came down last had mild attacks, and all recovered without developing pneumonia or other complications. The 7 who contracted the disease during the interval between the first and the last cases all had severe attacks; 3 died from influenzal pneumonia; 2 of those who recovered developed pneumonia, and 1 phlebitis of the leg; the fourth had a severe attack, but did not develop outspoken signs of pneumonia. The source of the infection was not known. From the dates of onset of symptoms in these cases, it seems that the

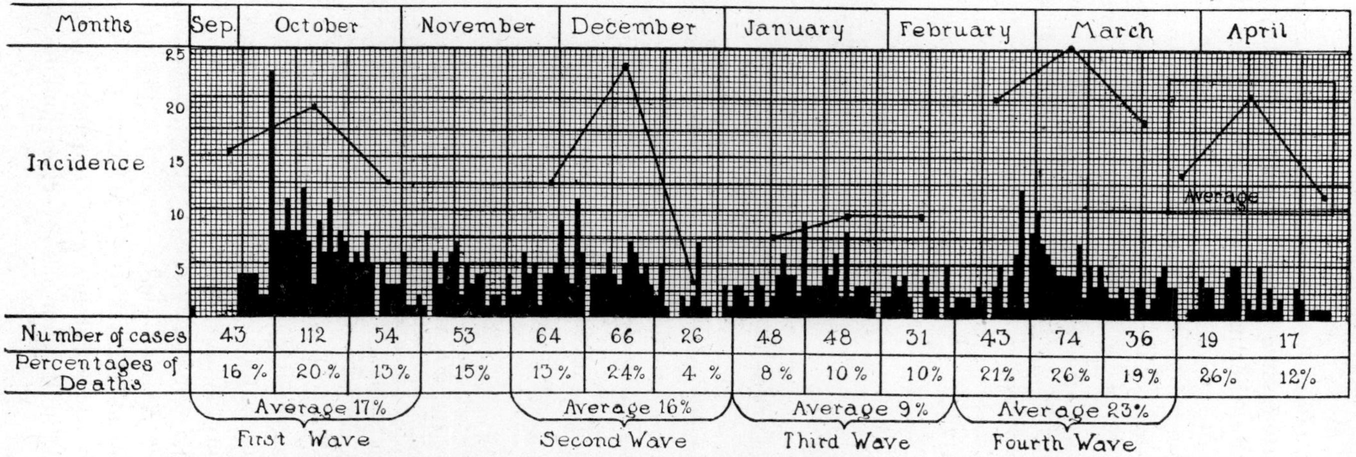

Chart 3.—Mortality from influenza in relation to the rise and fall of epidemic waves of the disease. The black columns show the number of cases of influenza. The curves show the percentage of deaths in persons who developed influenza during two weeks prior to the crest, first two weeks following the crest and second two weeks following the crest of the waves.

organism passed through five persons, and as this occurred the virulency, just as on successive animal passage on tracheal application increased during the earlier passages and then decreased, and was lost in the sixth passage.

CHART 4

THE RISE AND FALL IN VIRULENCY OF INFLUENZAL INFECTION AS IT PASSED THROUGH A LARGE FAMILY

William K., aged 31, farmer. Influenza Sept. 27, 1918; mild attack at first; would not give up work; then had severe attack. Recovered.

↓

Mrs. K., aged 60. Influenza October 1. Severe attack with influenzal pneumonia, but recovered.

Walter K., aged 30. Influenza October 1. Death from influenzal pneumonia, October 13.

↓

Laura K., aged 29. Influenza October 15. Death from influenzal pneumonia October 23.

Edwin K., aged 21. Severe influenza October 13, but no pneumonia. Recovered.

↓

Meda K., aged 17. Influenza October 23. Severe attack with pneumonia, but recovered.

Selma K., aged 26. Influenza October 23; extremely ill; developed phlebitis of leg, but recovered.

↓

Freda K., aged 21. Influenza November 4. Extremely ill and died November 17 of pneumonia.

↓

Hired Girl, aged 22. Influenza November 17. Mild attack.

Ben K., aged 25. Influenza November 19. Mild attack.

Ezra K., aged 16. Influenza November 17. Mild attack.

SUMMARY

The results reported elsewhere following the intratracheal injection of the green-producing streptococcus from influenza have been verified and extended in this study.

The virulency and mortality in animals increased for one or two successive intratracheal injections of this organism, and on further animal passage progressively diminished. At the peak of virulency the symptoms of respiratory embarrassment are frequently violent and often resemble those of anaphylaxis. Cyanosis and leukopenia are marked, and death from hugely dilated lungs filled with hemorrhagic edema fluid with relatively slight exudative pneumonia frequently occurs. Microscopically, necrosis of alveolar epithelium and endothelium of the capillaries of all grades with marked hemorrhagic edema and little leukocytic infiltration are the chief findings. In subsequent intratracheal injection respiratory embarrassment becomes less marked, reduction in leukocytes less pronounced or wholly absent, and as this occurs the dilatation of the lung becomes less, exudation of leukocytes in the lung more pronounced, and extensive pneumonia with little hemorrhage and edema is the dominant picture.

TABLE 1

EFFECT OF SUCCESSIVE INTRATRACHEAL INJECTION OF STREPTOCOCCI FROM INFLUENZA, THE LEUKOCYTE COUNT AND MORTALITY

Animal Passage	Strains	Animals Injected	Average			Percentage Showing			Mortality per Cent.
			Before Injection	After Injection (24 hours)	Reduction, %	Leukopenia	Leukocytosis	No Change	
First............	5	14	14,800	7,200	51	92	4	4	57
Second..........	5	8	12,300	4,200	66	88	0	12	100
Third............	3	7	17,100	8,500	50	70	15	15	57
Fourth..........	3	13	·14,700	13,300	9.5	47	25	25	38

From a study of the four epidemic waves as they occurred in Rochester, it has been found that a similar rise and fall in severity of symptoms, mortality and character of lung lesions occurred as the epidemic waves appeared and disappeared. The symptoms, cyanosis and leukopenia were most pronounced, and the mortality was the highest at the peak of the waves when the lungs were of huge size, and at necropsy hemorrhagic edema with relatively slight exudative pneumonia was the striking picture. Later as the symptoms became milder, leukopenia less persistent, and the mortality rate lower, exudative pneumonia became more common. Experimental evidence has thus been obtained to show that (1) the change in the type of the disease early and late in epidemics, (2) the rise and fall in mortality rate in the same epidemic and the virulency of different epidemics, and (3) the lesser tendency to leukopenia late in epidemic waves may be due, in the main, to changes in virulency and other properties of the green-producing streptococci isolated so constantly in influenzal infection.

These facts do not exclude the possibility that the influenza bacillus may play a rôle in the production of symptoms and lesions in influenza. In some cases they rather suggest the possibility that this organism may undergo similar changes, and that it may acquire peculiar and high infecting powers. Indeed the recent work of Blake and Cecil, in which symptoms and lesions simulating influenza have been produced experimentally in the monkey with the influenza bacillus made highly virulent by repeated monkey passages, supports this view.

Throughout the work the well marked examples in which green-producing streptococci suddenly acquired hemolytic power and hemolytic streptococci suddenly became green-producing streptococci, both in vitro and in vivo, suggest strongly that the complete or partial displacement of one type of streptococcal flora by another throughout, especially late in the epidemic waves, may be due to the development of mutation forms rather than the result of superimposed infection from the upper respiratory tract.

Since the mutants have been found to possess the power of producing the characteristic lesions in the lung and a sharp leukopenia on intratracheal application, might not the green-producing streptococcus isolated so constantly early in influenza and influenzal pneumonia, since it has high and peculiar invasive and other properties, be a mutation form of the pneumococcus-streptococcus group which humans normally harbor? Moreover, might not the sudden appearance and rapid "spread" of influenza among isolated groups and often almost simultaneously over wide areas be in part due to this cause?

1. Blake, F. G., and Cecil, R. L.: The Production of an Acute Respiratory Disease in Monkeys by Inoculation with Bacillus Influenzae. A Preliminary Report, Jour. Am. Med. Assn., 1920, lxxiv, 170-172.

2. Hirsch, E. F., and McKinney, M.: An Epidemic of Pneumococcus Bronchopneumonia, Jour. Infect. Dis., 1919, xxiv, 594-617.

3. Rosenow, E. C.: Studies in Influenza and Pneumonia. II. The Experimental Production of Symptoms and Lesions Simulating Those of Influenza with Streptococci Isolated During the Present Pandemic, Jour. Am. Med. Assn., 1919, lxxii, 1604-1609.

4. Rosenow, E. C.: Studies in Influenza and Pneumonia. VI. The Leukocytic Reaction in Influenza and Influenzal Pneumonia. (In press.)

STUDIES IN INFLUENZA AND PNEUMONIA

STUDY X. THE IMMUNOLOGIC PROPERTIES OF THE GREEN-PRODUCING STREPTOCOCCI FROM INFLUENZA

E. C. Rosenow

Division of Experimental Bacteriology, The Mayo Foundation, Rochester, Minnesota.

In a previous report it was shown that most of the green-producing streptococci isolated so constantly in influenza were agglutinated specifically by a monovalent immune horse serum; that highly agglutinable strains absorb the agglutinins for the other strains; and that during convalescence in influenza the serum of patients acquires the power to agglutinate many of the freshly isolated green-producing streptococci. Attention was directed also to the fact that these organisms possess well marked antigenic properties, the serum of persons developing specific agglutinating power after injections of a mixed vaccine.

In this study I shall detail further results obtained by subjecting numerous strains of the green-producing streptococcus from influenza to the action of various immune serums, especially to the monovalent serum prepared with one of the strains of the green-producing streptococcus. The monovalent serum was prepared by injecting a large horse (horse 15) with increasing doses of one strain of green-producing streptococcus isolated from the blood after death in a case of influenza and influenzal pneumonia. The symptoms and findings in this case, reported elsewhere, were typical. The thorax was expanded and immobile, the patient expectorated a large amount of bloody, frothy fluid. The lung after death was voluminous, extremely wet with a dark colored bloody fluid and the seat of numerous coalescing areas of lobular pneumonia.

The strain as isolated from a single colony from the blood and after one animal passage was put aside on blood-agar slants and in deep tubes of dextrose-brain broth. Both of these produced typical, rather moist, spreading, greenish colonies on blood-agar plates, both fermented inulin, but they were not bile soluble. Cultures for immunization of the horse were made from the stock cultures in bottles of glucose broth containing 150 c c each. These were incubated over night, or until heavy growth had occurred, centrifuged and the sediment suspended in salt solution so that 1 c c of the sediment represented the growth from 15 c c of the broth. Control blood-agar plate cultures were made of the material inoculated in the bottle as well as of the growth injected into the horse. The dense bacterial suspension was used for intravenous immunizations. The first injection, made Jan. 9, 1919, consisted of 6 c c of the suspension or the growth from 90 c c of broth. The injections were given on three successive days in each week. The first six injections consisted of the heat killed bacteria (60 centigrade for thirty minutes). After that live cultures were injected. The dose by March 3, when 3 liters of blood were withdrawn, had been increased to 50 c c of the suspension or the growth from 750 c c of the glucose broth culture. The injections were continued and the dose gradually increased until April 4, when 14 liters of blood were withdrawn. The horse was given a rest for ten days, and the injections were resumed, but owing to marked reactions and loss of weight the dose had to be diminished and finally was discontinued, April 16. In spite of the fact that no more injections were given the horse continued to lose in weight and strength, and June 4 it was unable to get up, and was bled to death under ether.

The serums obtained before the injections were begun, and on March 3, April 4 and June 4 after immunization, were titrated against freshly isolated strains of the green-producing streptococcus. It was found that the upper limit of agglutinating power of the serum obtained before the injections were begun was about 1 to 10; the serum obtained March 3, about 1 to 500; April 4, 1 to 1,000 to 1 to 10,000; and June 4, 1 to 500 or 1 to 1,000. The serum of the highest titer obtained April 4 was mostly used in the agglutination experiments herein reported.

The antihemolytic streptococcus serum (horse 9) was prepared by repeated injections with four strains of highly virulent hemolytic streptococci from cases of severe ascending infections and cases of cellulitis. The injections were given between December 18, 1917, and July 1, 1918. The serum during this time had acquired marked agglutinating power over the strains injected. It should be emphasized that all of these strains were isolated before the epidemic of influenza occurred.

The pneumococcus immune serums were obtained from Dr. Rufus I. Cole, of the Hospital of the Rockefeller Institute for Medical Research, and from Dr. Augustus B. Wadsworth, of the New York State Department of Health. These were titrated against known strains of type pneumococci and were found to possess marked and specific agglutinating power.

METHODS

The freshly obtained sputum was sent to the laboratory for cultures throughout the four epidemic waves of influenza in 1918 and 1919. The cultures and agglutination experiments were made and recorded without knowledge of the history of the patients. The diagnosis, days of onset and other data were ascertained later from the records. A series of preliminary experiments in which various dilutions of serums were used (from 1 to 10 to 1 to 10,000), showed that a final dilution of these serums of 1 to 20 had the widest range of usefulness. Accordingly, for routine work the mixture in each tube consisted of 0.2 c c of the various serums diluted 1 to 10 with salt solution, and 0.2 c c of the antigen. The antigen consisted, for the most part, of the dextrose-blood broth or dextrose-acacia-broth culture, or of a salt solution suspension of bacteria grown in these after they had been preserved in 50 per cent. glycerol for a variable length of time. In some instances the peritoneal washings of mice and guinea-pigs which had succumbed to injections of sputum or primary culture from sputum, were also used as antigen. During the first two waves dense suspensions of the green-producing streptococci from primary cultures of sputum or blood of animals dead from injection of sputum were filed away in 50 per cent. glycerol, so that 1 c c equaled the growth from 15 c c of the dextrose-acacia-broth culture. These were kept in the ice chest and diluted with 15 parts of salt solution at the time the agglutination tests were performed. The mixtures of serum and antigen were thoroughly shaken and incubated at 37 C. for from one to one and one-half hours and placed in the ice chest over night, before readings were taken. The amount of agglutination, as indicated in the tables, was recorded by from 1 to 4 plus signs, 1 plus indicating slight but definite agglutination, 2 plus decided clumping but with little sedimentation, 3 plus marked agglutination and sedimentation but with supernatant fluid, not entirely clear, and 4 plus complete agglutination with the bacteria packed quite solidly at the bottom and the supernatant fluid completely cleared.

"Specific" agglutination is the term applied to the serum which agglutinated a particular strain to a greater degree than any of the other serums.

In most cases only one or two samples of sputum were cultivated and the agglutination tests made with the bacteria thus obtained. In some instances the agglutination experiments were done with strains isolated from the sputum daily or on alternate days throughout the illness and with the strains isolated after death. In selected cases cultures were made simultaneously of tonsil and of the throat or nasopharynx, and the strains isolated were subjected to the agglutinating action of the serums under identical conditions.

TABLE 1

AGGLUTINATION EXPERIMENTS WITH THE GREEN-PRODUCING STREPTOCOCCUS FROM INFLUENZA

Case or Strain	Date of Experiment	Date of Isolation	Source	Day of Disease	Antiserums: Pneumococcus I	Antiserums: Pneumococcus II	Antiserums: Pneumococcus III	Antiserums: Streptococcus Hemolytic Horse 9	Antiserums: Streptococcus Green Producing Horse 15	Controls: Normal Horse Serum	Controls: NaCl Solution
3218.2	3/ 9/19	3/ 7/19	Sputum	4	0	0	0	+	++	0	0
3218.2	3/ 9/19	3/ 7/19	Sputum	4	0	0	0	0	++	0	0
3225^2	3/19/19	3/17/19	Sputum	3	0	0	0	++	+++	0	0
3225^2.5	6/17/19	3/17/19	Sputum	3	0	0	0	0	+	0	0
3266	3/25/19	3/24/19	Sputum	5	+	0	0	++	+++	+	0
3266^2.2	3/27/19	3/24/19	Sputum	5	0	0	0	0	0	0	0
3282	3/31/19	3/30/19	Sputum	2	0	+++	+++	+++	++++	0	0
3282	4/ 3/19	4/ 2/19	Sputum	5	0	++	+	++	+++	0	0
3332	4/ 7/19	4/ 6/19	Sputum	3	0	0	0	0	+++	0	0
3332.2	4/ 8/19	4/ 6/19	Sputum	3	0	0	0	0	++	0	0
3332	4/ 9/19	4/ 8/19	Tonsil	5	++	++	++	+++	+++	++	0
3332.2	4/10/19	4/ 8/19	Tonsil	5	0	++	0	0	+++	0	0
3332.6	11/18/19	4/ 8/19	Sputum	3	0	+	+	+	+	0	0
3334	4/ 7/19	4/ 6/19	Sputum	1	0	0	0	+++	++++	0	0
3334	4/ 8/19	4/ 7/19	Throat	2	0	0	++	+++	+++	0	0
3334.2	4/ 9/19	4/ 7/19	Throat	2	0	0	0	0	+++	0	0
3334.2	4/ 9/19	4/ 7/19	Throat	2	0	0	++	+	+++	+	0
3334.2	4/ 9/19	4/ 7/19	Throat	2	0	0	0	+++	++++	+	0
3334	4/10/19	4/ 9/19	Sputum	3	0	0	++	++	++	0	0
3334.6	11/11/19	4/ 9/19	Sputum	3	0	0	+	+++	+++	+	0
3365	4/14/19	4/13/19	Throat	3	0	0	++	0	+++	+	0
3365	4/14/19	4/13/19	Throat	3	0	0	0	0	++	0	0
3365.2	4/15/19	4/13/19	Throat	3	0	0	0	0	+++	+	0
3365	4/14/19	4/13/19	Sputum	3	0	0	0	0	+++	0	0
3365.2	4/14/19	4/13/19	Sputum	3	0	0	0	0	++	0	0
3365.3	4/16/19	4/13/19	Sputum	3	+	+	+	+	+++	0	0
3365.6	5/ 1/19	4/13/19	Sputum	3	0	0	0	0	++++	0	0
3365.6	5/ 1/19	4/13/19	Sputum	3	0	0	0	0	++++	0	0
3365.7	11/ 4/19	4/13/19	Sputum	3	0	0	0	+	+++	0	0
3366	4/14/19	4/10/19	Tonsil	2	0	0	0	0	0	0	0
3366	4/14/19	4/10/19	Throat	2	0	0	0	0	+	0	0
3366	4/14/19	4/10/19	Sputum	2	0	0	0	0	++	0	0
3366	4/14/19	4/12/19	Sputum	4	0	0	++	++	+++	+	0
3366.2	4/14/19	4/12/19	Sputum	4	+	+	+	+	+++	+	0
3366.3	6/17/19	4/12/19	Sputum	4	0	0	0	0	+++	0	0
3366.7	11/14/19	4/12/19	Sputum	4	0	0	0	0	++	0	0
3370	4/14/19	4/11/19	Sputum	2	0	0	0	0	++	0	0
3370.2	4/14/19	4/11/19	Sputum	2	0	0	0	0	++	0	0
3370.3	4/16/19	4/11/19	Sputum	2	0	0	0	+	++	0	0
3370.4	4/21/19	4/11/19	Sputum	2	0	0	0	0	++	0	0
3370.6	5/ 1/19	4/11/19	Sputum	2	0	0	0	0	+++	4	0
3370.7	11/22/19	4/11/19	Sputum	2	++	+	+	++	+++	++	0

RESULTS

In table 1 are summarized representative experiments indicating the results obtained with the green-producing streptococcus isolated from patients with influenza. In these and other experiments the following findings were noted:

1. The monovalent serum of horse 15 agglutinated specifically most of the strains isolated throughout short initial attacks of typical influenza (cases 3218, 3225 and 3332).

2. Specific agglutination occurred (often in duplicate) in the primary mass culture of sputum or throat swab and of material from animals dead from injection of sputum, and in the early subcultures of the green-producing streptococcus isolated from sputum, throat swab and animals injected with these strains (cases 3225, 3266, 3365 and 3366).

3. The immunologic condition of the green-producing streptococci, as manifested by their agglutinability in the various immune serums, varied between wide limits (cases 3282, 3332 and 3334).

4. Specific agglutinability of most of the strains was lost on prolonged cultivation (cases 3332 and 3370), but in some strains it was retained for a long time (cases 3334, 3365 and 3366).

In table 2 are summarized representative experiments with strains of the green-producing streptococcus isolated during life and after death in cases of influenzal pneumonia. The results with the strains isolated early in these cases were similar to those isolated in cases of influenza (cases 3206, 3207 and 3264), while late in the disease during life (cases 3265 and 3331), and after death (cases 3404, 3410, 3420 and 3436) the incidence of specific agglutination was decidedly lower, but even here the incidence was higher than that obtained with any of the other immune serums.

The agglutination experiments with the green-producing streptococcus isolated from the same patient throughout both the influenza attack and the influenzal pneumonia which followed showed that there was practically no difference in the immunologic condition of the strains isolated during influenza and during the early part of the influenzal pneumonia. Late in the pneumonic attack there was often a shifting of specific agglutination of these strains to one of the other serums, or agglutination to the same degree occurred in most of the immune serums; in other cases they might not be agglutinated by any of the serums. Thus in one case specific agglutination occurred in the serum of horse 15 of the primary culture from the sputum, and from the blood of a guinea-pig dead from an intraperitoneal injection of sputum, obtained on the third day of influenza. No agglutination occurred in any of the other serums. The colonies of the green-producing streptococci were quite moist and large, resembling type III pneumococci, but were not so mucoid in character, whereas on the

TABLE 2

AGGLUTINATION EXPERIMENTS WITH THE GREEN-PRODUCING STREPTOCOCCUS FROM INFLUENZAL PNEUMONIA

Case or Strain	Date of Experiment	Date of Isolation	Source	Day of Disease	Antiserums: Pneumococcus I	Antiserums: Pneumococcus II	Antiserums: Pneumococcus III	Antiserums: Streptococcus Hemolytic Horse 9	Antiserums: Streptococcus Green Producing Horse 15	Controls: Normal Horse Serum	Controls: NaCl Solution
3097	3/12/19	3/11/19	Sputum	1	0	++	0	0	0	0	0
3175.2	3/14/19	3/11/19	Sputum	4	++	+++	++	++	++++	+	0
3175^{3}.2	3/27/19	3/11/19	Sputum	4	0	0	0	0	++	0	0
3206	3/13/19	3/12/19	Sputum	2	0	0	0	0	+++	0	0
3207	3/13/19	3/12/19	Sputum	4	0	0	0	0	+++	0	0
3207^{2}.2	4/ 3/19	3/12/19	Sputum	4	0	++	0	0	+++	0	0
3264	3/25/19	3/24/19	Sputum	8	0	0	0	++	+++	0	0
3264	3/25/19	3/24/19	Sputum	8	0	0	0	++	+++	0	0
3264^{2}.2	3/28/19	3/24/19	Sputum	8	0	0	0	+	++	0	0
3265	3/25/19	3/24/19	Sputum	13	++	+	0	++	+++	+	0
3265.2	3/31/19	3/29/19	Sputum	18	0	0	++	0	0	0	0
3265.2	4/ 3/19	4/ 2/19	Sputum	21	0	0	0	0	0	0	0
3265^{2}.2	4/ 3/19	4/ 2/19	Sputum	21	0	0	0	0	0	0	0
3265.4	9/ 3/19	4/ 2/19	Sputum	21	+	++	+	++	+	+	0
3270	4/ 4/19	4/ 3/19	Sputum	12	0	0	0	+++	0	0	0
3270^{2}	4/ 7/19	4/ 3/19	Sputum	12	0	0	0	++	0	0	0
3270.2	4/ 7/19	4/ 3/19	Sputum	12	0	0	0	++	0	0	0
3270^{2}.2	4/ 9/19	4/ 3/19	Sputum	12	0	0	0	++	++	0	0
3331	4/ 8/19	4/ 7/19	Sputum	2	0	0	++	++	+++	0	0
3331	4/ 8/19	4/ 7/19	Tonsil	2	0	0	0	0	++	0	0
3331	4/10/19	4/ 9/19	Sputum	4	0	0	0	0	0	0	0
3404	4/18/19	4/17/19	Throat	1	+	+	+	+	++	+	0
3404	4/21/19	4/20/19	Sputum	4	0	0	0	0	++	0	0
3404	4/21/19	4/20/19	Sputum	4	0	0		+	++	0	0
3404	4/25/19	4/24/19	Sputum	8	0	0	0	+++	0	0	0
3404	5/ 7/19	5/ 3/19	Lung after death	..	0	0	0	+	+	0	0
3404.2	5/ 8/19	5/ 6/19	Lung after death	..	0	0	0	++	++	0	0
2602.2	4/29/19	11/16/18	Lung after death	..	0	0	0	0	++	0	0
2630^{2}.2	4/29/19	11/30/18	Lung after death	..	+	+	+	+	+++	+	0
3228	3/19/19	3/18/19	Lung after death	..	0	0	0	++	+++	0	0
3287.3	4/ 8/19	3/31/19	Lung after death	..	0	0	0	0	+++	0	0
3287.3	4/ 8/19	3/31/19	Lung after death	..	0	0	0	0	+++	0	0
3410	4/21/19	4/19/19	Lung after death	..	0	0	0	0	0	0	0
3415	4/21/19	4/19/19	Lung after death	..	0	0	0	0	+++	0	0
3420	4/24/19	4/22/19	Lung after death	..	0	0	0	0	0	0	0
3433	4/25/19	4/24/19	Lung after death	..	++++	0	0	0	0	0	0
3436	4/26/19	4/25/19	Lung after death	..	0	0	0	+++	0	0	0

second and sixth days of the pneumonia which followed, specific agglutination occurred in type III pneumococcus serum of the primary culture from the sputum in four tests. Less agglutination occurred in the serum of horse 15 in three instances, and in two instances in each of the type II pneumococcus serum and hemolytic streptococcus serum of horse 9. In another case of typical influenza the green-producing streptococcus in the primary culture and in the first subculture from the sputum on the third day was agglutinated specifically by the serum of horse 9, while on the second day of the influenzal pneumonia which followed, and after death, it was not agglutinated by any of the serums. In still another case specific agglutination occurred in the serum of horse 15 during influenza and early in influenzal pneumonia, whereas

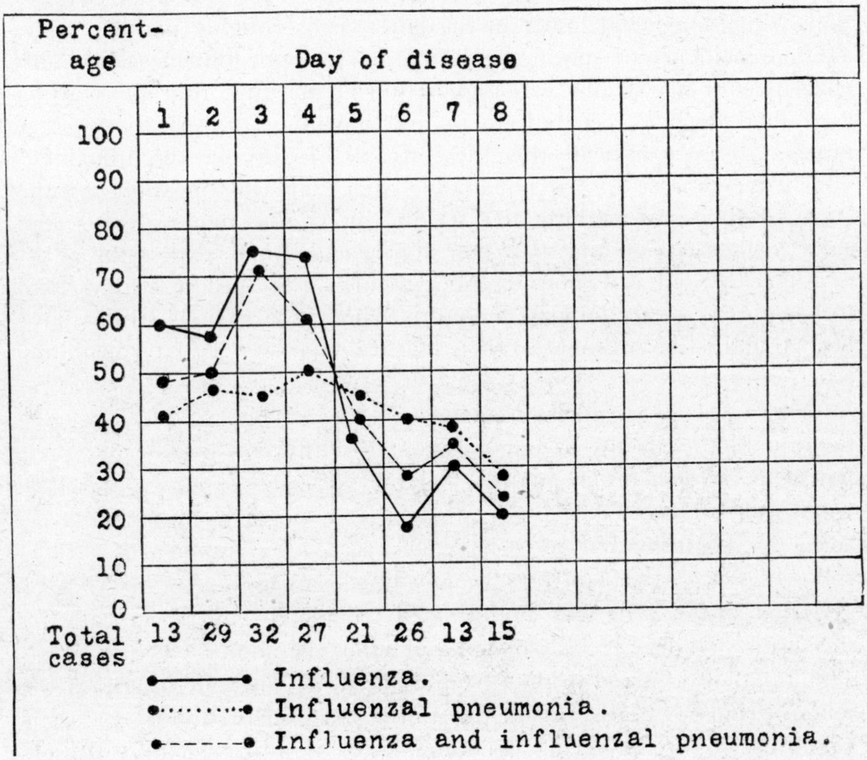

Chart 1.—Percentage of specific agglutination in the monovalent serum of the green-producing streptococcus from influenza and influenzal pneumonia according to the day of the disease.

later in the pneumonic attack specific and marked agglutination occurred in type II pneumococcus serum and lesser agglutination in the serum of horse 15.

In chart 1 is given graphically the average percentage incidence of specific agglutination by the monovalent serum of the green-producing streptococci from influenza and influenzal pneumonia, according to the days of the disease. The curves represent the results obtained on the days indicated. The antigen consisted throughout of the primary culture of the sputum in dextrose-blood broth or of animals injected with sputum irrespective of what the culture showed on plating, and with the early subcultures containing the green-producing streptococcus. The close parallelism between the strains isolated in influenza without frank signs of lung involvement and the cases of influenzal pneumonia is shown by the fact that the average incidence of specific agglutination, while somewhat lower in the latter, runs roughly parallel. The average incidence of specific agglutination for both influenza and influenzal pneumonia strains was highest during the first four days, when a gradual decline occurred up to and including the eighth day. A number of facts indicate that these strains of different agglutinability which appear late in the pneumonic attack are modifications of the strains which are agglutinated specifically by the monovalent serum early in the attacks, and that their appearance is not always the result of superimposed infections from without. The specific strains tend to lose this property on artificial cultivation. The various strains have been found to be unstable in their cultural character and fermentative reactions.

There was no parallelism between the occurrence of specific agglutination in the serum of horse 15 of the different strains and their power to ferment inulin, or their solubility in bile.

Moreover, marked changes in the immunologic condition as measured by agglutination tests have occurred in a number of strains following successive (intratracheal) animal passages.

Thus strain 2719 was agglutinated completely and specifically by the serum of horse 15, as isolated and after one animal passage. Less agglutination occurred in the serum of horse 9, but none in any of the other serums, whereas after the third and fourth animal passages agglutination in the serum of horse 15, while still specific, was less marked and some agglutination occurred in each of the other serums.

In strain 2749 a similar change in agglutinability occurred during the third and fourth animal passages.

In case 2800 the patient from whom the strain was isolated with which horse 15 was immunized, specific agglutination increased during the first and second animal passages over that noted before animal passage, and a marked diminution in agglutination occurred in the serum of horse 15 after the fourth animal passage.

In summarizing the agglutination tests which were made in a routine manner throughout the epidemic of 1918-1919 it was found that material from influenza and influenzal pneumonia, without regard to the time in the attack when the sputum or other material was obtained for culture, and without regard to the type of flora the cultures of the sputum or primary culture showed, was subjected to the agglutinating action of the monovalent immune serum in 567 experiments, representing 184 cases. Of these, 295 (52 per cent.) showed specific agglutination in the serum of horse 15. The primary culture of the sputum in many instances, especially late in the disease, and of the lung exudate after death, showed predominating numbers of hemolytic streptococci, less often staphylococci and rarely colon bacilli or bacillus mucosus.

Specific agglutination occurred in the serum of horse 15 in 29 instances (58 per cent.) of 50 experiments, representing 25 cases, and in 20 of the 25 cases in which the antigen consisted of a salt solution suspension of the primary culture of the sputum or blood of animals dead from injection of sputum, or of pure cultures of these after suspension in 50 per cent. glycerol for some months. All these were cultures from cases which occurred during the first two waves of the disease.

The relative significance of these figures becomes more apparent from a study of tables 1 and 2, in which it is shown that there is a relatively greater frequency and a greater degree of agglutination in the serum of horse 15 over those in the other immune serums; that the antihemolytic streptococcus serum (horse 9) ranks second, and that with few exceptions only a slight difference occurred between the type pneumococcus serums and normal horse serum. The exact figures of the total average incidence of agglutination from slight to marked agglutination in the different serums of the strains from influenza and influenzal pneumonia were found to be as follows: type I pneumococcus serum in 20 per cent. of 563 tests; type II pneumococcus serum in 22 per cent. of 525 tests; type III pneumococcus serum in 21 per cent. of 524 tests; horse 9 serum in 39 per cent. of 561 tests; horse 15 serum in 61 per cent. of 567 tests; normal horse serum in 23 per cent. of 556 tests; salt solution in 7 per cent. of 555 tests. It is certain that the high incidence of agglutination in horse 15 serum was not due to nonspecific effects, since its agglutinating power over 72 strains of green-producing streptococci or pneumococci from sources other than influenza was 25 per cent., or about that of normal horse serum. Moreover, the average amount of agglutination in the serum of horse 15 with the influenza strains was much higher than in the other serums. The control strains included, in addition to type pneumococci and hemolytic streptococci, green-producing streptococci from a wide range of sources, such as the nose and throat of normal persons, the nose of normal guinea-pigs, throats in simple nasopharyngitis, the central nervous system in poliomyelitis, ulcer of the stomach, and arthritis.

As I have pointed out, there was a tendency of the green-producing streptococci to become heterogeneous and to lose the property of specific agglutination after prolonged cultivation on artificial mediums. This varied greatly with different strains (tables 1 and 2). One hundred and fourteen strains after cultivation on artificial mediums (chiefly blood agar) for from 6 to 10 months were subjected to the agglutinating action of the monovalent and the other serums. In these only 26 strains, or 23 per cent., were agglutinated specifically by the monovalent serum. This low figure was no doubt due in part to the deterioration of the serum. It has been pointed out elsewhere (study III) that as these strains are cultivated on artificial mediums they tend to agglutinate spontaneously in liquid cultures, and many strains are unsuited for agglutination tests. This tendency was noted also in the strains which grew diffusely in that the incidence of nonspecific agglutination in the various serums was considerably higher than in the freshly isolated strains. Thus of the 114 experiments, nonspecific agglutination, usually slight, occurred in type I pneumococcus serum in 25 per cent.; type II, in 23 per cent.; type III, in 24 per cent.; antihemolytic streptococcus serum horse 9, in 54 per cent.; monovalent serum horse 15, in 78 per cent., and in normal horse serum, in 35 per cent.

The close relationship between the green-producing streptococcus and hemolytic streptococcus in influenza is shown by the fact that 18 per cent. of 44 strains of hemolytic streptococci isolated during life and after death in influenza were agglutinated specifically by the serum of horse 15.

Beside the time in the attack in which the cultures were made (chart 1) and the predominating flora at hand, the instability of the strains of green-producing streptococci had to be taken into consideration in properly interpreting the results of the agglutination experiments, for by plating the culture actually agglutinated it was found that nonspecific agglutination by the serum of horse 15 was often due either to the fact that green-producing streptococci were not inoculated, or marked changes had occurred in the culture. After these discrepancies, and the earlier experiments in which plates were not made of the cultures actually agglutinated are eliminated, there are in all 252 tests in which the culture subjected to the agglutinating action of the serum was proved to contain green-producing streptococci. Of the 252 tests, 120, representing 92 different cases, were made with the green-producing streptococci in the primary culture of dextrose-blood or acacia broth from sputum and throat exudate during life and lung exudate after death. In 72 (60 per cent.) specific agglutination occurred in the serum of horse 15. Of 27 tests, representing 16 cases, 19 (70 per cent.) showed specific agglutination in this serum in the primary culture of blood or peritoneal exudate of animals dead from injection of sputum, or primary culture of sputum. In the remaining 105 tests in which pure cultures of the green-producing streptococci in from the first to the sixth subcultures were used as antigen, representing 90 cases of influenza or influenzal pneumonia, 85 (81 per cent.) showed specific agglutination in the monovalent serum. Thus specific agglutination of the green-producing streptococci, which was proved to be contained in the antigen used, occurred in the monovalent serum in 176 of 252 agglutination experiments, an average of 70 per cent. Hence this figure may be taken to express roughly the percentage of the strains of green-producing streptococci which were immunologically identical and found throughout influenza and influenzal pneumonia.

Through the kindness of Major Fennell, of the Army Medical School, I have had an opportunity to test the behavior of strains of green-producing streptococci and type IV pneumococci, which he obtained from widely separated localities, toward the monovalent serum of horse 15. The source of these strains and their immunologic condition as measured by the various immune serums are given in table 3. Specific agglutination was obtained in 12 of 16 strains, or in 75 per cent. of the strains isolated from influenzal pneumonia, and in no instance in four other strains, one isolated from the normal mouth in Washington during the epidemic and three strains of pneumococci which Major Fennel isolated from spontaneous pneumonia in the monkey. A study of the results obtained with these strains in relation to their solubility in bile and their ability to ferment inulin shows that in these strains, as in those isolated in Rochester, specific agglutination does not depend either on whether they are or are not bile soluble, or whether they do or do not ferment inulin. Some of the negative agglutinations may be due to the fact that the strains had been cultivated for some time before the agglutination tests were made, all being in at least the eighth subculture. The incidence of agglutination of these strains by the other serums is about that of the strains isolated by us.

TABLE 3

Agglutination Experiments with Strains of Green-Producing Streptococci from Widely Distant Localities

Strain	Source	Antiserums					Controls		Solubility in Bile	Acid in Inulin
		Pneumococcus			Streptococcus					
		I	II	III	Hemolytic Horse 9	Green Producing Horse 15	Normal Horse Serum	NaCl Solution		
S 1	Influenzal pneumonia, Camp Wheeler	0	0	+	+	++++	0	0	0	+
S 3	Influenzal pneumonia, Camp Wheeler	0	0	0	0	++++	0	0	0	0
S 3	Influenzal pneumonia, Camp Wheeler	0	0	0	0	++++	0	0	0	0
S 5	Influenzal pneumonia, Camp Wheeler	0	+++	0	++	++++	0	0	0	0
S 6	Influenzal pneumonia, Camp Wheeler	0	0	0	0	++	0	0	0	0
55	Influenzal pneumonia, Camp Wheeler	0	0	0	0	+	0	0	+	+
S 14	Influenzal pneumonia, Chicago	0	0	0	0	+++	0	0	0	0
S 24	Influenzal pneumonia, Chicago	0	0	0	++	+++	0	0	0	0
S 17	Influenzal pneumonia, Walter Reed Hospital	0	0	0	0	0	0	0	0	0
24	Influenzal pneumonia, Walter Reed Hospital	0	0	0	++	+++	0	0	+	+
15	Influenzal pneumonia, Camp Sherman	0	0	0	0	++	0	0	+	+
S 19	Influenzal pneumonia, Camp Sherman	0	0	0	+++	++++	+	0	0	+
S 25	Influenzal pneumonia, Camp Sherman	0	0	0	0	0	0	0	0	0
S 27	Influenzal pneumonia, Johns Hopkins	0	0	0	0	0	0	0	0	0
113	Influenzal pneumonia, Camp Greene	0	0	0	0	+++	0	0	+	+
152	Influenzal pneumonia, Camp Greene	0	0	0	0	0	0	0	+	+
149	Normal mouth, Washington during epidemic	0	0	0	0	0	0	0	+	+
194	Spontaneous pneumonia, monkey	0	0	0	0	0	0	0	+	+
212	Spontaneous pneumonia, monkey	0	0	0	0	0	0	0	+	+
225	Spontaneous pneumonia, monkey	0	0	0	0	0	0	0	+	+
225	Spontaneous pneumonia, monkey	0	0	0	0	0	0	0	+	+

Owing to the instability of the green-producing streptococci from influenza, and the tendency to the development of mutation forms, it was found necessary to inoculate a blood-agar plate with the culture subjected to the agglutinating action of the different serums in order to interpret properly the results obtained.

Striking examples of the development of mutation forms as measured by changes in morphology in cultural characteristics and in immunologic conditions were noted in many instances. The source of the micro-organism, the culture medium inoculated and the effect of the various serums in some of the cultures which yielded mutation forms on plating are summarized in table 4. It will be noted that in the first nine experiments, hemolytic streptococci were obtained on the blood-agar plate in pure culture in eight and together with staphylococci in two when single colonies or groups of well isolated colonies of green-producing streptococci were inoculated, and that specific agglutination by the serum of horse 9 occurred in three, and in the serum of horse 15 in one instance. The rest were not agglutinated by any of the serums.

In experiments 10 to 13, inclusive, pure cultures of green-producing streptococci were obtained from the dextrose-blood or dextrose-acacia broth when single colonies of hemolytic streptococci were inoculated. One of these was agglutinated specifically by the hemolytic streptococcus, the other by the green-producing streptococcus antiserums. In these experiments it is assumed that the culture actually agglutinated contained the type of streptococcus homologous to the serum which agglutinated specifically. Proof that this was actually the case could not be obtained, because it is conceivable that mutation forms might develop not in the broth culture, but as growth occurred on the blood-agar plate, and the morphology of the two types of streptococci were so similar that differentiation in this way was not possible.

In experiments 14 to 24, inclusive, in which the mutant was a streptococcus, the morphology and immunologic condition were sufficiently different from that of the organisms inoculated to make it possible to determine where the mutation occurred. Specific or marked agglutination in the monovalent serum occurred in the dextrose-blood or acacia broth cultures in all but one of these strains. Smears of the cultures agglutinated in these showed no staphylococci, but typical elongated diplococci singly or in chains of variable length.

Smears of those in which agglutination did not occur (experiment 24) showed staphylococci, and agglutination experiments with streptococci from the sputum in influenza were not agglutinated by this or other serums (experiments 29 to 34). The number of staphylococcus colonies on the plates was often very large. Their number and distribution on the plates were such as to exclude the possibility of contamination from the air. Hence it is certain that mutation must have occurred on the blood-agar plates, and that many of the organisms in

TABLE 4

THE RELATION OF THE AGGLUTINABILITY OF BACTERIA FROM INFLUENZA TO THE DEVELOPMENT OF MUTATION FORMS

Number	Strain	Micro-organism Inoculated	Culture Used in Agglutination Test	Antiserums					Controls		Growth on Blood-Agar Plate of Culture Agglutinated
				Pneumococcus			Streptococcus				
				I	II	III	Hemolytic Horse 9	Green Producing Horse 15	Normal Horse Serum	NaCl Solution	
1	2698^2	Green-producing streptococcus from pleural fluid of guinea-pig injected with sputum	Dextrose-blood broth	0	0	0	+++	++	0	0	Hemolytic streptococci and staphylococci
2	3083.4	Single colony of green-producing streptococcus from sputum	Dextrose-blood broth	0	0	0	0	0	0	0	Slightly hemolytic streptococci
3	3270.2	Single colony of green-producing streptococcus from sputum	Dextrose-blood broth	0	0	0	0	0	0	0	Hemolytic streptococci and staphylococci
4	3296^2	Green-producing streptococcus from blood of mouse injected with sputum	Dextrose-blood broth	0	0	0	0	0	0	0	Hemolytic streptococci
5	3297.2	Single colony of green-producing streptococcus from sputum	Dextrose-blood broth	0	0	0	0	0	0	0	Hemolytic streptococci
6	3300.2	Group of green-producing streptococcus colonies from throat	Dextrose-blood broth	0	0	0	0	0	0	0	Hemolytic streptococci
7	3358	Green-producing streptococcus from sputum	Dextrose-acacia broth	0	0	0	++++	0	0	0	Hemolytic streptococci
8	3394^2.2	Single colony of green-producing streptococcus from blood of mouse injected with sputum	Dextrose-acacia broth	0	0	0	0	++	0	0	Hemolytic streptococci
9	3398.5	Single colony of green-producing streptococcus from sputum	Dextrose-blood broth	0	0	0	++	0	+	0	Hemolytic streptococci
10	3266^2.10	Single colony of slightly hemolytic streptococcus	Dextrose-blood broth	0	0	0	0	0	0	0	Green-producing streptococci
11	3048.3	Single colony of green-producing streptococcus from hemolytic streptococcus	Dextrose-acacia broth	0	0	0	++	+	0	0	Green-producing streptococci
12	3387^2.5	Slightly hemolytic streptococcus..............	Dextrose-blood broth	0	0	0	0	0	0	0	Green-producing streptococci
13	2698^2.2	Single colony of hemolytic streptococcus....	Dextrose-blood broth	0	0	0	0	+++	0	0	Green-producing streptococci
14	2719	Green-producing streptococcus from pleural fluid of guinea-pig injected with sputum	Dextrose-blood broth	0	0	0	++	+++	0	0	Staphylococci
15	2719^4.4	Single colony of green-producing streptococcus	Dextrose-blood broth	+	+	+	+	++	0	0	Staphylococci
16	2757^2.4	Green-producing streptococcus from blood of guinea-pig injected with sputum	Dextrose-blood broth	0	0	0	++	+++	+	0	Staphylococci
17	2800^2	Green-producing streptococcus from blood of guinea-pig injected with sputum	Dextrose-blood broth	0	0	0	++	+++	+	0	Staphylococci
18	3225^2.3	Green-producing streptococcus from blood of mouse injected with sputum	Dextrose-blood broth	0	0	0	0	+	0	0	Staphylococci
19	3241^2	Green-producing streptococcus from blood of guinea-pig injected with sputum	Dextrose-acacia broth	0	++	0	0	++++	0	0	Staphylococci

20	$3241^2.2$	Single colony of green-producing streptococcus from blood of guinea-pig injected with sputum	Dextrose-acacia broth	0	0	0	++	+++	0	0	Staphylococci
21	$3270^2.2$	Green-producing streptococcus from blood of guinea-pig injected with sputum	Dextrose-acacia broth	0	0	0	++	++	0	0	Staphylococci
22	$3296^2.2$	Green-producing streptococcus from blood of mouse injected with sputum	Dextrose-acacia broth	0	0	0	++	++	0	0	Staphylococci
23	3334.2	Single colony of green-producing streptococcus from sputum	Dextrose-acacia broth	0	0	+++	0	+++	0	0	Staphylococci
24	3434^2	Green-producing streptococcus from blood of mouse injected with sputum	Dextrose-blood broth	0	0	0	0	0	0	0	Staphylococci
25	2917.3	Single colony of hemolytic streptococcus......	Dextrose-acacia broth	0	0	0	0	0	0	0	Staphylococci
26	3211.2	Single colony of hemolytic streptococcus......	Dextrose-acacia broth	0	0	0	0	0	0	0	Staphylococci
27	3296^2	Single colony of hemolytic streptococcus......	Dextrose-acacia broth	0	0	0	++	++	0	0	Staphylococci
28	3334.2	Single colony of slightly hemolytic streptococcus	Dextrose-acacia broth	0	0	0	++	++	0	0	Staphylococci
29	$2608^3.2$	Single colony of staphylococcus from sputum	Dextrose-blood broth	0	0	0	0	0	0	0	Staphylococci
30	3175.4	Single colony of staphylococcus from sputum	Dextrose-blood broth	0	0	0	0	0	0	0	Staphylococci
31	3208.2	Single colony of staphylococcus from sputum	Dextrose-blood broth	0	0	0	0	0	0	0	Staphylococci
32	3302.2	Staphylococcus from sputum..................	Dextrose-blood broth	0	0	0	0	0	0	0	Staphylococci
33	3357.2	Single colony of staphylococcus from sputum	Dextrose-acacia broth	0	0	0	0	0	0	0	Staphylococci
34	3434.2	Staphylococcus from sputum..................	Dextrose-blood broth	0	0	0	0	0	0	0	Staphylococci
35	3334.2	Single colony of influenza bacillus from sputum	Dextrose-blood broth	0	0	+	0	++	0	0	Green-producing streptococci
36	3334.2	Single colony of influenza bacillus from sputum	Dextrose-blood broth	0	0	0	+++	++++	0	0	Green-producing streptococci
37	3341.2	Single colony of influenza bacillus from sputum	Dextrose-blood broth	0	0	0	0	0	0	0	Green-producing streptococci
38	3332.2	Single colony of influenza bacillus from sputum	Dextrose-blood broth	0	0	0	0	+	0	0	Slightly hemolytic streptococci
39	3332.2	Single colony of influenza bacillus from sputum	Dextrose-blood broth	0	0		0	0	0	0	Hemolytic streptococci
40	3248.2	Single colony of influenza bacilus from sputum	Dextrose-blood broth	0	0	0	0	0	0	0	Moist hemolytic streptococci
41	3283.8	Single colony of influenza bacillus from evaporated oil suspension	Dextrose-blood broth	0	+++	0	0	++	0	0	Green-producing streptococci and staphylococci
42	3201.3	Single colony (twice) of influenza bacillus from sputum	Dextrose-blood broth	0	+++	0	0	++	0	0	Staphylococci
43	3178.8	Group of colonies of influenza bacillus from sputum	Dextrose-blood broth	0	0	0	0	0	0	0	Bacillus influenza
44	3353^2	Influenza bacilli from blood of mouse........	Dextrose-blood broth	0	0	0	0	0	0	0	Bacillus influenza

the tall cultures of dextrose-blood or acacia broth took part in this process. The lack of specific agglutination when the cultures of hemolytic streptococci yielded staphylococci is also in harmony with this idea.

Similar results were obtained in many instances in which influenza bacilli were inoculated into the dextrose-blood broth (experiments 35 to 44). In most of these the culture of influenza bacillus was derived from a single colony on blood-agar plates inoculated with sputum, and in these it is conceivable, but not probable, that what appeared as a mutation might merely be the growth of this organism in the broth when inhibited on the blood-agar plate, the contact on the blood-agar plate inoculated with the sputum not being sufficiently intimate to allow growth of one or a few organisms.

Control inoculations from the colony fished in these as well as in the streptococcus experiments made in the immediate neighborhood of the colony or on another blood-agar plate showed only the growth characteristic of the colony from which inoculated. Moreover, similar results were obtained with some strains after many subcultures and after repeated platings from single colonies (experiments 41 and 42). The mode of occurrence, the immunologic condition, the control cultures of the blood used in the broth, and finally, the fact that the mutants were often highly virulent, rule out all reasonable possibility that we were dealing with contaminations, but, as pointed out elsewhere, final conclusions cannot be drawn until the pure line requirement has been fulfilled.

The suddenness and degree of the changes noted throughout these studies were similar to those I noted in a study on the transmutation of pneumococci and streptococci, and to those described by Clough in a study of pneumococci reacting with all of the three antipneumococcus type serums and in which a striking example of mutation occurred.

By the use of various immune serums, including the monovalent serum, it may be concluded that the somewhat peculiar green-producing streptococci noted at the outset of the epidemic and isolated so constantly since, both in influenza and influenzal pneumonia, are immunologically quite homogeneous. A high percentage of the strains, especially those isolated early in the attacks, are agglutinated specifically in the serum prepared with one of these strains. Highly agglutinable strains, as has been shown, absorb the agglutinins for other strains. The serum of patients recovering from influenza acquires agglutinating power over homologous and other strains. This finding is in accord with those of Tunnicliff and of Howell and Anderson, who also find immunologic evidence of the identity of green-producing streptococci from influenza. Specific agglutination occurred in the monovalent serum irrespective of whether or not they fermented inulin or of whether they were bile soluble or insoluble. After cultivation on artificial mediums, and after repeated animal passages, as well as late in influenza and influenzal pneumonia, the strains tend to become more heterogeneous.

The findings of immunologically dissimilar green-producing streptococci late in influenza is in harmony with the results obtained by Mathers in a study of pneumococci in reinfection in lobar pneumonia in which the type was also found to change. Evidence has been obtained to show that the mutation forms which develop in vitro and in vivo in animals are in general similar immunologically to the organisms commonly isolated in influenza. It has been shown elsewhere that they resemble these also in infecting power. Hence, it would seem that mutation may play an important rôle in the pathogenesis of influenza.

BIBLIOGRAPHY

Clough, Mildred C.: A Study of Pneumococci Reacting with Antipneumococcus, Sera of Types I, II and III, Jour. Exper. Med., 1919, xxx, 123-146.

Howell, Katherine, and Anderson, Ruth: Complement Fixation in Influenza, Jour. Infect. Dis., 1919, xxv, 1-5.

Mathers, G.: The Varieties of Pneumococci Causing Lobar Pneumonia, with Especial Reference to Their Biologic Differences, Jour. Infect. Dis., 1915, xvii, 514-521.

Rosenow, E. C.: Transmutations Within the Streptococcus-Pneumococcus Group, Jour. Infect. Dis., 1914, xiv, 1-32.

Rosenow, E. C.: Studies in Influenza and Pneumonia III. The Occurrence of a Pandemic, Strain of Streptococcus During the Pandemic of Influenza, Jour. Am. Med. Assn., 1919, lxxii, 1608-1609.

Tunnicliff, Ruth: Phagocytic Experiments in Influenza, Jour. Am. Med. Assn., 1918, lxxi, 1733-1734.

STUDIES IN INFLUENZA AND PNEUMONIA

XI. THERAPEUTIC EFFECTS OF A MONOVALENT ANTISTREPTOCOCCUS SERUM IN INFLUENZA AND INFLUENZAL PNEUMONIA

E. C. Rosenow

Division of Experimental Bacteriology, The Mayo Foundation, Rochester, Minnesota.

In this study I shall record the results obtained in the treatment of influenza and influenzal pneumonia with the serum prepared with one strain of the green-producing streptococcus, and a study of the immunologic condition of the streptococcal flora of the sputum made at the same time in the patients receiving the serum injections.

The serum was used in undoubted and, with one exception, in severe cases only. All injections were made slowly intravenously. The amount injected at one time varied from 25 c c to 100 c c of the undiluted serum. In some instances a desensitizing dose of 1 c c was given one hour previously. Twelve patients were given the serum. These may be conveniently divided into three groups according to the agglutination tests and therapeutic results.

Group 1 (*Four Patients*).—The sputum of all contained predominating numbers of green-producing streptococci which were agglutinated specifically by the monovalent serum. All four patients showed marked improvement and recovered promptly following the serum treatment. Three of the patients were experiencing the initial influenzal attack, and one had a recrudescence at the time of the serum treatment. The lung findings remained limited; none of the patients developed outspoken signs of extensive consolidation. In at least two, the improvement seems definitely attributable to the serum since the lung findings and symptoms were on the increase at the time of the serum treatment (cases 1, 2 and 3, and chart 1).

Case 1 (3283).—Mrs. H. C. L. came to the Clinic March 11, 1919, on account of nervousness, general weakness, fluttering of the heart and profuse menstruation. The symptoms followed a severe attack of influenza in October, 1918. Examination revealed a pelvic tumor for which a hysterectomy was advised.

March 28 the patient was admitted to the isolation hospital, with symptoms of influenza. She had been taken ill five days before with moderate headache, aching in the arms and back, sore throat, cough and slight nausea. These symptoms grew gradually less severe until the day before admission to the hospital, when she became worse with general aching, chilly sensations in the back, but no distinct chill or fever. The patient's throat was diffusely red, her tongue coated, she was cyanotic, and crackling râles were elicited over the bases of both lungs, especially on the right side. Findings of the heart, blood and urine were normal. On the day of admission the sputum was slightly blood streaked. No evidence of consolidation was noted at any time. A culture of the sputum showed predominating numbers of green-producing streptococci and a few staphylococci, and the primary culture in dextrose-blood broth was agglutinated specifically by the serum from horse 15 (table 1). March 29 the patient was given 50 c c of this serum; the aching disappeared during the course of the day, the cough lessened, and the following day the temperature dropped perceptibly and became normal (chart 1). The leukocyte count was 7,300 the day after admission and rose to 13,500 March 31 and April 1. The patient made an uneventful recovery.

Case 2 (3208).—A farmer of middle age, entered the hospital March 11, 1919. He complained of severe backache, headache, inability to sleep, sore throat and cough. The illness had begun the previous day with chilly

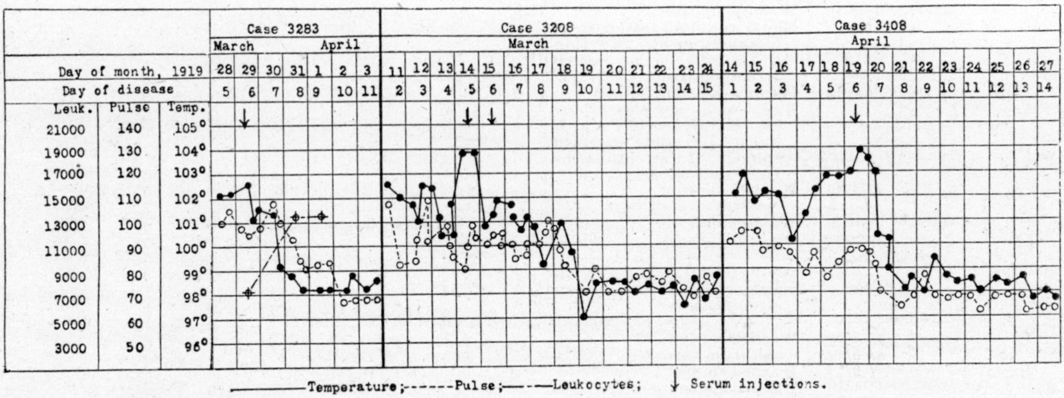

Chart 1.—Temperature, pulse and leukocyte curves in three patients in whom specific agglutination of the green-producing streptococcus from the sputum was obtained, and in whom marked improvement followed injection of the monovalent serum. In this and the following charts temperature is indicated by a solid line; leukocytes by a long and short dash line; pulse by a short dash line, and serum injections by arrows.

sensations but there had been no distinct chill. The patient's lips and fingernails were moderately cyanotic, he was mentally apathetic, although he complained of inability to sleep. His throat was diffusely red. The tonsils were also congested and the tongue was heavily coated. In the night of March 13 severe hemorrhage from the nose occurred and continued at intervals the following day. The lung findings were negative until March 17 when a small area of dulness was found at the inferior angle of the left scapula with slightly increased vocal fremitus and a suggestion of bronchial breathing. Later in the day dulness at the left base of the lung, fine crepitant râles in showers, and distinct bronchial breathing, especially at the inferior angle of the scapula near the spine, were noted. The sputum at first was mucopurulent, but March 13 it became serous in character and streaked with blood. Leukopenia was marked (chart 1). Blood-agar-plate cultures of the sputum obtained March 13, 15, and 17, showed countless numbers of green-producing streptococci, a

TABLE 1

AGGLUTINATION EXPERIMENTS WITH CULTURES FROM THE SPUTUM IN CASES OF INFLUENZA AND INFLUENZAL PNEUMONIA IN WHICH IMMUNE SERUM WAS USED

Case	Date on Which Sputum Culture Was Made	Condition of Culture at Time of Agglutination Test Dextrose-Blood-Broth Inoculated with	Antiserums: Pneumococcus I	Antiserums: Pneumococcus II	Antiserums: Pneumococcus III	Antiserums: Streptococcus Hemolytic of Horse 9	Antiserums: Streptococcus Green-producing of Horse 15	Controls: Normal Horse Serum	Controls: NaCl Solution
3208	3/13/19	Single green colony streptococcus	0	0	0	0	+++	0	0
		Green-producing streptococcus after one animal passage	0	0	0	++	++++	0	0
		Green-producing streptococcus in third generation after one animal passage	+	+	+	+	+++	0	0
3276	3/28/19	Washed sputum	0	0	0	0	+++	0	0
		Blood of mouse dead from intraperitoneal injection of sputum. Pure green streptococcus	++	++	++	++	++++	++	0
	3/30/19	Washed sputum	0	+	+++	+	++	+	0
		Blood of guinea-pigs injected intratracheally with moist, spreading greenish colony of streptococcus from sputum	0	0	+++	0	0	0	0
	4/ 2/19	Washed sputum	0	0	++	++	0	0	0
3282	3/30/19	Washed sputum	0	+++	+++	+++	++++	0	0
	4/ 2/19	Washed sputum	0	++	+	++	+++	0	0
3283	3/30/19	Washed sputum	0	0	0	0	+	0	0
		Single colony moist, green streptococcus	0	+	0	+	++	0	0
3338	4/ 7/19	Washed sputum	0	0	0	++	++++	+	0
	4/ 8/19	Swab from throat	0	0	0	0	+	0	0
	4/ 9/19	Washed sputum	0	0	0	+	++	0	0
	4/11/19	Washed sputum	0	++	0	++	0	0	0
	4/13/19	Washed sputum	+	+	+	+	+	+	+
		Single colony green-producing streptococcus from sputum	+	0	+	++	++	+	0
	4/16/19	Washed sputum	0	0	0	0	0	0	0
	4/17/19	Washed sputum	0	0	0	++	++	0	0
	4/25/19	Exudate right lung (hemolytic streptococci)	0	++	0	+++	0	++	0
		Exudate right lung (hemolytic streptococci)	+	+	+	+++	+	+	0
3341	4/ 8/19	Tonsil swab	0	0	0	0	0	0	0
	4/ 9/19	Washed sputum	0	+++	0	0	++	0	0
	4/11/19	Washed sputum	0	+++	++	++	++	0	0
	4/12/19	Single colony green streptococcus	0	+++	0	+++	++	0	0
3402	4/17/19	Throat swab	0	0	0	0	0	0	0
		Washed sputum	+	+	+	+	+	+	+
3408	4/18/19	Washed sputum	0	0	0	0	++	0	0

few staphylococci, but no hemolytic streptococci nor influenza bacilli. A blood culture made March 12 was negative. Dextrose-blood-broth cultures of the green-producing streptococcus isolated directly from the sputum March 13 and from the lung of a guinea-pig injected intratracheally with the sputum were agglutinated specifically by the serum of horse 15 (table 1). March 14 the patient's condition was very serious. Cyanosis was increasing, the sputum became more bloody and frothy, the mental apathy was worse, and prostration and epistaxis were marked. In the afternoon the patient was given 60 c c of the serum intravenously. The hemorrhage from the nose stopped, the patient's general condition became much better, and he was brighter mentally soon after the injection. The following day the injection of serum was repeated. The temperature dropped gradually to normal, and uneventful recovery followed (chart 1). The effect of the serum in this case appeared strikingly favorable, and probably was not coincident, since the symptoms and lung findings were on the increase at the time the serum was given. A slight urticarial rash developed ten days later. This patient was one of a group of five from the same locality who had severe attacks of influenza within a few days of each other after their arrival in Rochester; two of the patients died.

Case 3 (3408).—A middle aged man, entered the hospital April 14, 1919. He complained of severe aching, headache, malaise, weakness, sore throat, and slight cough. A general examination revealed moderate cyanosis, without manifest dyspnea, mental apathy, a diffusely red throat, and coated tongue. The chest findings were negative on the day of admission, but bubbling râles over both chests were elicited posteriorly April 15, 16, 17 and 18. The sputum obtained April 18 was mucopurulent. The cultures showed countless numbers of staphylococci and a moderate number of rather moist, spreading, green-producing and hemolytic streptococci. The leukocyte count on the fifteenth was 4,700. A blood culture made on the nineteenth proved negative. The primary culture of the washed sputum in dextrose-blood broth was agglutinated specifically by the serum of horse 15 (table 1). April 19, 25 c c of the serum were injected intravenously; the temperature and pulse rate dropped rapidly, and the general improvement was marked. The patient recovered promptly.

Group 2.—The three patients in this group were treated with the serum, and all showed marked improvement following injections during the initial attack of influenza when the green-producing streptococci from the sputum were agglutinated specifically by the monovalent serum. Later the patients developed bronchopneumonia due to green-producing streptococci that were not specifically agglutinated by this serum or by any of the immune serums tested (table 1, cases 4 and 5, and chart 2).

Case 4 (3282).—A woman, aged 48, came to the Clinic because of the recurrence of an abdominal tumor which had been operated on two years before. She was admitted to the isolation hospital March 28, 1919, stating that she had become ill the day before with a severe chill, sore throat, headache, and severe general aching. Her lips and fingernails were cyanotic, she was short of breath, even when lying quietly in bed, and abundant crepitant râles were found posteriorly at the left base of the lung and on the right side. A culture of the sputum obtained on the day of admission showed a large number of staphylococci and green-producing streptococci, and duplicate cultures in dextrose-blood broth were agglutinated specifically by the serum of horse 15 (table 1). March 29 and 30, 80 c c and 60 c c, respectively, of the serum of horse 15 were given intravenously. The patient's general condition improved following both injections, and her temperature and pulse rate dropped to normal (chart 2). The temperature remained normal for four days, and the abnormal lung findings almost disappeared. On the fifth day the temperature again rose and remained high for nine days, the pulse was rapid, and a sharp rise in the leukocyte count occurred. On the day following the rise of temperature an urticarial rash covered the entire body. With the increase in the temperature, dulness, bronchovesicular breathing and crepitant râles developed over the right side below the angle of the scapula. A culture of the sputum on the first day of normal temperature which followed the injection of the serum showed countless numbers of green-producing streptococci and staphylococci. The primary culture in dextrose-blood broth was

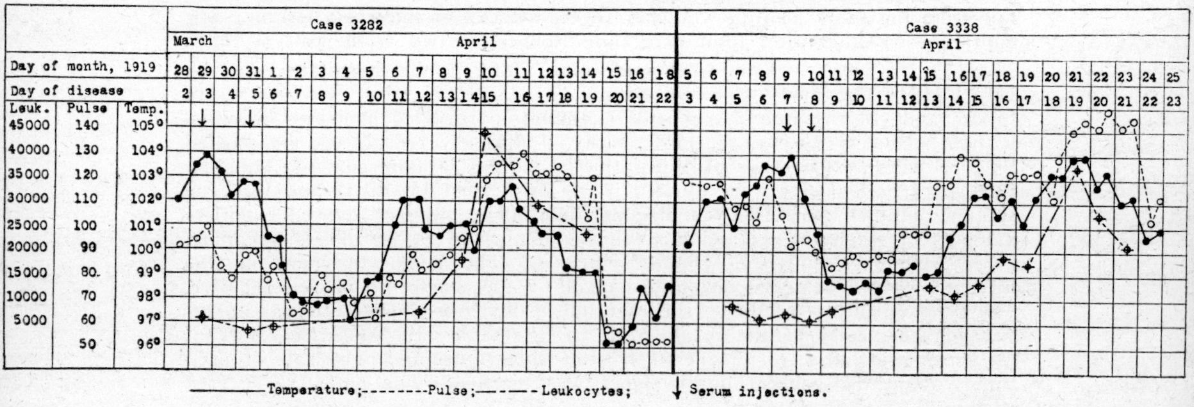

Chart 2.—Temperature, pulse and leukocyte curves in two patients in whom specific agglutination of the streptococcus was obtained during the initial attack, in whom there was marked improvement following injection of the monovalent serum, and in whom immunologically different green-producing streptococci were found during a reinfection.

again agglutinated specifically by the serum of horse 15. No cultures of the sputum were made subsequently. During the latter part of the attack of pneumonia, as the pulse rate crossed the temperature line (chart 2), the patient's condition was extremely critical for a number of days, but she finally made a complete, although slow, recovery.

Case 5 (3338).—A woman, aged 39, housekeeper, entered the isolation hospital April 5, 1919. Three days before the patient had felt chilly and could not get warm; she complained of moderate aching and was stiff in the joints and muscles. Two days afterward she developed a cough with a slight sore throat, and a moderately severe headache. If quiet in bed, she appeared well, but her lips and fingernails were decidedly blue. The examination of the chest was negative. On the morning of April 7 appeared a small area of slightly decreased resonance, bronchovesicular breathing, and a few râles below the angle of the left scapula near the posterior axillary line. The evening of April 8, crackling râles were heard on both sides in the lower axillae and posteriorly. On the morning of April 9 there were impaired resonance and crackling râles over the left base behind and at the side, and crackling râles on the right base posteriorly. The sputum was blood tinged and serous. By evening there was dulness over both lower lobes, but no definite bronchial breathing; crackling râles were heard over the entire chest. A culture of the sputum April 7 showed countless numbers of staphylococci and green-producing streptococci, a few hemolytic streptococci, and a moderate number of influenza bacilli. The primary culture in dextrose-blood broth of the washed sputum obtained April 7 and 9, and of a throat swab, showed almost pure cultures of green-producing streptococci which were agglutinated specifically by the serum of horse 15. Accordingly the patient was given intravenously 100 c c of serum April 9 and 10, respectively. The patient's general condition improved following both injections, the cyanosis became less marked, the expectoration diminished, and a drop in temperature and pulse rate occurred, the temperature reaching normal the day after the second injection (chart 2). The temperature remained normal for two days and then began to rise again, as evidence of a new involvement of the lung developed. The pulse rate remained high and continued unusually high throughout the fatal recurrence. Cultures of the sputum obtained on April 11, 13, 17 and 18 showed countless numbers of staphylococci, green-producing streptococci, an increasing number of hemolytic streptococci, and a few influenza bacilli. The green-producing streptococci, however, were no longer agglutinated specifically by the serum of horse 15 (table 1). The leukocyte count was persistently low throughout the first attack of fever, and at the onset of the recurrence, but then it rose to a high point, the maximum (43,000) being reached on the sixth day. On the two subsequent days the leukocytes diminished markedly and the patient died on the following day from what appeared to be cardiac failure from an overwhelming toxemia. After death the lung showed green-producing streptococci, hemolytic streptococci, and staphylococci, but no influenza bacilli. Duplicate cultures in dextrose-blood broth of the lung exudate showed hemolytic streptococci which were agglutinated by the antihemolytic streptococcus serum from horse 9. The reinfection in this case was clearly due to streptococci which were culturally identical, but immunologically were unlike those found during the initial attack. The anatomic diagnosis made at necropsy was: "Unresolved influenzal bronchopneumonia; marked enlargement of the tracheobronchial lymph nodes; purulent hemocatarrhal tracheal bronchitis; bilateral serofibrinous pleuritis; marked engorgement of the venous trunks of the body; petechial hemorrhages in the lining of the stomach and duodenum; hemorrhagic cystitis and marked hyperplasia of the spleen."

Group 3.—This group consisted of five cases in which no improvement followed the injection of the serum. In none of these was specific agglutination obtained at the time of the serum treatment, and all the patients died. In one case (case 3276) the agglutination of the streptococcus isolated from the sputum shifted from the serum of horse 15 to type III pneumococcus serum. In another case (case 3341) agglutination occurred in type II pneumococcus and hemolytic streptococcus serums. In the third case (case 3402) the sputum showed hemolytic streptococci which were not agglutinated by any of the serums (table 1). In two cases in this group countless numbers of green-producing streptococci were found in the sputum which were not agglutinated by any of the serums, and the patients were moribund at the time of the serum treatment. Cases 6, 7 and 8 illustrate the conditions found in this group of cases.

Case 6 (3276).—A farmer, aged 36, was admitted to the isolation hospital March 27, 1919. He had developed fever, backache, general aching, headache, dry throat, cough, and marked weakness the day before. On March 28 the throat was congested; the chest was negative except for a few scattered crackling râles. March 29 crackling râles and decreased resonance were found at the base of the left lung. The sputum was moderately bloody. On the afternoon of March 29 the patient was given 50 c c of serum from horse 15; the injection had no effect. April 1 there were definite signs of pneumonia on the left side, especially below the angle of the left scapula. The sputum was very frothy and bloody. The patient's condition grew rapidly worse, cyanosis and dyspnea increased, and he died from typical hemorrhagic pulmonary edema April 2. The leukocyte count was low at first, but it rose

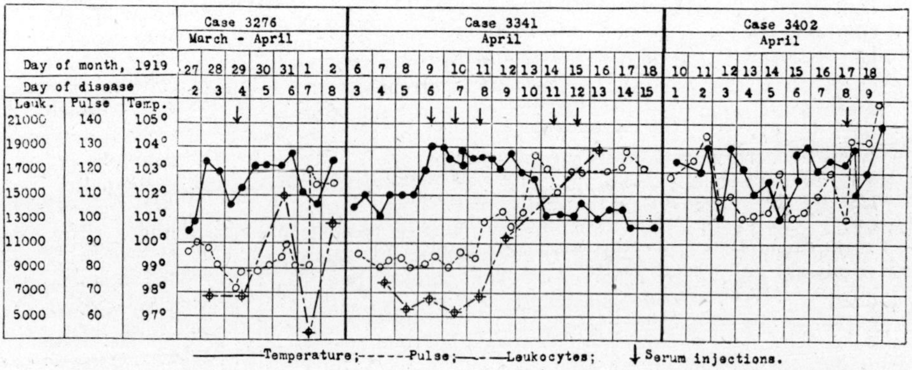

Chart 3.—Temperature, pulse and leukocyte curves in three patients in whom specific agglutination of streptococci from the sputum was not obtained and in whom the injection of the monovalent serum was without effect.

to 15,000 on March 31, and with the overwhelming toxemia showed a marked drop to 3,500 April 1, with another slight increase on the day of death (chart 3). Cultures from the sputum obtained March 28 showed countless numbers of moist, spreading, green-producing streptococci, a few staphylococci, but no hemolytic streptococci nor influenza bacilli. The primary culture in dextrose-blood broth of the washed sputum obtained on the twenty-eighth, and of the blood of a mouse, dead from intraperitoneal injection of sputum, were agglutinated specifically by the serum of horse 15. In contradistinction to this, March 30, the primary dextrose-blood-broth culture of the washed sputum, and of the moist, spreading, greenish colony of streptococci from the sputum was agglutinated specifically by type III pneumococcus serum. The primary culture of the sputum obtained April 2 was agglutinated slightly but equally by type III pneumococcus serum and antihemolytic streptococcus serum from horse 9 (table 1). The colonies on blood-agar from the dextrose-blood broth on all the days showed no change and resembled closely type III pneumococci, but they were not so elevated, and not so mucoid in character as pneumococcus mucosus.

Case 7 (3341).—A man, aged 38, undertaker, was admitted to the isolation hospital April 6, 1919. His illness had begun two nights before with a severe chill, vomiting, fever, backache, aching in the knees, general aching, slight nose bleed, and sore throat. The patient coughed and expectorated mucopurulent sputum. He was definitely short of breath and cyanotic. An examination of the chest was negative except for a few scattered râles. April 7 there were decreased resonance, and decreased breath sounds below the angle of the left scapula; April 8 decreased resonance and breath sounds and a few crackling râles were noted at the right base behind. On April 9 very definite signs of pneumonia were found on both sides. The sputum became bloody and serous. Cultures of the sputum and throat swab obtained April 7 and April 9 showed countless numbers of green-producing streptococci and staphylococci. On April 12 cultures showed countless numbers of staphylococci, a moderate number of green-producing streptococci, and larger, more moist spreading colonies resembling type III pneumococci. April 8, the primary cultures in dextrose-blood broth of the tonsil swab, and April 9, 11 and 13, of the sputum, were not agglutinated specifically by the serum of horse 15. Fermentative reactions showed that the green-producing streptococci from the sputum fermented inulin. The cultures of the sputum obtained on April 9 and 11 were agglutinated specifically by type II pneumococcus serum; those on April 13 by type II, and hemolytic streptococcus serum (table 1). The afternoons of April 9 and 10, 100 c c of serum from horse 15 were injected intravenously without effect. On April 11 and 14 injections of polyvalent antipneumococcus serums were given without effect. April 13 the urine showed a large amount of albumin and some red blood corpuscles. April 15 the patient was growing worse. He was bled 250 c c and was then given intravenously 250 c c of blood of a convalescent influenza patient, likewise without effect. The leukocyte count ranged from 5,500 in the earlier part of the attack to 19,200 in the latter (chart 3). The patient died April 18. The anatomic diagnosis was: "Bronchopneumonia, chronic cystitis with exacerbation, chronic parenchymatous nephritis, and old tuberculosis abscesses of the left lower lobe."

Case 8 (3402).—Woman, entered the hospital April 11, 1919; she complained of severe aching, fever, sore throat, and cough; she was toxic, cyanosed, and expectorated a small amount of mucopurulent sputum. The lung findings were negative. The heart showed mitral endocarditis with stenosis. April 14 and 15 crackling râles were elicited over both sides of the chest posteriorly, together with auricular fibrillation. April 16 the findings were definite for pneumonia of the left base. April 17 the expectorations became bloody, and profuse; the cyanosis and dyspnea increased. An injection of the serum of horse 15 had no apparent effect (chart 3), and the patient died April 18 with signs of acute hemorrhagic pulmonary edema. The sputum obtained April 17 showed countless numbers of hemolytic streptococci, staphylococci, and a few green-producing streptococci, but no influenza bacilli. The primary cultures in dextrose-blood broth of a throat swab and washed sputum were not agglutinated by any of the serums (table 1).

DISCUSSION

Of the twelve patients treated, all but one were critically ill at the time of serum treatment. Five recovered and seven died. Three of the patients who died were practically moribund at the time of the serum treatment and good effects could scarcely be expected. The two others that died showed green-producing streptococci immunologically different from the strain with which the serum was prepared, and in two, hemolytic streptococci caused death. In these cases also improvement could not be expected. In all cases in which specific agglutination was obtained, marked improvement followed the injection of the serum, and in no case were good effects noted at a time when agglutination tests were negative.

The influenza bacilli found in the sputum in two cases might be regarded as unimportant since both patients showed marked improvement following injections of the serum. The patients treated are of course too few to permit sweeping conclusions, but since the results were controlled by immunologic studies it would seem that diplostreptococci, closely related to pneumococci on the one hand and hemolytic streptococci on the other, bear important etiologic relationship to influenza and to influenzal pneumonia, especially early in the attack. The injection of properly prepared hyperimmune serums may prove curative in cases due to organisms immunologically identical to those used in the preparation of the serum, quite as has been found in the case of type pneumococcus infections in lobar pneumonia.

The changes which occurred in bacterial flora as measured by cultural and immunologic tests during the course of the disease, emphasize the complexity of the problem and the need for their consideration in the developement of specific methods of prevention and treatment of influenza and its complications.

GENERAL INDEX

A

PAGE
Acidfast bacteria - - - - - - - - - - - - - - 45, 77
Agglutination, grouping of B. influenzae by - - - - - - - 230
Anthrax bacillus, influence of beef serum on - - - - - - - 148
Antibody formation, influence of thorium-x on - - - - - - 330
Antitoxic serum, potency of concentrated - - - - - - - - 130
Antistreptococcus serum, monovalent, in influenza and pneumonia - - 614

B

B. aerogenes, fermentation of polysaccharids by - - - - - - 418
B. anatum N. S. cause of disease of ducklings - - - - - - - 217
B. anthracis, influence of beef serum on - - - - - - - - 148
B. diphtheriae, influence of brilliant green on - - - - - - - 179
B. diphtheria - - - - - - - - - - - - - - - 388
B. enteritidis in rats - - - - - - - - - - - - - 402
B. enteritidis-like organisms from feces in influenza - - - - - 16
B. influenzae, grouping by agglutination - - - - - - - - 230
B. typhosus, action on xylose and - - - - - - - - - - 52
Bacterial cultures, final H-ion concentration in - - - - - - 160
Bacterial cultures, phenol red-china blue as indicator in fermentation test of 43
Blood serum, colloidal state of normal and immune - - - - - 8
Blood serum, ultraspectroscopic studies on - - - - - - - - 1, 8

C

Cannon, Paul R. Bacillus enteritidis in laboratory rats - - - - 402
Chaulmoogric acid series in leprosy and tuberculosis - - - - - 238
Chemotherapy in experimental pneumococcus meningitis - - - - - 355
China Blue as indicator in bacterial fermentation tests - - - - - 43
Cholera immunization - - - - - - - - - - - - - 441
Clawson, Benjamin Junior. Varieties of streptococci with special reference to constancy - - - - - - - - - - - - - 93
Colon typhoid bacillus in case of furunculosis - - - - - - - 336
Complement fixation in diagnosis of tuberculosis - - - - - - 85
Connecticut, statistics of 1918 epidemic of influenza - - - - - - 185
Corper, H. J. See Hektoen, Ludvig - - - - - - - - - 330

D

Davis, David J. Fate of streptococcus hemolyticus in gastro-intestinal canal 171
Day, Alexander A. See Kendall, Arthur I. - - - - - - - 45, 77
De Kruif, Paul H., and Ireland, Paul M. Streptolysin - - - - 285
Dickson, G. K. See Small, Jas. C. - - - - - - - - - 230
Diphtheria bacillus, biologic studies of - - - - - - - - - 388

PAGE
Diphtheria bacillus, influence of brilliant green on - - - - - - 179
Disinfecting value, causes for variation in determinations of - - - 351
DOWNS, C. M. See SHERWOOD, N. P. - - - - - - - - - - - 16
Ducklings, B. anatum cause of disease in - - - - - - - - 217

E

Empyema, bacteriology of chronic - - - - - - - - - 29
Empyema, experimental streptococcus - - - - - - - - - 265
Ethylhydrocuprein in experimental pneumococcus meningitis - - - 355

F

FANTUS, BERNARD, AND RUMRY, FLORENCE. Causes for variation in determinations of disinfecting value - - - - - - - - - 351
Feces, nonlactose fermenting organisms from, in influenza - - - 16
Fermentation test, phenol red-china blue as indicator in, of bacterial cultures - - - - - - - - - - - - - - - 43
FRANKLIN, C. M. See HASLAM, T. P. - - - - - - - - - 424
Furunculosis, colon-typhoid bacillus in case of - - - - - - 336

G

GAY, F. P., AND STONE, R. L. Experimental streptococcus empyema - 265
GORDON, J. E. Bacteriology of chronic empyema - - - - - - 29
GRACE, LINWOOD G., AND HIGHBERGER, FLORENCE. Acid production by streptococcus viridans in different hydrogen-ion concentration - - 451
GRACE, LINWOOD G., AND HIGHBERGER, FLORENCE. Variations in hydrogen-ion concentration in uninoculated medium - - - - - - - 457

H

HASLAM, T. P., AND FRANKLIN, O. M. Immunization with pseudoblackleg pellets - - - - - - - - - - - - - - - 424
HAVENS, LEON C. Biologic studies of diphtheria bacillus - - - 388
HEKTOEN, LUDVIG, AND CORPER, H. J. Influence of thorium-x on antibody formation - - - - - - - - - - - - - - 330
HIGHBERGER, FLORENCE. See GRACE, LINWOOD G. - - - - - 451, 457
HIXSON, CHARLES R. Factors influencing the potency of concentrated antitoxic serum - - - - - - - - - - - - - 130
Hydrogen-ion, concentration of, in cultures, especially of streptococci - 160
Hydrogen-ion concentration in uninoculated medium - - - - - 457

I

IDZUMI, GORO. Experimental pneumococcus meningitis in rabbits and dogs 373
IDZUMI, GORO. See KOLMER, JOHN A. - - - - - - - - - - 355
Immunity in influenza - - - - - - - - - - - - - - 463
Influenza, factors in prevalence in Connecticut in 1918 epidemic - - 185
Influenza, gastro-intestinal - - - - - - - - - - - - 557

PAGE
Influenza, green producing cocci in - - - - - - - - - - - - 405
Influenza, immunity in - - - - - - - - - - - - - - - 463
Influenza and influenzal pneumonia, bacteriology and clinical features - 469
Influenza and influenzal pneumonia, leukocytic reaction - - - - - 492
Influenza and influenzal pneumonia, effects of monovalent antistreptococcus serum in - - - - - - - - - - - - - - 614
Influenza, nonlactose fermenting organisms from feces in - - - - 16
Influenza, statistics of 1918 epidemic in Connecticut - - - - - - 185
Ireland, Paul M. See De Kruif, Paul H. - - - - - - - - 285

J

Jackson, Leila. Intracellular protozoan parasite of ducts of salivary glands of guinea-pig - - - - - - - - - - - - - 347
Jones, H. M. Limiting hydrogen-ion concentration of various pneumococci 435
Jones, Horry. Factors influencing final hydrogen-ion concentration in bacterial cultures with special reference to streptococci - - - - 160
Jordan, Edwin O. Differentiation of paratyphoid-enteritidis group. VII. Irregular and variable strains - - - - - - - - - - 427
Jordan, Edwin O., and Sharp, W. B. Influenza studies. I. Immunity in influenza - - - - - - - - - - - - - - - - 463

K

"Keel," disease of ducklings caused by B. anatum - - - - - - 217
Kendall, A. I.; Day, A. A., and Walker, A. W. Metabolism of virulent human tubercle bacilli. Studies in acid-fast bacteria, XI - - - 45
Kendall, A. L.; Day, A. A., and Walker, A. W. Metabolism of bovine tubercle bacilli. Studies in acid-fast bacteria, XII - - - - - 77
Koehler, M. E. See Kolmer, J. A. - - - - - - - - - - - 148
Kolmer, John A., and Idzumi, Goro. Chemotherapeutic studies with ethylhydrocuprein and mercurophen in experimental pneumococcus meningitis in rabbits - - - - - - - - - - - - - - 355
Kolmer, J. A.; Wanner, D. C., and Koehler, M. E. Influence of beef serum on anthrax bacillus - - - - - - - - - - - - 148
Kolmer, J. A.; Woody, S. S., and Yagle, E. M. Influence of brilliant green on diphtheria bacillus - - - - - - - - - - - 179

L

Laybourn, R. L. Fermentation of polysaccharids by B. aerogenes - 418
Leprosy, chaulmoogric acid and other fatty acids in - - - - - 238
Leukocytes, effect of leukocytic extracts on phagocytic activity of - 447

M

McNaught, J. B. See Sherwood, N. P. - - - - - - - - - 16
Meningitis, pneumococcus, ethylhydrocuprein and mercurophen in experimental - - - - - - - - - - - - - - - - 355
Meningitis, pneumococcus, experimental in rabbits and dogs - - - 373

PAGE

Mercurophen in experimental pneumococcus meningitis - - - - - 355
MORISHIMA, KAN-ICHIRO. See TEAGUE, OSCAR - - - - - - - - 52
MORISHIMA, K. Phenol red-china blue as an indicator in fermentation tests of bacterial cultures - - - - - - - - - - 43
MOURSUND, W. H. Complement fixation in diagnosis of tuberculosis - 85

N

NAKAYAMA, Y. See TADOKORO, T. - - - - - - - - 1

O

OLIVER, WADE W., AND SCHWAB, ALMA F. Bacillus of colon-typhoid group from a case of furunculosis - - - - - - - - - - 336
OPPENHEIM, C. J. Human fecal streptococci - - - - - - 117
OTTERAAEN, A. Hemolytic streptococci in throat in certain acute infectious diseases - - - - - - - - - - - - - - 23

P

Paratyphoid bacilli, effect of pasteurizing temperatures on - - - 165
Paratyphoid-enteritidis group, differentiation of - - - - - - 427
Paratyphoid bacilli recently isolated from animals - - - - - - 340
Pasteurization, effect on paratyphoid bacilli - - - - - - - 165
Phenol red as indicator in fermentation test of bacterial cultures - - 43
Pneumococcus meningitis, experimental - - - - - - - - 373
Pneumococci, concentration of, limiting H-ion - - - - - - 435
Pneumonia, influenzal, see influenza
Protozoan in salivary glands of guinea-pig - - - - - - 347
Pseudoblackleg, pellets, immunization with - - - - - - - 424

R

RETTGER, LEO F., AND SCOVILLE, MARGARET M. Bacterium Anatum, N. S., etiologic factor in disease of young ducklings known as "keel" - 217
ROGERS, J. F. See WINSLOW, S.-E. A. - - - - - - - - 185
ROSENOW, E. C. Studies in influenza and pneumonia:
Bacteriology and clinical features - - - - - - 469
Leukocytic reaction - - - - - - - - - 492
Effects of injection of bacteria found in influenza, etc. 504
Etiology of gastro-intestinal influenza - - - - - 557
Changes in green producing streptococcus by animal passage and their significance in influenza - - 567
Immunology of green-producing streptococcus from influenza - - - - - - - - - - 597
Monovalent antistreptococcus serum in influenza and influenzal pneumonia - - - - - - - - 614
RUMRY, FLORENCE. See FANTUS, BERNARD - - - - - - - 351

S

PAGE

SCHWAB, ALMA F. See OLIVER, WADE W. - - - - - - - - 336
SCOVILLE, MARGARET. See RETTGER, LEO F. - - - - - - - - 217
Serum, antitoxic, potency of concentrated - - - - - - - - 130
Serum, differentiation in colloidal state of normal and immune - - 8
SHARP, W. B. See JORDAN, EDWIN O. - - - - - - - - - 463
SHERWOOD, N. P.; DOWNS, C. M., AND MCNAUGHT, J. B. Nonlactose fermenting organism from feces of influenza patients - - - - - 16
SMALL, JAMES C., AND DICKSON, G. K. Grouping of Bacillus influenzae by specific agglutination - - - - - - - - - - - 230
SPRAY, ROBB SPALDING. Observations on paratyphoid bacilli recently isolated from animals - - - - - - - - - - - - - 340
STONE, R. L. See GAY, F. P. - - - - - - - - - - - - 265
Streptococci, constancy of varieties of - - - - - - - - 93
Streptococcus empyema, experimental - - - - - - - - 265
Streptococci, fecal, human - - - - - - - - - - - - 117
Streptococci, green producing, in influenza - - - - - - - 405
Streptococci, final H-ion concentration in cultures - - - - - 160
Streptococci, hemolytic in throat in infectious diseases - - - - 23
Streptococcus hemolyticus, fate of, in gastro-intestinal canal - - - 171
Streptococcus viridans, acid production by - - - - - - - - 451
Streptolysin - - - - - - - - - - - - - - - 285
Sugars, action of B. typhosus on - - - - - - - - - 52
SWEENEY, MARION A. See WALKER, E. L. - - - - - - - 238

T

TADOKORO, T. Ultraspectroscopic studies on blood serum. I. Antagonistic action of salt in blood serum - - - - - - - - - - 1
TADOKORO, T., AND NAKAYAMA, Y. Ultraspectroscopic studies on blood serum. II. Difference in the colloidal state of normal and immune serum - - - - - - - - - - - - - - - - 8
TAKENOUCHI, MATSUZIRO. Sensitized and nonsensitized vaccines in cholera immunization - - - - - - - - - - - - - - 441
TEAGUE, O., AND MORISHIMA, K. Action of B. typhosus on xylose and some other less frequently used sugars - - - - - - - - 52
Thorium-x and antibody formation - - - - - - - - - 330
Tubercle bacilli, metabolism of virulent human - - - - - - 45
Tuberculosis, chaulmoogric acid and other fatty acids in treatment of - 238
Tuberculosis, complement fixation in diagnosis of - - - - - - 85
Tubercle bacilli, metabolism of bovine - - - - - - - - 77
TUNNICLIFF, RUTH. Action of leukocytic extracts on phagocytic activity of leukocytes - - - - - - - - - - - - - - 447
TUNNICLIFF, RUTH. Observations on green producing cocci of influenza 405
TWISS, EDITH M. Effect of pasteurizing temperatures on para-typhoid group - - - - - - - - - - - - - - - - 165

PAGE

V

Vaccines, sensitized and nonsensitized, in cholera immunization - - 441

W

WALKER, ARTHUR W. See KENDALL, ARTHUR I. - - - - - 45, 77
WALKER, ERNEST LINWOOD, AND SWEENEY, MARION A. Chemotherapeutics of chaulmoogric acid series and other fatty acids in leprosy and tuberculosis. I. Bactericidal action; active principle; specificity - 238
WANNER, D. C. See KOLMER, J. A. - - - - - - - - - - - - 148
WINSLOW, C.-E. A., AND ROGERS, J. F. Statistics of the 1918 epidemic of influenza in Connecticut, with a consideration of the factors which influenced the prevalence of this disease in various communities - 185
WOODY, S. S. See KOLMER, J. A. - - - - - - - - - - - 179

X

Xylose, action of B. typhosus on - - - - - - - - - - - 52

Y

YAGLE, E. M. See KOLMER, J. A. - - - - - - - - - - - 179